The Garden of Earth

~ volume two ~

The Garden of Earth

~ volume two ~

WILD PLANT SECRETS & PRACTICAL NATURAL SKILLS

Laura Lamun, C.A.

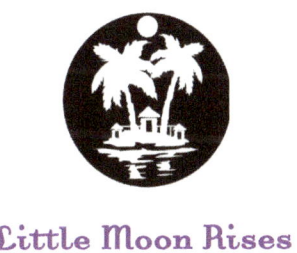

Little Moon Rises

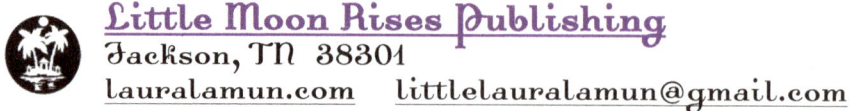

Little Moon Rises Publishing
Jackson, TN 38301
lauralamun.com   littlelauralamun@gmail.com

Copyright © 2025 by Laura Lamun & Little Moon Rises Publishing

All rights reserved, contents protected under copyright law. However, the author respectfully requests you spread this information around to others. Please refer to this information and quote, please distribute widely, please give credit and attribution. Sincere Gratitude is given to all the supportive mentors quoted here, and the ideas shared from others within this book, and every effort has been made to assure credit is attributed.

Any suggestions given in this book should be used with caution and prudence, and **all emergencies, heart attacks, asthma attacks, serious illness, allergic reaction, bites or stings require medical assistance.** Please seek appropriate urgent care professionals. The publisher and author waive any responsibility for the mis-use of any of the ideas presented in this work. Please take care of yourself and others, confirm wild plants several times and use common sense. We DO take responsibility for the wonderful and miraculous things that may happen as a result of reading this material.

ENORMOUS THANKS TO EVERYONE WHO SUPPORTED THIS EFFORT!

Editorial Support: **Paula Kalustian, JoAnne Lamun**
Interview: **Pepper Keen Lewis & GAIA,**
             thepeacefulplanet.com, pepperkeenlewis.com
Design & Typeset: **Annie Dore   beespringdesigns.com**
Special thanks to **Don Kinney, motherearthimages.com** for stunning photos

**Will there be a *Volume Three*? It is already written!
Stay in touch - it will be available SOON!**

Library of Congress Cataloging-in-Publication Data
Lamun, Laura Anne 1964-
    The garden of earth: wild plant secrets & practical natural skills / Laura Lamun

Includes bibliographical references and index.
ISBN 978-0-9801513-1-2   0-9801513-1-7
1.   Nature - Plants - Spirituality - Handbooks - Weeds - Natural Remedies - 1. Title

"Whoever educates the people without uniting them in a loving way of mind, is like someone who weeds without wanting to harvest.

Whoever unites the people through a loving way of mind without calming them with music, is like someone who harvests without wanting to eat.

Whoever calms the people with music but does not perfect them in harmony with the Law of Nature, is like someone who eats but does not thrive.

~ Confucius

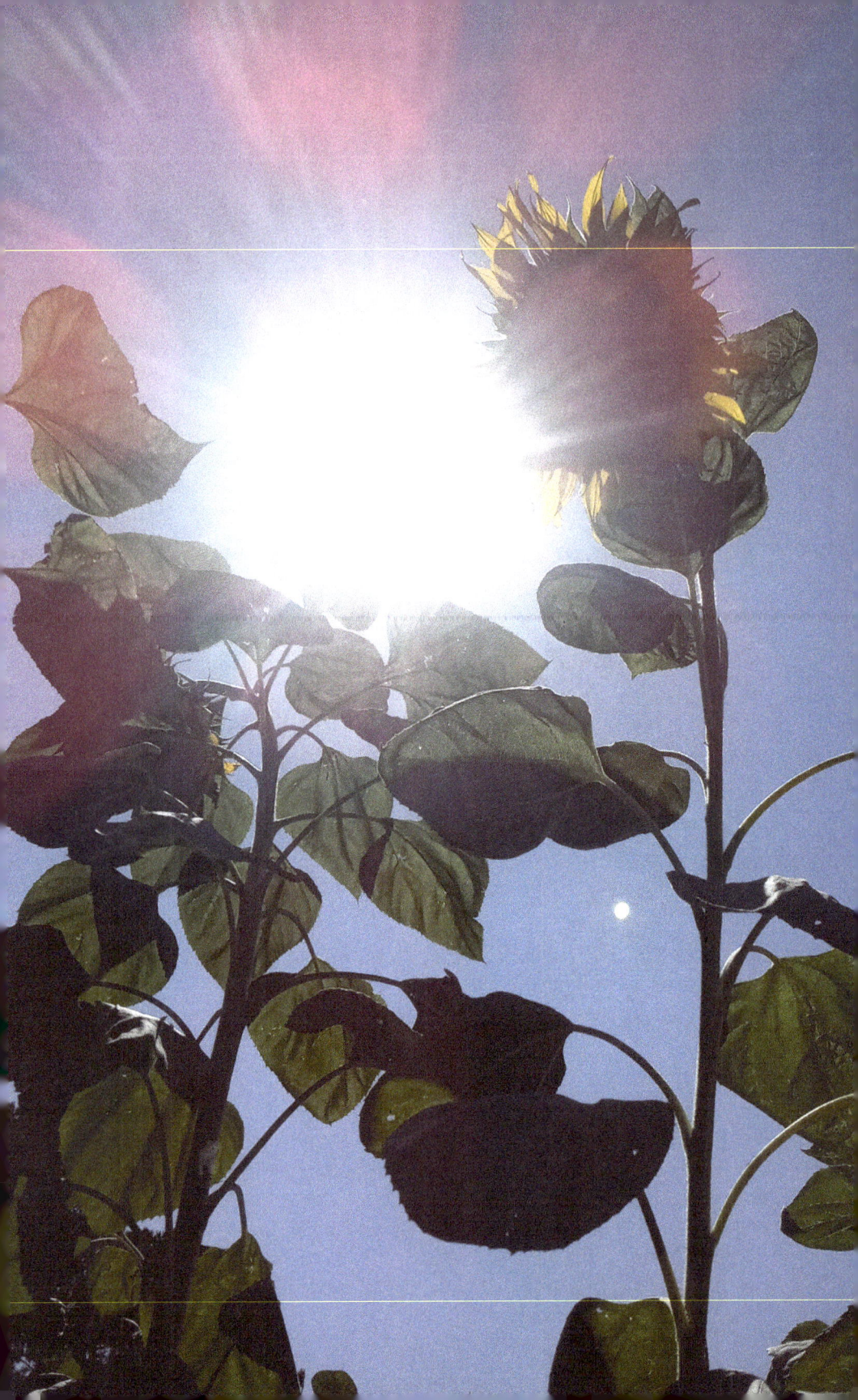

~ the garden of earth ~

Table of Contents

Foreword by Brigitte Mars 1

Introduction 2

Chapter 1   WELCOME TO THE GARDEN
In which we become reacquainted with the Earth & Laura 7

Chapter 2   PARTNERS IN THE GARDEN
In which we appreciate Gaia's Champions & Grow Our Own Food 49
- Pollinator-Attracting Plants 54
- Vegan Protein Sources 65
- Gardening 67
- Sprouting 88
- Fermenting & Yeast Creation 97
- Composting 106

Chapter 2.15   OUTLAWS OF THE GARDEN
In which we meet the **Weeds**, Free Food for Feeding the World 113
- Plant Families 121
- **MATERIA WEEDICA: Secrets of 25 Wild EDIBLE Weeds** **140**

Chapter 3   GIFTS OF THE GARDEN
In which we learn Cool Facts to Nourish Ourselves & Others 245
- Food Sources for Major Nutrients 250
- Life-Saving Practices 268
- **LAURA's LISTS:**
  - Mental Energy & Focus 275
  - Hangover Remedies 278
  - Viral Immunity 280
  - Lactation Support 284
  - Pregnancy Safety 287
  - Effortless Sleep 289
  - Testosterone Boosting 292

Chapter 4   REBELS OF THE GARDEN

In which we celebrate Plant Pioneers & their Discoveries 297
     James Lovelock 298
     George Washington Carver 301
     Cleve Backster 306
     Monica Gagliano 309
     Bruce French 313

Chapter 5   PRESERVING THE GARDEN

In which we revive the Skills of our Ancestors & Provision Our Pantries 317
     Canning 321
     Drying 325
     Extracting Medicines 328
     Freezing 334
     Root Cellars & Fridge Holes 338
     Preparing For Everything 342

Chapter 6   MOTHER OF THE GARDEN

In which we listen to Our Mother and Continue On 349
     Gaia Interview 350

Chapter 7   WISDOM OF THE GARDEN

In which we revitalize Our Personal & Planetary Broadcast 365

Heartfelt Acknowledgements viii
Footnotes xvi
Sources xviii
Image & Illustration Directory xx
Index xxvi
About The Author xxxiv

> "You have to touch the Heart
> to reach the Mind."
>
> ~ *Jack Hanna*

> "My love affair with Nature is so deep that I am not satisfied with being a mere onlooker, or Nature tourist. I crave a more real and meaningful relationship. The spicy teas and tasty delicacies I prepare from wild ingredients are the bread and wine in which I have communion and fellowship with Nature, and with the Author of that Nature."
>
> ~ Euell Gibbons

> "It is an incalculable added pleasure to anyone's sum of Happiness if he or she grows to know, even slightly and imperfectly, how to read and enjoy the wonder-book of Nature."
>
> ~ President Theodore Roosevelt

> "The love of wilderness is more than a hunger for what is always beyond reach; it is also an expression of loyalty to the Earth, the Earth which bore us and sustains us, the only paradise we shall ever know, the only paradise we ever need, if only we had the eyes to see."
>
> ~ Edward Abbey

~ the garden of earth ~

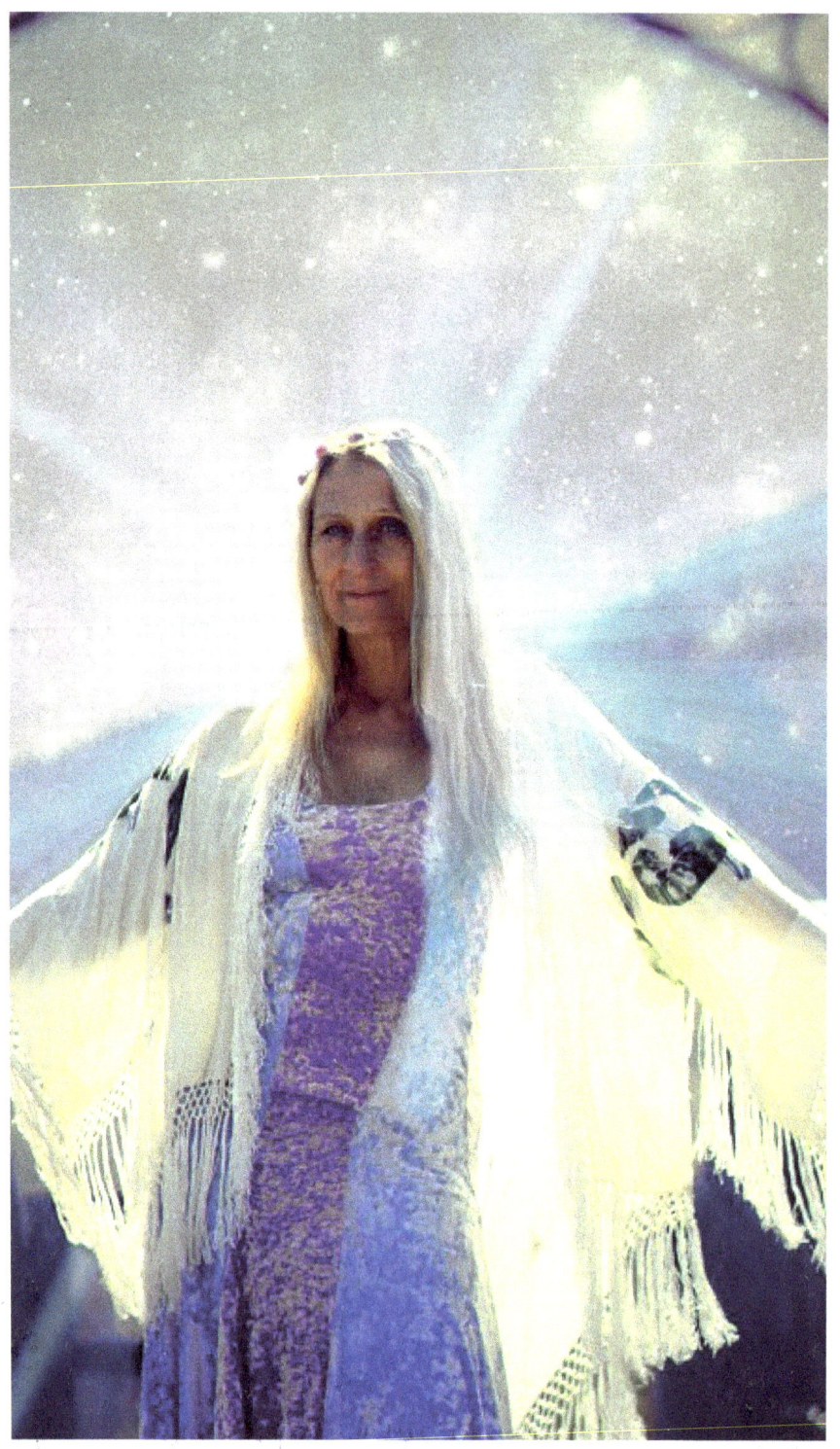

Foreword

by Brigitte Mars

Greetings Dear Readers,

I have known Laura Lamun for over 36 years. We worked together at a legendary natural foods store in Boulder, Colorado called Alfalfa's Market, in the herb and nutrition section. Here we helped people with herbs, supplements, & essential oils, and were delighted to see if we could make a difference in helping people and the Planet.

When Laura applied to work at the store, her resumé included some of her theatrical performances and since then, I have seen her in many: *Beehive, Into the Woods, Meet Me in St. Louis* and *Nunsense*, as a leading lady. All of her performances were thrilling, and she now offers her voice again, to lead with a simple script she has created that is just what the World needs.

I have just read through *The Garden of Earth, Volume Two*, and though I did not think I needed any more books in my already vast library, this is certainly one to include that well deserves a prime placement! Thank you, Laura Lamun, for sharing so much time-tested wisdom in such a beautiful way. Here is a book that can help us live with more grace and ease, adding to our skills of survival, personal and planetary health. Shared here are an abundance of ideas and life-enhancing techniques.

We may face dire news in the media, about our country, the world, climate change, and impending crisis, but **solutions** are what we need! *The Garden of Earth Volume Two* offers practical, simple and delicious remedies, recipes and insight about how we can live more in harmony on every level of existence.

This collection of inspiring information offers what we all need to know more about: food, herbs, wild edible plants, seed-saving, food preservation, fermenting, weather wisdom, mentor-honoring and better ways we can live on this Planet with less impact. This is what we really should be teaching in schools! But starting at home is imperative.

Laura Lamun's effervescent personality shines through with tips and tricks, so that you can get started right away. Here is a book that enhances our connection to Nature, awakening us to the connectedness of all life, and how body, mind and spirit intertwine with divine evolutionary purpose. *The Garden of Earth Volume 2* is a tribute to the arts of our ancestors! These can easily be re-learned in this inspirational book on how to get started and increase our life skills to help ourselves, our family, neighbors, and the Planet. With this one small volume (though perhaps more will come) we can begin the journey.

Many Blessings,

Brigitte Mars   *Herbalist, Author, Professor*   www.brigittemars.com

~ the garden of earth ~

Introduction

HELLO FRIEND, I WROTE THIS BOOK FOR YOU.

Somehow, out of the millions of books in the World, you have *this one* in your hands. Serendipity is real, and I am so happy it brought us together. Now we get to make a connection, and I know this has happened for a reason. There is something in these pages that you need, and I need *you* to read this, so thank-you for meeting me here.

Writing this book was a beautiful escape for me during a rough couple of years. And although I would *wish* to, there is no way I could pretend 2020-2023 didn't happen and write only from the perspective of the Joy of Nature, without acknowledging the elephant in the room. Our Human Race lived through a mountain of harsh health experiences in the early 2020's. **Worldwide, we were all united** in a very real and very weird way, by a strange set of health, social, and economic circumstances which touched everyone differently. I am so sorry to those of you who lost loved ones, or your businesses. I feel genuinely sorry for all of us whose lives were altered as a result.

I imagine we all have our thoughts and theories about what happened. Regardless, it was a very dark time for Humanity and something from which we are still in recovery. I have tried not to let it commandeer my writing, although for awhile it was very healing to speak my mind in this book process (much of it revised later). There is no doubt I needed the information I was researching and writing and venting about, so did *everybody*, but it was literally not safe to broadcast it on social media. You are holding the fruit of my labor from this time, but also the work of the rest of my life. I tried to concentrate on the most helpful topics and steer clear of censors, blame and triggers.

What kept me going were the people asking for *Volume Two*. I offer my great thanks to Dave Allen, my Family, Brigitte, Catay, Deelicious, Rachel, Paula, Caden and all the friends and strangers who wrote to me, cajoled and convinced me to keep going, get the second book finished. And I give great gratitude to the many non-physical Beings, my Book Angel, the Plant Spirits and Angels who were constantly enticing me to get busy writing about what I LOVE.

I actually *did* write this book for you, for *all* of my Friends and Family. I reached out in companionship to feel you as I wrote, and specifically tried to connect with you and wonder what you might need. I wrote it because I wanted to do ***something*** to support, nourish, and encourage YOU to make it through, during hard times and good. We all need inspiration and something to hold onto, something to get excited about. This was written during one of those times. Hopefully this book can continue to be there for you, can help you feel more secure, with suggestions to support your health, increase your bounty, offer you means to self-sufficiency, and just plain inspire you to **make Life more beautiful every day.**

What knowledge would help all of us to live more comfortably through ANY strange and challenging time, what could keep us well, put food on our table? **What ancestral skills have we lost that might be important in our shared future?** How could I create a natural companion to healthier living, and be of service to my friends and All the Beings of the Garden at the same time? I compiled it all into this book: **radical, revolutionary and important self-sufficiency skills and techniques for your Universal Survival.** Personally, I learned so much from writing this book, and I refer to it often.

I offer *tons* of information for you to pore over, ideas you can use to enhance your life **right now**, and many new things to think about. There are practices and skills you can refer to later, if and when they become needed. There are lots of nutritional suggestions that could make a radical difference to your health. I expect your mind will be blown a time or two by the **miracles of Nature** I report about, as well as some wonderful new scientific findings. If just one thing you learn in this book helps you or someone you love, I will have done my job. If you possibly get sparked into a new NATURAL connection with the beautiful Planet Earth and her abundant Garden - then I'll be so happy because **the book totally worked.**

As a confessed book junkie, I grew up with the hope that someday I might be able to write books that would truly help people. I was so excited to write and self-publish my first *Garden of Earth* book in 2008. It won a few (very minor) awards, most notably the *Green Festival Book Award for* **Best Spiritual Book.** That accolade surprised me, woke me up to the fact that I was writing books about the **Spirituality of NATURE**, beyond just what plants were *good for* or which ones to choose. Because I knew there was a such a **Spiritual, MAGICAL aspect** to engaging with the Natural World, I *did* want to reveal something that was beyond just the physical - *the Spiritual Secrets of Plants!* This gave me a mission to teach everyone that by tuning-in to Nature, to Gaia, you establish a blessed higher connection with one of the Perfect Systems of the Divine Source, The Creator of us All.

Volume One was about **Living Remedies and Earth-Honoring Practices**, and included a *Materia Medica* highlighting the **Raw Aromatherapy of 33 Scent Plants**. That book contains a bunch of body care recipes, a list of edible flowers and aphrodisiac foods, wild anecdotes, theories from my brilliant friends, and some beautiful ways to connect with Gaia, the sentience of the Earth.

Volume Two demonstrates a deeper dive into **Survival and Self-Reliance**. It contains many tips for growing your own food and offers age-old as well as innovative new preserving techniques. This book's *Materia Medica* is a **"Weedica"** detailing the free wild **Weeds** that grow everywhere, how to use them for food and make wild medicine. You will find **essential oil and plant remedies** that can deeply enhance your life and personal wellness, as well as pertinent (in any time) guidance about **immunity** and **medicine-making**. This book ends with another beautiful interview with the soul of Earth, our **Gaia**, and contains some excellent additional advice for living more joyfully.

Volume Three *(which I have already finished)*, contains valuable information about the **Elements**, their representatives on Earth and how they explain our health perfectly. There is a section on **Mineral & Earthen Remedies** which will blow you away. Expect more illumination from the Soul of our Earth, **Gaia**, in another nice long interview. And the last section offers a *"Materia Planetica"* with great detail about our Celestial Neighbors the **Planets**, their influence mighty. It's a very exciting and magical book just edging over the horizon.

With luck and divine timing there will be a fourth in this series, as ***Volume Four*** has already bloomed deeply in my consciousness. There's always material left over from the process of crafting a book. In this case, I believe I have enough for several more books! I am feeling inspired with cosmic information about **TREES**. They are so magical and helpful and are clamoring to me to be written about. So far, I plan to concentrate on **Trees, Mushrooms,** and **Colors** in *Volume 4*, and have reserved lots of my latest cool research for the next book. My plan is to keep adding volumes to the *Garden Of Earth Series* so it can be a **GROWING NATURAL TOOLBOX** to make your Life ever better.

But back to *this* book - it is chock full of information you can use right now. Need some help making your **Garden yield more food**? *Check out Pleasing Partners on page 82.* Want to look up **Foods that contain Zinc**? *Check out page 266.* Want to try **Sprouting**? *Turn to page 91.* Need to know how to **make your own Yeast**? *Check out a few methods on page 103.* Want help getting to **Sleep**? *Find it on page 289.*

Or skip all this stuff and go right to **Gaia's Message** on **page 350**. She has the *most unique* perspective of all regarding our Earthly experience. She helps us tune-in to our *Gaian Library of Information*, our very *Planet's* experience and perspective. She wraps her information in layers of communication, which upon re-reading open even further to reveal her timeless wisdom. Like any good teacher, her guidance requires participation on our part, as we have to think deeply to puzzle it all out, and unpack it again and again, each time revealing more. Years later I am still working through the guidance she offered for this book, realizing how right-on and time-looped she was.

I tell a lot of my personal stories here, in the hopes you can derive insight from my experiences, both challenging and wonderful. So the book is **part memoir, part guidebook, part reference book**, all for your education and inspiration. I hope to enliven your sense of humor, too! I hope the support you find here will give YOU the strength to keep going no matter what challenges you face. May you keep your health, and ensure your Family is always fully nourished.

As in all of my books, the overlighting message is the same -

The Garden of Earth grows for YOU.

Let's experience, explore, and learn to utilize ALL of it! Most people don't even scratch the surface of knowing what this Planet offers, what the many diverse species upon her are providing. These books are meant to educate you (or remind you) of all the many, many **resources** Gaia has given you to care for your every need. Most importantly, I pray that reading these books helps you to personally experience the Joy and Self-Sufficiency that comes from **KNOWING Nature better**.

But then, I dream that you put the books down, because YOU have found a way to experience Gaia and Mother Nature for yourself! You discover how to connect and communicate. And suddenly, you are the recipient of what was always there in the first place - **Everything You Always Need in Each Moment.** You recognize knowledge is flowing all around you, and *living each day* is how you are taught. You LEARN to see the signs, and know the phases, and live in the cycles that bring you what you need. You find ways to communicate with all of Life around you. You pay more attention to Nature and Weather and the Plants and your Feelings...**and you KNOW stuff**.

Helpful Stuff! Good Stuff! More than you ever did before. ***Knowing better information makes Life easier!*** It brings you a new sense of personal confidence and makes you HAPPIER, which causes you to get stronger and your ENERGY to rise. This frequency shift helps you subsequently broadcast a more Compassionate, Loving, Peaceful Vibration to our Planet Earth and All People.

We all live so that we may be inspired, happy, and add our personal experiences and MASTERPIECES to the Earth Story, giving back to the Garden ourselves! **We each have a lifetime of opportunities with which to create Benevolent Solutions and Beautiful Creations for our Earth!** What a sacred and important task. Let's all do our best to make a worthy contribution, and have one Heaven-of-a time!
Thanks for reading,

~ LAURA

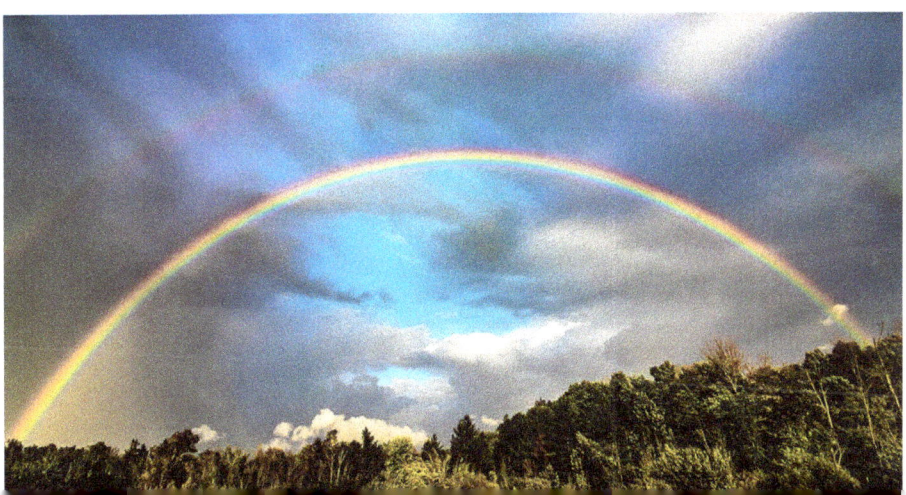

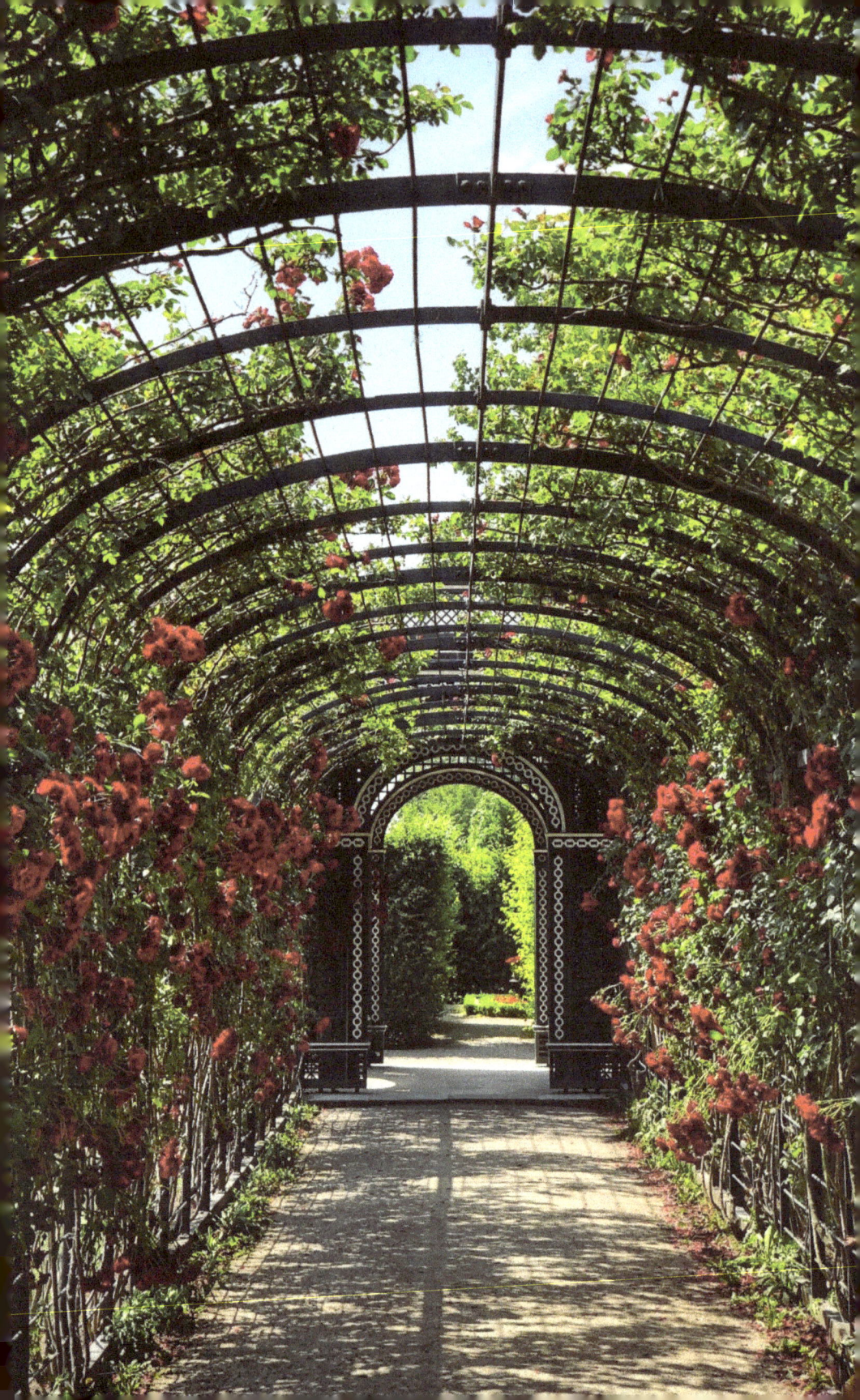

~ Chapter 1 ~

WELCOME TO THE GARDEN

> "The best remedy for those who are afraid, lonely or unhappy is to go outside, somewhere where they can be quite alone with the Heavens, Nature and God. Because only then does one feel that all is as it should be - and that God wishes to see people happy, amidst the simple beauty of Nature. As long as this exists, and it certainly always will, I know that then there will always be comfort for every sorrow."
>
> ~ *Anne Frank,* The Diary of a Young Girl

COULD WE *BE* ANY MORE LUCKY?

We LIVE in the Garden of Earth.

We are blessed to exist on such a miraculous, varied and verdant Planet. Our Earth is a **True Provider** - we have our sustenance, our remedies, and everything necessary for Life including our natural resources, all right here. So far, we can survive without the need to leave our home (not all planets are this way). Even though we may not be aware or always act like it, *we are being provided* with the means to feed our Whole World, and to keep it radiantly healthy. Much of this is ancestral knowledge, and is not widely known these days. But some of it is information living within the Plants! It can be discovered, explored and taught. The value of Earth is greater than we thought. We all must realize how precious these natural resources are, and how important it is to sustain them, without destroying their source. **Learning to recognize value and work WITH Nature is a requirement for our future**; it is a teaching mechanism, as well as a survival skill we all need. This is exactly what this whole book is about.

I am going to reveal some of Mother Earth's magical patterns, and expound on the wonder and the unending practicality of her extensive offerings. Here you will learn new ways to think about your Planet, and will develop new ways of seeing. I will prove it to you, with every page, that you are being **constantly supported by the Natural World**. I intend to reveal some of its mysteries, and return to you some ancestral knowledge you can really use right now. We will journey together into a deep communion, where you will find, remember, and be reminded again and again, that **NATURE HAS THE ANSWER FOR EVERYTHING**.

By design.

You live within a beautifully orchestrated and highly organized *Natural System*, that has been designed to **provide a remedy for every imbalance.** This System is always seeking **Wholeness**. This means the Earth was *engineered* to be perfectly habitable for ongoing Life, and therefore must have the ability to be **self-healing**. This means you (as a microcosmic fractal of the Macrocosmic Planet), YOU were also designed to be self-healing. If you need help with that, the remedy you seek is already here - or out there, somewhere in the fields of Weeds, waiting to be discovered, learned about, and utilized. If you know that your body is designed to find a way to heal, and that your Planet has everything you need to do just that, **you have found the REAL secret**. What a genuine comfort to know this! Can you believe it and work with it? The system is **so practical** and **so magical**, and **so designed for you**, all at the same time. It was purposefully and masterfully built to sustain you.

We do trust the Earth (and a few million Farmers) to feed us. We count on the mysterious Forces of Nature to heal our bodies and restore balance within our immune systems. We rely on native species to balance and protect our ecosystems. We witness changing seasons as a metaphor for shifts in our lives. We have experienced Mother Nature as a joyful friend in good times, and a nurturing partner to ease the bad times. But there's so much more! Every one of us has an All-Access Pass to her Earthly Wisdom, it just seems like we have misplaced the virtual password.

Let's see if I can help you to recover and preserve some of this age-old wisdom. Here's a perfect secret to begin with - **we have Food in places we never even thought to look!** We have Medicinal Herbs growing by our fences, Protein Sources covering our fields, and Helpful Remedies hiding all over outside, just waiting to be utilized. We have this genuine and abundant FOOD SUPPLY support from our Planet that will never run out. Unless we destroy it - which we do every time we spray the Weeds or our yards with pesticides and herbicides. Humans need to understand what's here first, before eradicating it! They need education in order to realize what they are doing wrong and then face up to their brutal impact. They *need* a wake-up call, what some people are calling a "Great Awakening," to understand their **automatic and programmed actions** in every facet of Life, including food eradication. Now each of us must learn and share what we can improve upon, so we can all do better. As my native Brother, Robert Stroud said, *"It's Grow Time."*

I have never been more convinced of the power and the wonder of the Natural World than I am these days. *Every time* I needed a lift, a change of heart, or an attitude adjustment, the Plants, Animals, Sunshine and Blue Sky, and even the Planets were there for me. Special Herbs and Foods showed up to keep us well. Remedies were easy to find if you looked for them. Our pets and the natural wildlife kept us centered. We watched the seasons change and the trees restored to full glory in the Spring, and the Sun came up every single day to greet us with renewed promise. The Flowers and Weeds blossomed abundantly. In the dead of Winter in 2020, even the Cosmos treated us to a show. We, along with the rest of the World, looked up into the heavens to watch a glorious and visible Conjunction of Jupiter and Saturn. It was a beautiful distraction from a hard, strange year and it was wonderful to witness this celestial meeting make the Nightly News! Nature and her cycles continue on, regardless of what we are all going through, and in that we can always to find comfort and solace.

If someone like Anne Frank, who endured hiding from the Nazis in an attic for **761 days,** could emerge with hope and faith in the **Healing Power of Nature** - *so can we*. If she could make these powerful statements *without being able to go outside at the time*, we should revel in our freedom to wander wildly through Nature. We get to utilize Earth's many gifts now, when we all need them the most. We are free to explore and discover what has been made for all of us. We have always counted on Nature to heal us, this moment is no different. Let's always return to our Mother Earth for support.

CHANGES UPON CHANGES

As we turn our attention to our beautiful Earth, we see lightning fast changes happening to our Planet, as well as to our People. Landscapes are altering and climates are shifting. Volcanoes are waking up after centuries of slumber. Weather is wild and unpredictable, floods, fires, and natural disasters changing lives and locales forever. We all lived through a major health crisis which consumed the attention of the *entire World* at the same time, and altered (probably forever) our habits, our sense of security, our educational system, our children, our access to food and our economy. We have all had to adapt, and we continue to seek new ways to restore our lives. **Change** has become our new normal. All this change can be more than a little unsettling, like being pulled up by our very roots, out of the world we always knew.

What on Earth is next? Has any generation ever witnessed so much growth and so much change? Do you suppose they all feel this way? Where are we headed, and what do we have left to be excited about? What is there to live for?

SO MUCH, trust me. This whole book is dedicated to restoring your Excitement! I am excited to share the many ways I am certain **everything is going to work out for us.**

Nature will provide *this* remedy, as well, but we each must play our part. Our Planet is adaptive, intelligent, and ALIVE, and will continue to work for us. But we need to participate, and we will create **exponentially better results** when we work *with* her. I know in my heart we will invent ways to clean up the messes we have made, and honor her again. I believe, with our devotion and hearty efforts, she can thrive, we can thrive, and we will learn volumes about how to do better in the process.

Keep in mind that Mother Earth does not get mad at us. She is not *changing out of spite or punishment*, or creating havoc as revenge for our "crimes against her." No, not at all. Nor would she ever give up on us. **She loves us unconditionally like a Mother,** regardless of our ignorance. She *evolves* with what comes, she adapts, she grows, even through what Humans have done to her, in an effort to support all Earthly Life. We are not being punished by her, but we are *daily* being made more **AWARE**. Her body shows our impact and we must see it. Like the ultimate Mother, she seeks to inspire solutions and success in all her Creatures by living the example. Watch the many ways she supports and educates you everyday.

Anne Frank also said, *"How wonderful it is that nobody need wait a single moment before starting to improve the World."* She is right! We are each on a personal mission to make Life work, **right here right NOW**, no matter what. We are all here at this time to create a beautiful, natural experience for ourselves, our children and their children. Along the way, there are *always* mountains to climb and rivers to cross that teach us about ourselves and our World.

As Gaia told me, transcribed in our interview in Chapter 6, **"Now is the time to Trust the Process of Life."** And to "*know that we are sitting within paradigm shifts that are necessary and helpful.*" What could that mean? A paradigm is defined as a *"system or typical example of a model or design."* Well, our design is definitely showing signs of altering! We *are* shifting our thought systems and beliefs and models of the Universe, and with all that, we are shifting our very consciousness! We are living in a World we could not have recognized ten, twenty, or thirty years ago. Old concepts are being examined and redefined (and forgotten!). Much of this process is happening directly *as a result* of all the strange times we are living through. She's right, we should trust it.

Cultures and Beliefs, Money and Governments, Health Care and Media, all are altering before our very eyes. Policy is changing, and not just in the US, but all over the World. Humans are standing up for what they believe in the name of **Integrity and Freedom**. Protests are being witnessed worldwide, alternative voices are being heard. Since we have tools that connect every household, and phone cameras in every hand, nothing can stay hidden in the dark for long! Abusers are being punished, and Heroes are being revealed. Science is revising. Traditional roles are being examined and redefined. Opinions and trends are being made as fast as they are changing. Karma is being transmuted, revolution is afoot. Think what you have lived to see and what might be next! If we are shifting on all those levels, then yes, a lot is going on. But, let me remind you, this is a natural process.

The really good news is that all Earthly Creatures contain an ingenious program that codes for Survival and turns on when needed. We see this in the Plants, who flower and set their seeds when they begin to feel threatened by weather or some outside stressor. Their mission is to continue the species and to keep growing, and they will alter their growing habits in order to reproduce. You can witness this in any seed you've seen planted deep in the dark soil, that grows to the Light against all odds, to survive. Life has a relentless mission to fulfill, and it is shining brightly in you.

People also become more efficient and potent when they are challenged. I see us finding ways to come together, work with Nature and each other to create positive changes that grow into a whole new blossoming. Someday, this time will be remembered for enabling nothing less than a **Personal and Planetary Renaissance!**

I believe we are ALL headed for more glorious times right here on *Earth*, based on what we learn. I think Humans are in a crucible now, pressured and stressed so we will **choose to discern and grow** in this Garden of Earth School. Like Lead being transformed into GOLD, in a true alchemical process we are being separated, altered and recombined into something more valuable. Our challenges are *designed* so we must seek their solutions, with every natural and supernatural ability we possess! Once we have solved enough of our own problems and cease to create more - maybe *then* we can then go out and explore other worlds.

DON'T BELIEVE ALL THE BAD NEWS

Our Mothers used to warn us, *"Don't believe everything you hear."* I want you to keep that in mind with the News! Don't believe it all, don't let too much of the bad news get inside you. Don't let it harm you, and put you into a fear state that is dark, unproductive, and negatively impacts your immune system. TURN IT OFF. Now is the time to keep your Peace and perspective, maintain healthy detachment and keep your sense of humor. Watch more comedies and laugh more!

I believe **Information** is having an identity crisis - people are *classifying* it as "good" and "bad," "misinformation" or "disinformation." **Judgement** is at an all-time high, and Information is being used in the conflict to divide people. No one knows what to think, whom to trust, or what exactly the Truth IS anymore! The "News" and what Mainstream Media is doing with it, has become a commodity, and we are watching this "information" be advertised, traded, hidden, censored, bought and sold. **We must all remember that just because a viewpoint is on the News, or on Social Media, it does not automatically make it accurate or true - on any channel - and that it very possibly was paid for by someone who wants you to believe it. Just be aware.**

Dramatic bad news excites something primeval in people, and we know it can be very addictive. Some social media platforms take advantage of this, they use algorithms everyday to provide negative stories to engage readers for longer amounts of time. Additionally manipulative, *censorship* and *engineering of information* are rearing their ugly heads again. Book banning, book-BURNING, de-platforming, search engine programming, and content judgment must have crept in the side door while we weren't looking. I never thought we'd see those things again in our lifetimes. I absolutely do not comply with the notion that any viewpoint, creation or broadcast should be destroyed or censored. I would hope we are evolving enough to see everything, and then be able to discern and decide for ourselves what we need. We deserve the chance to make the choice. Uncensored Free Speech is Vital.

What bothers me the *most* is that I believe an enormous amount of **valuable and uplifting** information - **Good News** - was being banned or "removed for content." What kind of nefarious energy doesn't want people to know about the value of Vitamin C? Why remove badly-needed doctors from service because of their remedy choices? Who exactly is doing the "deciding" and why do we trust them? Why silence the people who are thinking for themselves? I am certain that in this process we are being denied a great deal of the Good Stuff. And I am pleased that the trend is building to find out why, and free our valuable, positive, natural information.

> "The omission of Good is no less reprehensible
> than the commission of Evil."
>
> ~ *Plutarch*

Most importantly, when making health decisions, don't let anyone's "omission" or "curated information" convince you to do something you don't feel right about. You must study, and search deeply for what Information rings TRUE to you. Do your own research. Look to your trusted experts, but feel if what they say resonates with you, and is for you. Your **heart** must be your guide now, and you must *feel* your way, following your Inner Guidance, through the Information Field.

TRUTH HAS A FEELING

Ronald Reagan was famously quoted for saying, *"Trust, but Verify,"* although the phrase was actually coined from an old Russian proverb. While I seek your *trust*, in offering my opinions and ideas here in my book, I want you to search for how they make you feel, too. In order to help you to **verify** in your truth-seeking, I offer you information in the Footnotes in the back of the book, and References on my website, so you can learn more if you are interested. Keep in mind that it may not be wise to rely solely on your internet browser or "fact-checker" websites for your **Truth**. Many of them are hasty to post and have proven to be funded by the very people on whom you are checking![1] *(Footnotes will be found on pg. xvi)* It may not be possible anymore to rely on a singular news source on television, even if it is one you always trusted, for times have changed. And it is definitely not wise to allow any government, mainstream or social media outlet to censor, manage, define, or manufacture your Truth.

Truth has a frequency you can see, hear and feel. *Search Yourself For Sensations.* Get in touch with what Truth feels like. Examine how your body is expressing its feelings to you (goosebumps, chills up your spine, impending dread or feelings of elation). Notice how it feels when you know something to be true in your core. There is a real certainty that comes from inside, in your heart of hearts, when you know, that you know, that you know it is true. I remind you to always choose for yourself based on this heartfelt counsel. Ask your *Body* for the answers and feel what it says, even if the ideas don't agree with what you hear on the outside. I will remind you many times in this book to **trust your own Heart and your Gut Feelings to verify Information.** Here and *everywhere.* Some people call that listening to your Bullshit Detector!

I see it like a window my heart that says *yes* or *no*. Some people say it is the voice of your Higher Self, or the whisper or voice of God. Some would call it your Inner Light or your Consciousness. Whatever you think it is, it is *standard* on all Human models! Everybody has one. I have learned to call it your **Innate Knowing** - something that comes from the Inside. We are ALL learning *how* to feel, recognize, and understand more about Inner Guidance and Truth. If you have dealt with people who tell a lot of lies, you begin to hear patterns and see body language that tells the real story and you take note of those sensations. Trust the Truth you feel from *all* the impressions you receive.

And I will tell you this: your **PERSPECTIVE** of Truth is personal and changeable. Your Personal Truth can *evolve and alter*, just as you do, with different experiences, choices and discernment. We don't all need to have the same Personal Truth or the same perspective at the same time. It is okay if you agree with some of what interests me, but not all of it. I am here to offer a different perspective, another SOURCE of knowledge for you to feel and think about. You decide for yourself. As with all things in Life, you get to feel it, choose what resonates with you, and release what doesn't.

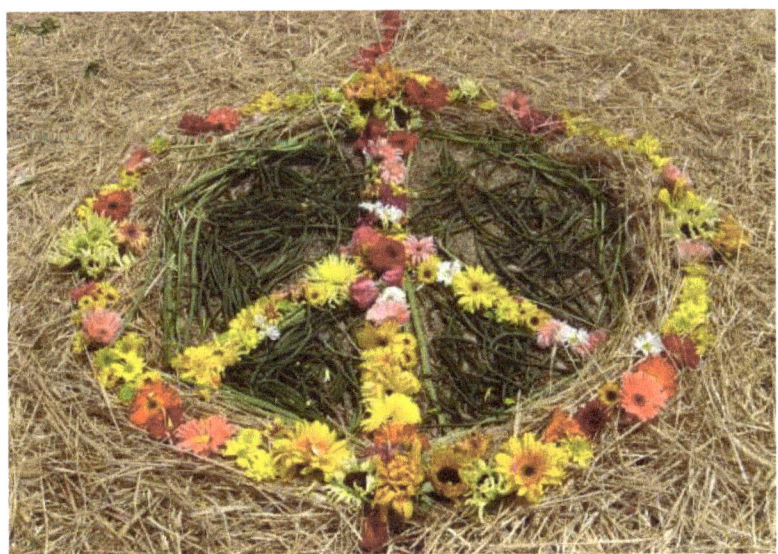

WHAT IS YOUR PEACE?

As a foundation, as a practice everyday, you must "do your job." And you may not know this - but your job is to **FIND YOUR PEACE** and **STAY HAPPY!** Don't underestimate the simplicity of this advice. Find a way to work in the World that makes you *happy* most all of the time. This is one thing that is absolutely within your control and the perfect place to find your Peace. Find what makes you happy and do *that* until you are abundant and shiny and joyful enough to help others get there, too! **Be kind, be of service to others, do your part, find and keep the peace, lighten up, and trust that it is all working out for a greater good.** We have to help each other. We are all meant to be a peaceful part of the One, Divinely connected, cooperating and lifting each other up. Especially in the most unpeaceful of times, we must work together to make the World better with our actions. But it does start with YOU working on *you* - the only person you *can* control - and the only person who controls your own personal happiness, which is solely in your hands.

There is something very magical about working on yourself. When you concentrate your efforts to find **YOUR OWN HAPPINESS**, you naturally create more **harmonious interactions with others**, and you really do influence the World around you. As a matter of fact, *this is the very way* we can all create a better World! This is where our responsibility lies, in maintaining our own high frequency emotional charge, created from Love, Peace, Gratitude, and Positive Energies.

This is the way we work with **Energy,** as well as physicality. We are designed to be *Spiritual* as well as physical Human Beings, and this is exactly what that means. All cultures and religions have practices to explore the Self, and raise our personal frequencies: **Meditation, Prayer, Ritual, Service, Self-Exploration, Forest Bathing, Intention Setting, and Practicing Loving Kindness.** Each civilization before us had to find ways to do this, no matter what was going on, and many credit their spiritual belief systems with success in challenging times. In the midst of the storm, we can choose to be the Lighthouse! Our positivity is nourishing to everything. It is actually **up to us** to feed our most positive energy manifestations into the System. **Our Emanations Matter!** Every positive creation or uplifting thought we can come up with contributes to the whole, and is magnified by joining with other similar frequencies. Before we know it we have shifted the energy of a room, of a town, of a Planet.

> "Let your Light shine through this in such an amazing way that there is no longer a horrible, controlling four-letter word called fear. It doesn't even exist. March through these times and remember them, for you expected them and were working towards them. Work toward the new four-letter word - LOVE."
>
> ~ Kryon

Love and Trust are quantum energies (meaning they vibrate and resonate *beyond* the physical) and can be **added** to every system we live within! This high vibrational energy is the ***Light*** that simply and effortlessly illuminates the darkness, so that evil can no longer hide. It brings problems to the forefront to be solved. And it helps break down outmoded ways of thinking and behaving. Wildly enough, when things fall apart, they often get rearranged in a better fashion, benefiting more people than ever. We are certainly living through this now. Hold steady. I know it feels unsettling, and there is still more to come. But we are getting somewhere. A Shift is Happening.

In the midst of any madness, our mission is to keep trying to do **Good**. Keep finding ways to laugh at it all! Continue to practice daily kindness, generosity, and helping others out of joy as well as necessity. Explore the freedom to be "unique" and "original." Invent new ways of communicating without censorship and engage in research and activism. Join people marching in the streets all over the World. Raise your voice so it can be heard while you fight for what is right. We must realize there are some Freedoms we maintain, but some we will lose if we don't pay attention and speak up. Make informed choices for the World we will leave to our children and our children's children. What is **most important**? In what or whom do we believe? What could we be growing and nurturing if we tried a little harder? How can we work to benefit all of Humanity in our Garden?

I look forward to what we have yet to learn. We might find our history books become obsolete overnight! Our very firmament of technology could be revolutionized! I can't wait to learn and discover more about the enhanced Human abilities that come with such consciousness shifts. I believe our ability to work in tune with Nature will be revealed and will greatly enhance our lives. We will be able to do things we only dreamed of: cooperatively clean up the oceans, remediate nuclear waste, control diseases, prevent famine, and prolong life. What if we learn how powerful we really are - and *what is really going on around us* - and we have to create **a whole new idea of ourselves?** What would happen if everyone had to change, open up to and invent a whole New Kind of Civilization, a New Human on a New Earth? Well, welcome to the Show! Get the popcorn, it's all happening.

BUSTED AND AWAITING IMPROVEMENT

Why is so much being revealed now? Because we can no longer ignore the fact that we have been operating within a **chronic disconnect from Nature and what is REAL!**

Humans have solved problems we are still living within. Scientists and inspired geniuses have discovered more solutions than we are aware of, thanks to the News and our Leaders. At times, we have been purposely misled in order to "keep the peace." *Because of this disconnect we are continuing to do harm to our Planet and our People!* We are keeping outdated systems and practices in place for too long when we could be doing better. We continue to allow corporations to do terrible things to the environment. Because of this disconnect we are not only missing out on some of Humanity's greatest inventions, but we are maintaining an unsustainable and unnecessary way of life (that is harmful to our Planet and all People). Much of this is done for the sake of the "almighty dollar." Unproductive, soil-depleting, health-compromising, trash-accumulating, environment-collapsing, inhumane choices are being made everyday for the sake of *business*. **We must notice this, stand up and take action against it.**

Nicola Tesla solved the energy problem for the World in 1891 - yes, 1891. Not only was his Free Energy technology hidden by the electric and gas companies, he died penniless because he would not go along with the military's aims to weaponize his inventions. Can you imagine a Planet *without* electrical wires everywhere, but everyone has power? Where energy naturally provided by the Earth was freely channeled *and given for free*, to all? He solved our biggest energy needs, his designs were brilliant and effective. But contrary to a public **misinformation campaign**, we were told they were unproductive or even dangerous. You better believe the government seized every bit of his ground-breaking research within hours of his death. Of course they would carry to fruition (and utilize) some of his inventions for their own use. But we know relatively little about them today, and certainly don't benefit from them.

I want you to understand that this is merely one example of the control mechanism we have been living within. Think about how food companies overpackage what Nature contained perfectly the first time, like plastic wrap on produce! Imagine what chemical poisons have had to be invented to take the place of our perfect Herbs and Weeds. Notice how much money is spent killing Dandelions, one of our most powerful Medicines. Investigate how geneticists are splicing fish cells into Strawberries to genetically modify our food to have thicker skin. You can witness *many* examples of how **UNNATURAL** our system has become, and why in some cases it fails us.

And why it needs us.

Each one of us must take our own smart and important steps for **NATURE-SUPPORTIVE AWARENESS AND ACTION**. Each one of us has a powerful voice, and it is time we raise it for our Mother Earth and what she provides, for all of our Brothers and Sisters here. I want you to study what is going on with the Planet. I want you to ask questions, wonder why things are the way they are, rebel a little and seek out deeper Truths. I WANT you to question dishonest authority and bad business and poisonous practices! I want you to engage even more. I want you to become a Champion for the Earth.

I want you to have the very best of what Nature provides. I want YOU to profit from the many discoveries we Humans have ALREADY made. I want us to have Free Energy! I want you to live in Harmony with all People, working for the same helpful solutions. I want you to feel the unique Humanity that connects us the World over, and can enable us to enjoy working together. I am asking you to make a difference with your awareness and abilities, your thoughts and actions, your free time and work, your causes and choices, your pocketbook and your vote. I am asking you to join with people of all religious beliefs and political affiliations, colors and creeds to work together for our Earth.

> **"Like Music and Art, Love of Nature is a common language that can transcend political or social boundaries."**
>
> *~ President Jimmy Carter*

Let's release the need to fight behind party or team lines and work together to make real progress. It is time we study together the ways we can clean, restore and preserve our Environment, and spread these life-saving techniques far and wide. It is time we take polluters to task and support organic farmers. It is time we demand declassification of "secret technology" so we can all profit from information heretofore unknown to the public. It is time we understand our planetary neighbors better. It is time we teach our children to meditate and explore their inner worlds. It is time we learn how to operate with Gratitude for the Earth, and make Compassion and Peace and Harmonious Relations a premium. It is time we focus on LOVE. It is high time we all care for Others a little more. It will be our *mutually beneficial* choices, with the correct motivation (*health not money*), working with (*not against*) Nature, that will create the World we are envisioning. Imagine and feel *this* World powerfully until it exists.

Most obviously - it is PAST TIME all of this happened. For **many** decades now, there have been tireless heroes crusading on behalf of our People and Planet. I guarantee you there is someone living nearby who you could connect with, who would inspire you, right in your town. Write to your environmental heroes, your Leaders, your teachers, your heroes - send them direct messsages! Write your Congress-men and -women! Now is the best time ever to find powerful people of like minds, to contact them, go meet them, and join them.

I remind you again to *investigate*, research, and seek out *alternative sources* of information. Read books and papers and websites and stories and be social and correspond with others. Bring your **awareness** to a new level. Explore new social platforms and community organizations. **Study Nature**, seek her Information Field, dare to think and feel for yourselves. I am engaged and excited, right here with you, because I know MUCH more revelation, adventure, and innovation is in store for us.

SPHERICAL REMEDIES

I have heard it said, *"The solution is created at the moment the problem is created, it just needs to be found."* **The solution is the other half of the circle!** It is the Yin to the Yang, the high point of the next cycle. Herbalists teach this truth in the field, that the **"Remedy" grows right next to the "Poison."** We only need to find it and use it. When we need it, it is right there. The remedy plants of Jewelweed, Plantain and Yellow Dock grow right next to the Poison Ivy and Stinging Nettle that cause so much pain. Aloe Vera grows in the hot desert where we are likely to get a sunburn. Soapwort grows next to streams with which it can be used to wash.

Nature offers these examples so we can all trust that **there is a solution somewhere**. That eventually the unhealthy, uncomfortable (or even unjust, or evil) energies will be revealed in their cycle, and that a new way of being will balance those conditions with Goodness, Justice and Light. That *right nearby there will be provided a remedy*, and a more *organic* way of life will always be restored. It is, again, the reflection of our natural, self-healing and adaptive Earth design, reminding us to trust.

We all will have a role to play in this latest phase change. Since I believe our more *natural state* is one of **Peace, Cooperation, and Love**, I think it could be more effortless than it has been. It shouldn't be so hard to "just be nice." I feel that we are already moving in the right direction, regardless of what the evening news has to say or how it may look at any moment. I think our natural progression on Earth is *biased toward* the Good, toward the Light, toward what is truly **natural and unaffected.** And that we won't stop until it feels right.

I believe The Light Wins, and that Love (not fear) will be the sovereign emotion on this Planet.

This is why I am certain that when the system rights itself from the swings of the pendulum, we will see a much more cooperative and mutually benevolent World. I believe we are living through, on many levels, the chaotic growing pains of that very process right now.

The secret to better times, to having the life you want, to being in a higher dimension, or to feeling successful - is to **LIVE THERE RIGHT NOW** - *while* things feel so chaotic. Find that happy place, stay in that peaceful mindset, insist on positivity, and utilize Nature to keep you well and help you stay inspired. The positive energy you generate is what eventually brings your desire into form, and **causes the system to rebalance**. You need to *create* and *be* the **frequency change** you wish to see, and you can live *within* it right this very moment.

SELF-HEALING STATE OF MIND

Nature will go to *ultimate* lengths to heal itself. You need only to look at your own body, as you read this, to prove it to yourself. You have (most-likely) **successfully recovered** from every virus and bacteria that ever made you ill, and millions more that are thwarted by your very powerful immune system every day. Your scars from even deep wounds have all healed. Your broken bones have grown together and recalcified. You have recovered from many of your addictions and bad habits. You have healed every wound you ever received. **YOU ARE A POWERFUL HEALER!** Even if you were very ill at one time in your life - you likely recovered. Life Goes On, by design, and so did yours. Your body works with whatever you give it and still produces a reasonably long Life for you. Even when people do succumb to major illnesses, it takes the body a long time to die. **Your Body wants to survive and is designed to do so against all odds.**

A diseased Human heart will grow to two times its own size just to continue to provide blood to the body. Entire new circulatory networks grow in the bodies of people who have clogged arteries. Parts of the brain assume new duties to compensate when a brain injury occurs. People who lose one of their senses develop other enhanced abilities to meet their needs. Damaged skin and liver cells completely regenerate. Every day the body protects and heals itself.

FOOD - the quality of the "fuel" you use - plays an enormous part in helping your body recover. I watched my dear friend **Doug Rosen**, with *years* of healthy eating and an incredible attitude, reduce his viral load to the point where he was HIV-negative. Diabetes can reverse when a person is put on a healing raw food diet. Terminal cancer could vanish altogether if we would remove the toxins that feed it (like white sugar, preservatives, pesticides, chemical-laden, non-organic food). Imagine what we could heal if we would just give the body exactly what it needs.

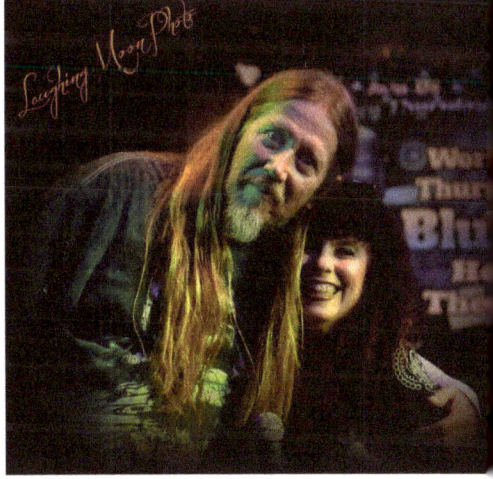

We watched our friend and Blues Legend **Donnie Miller** beat cancer back with a much-improved dietary regimen, Rick Simpson's Oil, MUSIC (of course, the *great* healer), and the Love of his life, Deanne. Donnie decided he had **too much to do** to go right then - and his body responded. We were elated to witness this miracle while it lasted, he got extra (but never enough) years for sure. But he had a gig to play in Heaven; they needed the best guitar wailing, hard-singing Son of Two Mothers in America. So now Donnie Miller is back on Cosmic Tour, Bluesing Up the Great Beyond. Thank God he left his Music with us. His latest record *"Dig"* is his best ever, and my very favorite.
https://www.donniemillermusic.com/home

GOOD TO KNOW

I always teach people to **trust their bodies** - but every now and then you need verification and expert diagnosis. One of my favorite herbal wizards, Scott Storrie once told me, *"Don't be an herbal martyr."* In other words (coming from a devoted natural medicine doctor) it is sometimes necessary to trust allopathic, conventional medicine. Many wonderful advances have been made in modern medicine, medical diagnosis, education and care, and I respect such noble professions. We all know emergency practitioners save bodies everyday, that may not have been capable of healing themselves. So when you know something is not right it is important to find out for sure. **Go see a doctor if you know you need to** - DO listen to your Innate Knowing about this, so you don't regret it later. Besides, just getting a diagnosis, with several different opinions, makes it easier to know what to do to treat it naturally.

> **"These pains you feel are Messengers. Listen to them."**
>
> *~ Rumi*

I tell you now: **even the *very worst diagnosis* has ABSOLUTELY been miraculously overcome by someone**. You've probably heard stories of just such kinds of miracles! Having a diagnosis arms you with data, so then you can go to work on it nutritionally, emotionally, and spiritually. Don't be afraid to find out what's up with your complex body. **Knowing makes it better and gives you a mission.** Now your body can stop giving you desperate pleas for attention, put its red flags away, and get to work healing. There's no need to hide from what you and your body need, or to feel shame for not acknowledging it sooner. I am here to remind you, **the body wants to heal** and it will do everything in its power to do just that. When we listen, heed early warning signs of trouble, and take the best actions, we honor the Message and the Messenger. We are each in possession of a **remarkable healing body**, on a remarkable healing Planet. **Trust it,** believe it and support it every way you can.

> **"There is more wisdom in your Body**
> **than there is in your deepest Philosophy."**
>
> *~Friedrich Nietzsche*

Your body, by the way, is CAPABLE of accomplishing such **miraculous healing** *without* any chemical or pharmaceutical interference. **It can heal itself completely given the right food, conditions, and state of mind**. Natural support, with Herbs and Superfoods, can speed and enhance every healing process the body initiates.

The importance of **detoxifying** cannot be overstated. You must rid the body, environment, and Spirit of poisons, parasites, toxins and triggers, to give it a better fighting chance. Finding ways to let go, purify, be open to the healing process (and happy with the new self you reveal within it) will definitely help deliver the results you need. Accepting and loving yourself helps you heal, re-lease, and become strong.

QUIET TIME REVELATIONS

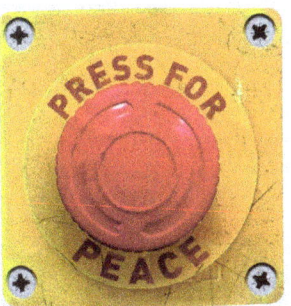

> "Peace is not something you wish for;
> it's something you make, something you do,
> something you are,
> and something you give away."
>
> ~ *John Lennon*

So much of living a healthy, bright and shiny Life starts with being at PEACE with everything! *Seek out* that promising Peace I am talking about - be in the feeling of it everyday now. Seek to live it and embody it. Find it in the present moment. Find it OUTSIDE! Close your eyes for a few minutes several times a day and just feel for Peace with your inner senses. With all the wild advances in machines, we Humans need to make our own personal advances to **preserve our connection to Nature, to Peace**, and to **our Inner Selves**. I would love to see many more people **go within**, or go outside, or begin to meditate. It is wildly helpful to have more time to devote to individuation, self-reflection and self-improvement. To be able to seek and read - and have actual time to "Just Be" with Source, The Great Spirit, your Creator, radiating Peace - is priceless.

If you haven't had enough time for delving inward, **make some time now**. Start today. You don't need any excuse to make time for YOU, and should never feel guilty for needing it. It's actually really important right now, to take a flipping moment to feel it all going by, and find your Center. You need your own time to go deep within yourself to notice what is happening, changing and upgrading. There is new revelation to be found in Inner Exploration. Things are certainly altering there as well.

You have always heard people speak about how the Earth plane is one of "duality." It is true that **your very Being has a dual Nature**. You are more than the physical part of you that exists here in 3D (the Third Dimension). You also have a *multi-dimensional* Higher Self that holds the rest of your Spirit, too big for your body, that resides in many other dimensions. This is the energy from YOU that lives on after death, your Soul, which will continue to exist on other realms. **You are *connected* to your Creator (your Source Field) through this energetic, spiritual part of you.** Through it you have a direct line to higher truths and a completely different teaching perspective, *because* you are connected to a *higher vibrational Source*. It is the Smart Voice in your head that knows best, because it has **ACCESS**! Use it - find closed-eye time, or go back to a Meditation Practice, seek your Higher Self, or connect with Gaia. Ask to speak with Plant Spirits, Ascended Masters, seek the Angel of your City, talk to God. Ask for help and support and information. See if there is any new development or helpful guidance flowing in from acknowledging these wise teachers and perspectives. Always give Gratitude and Love for what you receive, and do write down your conversations.

My personal experience when I meditate these days is very different. I see new geometric patterns, visuals and more complex colors and light when I close my eyes and go within, and I feel my *internal senses* strengthening. I can get into deeper states of altered consciousness in a shorter time. I feel a Peace I can **ALWAYS access** if I will literally **just close my eyes for a second**. I am always so relieved when I do.

I find it is *not very hard at all* to release fearful, anxious or worried feelings when I take the time to close my eyes and center myself. I consciously ground my energy down into the Earth. I call for Nature, and instantly feel the support. I reach inward for my Higher Self, opening my heart, and outward to all my Friends in Spirit and Space, to the Love of my Angels, Guardian Angels, Guides and Protectors. Every time I tune-in to Source/God/Creator I experience a **Field of Love** all around me, and it is of great comfort. It seems like new communications are coming in, so I always keep a Spirit Journal and a pen handy. I hear the personal voice of my Higher Self more clearly and I have been feeling a palpable change of energy deep inside. Often, the words I write down while meditating turn out later to be quite inspiring in their guidance. I always communicated with the Plants and all living things - and even the Rocks and Minerals other people assumed were not alive. But lately, I am feeling more than ever wise support from **EVERYTHING**, and I know that I am not alone. I feel *every living and supposedly non-living thing* broadcasting energy my way, as well as a whole inner world willing to communicate with me. I simply need to make the time to tune in.

Dreams are another way you receive helpful guidance. Before you go to bed, command yourself to *program your sleep for dreams you can remember*, and whatever else you need. Sometimes I will say, *"Okay, tonight I require 12 hours of sleep in the next four hours, and that my dreams will be plentiful and easy to recall when I awaken, refreshed and fully rested."* I'm telling you, *Sleep Programming* really works! I have made it through many a long night by telling my body I will get more sleep than I really can, and it turns out I DO wake up rested! Pay attention to the FEELING you have when you wake up. Before you move, just reflect for a minute about what you were dreaming, and the feeling with which it left you. Write your dreams down if you can, sometimes they are predictive and revealing. Sometimes you may just feel reassured by them - but whatever you glean, this is another avenue of inner communication.

There's much to receive to in quiet contemplation of the outer natural world, too. Outside the high vibrational Birdsong is raising everyone's energy higher, and creating the frequency that instructs the Spring grass to grow and the trees to bud! Enhanced Light from the Sun is beaming **new information** directly to us every eight minutes. The Planetary Motions and alignments are sending us supportive energy at all times. Our Dreams are launching us into new energetic realms. The new expanding colors of Plants, Flowers, and Grasses seem especially vivid. Everything is changing and growing. Nature is calling louder than ever before! I think this is a **revealing of** the balancing point we all are working toward. We need Nature's guidance and support now more than ever. Let's work with the healing potential of our dual Nature, trusting it, trusting we are well-made, and can be peaceful, content, free of fear and worry.

PLEASE BELIEVE THE GOOD NEWS

Whatever is happening out there in the World, I want you to hear some Good News; **YOU are being HELPED.** Your prayers are being heard and answered. Solutions are being prepared for you, and wonderful synchronicities are coming to prove it to you. YOU ARE NOWHERE NEAR ALONE IN THIS. Keep a watchful eye out for the **support you *are* receiving**, whether it is green lights all the way to work, or the check in the mail at the perfect moment. When you witness strange and wonderful things happening to you, recognize that it is the work of what I call your **Spiritual Entourage,** working with your **Creator**. It's all real, and it's all happening to encourage you, keep you going! Interesting, it seems like the messages increase as you notice them, so say *thank-you* and stay tuned!

Your life matters to Creation! You are an important part of The Plan. You have a mission to accomplish and only *you* can do it. Your have planned with and been gifted Guardian Angels, Guides, the Archangels, your Family of Loved Ones in Spirit, Ancient Sisters and Brotherhoods, Gaia, the Cosmos and your ultimate Creator who are all assisting you in your purpose. Every single day, you are being given **Guidance, Support** and **Love** from this enormous Spiritual Entourage - *specifically* so you can make it through these times! Feel them, so you can be comforted by this.

If you only knew how LOVED you are! If you only knew how much help and protection you are being given. Your voice matters, and *you will make a difference* while you are here, **they will see to it that you do**. It is a perfect time to open up to even more of this Divine support. My experience is that your Guardian Angel, and any kind of Angelic Support, can only work for you when you **ASK.** You must engage it, work with it, and specifically request help. Just like *people* appreciate being ASKED to help and enjoy being recognized and given thanks and gratitude, so too does your Spiritual Entourage. They love to co-create with you if you will simply authorize their help. But, like the Prime Directive in *Star Trek*, they cannot interfere unless you *DO ask*, so they do not infringe upon your Free Will. They must have your authorization to proceed. **Ask and it is always given.**

Life is much more *magical* than we have been led to believe! We are *all* being SEEN and guided by a **Spiritual Support System** that operates much the way our bodily support systems know how to heal, on yet a whole other level of our programmed design for Life. We are all being given assistance and guidance on higher dimensions by the Natural System of the Logos **because we are a vital part of a design that goes way beyond just this Planet.** Our success here on Earth really DOES affect the rest of the Galaxy and beyond. So it is only natural that there may be *support from*

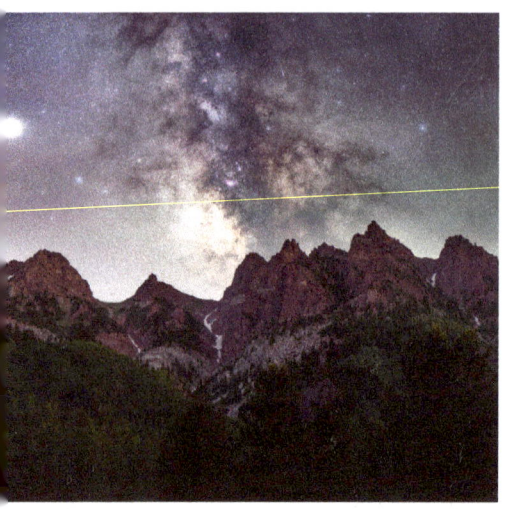

beyond our sphere and Solar System for our process. Turns out that there is a whole other World of support - the Galactic news is very encouraging, according to insider sources. We are receiving *real help* from beyond Earth, from the very ancient energy of our Creator and quite probably from ancient **Star Races** that originally seeded Life here - our Celestial Family, our Otherworldly Neighbors (explored more in *Volume Three*). Revelations are coming out about UFO's and our celestial neighbors right now, in recently declassified government documents! Expect to learn much more soon.

SHE'S ALIVE

Speaking of being open to new realizations, have you received this one? You are learning and growing on a **Living Being** that our modern culture has simply designated as a **Planet** (and may even be a Plane, who knows?). Our Earth is very much **ALIVE** just as you are. *Everything Is Alive.* And while she expresses differently than Humans, the Earth also has a **Body** and a **Soul**. You are actually on this physical and spiritual journey together, companions, living through it all in cooperation, relationship and vibrant co-creation. You may have recognized this always and speak with our Mother Earth daily. But if not, chances are good that it *feels right* to you, in your heart, that she is living, too. Even though it is a little mind-blowing, it makes her more REAL.

> "Nature is alive and talking to us. This is not a metaphor."
>
> ~ *Terrence McKenna*

We call her GAIA, Anima Mundi, Mother Earth - and she is in right now in constant communication with you. She is a Sovereign, Ensouled Being just like you, but she expresses her energy through the medium of Nature. Her Body is our Earth, and what she experiences we can relate to our *own* bodies, as they both go through many of the same processes. She is your **primordial Mother** and she is available to you. Tune in to your body, open your Heart, and then ask to connect with and **feel Gaia**. Reach down into the Earth until you feel her energy rise from below you to greet and embrace you. You will feel her in your heart and she always answers when you call, usually before you finish speaking a question. She also lovingly speaks in the Birds and Flowers and Trees or even the Weather that sends signals your way. You can experience her teachings in many ways.

You can send her Love every day, *pray for her* balance, visualize her radiant health, ask for pollution remediation for her, talk to her, and even ask ***her*** for assistance with weather, protection and help. **Flip to page 350 to hear her tell you so, in her own words, in my interview with Gaia though Pepper Keen Lewis.** Connecting with our beloved Mother Nature has been a remarkable opportunity for me, and this interview offers a unique opportunity to give her a voice that YOU can hear. She has some great information to impart, and I think her words will encourage you. Just remember, you can connect and hear her, too!

Beyond a channel, a book, or a screen on an electronic device, at *every moment* there is **Gaian, Divine information** coursing right toward you, sending you moment-by-moment input with her natural signals. From the life stage of every plant to the physical condition of every person, from the quality of the wind to the sounds of the birds, from the Lightshow in the Heavens to the Fakeshow of the Media - there are signs everywhere. You can see symbols and conditions, colors and feelings. ***This is a system that does communicate*** and information is being indicated to you everywhere, all the time. It is helpful to consciously *slow down* and become very still, to open up to it all, noticing again what sensations you feel. Come to Gaia *lovingly*. Greet her, send her love, and then tune in to the feelings and words and images you receive, to experience what is there to be LEARNED.

At all times the Information is there (here). Once you realize that much more is coming your way than "meets the eye" - it's easier to rearrange your vision to see it, and your other senses to deeply feel and receive it. Perhaps you can even open up *new* senses, develop your **extrasensory perception**, through which even more Information streams in! You are cultivating a Loving, *evolving* Earth Connection, which offers you the opportunity to work with it , evolving yourself and your abilities.

- **IN AND OUT MEDITATION:** I like to have a journal in my lap when I tune in to connect to Gaia, or the Sun or my Higher Self or my Daddy, whomever I am seeking at the moment. I ask if they will come to speak with me, say hello and open my heart, and then ask questions which I write down in shorthand. Then I close my eyes, and wait for some words to come into my head. I open my eyes when I hear something fairly complete, simply write the words down, and try not to think about it all too much. I just grasp the feelings these word bursts give me, and then I write them down as best I can. Then I reply, close my eyes and go inside again to listen, and repeat. Before I know it, there are a few pages of dialogue and some actual helpful information there! Many times, I personally did not know the information that the pages contained. Where did it come from exactly? Am I just counseling and teaching myself? If I am being supported in a loving way, by our Loving Universe - who cares?

Gaia counsels us to remove the boundaries between us all, and blur the edges that divide us. She implores us to join our energy into One, in the hopes of understanding and FEELING that we are Equals. We are Family. We are **all parts of a Whole**. We are connected and All One in the creative energy of **LOVE**. We get to work with each other co-creatively to make amazing things and find radical solutions, and that's why we are here! This is the same inclusive, loving, rejuvenating feeling that we get from connecting with the Divine - **The Great Spirit, One Infinite Creator, Source, The Universe, God** - our **Creator**, in which we are all united. We're all the same stuff.

TUNE-IN TO THE LIGHT CHANNEL

Take the advice of George Washington Carver, someone with whom I was fascinated as a child, *"I love to think of Nature as an Unlimited Broadcasting Station, through which God speaks to us every hour, if we will only tune in."* So, find your way to listen! You can read more about George's revolutionary thinking, as I feature him, with some other rebellious geniuses, in Chapter 4.

Dialing up the Light Channel - tuning-in to your Higher Self, Nature, or God - imparts Information. When you expand to *allow in* this extra Divine energy, it creates a super high vibration within you: **LIGHT!** You literally *shine* with the extra vibrational energy, as the increase of **Photons** (light particles) are received and emitted. **Divine Light** works like an extra nourishment source, like a supervitamin, infusing every one of your cells with energy. So what changes are happening to *all of us* with this dramatic increase of Light? And why NOW?

It is all a set-up for **ENLIGHTENMENT**. Adding more Light to a system (or a person) *advances* it! We on Earth are preparing for a major shift, a leap in consciousness, an expansion of Light of epic proportions. This is a repeating design of this Solar System, it has been a set-up all along. It is simply Earth's turn again.

COSMIC EVOLUTION AND THE PHOTON BAND

As it turns out, our Solar System is currently traveling through a very charged, and very bright, Light-filled place in Space, a cloud of high temperature glowing particles some experts call the **Photon Band**. It is also referred to as the Golden Nebula, The Manasic Ring, and the Cosmic Fluff (more in *Volume Three*). It is another influence that is causing Life on Earth to be very stimulated, fast-evolving and new! **Light is increasing exponentially in our Solar System**, and this new energy is making every Planet change, is raising our Body's frequency, and has probably even increased the Speed of Time. Some scientists believe what we are experiencing now is more like the equivalent of a 16-hour day, instead of twenty-four! Whether or not this is provable, I know you sense the obvious quickening of time and frequencies.

Since no one alive now has ever lived through this new influence of Photons, we have no idea what will happen. But we are beginning to see the effects on Earth, as well as all the Planets of our Solar System. They are ALL getting *"hotter, brighter and more magnetic,"* says David Wilcock, citing many scientists who have proven we are going through a Solar-System-Wide Warming. As if being affected by all this *new Light* from our **Galactic Location** in space was not enough, the radical **Change to the Aquarian Age** is upon us as well, with a Revolutionary Code we are living through. ALL of this contributes to the many natural cycles meant to uplevel Planets and People with Light and Cosmic Energy - and it has been going on for eons. This Photon Band location in Space plays its **evolutionary** part in programming the changes that ride on its Light.

LIGHT MAKES RIGHT

Light can be directed. *Every time* you make an Intention or Prayer or have a Positive Thought, you are actually *programming the Light* - the Photons - to work for you, to create your blessing in the World. You can imprint them with intention, and charge the Light to produce your desired results. The healing implications of this Light Technology are greater than you can imagine.

This is no different than the intentional sending of White Light and Love. **Rupert Sheldrake, Dr. Bruce Lipton, Dr. Joe Dispenza, Lynne McTaggart** and many more Field researchers have proven that people who are prayed for, or sent healing energy, actually **DO receive the Photons of Light** being sent. Their proof will blow you away!

> "A scientifically controlled study, conducted by German researchers at the University of Kassel, has shown that while the chest area of an average person emits only 20 Photons of light per second, someone who meditates on their heart center and sends Love and Light to others emits an amazing 100,000 Photons per second. That is 5000 times more than the average human being. Numerous studies have also shown that when these Photons are infused with a loving and healing intent, their frequency and vibration increases to the point where they can literally change matter, heal disease, and transform negative events. Ten minutes of meditating on Compassion, on Kindness for others, and you will see its effects all day. That's the way to maintain a calm and joyous mind."
>
> ~ *Dalai Lama*
> from *"The Book of Joy: Lasting Happiness in a Changing World"*

It is common knowledge now that many people are miraculously healed by the frequency of prayer. You probably have stories of family members or friends who made complete and miraculous recoveries when so many people were praying for them. Prayer and Meditation align you with an energy field of Light (frequency). Your Concentration and Intent will **magnify, potentize and direct** that Frequency Field to create Healing. When more than one person meditates (or prays) at the same time, this energy field is increased *exponentially*. Because of this dynamic effect, many Prayer Groups witness the person they have prayed for being spontaneously healed, or miraculously recovering when the diagnosis was dismal. The Light is WORKING!

Meditating in *groups*, with directed intention, has **stunning. provable results**. When a group of Japanese Buddhist Monks prayed and chanted for a very smelly, polluted water source from the Fujiwara Dam, it cleared and became fresh again. Dr. Masaru Emoto has done amazing research with photos of the crystallization of Water after it has been subjected to positive (or hurtful) words, images and music. He has unequivocally proven: **Water absorbs and retains intent and information**. His snowflake crystals of the Dam Water before and after prayer tell the whole story. The "before prayer" crystal is misshapen and discolored, with no geometry, form or symmetry. The snowflake crystal of the Water that was **prayed for** is a perfectly formed symmetrical beauty, a geometrical wonder, stunningly complex & pristine. This is just the beginning of what directed thought can accomplish - and your body is 70% water!

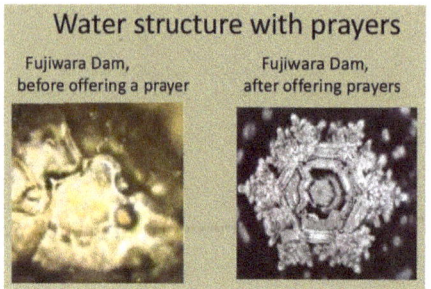

Water structure with prayers
Fujiwara Dam, before offering a prayer
Fujiwara Dam, after offering prayers

> **"In 1960, Maharishi Mahesh Yogi predicted that one percent of a population practicing the TM technique would produce measurable improvements in the quality of life for the whole population. This phenomenon was first documented in scientific research in 1976 when it was found that when 1% of a community practiced Transcendental Meditation, the crime rate was reduced by 16% on average."[2]**

This group meditation phenomena has been named "The Maharishi Effect" after the ground-breaking research he inspired. Since the early days of its realization, this Effect has been rigorously studied, practiced, and perfected. Recently, larger groups in deep meditation have been proven to **lower crime, violence and negative Earth change events by significant amounts**. In a particular study of this meditational effect, involving a group of 7,000 praying monks, there was a **72% change** in before and after crime statistics. Now *that* is altering reality and truly making a difference with your life and your energy.

This is something we should practice Worldwide with our fellow Humans!

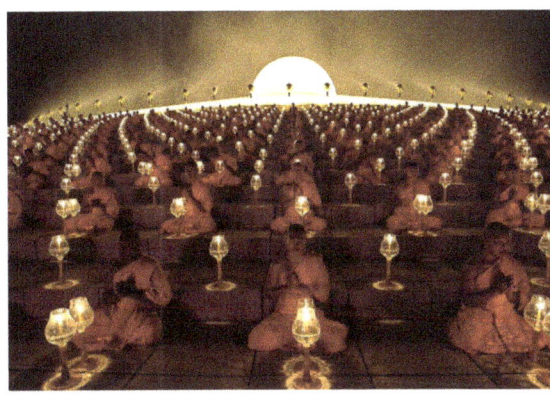

Let's Do It. Let's meditate in groups for all the best causes. Gatherings of like-minded individuals can send positive energy to all beings and to Gaia, creating powerful **Life Support.** When we do find ourselves in a group, let's end our meetings and videos and calls with a short meditation or prayer for World Peace and Planetary Cooperation. What could we do with our positive thoughts and prayers? What could we send **on** the Light? We will all need to *explore* creative ways to gather and utilize this amazing power we have been given.

What environmental disasters could we repair or redirect if we ALL meditated on them together? Could we change the weather? Could we move a hurricane? Could we split a storm around us? Could we heal the Water? Our Atmosphere? Soothe our collective pain or control oppressive viruses? What could our powerful, intentional thoughts and prayers for the Future of our New Earth create? How can we use this Collective Light Technology for GOOD? I can tell you, I have done it with a tornado in our neighborhood, we could see it in the back yard and we prayed it up and away.

You have power and abilities you have yet to understand. Each one of you can channel your own humble, personal **prayers** for restoring and healing yourselves and our Planet. **Speak them daily.** I write myself new daily Prayers (or Decrees or Meditations, whatever you like to call them) every few months, and speak them with passion everyday if I can. Also, when you see weather disasters looming, pray them away, command for them to be moved, pray for early warning, pray to save the people and animals nearby.

"The momentum of all subjects increases when you focus upon it."

~ Abraham, through Esther Hicks

The KEY with a practice like this is to **imagine your desired result vividly in your mind**, see it in detail, *witness* it happening and accomplished perfectly. I enhance my prayers, supercharging them and **speaking my miracles into existence** by saying, *"I command that my request manifests effortlessly. May this or an even more benevolent outcome, better than I could hope for or imagine, be created!"* Practice this type of CREATION focus often. We make great strides when we meditate together in groups, but we can be so very powerful when we work with the Light individually. Why wait? Let's all pray and meditate together right now. Open your heart and receive the Love of the Divine Light in your own way. Speak or read the following Benevolent Prayer:

I open my heart and tune-in to my Creator, greeting my Angels and Great Spirit. I ask for my Highest Light to enter and surround me. I receive, and can feel Loving, Healing Frequencies coming to me from Divine Source, my whole body filling with this Holy Light of Love. I receive with great gratitude all of my Friends in Spirit and Space. I open to the Protection of the Archangel Michael, and we allow only the highest vibrational energies near me. I feel my body *shining*, as all the vibrant energy is coursing through me, lighting me up. I visualize myself, living in **Radiant, Renewed Health** and my Body is now healing dramatically with the support of all the Light. I request and imagine **all health issues resolved, and all ailments reversed to pristine, optimal, original-blueprint Health**. I see my perfected design updating. I witness a sparkly River of Healing Light expanding out *beyond* my body's border. These Loving Healing Vibrations expand outward to nourish my Beloved Family. I see every one of them shine with the Light of True Radiant Health. I witness as the Light spills out over the entire neighborhood, filling my Neighbors and their gardens with Abundant Joy. Further still, the Light of Love spreads over my whole state, my whole country, all countries and oceans and our whole beloved Earth. I imagine my Body and the beautiful Earth surrounded in the Light of Love until they both glow brightly. I witness, while I heal, that every single Person, Animal, Mineral and Plant is also renewed, and the Planet Earth is thriving and rejoicing, glowing with healthy and joyful Life.

I join with all my Brothers and Sisters, and together we work on **Solutions**. We see the Water clean again, the Air full of Light, and the Earth and her People renewed. We pray for the healing of the Plant Kingdom, and the Animals, Insects and Elementals. We pray for the Soil and the Minerals, and give genuine thanks for the Abundant Food we are all gifted with that grows just for us. We give our Gratitude to Fire and Ether, and their Elemental Creational Forces, without which we could not survive.

We include ALL People in our prayers. All People deserve *all* the LOVE we can possibly create. **We send up a prayer for the *evil ones* who may need it the most.** We pray to see the difference that our positive concentration makes, in a brighter and more Loving World. We all pray for a Most Benevolent Outcome for Earth, invoking Executive Function to utilize and enhance the Highest Optimal Timeline. We pray for **PEACE** that we can *feel* right now, here and all over the World. **I am renewed, you are renewed and the Earth is renewed. May we all increase in Peace, Love, Health, Harmony and Abundance.** Aho, Aho, We Are Light, We Make It So. Thank-you, thank-you, thank-you - it is done, it is done, it is done.

I know that even this small moment we shared together makes a genuine difference. Come back to this meditation and practice or speak it aloud often! Thank-you.

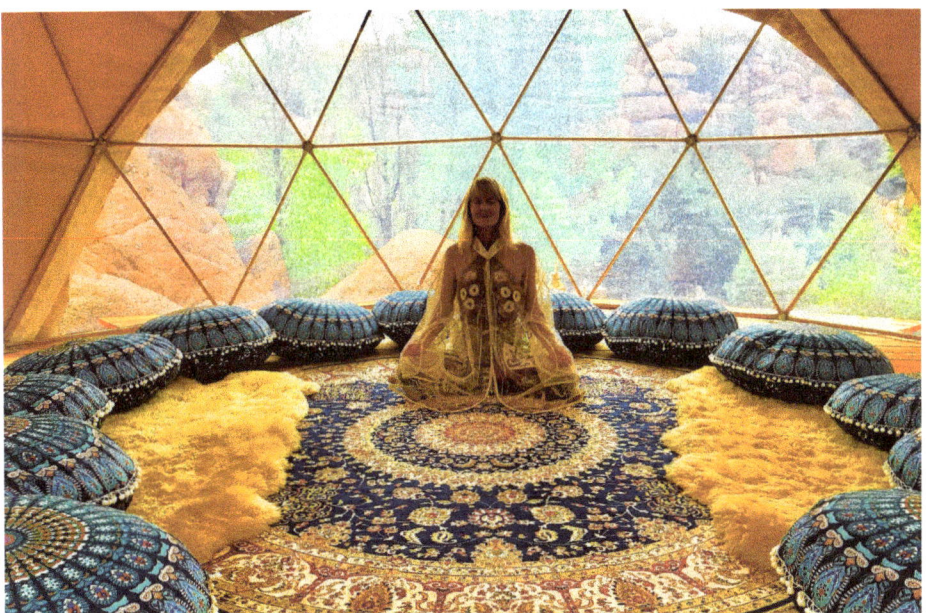

THE NEW HUMAN

I believe we are, each of us, quite literally transforming with every breath. As Dannion Brinkley says, *"The whole world changes and is completely different from the moment you breathed in, to the moment you breathe out."* This gives me HOPE! We always have a chance to make it better, even breath by breath. And I remember Louise Hay always said, *"The Point of Power is in the Present Moment."* Each and every moment, we can take steps to make things right, we can make changes to benefit ourselves and Humanity. And it is NOT too late.

> **"There is a dawn of a New Human happening right now.
> Your neighbors are changing, your kids are changing, your
> parents are changing, your nephews, your nieces, your sisters
> and brothers. Everybody is changing right now.
> Why not you?"**
>
> *~Allison Coe*

We **remake ourselves** with our new choices, new positive thoughts and prayers. It matters how we spend our energy, each second, each breath! **We have the power and the will to change anything right now.** We do not need to be bound by old definitions or probable disasters, history or genealogy - we can rewrite our lifeplan at any time. Courses can be changed! Our **choices** are the very way we create what comes next. And what YOU decide to create, influences the Many, so CHOOSE WISELY.

What it means to be Human is even changing. We are morphing, and we must be cognizant of all the changes we **authorize** and accept. It takes personal responsibility to run one of these bodies and all the power inherent! We are not all in agreement about how to utilize it. We might not all believe, for instance, that Transhumanism is a good thing - we might not all want a microchip in our finger that unlocks our cars, or buys our food or identifies our location at work. However, that same technology might help someone to see or walk again. We might not all believe in chemical remedies filled with poisons and technology, but in some cases they could be life-saving. Above all, we must maintain **choice!** We have to **stay aware** about changes anyone OUTSIDE of us might want to make to our personal biology and preserve our right to choose. This is exactly why we need to follow our own moral compass and listen to our **Innate Guidance** more than ever.

Search your feelings. Don't be herded into believing or doing something because others do, or because you saw it on the news, because someone shamed you into doing it, or because it follows a "party line." **Never grant permission for something that takes away your free will, power to choose, compassion, health freedom or personal peace.** No individual (or party) that usurps this is worth following.

ALL People have a voice, ALL Lives Matter, and many more people are realizing we can **create change when we band together** - look what happens when we take to the streets! Nothing goes unseen, and rightly so. This **New Human** will not be lied to, lorded over, muzzled, fooled, discriminated against, abused, treated unfairly, or enslaved. "*Been there, done that,*" we see it now; time for a new program, a new era, a new, more inclusive operating system upgrade.

Pepper Keen Lewis said something that keeps coming back to me. With all the wondering about information and biased media sources, it becomes more important than ever to rely on your **"in-house information."** What do you **feel in your gut?** How does your **heart** respond? Your heart is your most important discerning organ that helps you feel your correct path, and you know you also have your "gut feelings." **This is because the intestines and heart both include brain tissue for linking and quickly processing those exact kinds of instinctual decisions.** If a piece of your brain is there, it makes sense to pay more attention to **how things feel** in these energy centers of your body. **Feel your way** through the fast-paced changes, and trust that your Emotional Guidance System will never let you down. Act according to how GOOD something makes you feel and pay real attention to the stuff that's just not right! Your in-house feedback, your feelings, will help point you in the correct personal direction, every time. The more you trust yourself on this, use this guidance EVERY TIME, the faster it proves completely true and always reliable.

NEW IMPULSES: STAIRWAY A

There was a man named **Brian Clark** who was working on the 84th floor of Building 2 of the **World Trade Center on September 11, 2001**. When the first explosions hit the nearby North Tower, there were crashes and glass blowing out and a terrible cacophony, and the people in his office watched as flames grazed their windows and paper was falling from the sky. They had no idea what had happened.

Seventeen minutes later, a second explosion tore through the WTC South Tower 2 where Brian was, impacting directly between the 77th-85th floors. Suddenly it was sheer chaos, as his office was right in the blast zone. Stunned, but somehow unharmed, he regained his senses and stumbled his way through the falling structures to find the stairways.

Once he reached the end of a long hallway, he stood with the choice of three stairways to take - Staircase A, B, or C. **Just then, he heard a voice.** Not anyone special, or his voice, but a voice, a deep feeling, and then a real *physical* nudge, that pushed him to "*Go to the Left, to Stairway A.*" He couldn't explain the feeling, but he went with this guidance and followed his deepest gut impulse, hoping to survive.

Miraculously, while in the staircase, he heard and then found a man named Stanley who was completely buried in rubble, with only his hand sticking out to be seen. Brian rescued him, and pulled him from the wreckage. The two of them were able to make it all the way down Stairway A to the Plaza level, and **exit the building** together, heroically and triumphantly. As it turns out, they were *two out of only four people* who survived from their impacted floors, where hundreds of people had worked. Later, they would find out that both staircases B and C were *impassable*, as a result of the location of the damage, and would have only led them to their death. And of course, not long after their daring escape, both Towers collapsed altogether. This man, **trusting his inner voice**, saved both of their lives.

Trust your body to inform you. You get instinctual messages all the time. YOU ARE BEING TOLD WHAT TO DO by your Feelings. The hardest part is listening to everything that the *very smart* intuitive voice inside your head suggests! Listen - that you take a raincoat, or drive a different route, or leave a few minutes early. Sometimes the voice tells you to take something with you that you will find you need later that day. Pay attention, trust this guidance (and just do it). This is again what many call your **INNATE KNOWING**. It's a very well-informed sense. Don't resist its wise guidance.

Your sense of Innate Knowing has always been there for you. We will talk more about it throughout the book, but you **all** know what I mean. You know the voice, you recognize the guidance, and following it is always in your best interest. How many times after something bad happens do you say, "And I *knew* it, too! **I should have listened to myself.**" Each time is another lesson in listening to your Innate. Don't let the lessons become more serious, just follow your Inner Voice when you hear it the first time! You may receive *multiple* signals in order to avoid disaster. But sometimes there's only time for one little nudge. **Follow it.**

I believe these extrasensory perceptions and clues from our Innate will continue to become stronger the more attention we pay to their voice. We become altered ourselves in our own spiritual Evolution. We are in the process of becoming much more sensitive, much more perceptive, with far greater knowing than we ever had before. It is time we appreciate and **cultivate the wisdom** that is coursing into us daily!

UNPRECEDENTED EXPERIENCES

The past few years brought with them a host of unusual happenings. Most of us have never been through such strange, unexpected and even tragic times. I was reminded that many of our ancestors, even our parents and grandparents, had pivotal, sometimes tragic, life-altering things happen to them, too, which forever changed their lives and cultures. But **they survived** and became stronger and wiser for the experience. It may help you to reach back into your lineage and pull strength from the families who came before you, who experienced so much transformation through their challenges, and still went on to **succeed and overcome**. Ask your living relatives how they were able to cope, and learn their heroic stories of overcoming to add to your own.

Call on your *Ancestors in Spirit* for guidance! Seek your Soul Family in your prayers and meditations, try to connect with them and learn their stories. They may be available to offer you some energetic support. In Physics, courtesy of Albert Einstein, we know that **energy does not die or disappear**, it is neither created nor destroyed, it is only *transformed*. So your Loved Ones are still very much "there" - somewhere in another etheric realm to which your Higher Self *does* have an all-access pass. You can sit within their energy and feel their deep love for you when you reach out to them. Look for messages from them in daily life, in the bright red cardinal that stops to look you in the eye, the butterfly that lands on you, the enormous murmuration of

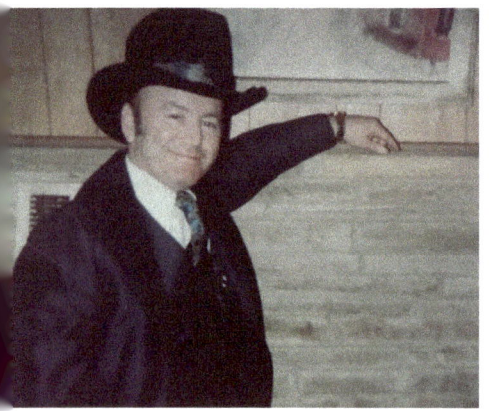

birds you see over your house. This is one of the secret and beautiful ways Nature helps them communicate with you. The many beautiful synchronicities that make you think of your loved ones, and help you FEEL them, I believe, are **proof of their contact**. What a joy it is to acknowledge them and communicate back. I am thrilled every time I get the feeling my Daddy is still very much here with me, and I love talking to him. Without fail, his voice and his guidance still exist and continue to nurture me. This helped me with my grief more than anything, because I realize **he lives on Unlimitedly** as Energy and as a Guide for me now. And he can still crack me up and laugh his way loudly through my life! He says he will still be there anytime I call.

BRING IT ON

You will hear Gaia herself say, **"Humans Are Evolving."** This means we are in the *middle* of the process, and can take an active role in manifesting exactly the Life and the Planet we want. What kind of influences are we under? It could be very helpful to understand that, always good to know what we are working with. What kinds of new freedoms are we looking to **include** in our new vision of ourselves? As individuals, what matters most to us? It is time to face ourselves, question ourselves, and feel our genuine answers in order to create a path to transformation.

What kinds of strides will people make for their personal health if it is threatened? What will we want to fight for, or be passionate about? Who will we march for next? Or even better, **when will we want to STOP fighting?** When will enough people realize the cost of separation and war and violence is too great? When will WE create something better? When will we Unite?

Here is where it starts. **Transformation requires Energy, Awareness, and Intention.** If you get inspired by anything, it creates a positive shift in your **Energy** flow RIGHT NOW. Your inspiration will produce brand new Energy. Taking time for yourself for inner focusing, meditation and contemplation offers you the gift of **Awareness**. Intending is fairly effortless, it takes only a moment to know your heart's desire, and to **set and send** out a most benevolent **Intention**. That is all it takes. Perfect, you are now transforming!

Michael Hamilton, one of the previous owners from Angel Valley outside of Sedona, Arizona gave me the advice to **"Follow Your Greatest Excitement."** He traveled the world doing this alone, basing his journey on which choices FELT more exciting, beautiful, sparkling and attractive. At each crossroads he would ask himself, "Which direction is *more* exciting?" *Every* time, the road and the experience he chose in this way proved synchronistic, life-altering, more educational and just plain FUN. He found that when he **listened to his gut feelings and intuitions** about what *felt* most exciting, he was not only never disappointed, but actual rescues came a few times from trusting his inner guidance. Michael left us (went Unlimited) early in 2021, at 3:33 am - and I know he is so happy because he really DOES know everything now! I am grateful for this legacy concept he left to all of us.

It is so important to explore what **inspires** you, excites you, what wakes you up to your current "NOW" moment. What makes you stay up all night wanting to learn more? This is a clue about YOUR evolutionary contribution! When you feel your Energy light up and you get really excited, you are perfectly in the flow of this transformational power. You lose time. You create out of thin air! **Your *Excitement Energy* is your most potent gift to Human Consciousness and can and should be directed.** It is the key to making positive changes in your life and the lives of those around you. Find it, and you will know yourself and your mission better.

How are you going to express all of your greatest thoughts and desires, and in what way will YOU become The New Human? **Your life is yours to work with.**

Be conscious about the energy you are offering *others* in finding your best and most authentic expression. Be Kind and Tolerant and Loving with those around you. Love them unconditionally, regardless of what they believe. Remember, when we are all **transforming at the same time**, at different rates, sometimes it gets a tad bit messy! It is wise to realize we don't all become enlightened at once, like *"the rainstorm doesn't stop all at once,"* as Josh White, Jr. used to say. Be patient with each other's progress and the awakening Mass Consciousness of Enlightenment. Seek to spread Benevolent Energies everywhere you go, to everyone you meet. Be supportive, inclusive and not divisive. **Kindness and Tolerance** are our new goals. Becoming this type of Radiant New Human is Blissful, Peaceful and Positively Light! As well as *Essential*.

This next section is purely a personal update about my journey. If you like, you can move forward to Chapter 2 and skip this autobiographical material.

THE (LATEST) NEW ME

Our life stories are **teaching devices**. You may learn something valuable from my experiences, so I like to share them. I personally have learned so many things by watching what happened to my friends and mentors throughout the years. Maybe you will read something that reminds you of issues you have been through, and you can consequently understand them better, or at least feel like you are not alone! It is important we all realize that success comes with many LESSONS. What has happened to me in the last 16 years has been full of them!

In the early part of my life, I was a professional actress in the Musical Theatre, and traveled literally all over this country, singing and performing. But I was always fascinated by the workings of the Natural World, losing myself out in Nature, chasing flowers and butterflies and colors since I was a little girl. I used to steal Coleus leaves from the neighbor to grow in my bedroom. I fed squirrels on the roof outside my window. I made my own little bowls of incense, with cloves and orange peels I would sneak out of the kitchen. I surrounded myself with flowers.

When I got old enough to travel alone, I road-tripped across the land, from coast to coast, watching all the PLANTS zoom by my windshield. Once, on my first foray to the Pacific Northwest, I even fell in love and decided to marry The Forest! Ever since those early adventures, I've lost (and found) myself in Nature, journeying, taking classes, gathering certifications and constantly researching Plants and Natural Remedies.

In 1988, after a lot of soul-searching, I heeded the call from the Plant Kingdom, and moved home to Colorado, where I was born. There, I grew even further enamoured with Nature, and absolutely blown away by her resources, with which I started to craft things. I researched and studied, experimenting until I founded and formulated enough products to start a body care company that I called **Little Moon Essentials**, acting as CEO for more than 20 years. I invented upwards of 400 different natural recipes and products for Little Moon, for the mass market and private clients. I loved to take my beautiful Little Moongirls to trade shows and retreats hawking our wares, and we made quite a splash, riding up in limousines, dressed in hemp, creating a buzz, spraying our Theramists and turning people on daily to natural body care. I loved my time educating people about the value and ease of using topical essential oil remedies. But, I found there were still many people who did not know the *necessity* of using CLEAN Natural Remedies that are free of chemicals, carcinogens, and hormone disrupters - for our bodies and the body of our Mother Earth. So I had a real mission.

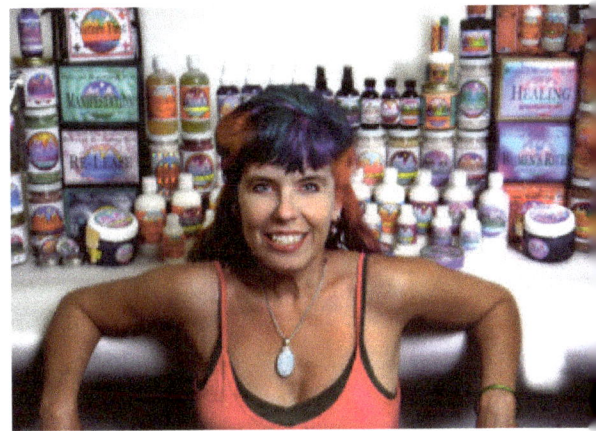

In my spare time from Little Moon, I decided to branch out a bit. I had a blast performing music with Dave Allen and several other bands, writing articles for The Local Magazine, teaching at raw food retreats and exhibiting at natural product events. I watched my friends Brigitte and Avo write books, and many of my contemporaries start retreat centers and release worthy personal projects. So I decided to write my first non-fiction book about Little Moon's journey and Raw Aromatherapy. At the time of *Volume One's* release in 2008, I assumed I would start *Volume Two* right away. But the country had just started to take a major economic downward spiral. I had hoped my company would somehow be immune to the economic tanking, and the resulting financial set-backs that so many were experiencing.

We made it through several years fairly unscathed, but eventually it affected our business too, as the economy finally caught up with all of our customers. Overnight, I lost future sales from my largest client, responsible for 75% of our income (which drove the lesson home about putting too many eggs in one basket...remember?). Little Moon had been a super-thriving business with 14 employees, an international reach, and **more than a million dollars** in sales every year. But with this loss, on top of the economic downturn and my customers' struggles, it all radically crashed down. Suddenly, Dave Allen and I, with a swiftly reduced staff of only two dedicated Little

Mooners, had to hold it all together. We had to learn to function with one-third of our normal sales, with rent and raw material prices going up, up, up. Such were the times. I had to work too hard to simply survive and save the business. The book had to wait.

I am sure anyone who was financially affected then (and lately) can relate! I called it my Dark Night of the Soul, further darkened by Dave Allen moving to Austin to play music for six months. I sank into a depression and lived through some low, dark days, and too many late nights of Stella Artois and "Twilight" movies! My frustration was increasing, my passion was waning, my normally rigid raw diet had floundered, my drive to push the business was simply not there. I began to feel I was no longer a great steward for my company. I am not usually one to despair, but I was getting low. As I have said, I believe the answers are always created *with* the questions, the solutions are always created *with* the problems. But this was pretty hard, and I could not see or feel the remedy I tried to believe was there. Not to mention, I had been mysteriously visited by three BATS while living alone, my nerves were shot, I missed my partner, and I was feeling pretty fragile.

Late in 2010, I attempted to sell the business and move to Austin, but the Fates just wouldn't have it. So, my beloved Dave Allen heard my call for help and came back home to Steamboat. If you know my husband at all, he is a truly dedicated, hard-working and thoroughly helpful man. It was just like him to see what needs to be fixed and create a system with which to do so. He dropped everything he was doing to rescue me and helped tirelessly to rebuild Little Moon.

For four years, you could find both of us, EVERY single day, holidays and all, at the Magic Factory, endlessly labeling and making full pallets of **Tired Old Ass Soak,** and all our other "children," until we nearly dropped. With 144 different products going strong, we rededicated and rebuilt the business, the public interest, and the Little Moon Magic. I never worked so hard in my whole life, and I'm supposed to be somewhat of a Diva! No applause this time, just saving a business was at stake. I am still forever grateful to those true blue Little Mooners and our dear loyal customers who pulled us through that time.

It was a wonderful sensation to build up a company to the point where there were so many employees, *I* was not needed for anything! I could be the spoiled brat, the angelic absentee owner, sleeping late and living it up. How disappointing and totally unsettling it was to realize that, fourteen years later, I would have to go **BACK to doing EVERY little thing by myself**, just like the early days! *Once again*, I was swamped performing every duty, as the production manager, the shopgirl, the bookkeeper, the inventor, the order-girl, and the cleaning service, all in one. **I never expected a boomerang in my success curve.** Turns out, Business is a *wavy* line, not always some ever-increasing angle upwards, like they'd have you believe! *Many* business owners have had to experience setbacks, move out of the giant corner office, work for someone half their age, or find themselves deeply **humbled,** sometime in their stellar careers. It happens to the best of us, and it's nothing of which to be ashamed.

But things have a funny way of working out all right, and you can be sure we had a lot of fun seeing to it! All these many years later, and any perceived failure forgotten, I realize it was all part of a great plan that did set us up perfectly. We did miraculously recover. Abraham likes to remind me to say, and I believe, **"Everything Always Works Out Great For Me."** It sure does. I am so grateful we DID sacrifice for the entity of Little Moon then, because it was to benefit both of us very soon.

MUSIC SAVES THE DAY

While being high performers at Little Moon by day, we were still following synchronicities in our long-term music careers by night. In 2008, the two of us gathered together a blues group we called **Little Laura & the Nude Blues Band**. The idea of "Nude" was that the *Blues* sound was really stripped down and naked - not the musicians! The name just *perfectly* described the spirit of our music, a little raw, a little wild. I personally was new to all the "rules of the Blues," and found it was nowhere near as easy as the music I had sung before, including jazz. So this early band was a great training ground for me. Except how many times did we field the question from booking agents, *"But you guys all wear clothes, right?"* Time for a new band name! We did some great shows with that band, opening twice for my favorites **JJ Grey & Mofro**.

Around this time, I got to open for **Todd Rundgren** at the Boulder Theatre with Grammy-nominated **Nick Urata** and **Tom Hagerman** of **DeVotchKa**. Nick had been a treasured part of our family for a long time. DeVotchKa's music is so completely raw, Eastern European, original, and emotional, and makes the gypsy in me dance around wildly. Singing with Nick and Tom was very special, I was beyond stoked to be able to perform with them for this show! But *Todd Rundgren* is my all-time, most favorite musician ever (thanks to many albums worth of his music I'd collected while at Interlochen, and beyond). I was in awe that night, thrilled that Todd had come right to me in Colorado, and that I was *on the gig* at such a beautiful venue!

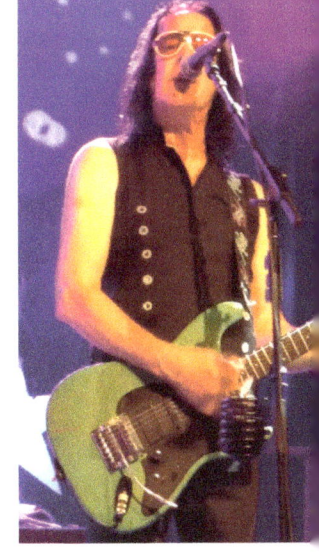

Backstage that fateful night, **two of my most precious Life Moments occurred**. During one portion of the show, Todd sat down at the piano to play *"Compassion."* I was standing backstage, very close, just across the piano from him. My dear sister LeeLee came up behind me and hugged me, and we swayed and cried and sang every word of the song to ourselves, remembering it as part of the soundtrack of our lives. I will never forget that sisterly bond and that moment of love with her, connected through Todd's music - and how she made the whole righteous and life-altering experience happen for me. I was, and still am, so grateful for that night, my musical heroes, and my sweet Little Sister.

The second moment was downstairs in the dressing room next to Todd's. I tried to be cool and get myself ready for the show, but I got to listen to Todd **warm up his voice**, which totally intrigues all professional singers! Later, I was at the band hospitality table and Todd walked up and said to me, "*That was YOU singing up there? WOW, that's some voice out of that little body. That long note you held? Wow.*" I don't know when I have ever had a compliment mean more. I respect his musicianship and opinion so much - you can just imagine my *smile of the century*. I had brought a bunch of my Little Moon products for him, **Tired Old Ass Soak** and all, displayed on the table. He cracked up, out loud, as he read the labels. Oh yeah, just me and Todd standing around laughing and joking about Music, Life, and my wacky company. PRICELESS.

HIGH NOTES

I was lucky to sing for several years with a killer, note-for-note **Pink Floyd** tribute band called **Wish You Were Pink**, belting out harmonies, and wailing the quintessential *"Great Gig in the Sky."* And yes, that *is* the hardest song in the world to sing, and

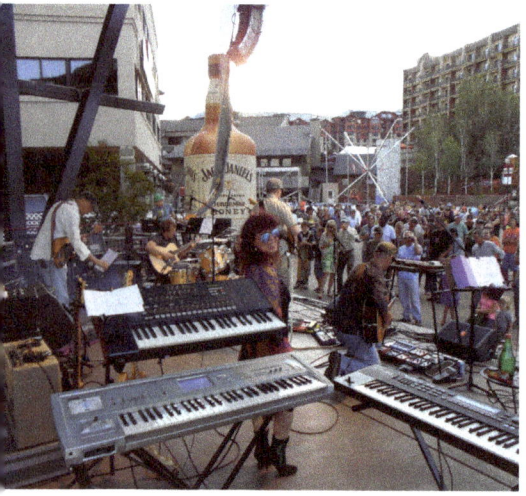

NO, it does NOT always go off perfectly each night! But we were a wonderful band of musical Brothers, each member meticulously recreating exact solos to perform the Floyd sound LIVE, with the ripping laser light show and all. It was remarkable to be in the middle of that onstage, it absolutely felt and sounded like the real Pink Floyd. Kudos to those guys. We played *full album sets*, just like on the records, usually four albums to a show. The feeling, with the crowd singing every word of every song, the hypnotic lights, sharing the mutual love of the music, layered with each of our own personal histories with Pink Floyd's tunes was intoxicating. It was real rockstar stuff and I loved it - shades, sparkly outfits, and all.

Dave Allen was busy playing with his own legendary bands, **The Worried Men**, and the **Smokehouse Band with Greg Scott**. In 2014, he was invited to work on a special project recording and playing drums with jazz fusion pioneer **Jeremy Wall** of Spyro Gyra and Broadway's **Phil Hernandez**. What a combo to watch! Listening to Dave Allen play the most difficult Leonard Bernstein and Stephen Sondheim Broadway standards, then switch to Jazz Fusion for the Spyro Gyra stuff was remarkably impressive. He really can play *anything*, because he works so hard at it. I watched him practice relentlessly to be ready. I love having him as a role model in music! Their concert at the world-famous Strings Music Tent was stunning. I was so proud of my Dave Allen.

But we very much wanted to play our gigs TOGETHER. Serendipitously, our buddy and local guitar genius, Steve Boynton, wanted to try out some new equipment in his recording studio in Steamboat, and asked if we had any material to record. In 2013, we formed the **Allen-Lamun Band** with Steve and Willie Samuelson, musicians we loved and played with for decades - and made our first record together at Steve's studio.

We also recorded some of the tracks for that album with world-famous studio engineer & producer Scott Singer who has earned his real gold records on the wall. Scotty recorded us with some of the priceless "equipment relics" he'd picked up from the old days at Capitol Records. **I got to sing into *the very same* microphone that Frank Sinatra used** at the epic Capitol Studios/Studio A sessions in Los Angeles! Not to mention the opportunity to work with such a top-level engineer in Scotty, we had a great experience at his awesome studio. Our first record, called ***All in the Numbers***, was a worthy project that distracted us from how hard we were working at the Magic Factory, and truly did rescue us, landing us right back in the Music Business.

FIRST RADIO PLAY - IN THE UK

The first time we "heard our song on the radio" was when **Kevin Beale** played us on his station outside of London, streamed live to our Magic Factory in Colorado - how times have changed! We definitely danced around and screamed and had a joyous affair nonetheless! It was a great moment that proved the hard work we'd put in locally had started to reach out globally. Our first album began to get a bit of traction in the Blues Radio world, we got some good reviews, and had airplay in wild places like **Argentina**, **Amsterdam** and the **Netherlands**, **Europe** and **New Zealand**. The new **Allen-Lamun Band** was quickly becoming an entity that needed a website and e-commerce and social media and pushing just like Little Moon. *What was I doing to myself?!* The difference was that running the band was fresh and exciting, it involved my first and deepest love for *singing,* and I got to do it with my beloved husband.

We began traveling to Memphis every year for the **Blues Music Awards** ceremonies, and became friends with some of our Blues Heroes! In Memphis, we connected with amazing musicians from all over the World, as well as fans we had acquired, and DJs we had come to know from many countries. It was glamorous and loud and lively and fun! We had amazing musical nights on Beale Street, played in killer jams, took fun trolley rides, and explored Memphis with our Blues Family which was thrilling. Thanks to our great buddy and music promoter, Peter "Blewzzman" Lauro, we got to travel to Helena, Arkansas to appear several times on the **KFFA's King Biscuit Time Radio Hour** with the legend **"Sunshine" Sonny Payne**. He was a HOOT, a real Blues aficionado and a true

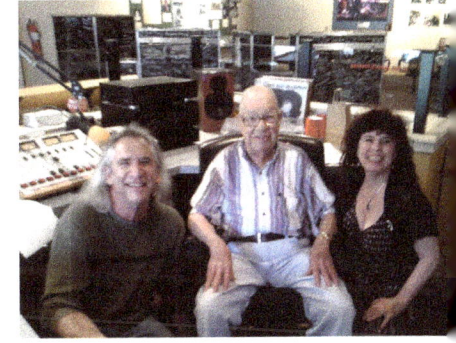

music lover. His show was the longest-running Blues Radio show in the country, and probably the World. Sonny asked us to hang out after the show, and played us *his* favorite music for over an hour, sharing stories about the upright bass he used to play. Sonny is gone now, too, but we have his voice and his memory archived in those shows forever. It's easy to understand that we started to dream about what we might be able to do with the band, if we could **rededicate to music** full-time. We had all of these amazing contacts, if only we could sell Little Moon and move forward. *I WAS SHOCKED* to watch this new plan evolve from an idea that had (heretofore) been **unthinkable** to me. I never thought I would let go of my company, never. Fast changes!

LET GO, LET GO MORE

Before the Blues called, I guess I thought we'd go on with Little Moon until some big company came begging for us to sell for some enormous amount of money. But in those days, literally **no one** was investing in a small natural business, especially if its leader wanted to go off somewhere and be a rockstar! I wish I had been trying to sell today, as I see many similar businesses being offered huge sums to sell, consumed by the big corporate players trying to pose as "natural" now. You want to say you would never "sell out" but you never know what you will decide until you are faced with the option. In late 2007, Burt's Bees sold to Clorox for $950,000,000 (yes, million) dollars.[3] It was a ridiculous windfall for a small natural company (and remains one of the industry's most oddly generous). But as a result, the brand lost most of its loyal natural health food store support, and its home-grown authentic reputation has never been quite the same. I didn't want some evil empire company to swallow us whole and compromise our values. All we wanted was the opportunity to make a life change for ourselves, and a positive sea change for Little Moon. I was hoping for an authentic transition to someone who would truly care for what we had grown.

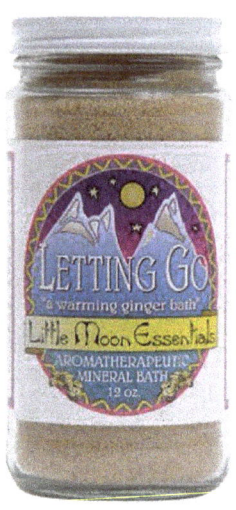

I did eventually sell *Little Moon Essentials* in 2015 to a loyal fan of the company who had been trying to purchase it for years. He seemed sincere, truly loved the products and used them daily. He had the money to promote the brand, which I loved watching. I went through a series of "Letting Go" experiences (especially ironic as **Letting Go** was the name of my very first product for Little Moon). They rebranded, of course, changing the very image I'd worked so hard to create, and systematically removed me and my creation story from the website, socials, and the history of the company. Ouch. The "new look" was beautiful, very current and still colorful, but I did relish in the fact that some people loved (and still miss) the original label. I had watched this happen to my friend Brigitte Mars, as the man who bought her tea company, *Unitea Herbs,* put *his face* on the label of *her teas* when he bought it! **But this is what you need to expect**

when you sell your creations. Like children, they grow up and have a life of their own that you can no longer control. Someday they may even become someone else's, to do with completely as they like! In 2020, the new owners closed the Magic Factory in Steamboat after 26 years, and moved Little Moon to Miami. Let Go! Let Go More. My "baby" had grown up and was far, far away at college, in no more need of me. Time for my next blossoming.

CALIFORNIA HERE WE COME

After we sold the business, we bought a used but spectacular Airstream Sprinter Van (a dream of mine fulfilled). Two days after my last day at Little Moon we took off in our magical "Streamer" for California. On the road again and it felt so good! Suddenly we were both very free, with **any possible future**, a little bit of money, and miles and miles of the journey to think about it. We stayed for many weeks with my

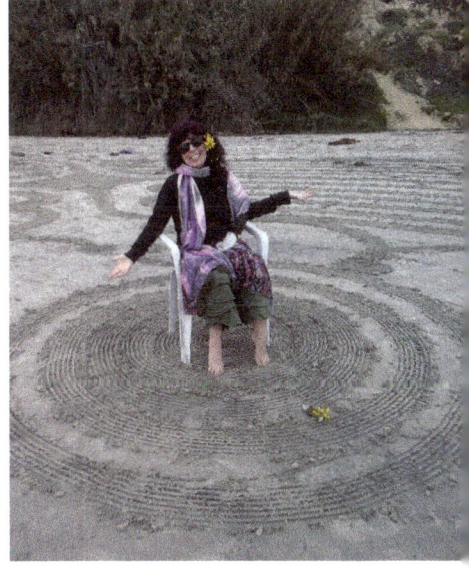

Second Family in California, Jill, Stevie and Paula, Aleka and Sean. We played at the beach and in the markets, with the flowers and palm trees and the ocean. We celebrated my birthday that year with a sunset at the Beach, only to find that a beautiful, enormous and intricate Labyrinth had been raked into the sand by the legendary **Leucadia Labyrinth Maker, Kirkos**. When I told him it was my birthday, Kirkos told me he had drawn this enormous work of art JUST FOR ME! I remember the back of his truck was filled with rakes of all sizes, and buckets of found art objects and marbles and beads. Kirkos gave us handfuls of treasures, offerings and flowers, instructing us to leave them all around the labyrinth to beautify it - are you kidding me, decorating my birthday mandala, how totally magical! Jilly and I ceremonially walked his Labyrinth Masterpiece, bedazzled it, and meditated inside of it. What an outrageously LARGE sign from the Universe that my New Life would be okay! Perhaps even *perfectly designed* with flowers and sparkles and magic - before I even got there.

VAGABONDS LAND IN NASHVILLE

The more we spoke with our foundational friends, the more a plan began to surface. Since we had considered carefully where we would *like* to be in the country, and we knew we were moving for music, we decided to check into **Nashville**. My dear friend Jenn Grinels had been doing super well there in her singer/songwriter genre, and she assured us there was a healthy Blues scene there as well. We got back on the road, and continued on to follow the many signs to our future!

Miraculously, we found a perfect place to rent in East Nashville, the trendy, Bohemian, artsy area, east of the city proper. Through some cool synchronicity - the realtor we engaged was about to move, and she rented HER house to us - we signed a lease for May 1, 2015. We sprinted back to Steamboat, packed up our whole lives in twenty-three days, and hit the road in the Streamer again, this time for good. **Leaving Colorado was so hard, truly heartbreaking and uprooting** - continues to be! But we really *loved* Nashville. We moved into a perfect little house on the corner of Rosebank and Welcome. It was an adjustment dealing with highways all the time, parking in a big city, and dealing with the huge DMV and the enormous scale of everything in general! But within our community we found vegan restaurants and places we loved, including the giant Shelby Bottoms Park within walking distance, to bike and walk and see the Big Trees, Cumberland River and all of Nature coming up through the cracks of the city.

We didn't have much spare time though, because we had a new determined focus: becoming KNOWN in a brand new town. We went to sit-in at Nashville Blues Jams *literally* six nights a week and also on Sunday afternoons! One week we played out *eleven nights in a row*. I remember Dave Allen saying, "We didn't come to Nashville to sit around and watch *"The Voice"* on TV. We are going out to Live This." Oh, how we did, and it was so exciting! Our timing seemed perfect because there were several Nashville legends we got to befriend and play with before they died (like our beloved

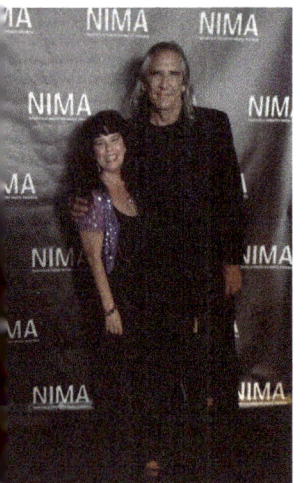

soul legend Nick Nixon, wizard on the B3 Moe Denham, keyboard wildman Larry van Loon who played on our record, Big Mike Griffin on the guitar, legend Johnny Neel on B3, and the Memphis superstars Jack Rowell, Russell Lee Wheeler, and saxophonist Dr. Herman Green). And we even got to know, and be a part of honoring the legendary Stax drummer Howard Grimes before he passed, who told me he *loved* Dave Allen's groove in his drumming!

Everybody in Nashville was welcoming and warm, and we quickly made lots of Blues musician friends, and got in deep with all the cool people. We found some badass musicians we wanted to record with at "The Colemine," with owner Randy Coleman on bass and at the board. The **Allen-Lamun Band** had begun work on a new album project right before we left Steamboat, and we brought some tracks with us, with guitar performances from our old pal Steve Boynton that we just loved. Randy managed to work everything together and soon we were adding finishing touches on all **12 original songs**, some of which completely evolved in the studio due to the A-Team of Randy Coleman, Kenne Cramer, and Jake Hill. The record also featured a few special guests and Nashville legends, guitar wizard Donnie Miller, the legendary Larry van Loon on B3 Hammond Organ and the absolutely crazy sax man, Miqui Gutierrez. Our Nashville contingent were some of the true legends of that town. Dreams Come True.

Our second record was called *"Maybe It's A Good Thing"* and this one brought us lots more recognition, with **ALL 12 songs receiving radio airplay all over the World**. It debuted at #1 on the Blues chart on iTunes, charting high on Roots Music Report, Airplay Direct and other platforms. This album was also nominated for *"Album of the Year"* by the Nashville Independent Music Awards (NIMA 2016) which included all genres in Music City. At one point, BOTH of our Allen-Lamun Band records were on the **"Top 100 National Blues Albums of 2016"** on the RMR Chart.

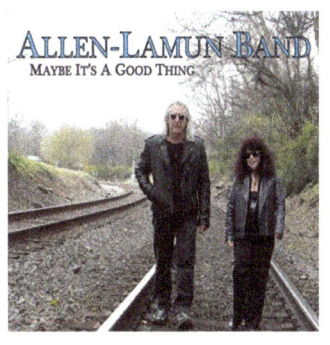

In the old days of the music business, this kind of success would have *meant* something more, this would have been the record that really made us! But while we were busy finding it this latest time, the music business had shifted and changed yet again. It was harder than ever to make a living or real *money*. And in a strange turn of the business, it had become impossible to reach the stellar heights of success without participating in a television talent show competition! Reality shows made superstar celebrities out of talented amateurs, while we watched so many brilliant *lifetime* musicians who could never even get seen or heard. Strange times, indeed.

Trying to find good, high-paying and steady music work in Nashville was difficult - like being a piece of chocolate in an enormous FREE chocolate factory. There are *so many* hopeful wanna-be musicians per capita there, most of whom would play for tips or even for FREE just to get noticed, people who had never played music in other cities to know they were supposed to get PAID. The clubs spoke about *exposure* a lot, tips as pay, and money very little. I wasn't prepared for that - we always made great money in Colorado as musicians, *nobody* played for free! In Nashville, MUSIC CITY, where musicians were supposedly celebrated (and pimped out with live music performed everywhere for the city's brand, even at the airport), **no one I knew could make a living at it**. Or very few let's say, and most had to do bus-tour work for big names, run studios of their own, or have day jobs to make ends meet. Plus, most everyone in Nashville seemed to want to work as a sideman only, mostly because *great* gigs, life-changing gigs could always come around and they wanted to be available, just in case. We had a hard time finding anyone who wanted to dedicate to create and sustain a band, although we played with some of the greatest we could find in the process! I am so happy for the musicians there who *have* found their niche, their bandmates, and have been able to create real success in their life's work. But for us, not being able to get a real sustainable group together was just a sign to keep moving.

GETTING OUT OF DODGE, GOIN' TO JACKSON

Through some cool synchronicities I got wind of a day job in Jackson, Tennessee - as Nutrition Manager at a health food store called Grubb's Grocery. Jackson is two hours to the west of Nashville, and only an hour from Memphis. When we went to look at the town, it was so much smaller than Nashville, and the trees were so much BIGGER! Jackson reminded me of Colorado, it was beautiful with a small-town, cozy feel. Plus, I relished the opportunity to bring more health information to the people of the South!

The owner hired Dave Allen part-time too, so we could both make a living while enjoying the experience of getting to regularly play music in our mecca of Memphis. Working at the store brought me a new Best Friend in Sarah Jones, and I was so grateful to find a kindred spirit and kick ass together at the store. Another unexpected miracle was the price of the homes in Jackson! With the last of the Little Moon money we were able to put a down payment on an enormous home of our dreams on 1 ½ acres - the Big House in the Little Forest. It had been our master plan to find a nice house of our own in a music town, somewhere in the middle of the country, from which we could go anywhere, like the center of a wheel. Now we had room for gardens and some of those Loblolly pines in the back yard and a big music room! Plus it doesn't really snow here, so after years of a foot-of-snow-every-day-Steamboat, I am happy to see those January Dandelions growing in Jackson!

Two years after moving here, my beloved Daddy passed away. I am so grateful for Christmas and the birthdays and the precious, beautiful moments I got to share with him before that happened, made possible because we moved so much closer. Dave Allen's Mother also moved on earlier that same year, and he was able to be with her as well. Thinking about aging Family was part of the counsel we received when searching our hearts about where to go. Again, our Innate Knowing proved right. And i am thankful we do have some great memories to show for it.

MEMPHIS BLUES & CONTENTMENT

Dave Allen was the first to hit the Blues Jams in Memphis, to be recognized and hired for his awesome drumming. When I joined him, soon WE were the ones playing in clubs on Beale Street, a total dream come true! We had written a song back in 2013 on the first record, called *"Delta Dream"* - about "playing a little room down in Clarksdale" and we got to LIVE that dream! Dave Allen got to play at **Morgan Freeman's Ground Zero** club in Clarksdale, Mississippi with *David Daniels & Soulbender*. I got to sit in, wail a bit myself on the Ground Zero stage, and sign the wall in the green room! If those walls could speak...everybody you'd ever dream of played there.

Soon we became known in Memphis, and were accepted into that Blues Scene which was a real honor after watching from afar for so long. We were thrilled to join **Brad Webb & Friends**, as the House Band for the **Memphis Blues Society's** weekly Thursday Blues Jam, and many special events for more than four years. **Brad Webb** is one of the very few (and maybe only) Blues LEGENDS to be honored with a *Brass Note on Beale Street* for his immense contribution to

Memphis Blues **while he is still alive**. I am so glad we got to play, jam and record with him. And that continues on. The amazing part of playing in Memphis is all the special guests who walk in the room! You never know which Blues Legend or celebrity we will get to watch, play with, and learn from next. Just another unexpected blessing from Tennessee for which to be exceedingly grateful.

In Jackson, I had a **weekly featured Talk Radio appearance** with local heroes SeaBass, Dan Reaves, Keith Sherley, and Chuck Walker. I spent more than six years on their various radio programs, offering health advice and my personal propaganda live on the air. I worked by day, played by night and even built myself a new website to house my many new inspirations at **www.lauralamun.com** (I include *Garden of Earth* extras and bonus content that could not make this book, so look for lots of **cool stuff** there).

In the middle of enjoying it all, the music business took another big hit during the health crisis - all our venues closed. Like many people, I struggled when I became unemployed after I was no longer "affordable" at the store during hard times. I was really searching for what I could do for money and to stay relevant and vocal. Ironically, I had been reading Tarot Cards for friends privately for years. In an interesting development, my friend Melanie said, "*You should do Tarot Card Tuesday at The Tavern!*" (which was coincidentally her bar). I tried reading in public there and I loved it, what a trip reaching clients who might never get a reading in the metaphysical store - but in a bar - yes!!! Before I knew it, I was booked doing Tarot readings, consulting and performing my other therapies for private clients six days a week. Working for myself saved my life again when I had to return to Colorado nine times in one year to care for and say goodbye to my beloved Mother. Flexibility is the blessing of the self-employed.

These last few years at home have been some of my most precious, with Dave Allen at my side, writing and studying, playing with our kittens and sleeping as late as we want. And although we aren't performing live as much, you better believe when we do, true Memphis Blues is always going down! We spend time at home practicing, writing songs, and in our own studio singing them and laying down harmonies until they stack up like old Christmas cards. We read and write and study and meditate and pray for World Peace! We are content, surprisingly - amidst political revolution, musical weirdness, viral living, weird weather, and fast changes in society. I know we both feel lucky to have been able to settle down and put down roots, even unexpectedly in Tennessee, finding new ground available for every seed we plant. Life is a beautiful, and often surprising, growing Garden of Joy. I know someday we will go back home to Colorado, but we are content for now, eagerly awaiting the next development.

*****

Now that you have been fully updated and know where I am coming from, let's dive right into the many wonderful Co-Creators we have in our **Beloved Garden**.

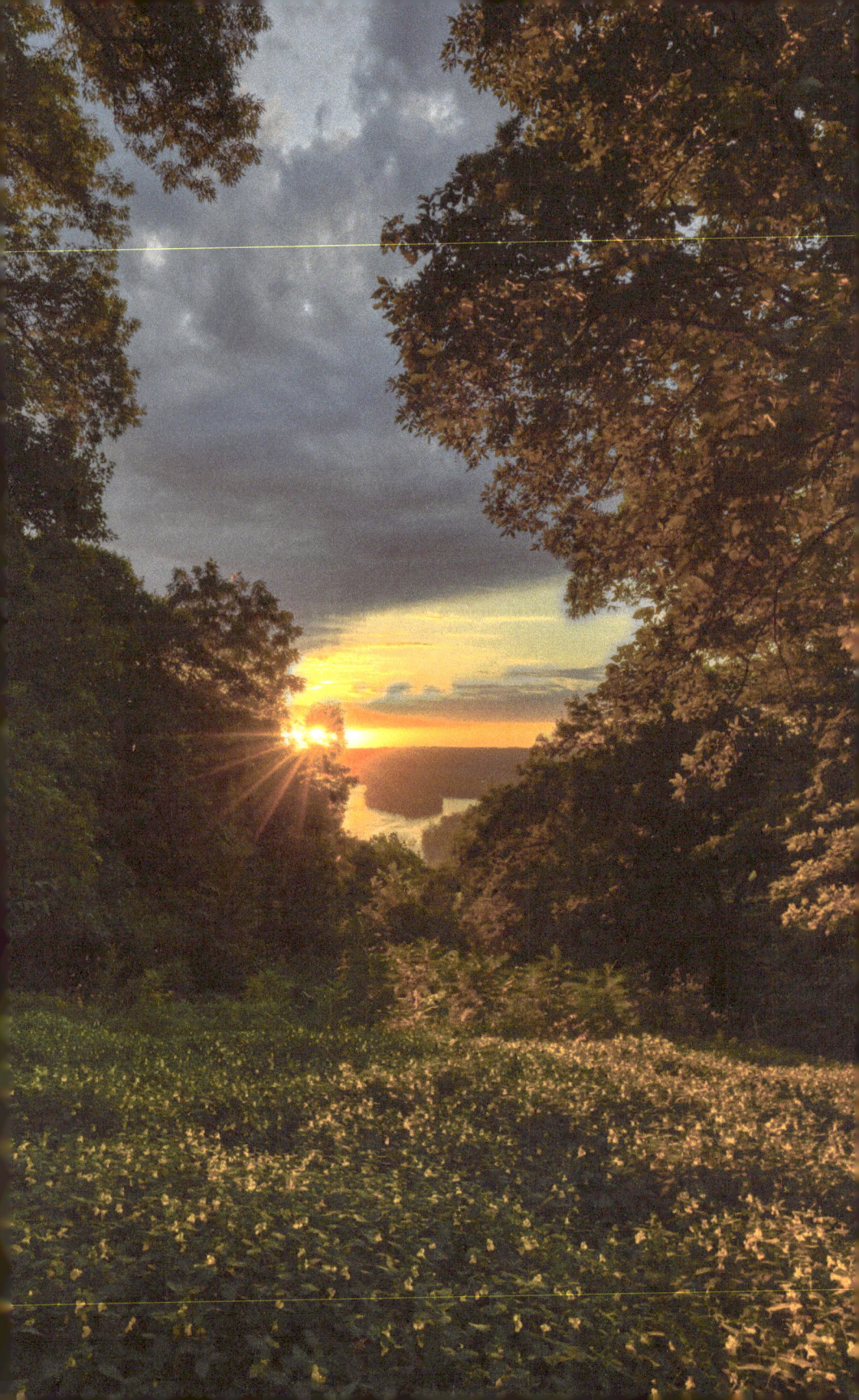

~ Chapter 2 ~

PARTNERS IN THE GARDEN

> *"When you choose to work in partnership with another, it's saying you recognize your partner's worth and what you bring to each other, and that essentially They Are You. You recognize your growth within them, and their invitation for you to grow to your highest aspect."*
>
> ~ *Victoria L. White*

INSPIRATION FROM EVERYWHERE

It is very engaging to write a book, because so much of what you think about, everything that happens in the World, everything you see, influences the writing. I recall being relieved I read a mentor's book, learned a new skill, or took a particular class *first*, before I finished my book, because it inspired me so much. I am wildly grateful for the many People and Plants and Pollinators who showed up to **partner with me**, inspiring me to tell their stories, and write about the very cool stuff they teach.

While I was researching, we experienced a few relatively minor (but first of their kind in my life) FOOD SHORTAGES, making the Garden and our Food Stores of even greater importance. And, moving to the South, living here through some of the strangest times ever, sparked in me a rather strong desire to learn more about what people need, to speak up, educate and *write* about **FOOD, HEALTH** and **SURVIVAL**! I realized I wanted to be in partnership with all the many heroes who actively, everyday **Ensure Our Food Supply**.

Seeing changes at the grocery store, and rising prices, made it ever more clear that we are all somewhat **at the mercy of others**, for many of our basic needs. Most people are totally *not ready* for food supply interruptions, empty shelves, or even power outages from inclement weather. Recent health scares revealed many people need better nutritional support to stay well. Unpredictable fires, and storm damage revealed our infrastructure weaknesses and caused supply chain disruptions. While we were being lulled into a false sense of security by the well-oiled machine of commerce and comfort, flaws were showing! And in the process, it seems some of the skills of our ancestors are slipping away. We can barely hear their guidance anymore to *"Be Prepared."* What do people really need to remember, cherish, preserve? What could we ALL utilize and count on to help us to not only survive, but THRIVE?

Plants (and those who tend them) are a huge part of the Solution! Plants truly are our Partners on Earth. Even beyond their amazing capacity for nourishing life and providing sustenance, it is likely Plants will supply the *most effective medicines* for the varied conditions that plague us, physical and mental. **Nature ALWAYS has the Remedies,** part of the design I speak about, and they come to us riding on the leaves and flowers of our beloved Plants. Through them, we see how perfectly vital our Planet truly is - **we have a very valuable Garden here.** Let's learn how to better partner with it, appreciate it and remind ourselves how to preserve it.

WE HAD IT ALL

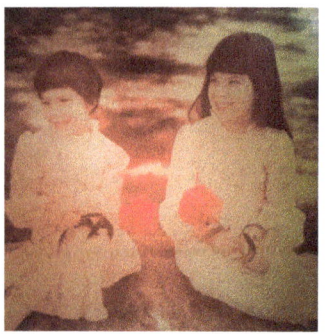

I loved growing up in the 60's and 70's, and I often look back on how easy things used to be. We grew up with everything we needed, literally. I was personally very lucky and had great opportunities, thanks to both of my hard-working parents. Everyone I knew always had enough to eat, had good places to live, we experienced very little REAL change or challenge in our lives. We were always lucky enough to grow a Garden for pleasure *and* for Food. We were totally accustomed to the "systems" our grandparents had in place, because they worked for so many years.

We may have *learned* from our history books about "wartime rations" and *shortages* of butter or sugar, or tea or coffee during World Wars. But NEVER in my life did I see empty shelves in the grocery store. I did not even realize it was possible! I never HAD to grow a garden for my family's own subsistence, or worry about a food supply.

Never until recently, when it became entirely clear that **food shortages** could happen any given week, and an entire city could be without something, or sold-out of many foods or vitamins, because the trucks just couldn't make it, drivers were sick, or the plants shut down (or were burned down). And it is still happening today. Cyberattacks on gasoline pipelines and food processing plants are the new warfare. Our *survival* may not be completely threatened, and I pray it never is - but it proved **it sure could be challenged**. Right here in the opulent and abundant USA there was a signal of weakness in the Food Supply. Add to that the private corporatizing of farmland and the patenting of seeds, requirement of pesticides and overregulation of Farmers.... It made me think it might be high time we all grow some Gardens of our own. And kiss a Farmer or two for their part in saving our lives.

> "There are two spiritual dangers in not owning a farm. One is the danger of supposing that breakfast comes from the grocery, and the other that heat comes from the furnace."
>
> ~ *Aldo Leopold*

WHAT ABOUT THE FARMERS?

Recent conditions (and successful protests) reveal the fact that we COMPLETELY rely on **Farmers**, trucking systems, factories, supermarkets, and even grocery workers to feed us. If any link in this chain fails, we may find ourselves looking at those empty shelves, staring at empty pantries with hungry bellies. **These Farmers are our Heroes, too.** *Thanks to them*, and to all the truckers and pickers and migrant workers and grocery clerks, all of you who are providing us with FOOD and survival! Thank-you.

And as we found out in 2020, **shortages** are not the only problem. Farmers were forced to dump perfectly good food because the stores were not able to buy it all, and because all the restaurants had to shut down. An overabundance of popping corn, resulting from the crash of the movie theatre business, left all the Popcorn undelivered, unpaid for, and unpopped. Many growers were forced into terrible choices with little support. **No infrastructure is in place to deal with food shortages as well as food overages!** We need systems to deal with the **overabundance of food** and the compensation for the Farmers who grew it, but could not sell it as well. Take away their *buyers*, and their entire cash crop may become a trash crop!

How can we reroute this food to feed the **needy**? These days there are people who do not have enough food to survive in nearly *every* community. Let's find solutions to **THAT** problem at the same time. We need **equanimity of food distribution and healthy, life-sustaining meals for all**. This is where health starts, this is our most important goal. We can find so many ways to help if we try, and hopefully this realization will give birth to ideas you could implement. Check in with the Farmers in your area and see how they are doing - maybe there is something you can do. Maybe you could *help them* give their food to charities or soup kitchens or homeless shelters or needy families? Maybe you will dream up an answer to this quandary or create some brilliant solutions for them. Find out what they need.

> **"My grandfather used to say that *once* in your life you need a Doctor, a Lawyer, a Policeman, and a Preacher. But *every day*, three times a day, you need a Farmer."**
> ~*Brenda Schoepp*

Some of the Farmers I hear from say equipment costs are rising every year and many can't even afford their most basic necessities. Mortgage debt, licensure costs, fertilizer shortages, failing crops and weather challenges have many questioning their profession. President John F. Kennedy said, *"The farmer is the only man in our economy who buys everything at retail, sells everything at wholesale, and pays the freight both ways."* Farmers have been struggling for decades under the weight of Monsanto telling them *what* to grow and how, seizing their seeds, and ruining their crops (not to mention developing poison products and enforcing shady, overlording, monopolistic patent control). I am overjoyed to finalluy see the lawsuits coming against this long-time polluter and bully of a company. **It is high time Farmers are given their SEEDS and their freedoms back**. They need real support.

A miracle struck in the form of **Willie Nelson.** Along with son **Lukas Nelson,** and friends **Dave Matthews, Neil Young,** and **John Mellencamp** (and eventually many more musicians) Willie began raising public awareness about farmers' challenges. Their brainchild, the *Farm Aid Music Festival* began in 1985, with a big Superstar lineup and an opportunity to bring real awareness to the farmers' plight. The boys had optimistically hoped they would raise **all the money the farmers would ever need**. Even *they* were surprised to realize the amount of help that is <u>**actually**</u> needed, and they swiftly realized the necessity of making this fundraiser an *annual* event. Every year, even in 2020 remotely, they put on a shindig of epic proportions with booths and food trucks and resources, inspiring music and many wild stories, shining the light on FARMERS. **You can donate any day of the year**, not simply during the Festival, and your spare change will definitely make a difference to some Hero out there trying to feed America. **Farm Aid** also has a hotline to assist Farmers and a website to help them connect with the heroic resources and support they dearly need.

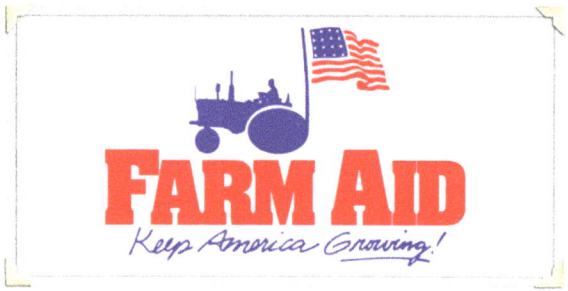

Call 1-800-FARM-AID (1-800-327-6243)
www.farmaid.org
https://farmerresourcenetwork.force.com/FRN/s/

Because of this **inspired idea** (and some compassionate and generous musicians) *millions* of dollars have been raised in extensive donations, while we all have been treated to some exceptional musical collaborations. True human camaraderie and service to others has proven **profitable** yet again. MOST importantly, the plight *has* been lessened for some of our dear Farmers, our critical food providers, our Plant Heroes. If you know a Farmer who is in trouble, point out these resources. Take a personal stand for Farmers. Donate! Volunteer! Participate! Grow Food! We all need to *befriend* a Farmer. Or BECOME one! Be like Willie.

"Greed doesn't rest, so neither for now does Willie Nelson."
~*Dave Matthews*

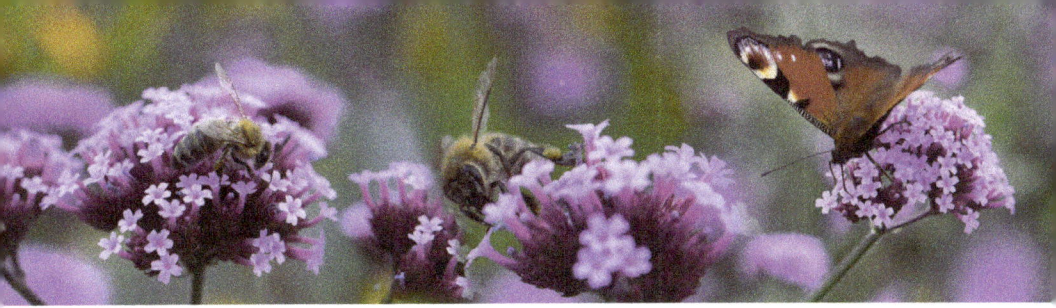

SAVE THE BEES, GROW FLOWERS

Another supercritical, **Heroic Partner** in the plant food chain is **The Bees**. As you may know, there are troubles within their environment. Many factors are contributing to a population crash in Bee colonies: pesticides, 5G, habitat loss, construction, weed and flower destruction, chemicals in the air and on flowers, magnetic disturbances, hive mites and diseases. Many have experienced *hivewide* die-offs, and in some parts of the world, Bees have simply disappeared altogether. **The Pollinators that assure the very Life of our Plant Kingdom, and our very Future, are in peril.** If we continue to decimate the Bee population we may see the most **critical, essential** part of our food chain *collapse*. In a domino effect, OUR FOOD PLANTS, needed to assure the lives of ALL OF US, are in dire jeopardy.

> **"Pollinators are said to be responsible for *one out of every three bites* we eat, and for decades, Ecologists have been sounding the alarm over their disappearance."**[4]

I beseech you to do everything you can to promote *habitats for Pollinators*. Our beloved **Bees, Beetles, Butterflies, Birds, Moths, Hummingbirds and Dragonflies** need you to grow **FLOWERS** for them! Plant fruit trees, wildflowers, & bushes, specifically seek out the ones they like the best and try to stick with *native* species for your area. Equally important is to allow **wild places** to grow in your yard that they can frequent - they actually like the natural messy look. Some gardeners recommend a spot specifically for the Nature Spirits that has a small fence and cannot be messed with by predators both animal or human! Pollinators will love that.

Leave the Clover Flowers and the Fleabane and the Dandelions in your grass in the early Spring to provide food sources for the Pollinators. If you must mow your yard, wait until the flowers fade, or leave patches of flowers for the Bees. Every time you see a Bee, consider it a victory! It is essential that we *stop spraying chemicals* to kill these beneficial bugs and their essential weeds, and give them back some habitat in which to flourish. These Pollinators are our **"Keystone Species"** which means **the entire ecology,** *and all of the other species*, depend on them. This includes Humans!

Last Summer, I had abundant growth in my vegetable garden, but very few Cucumbers and Tomatoes actually came to fruit from the flowers. This can be traced to an absence of **Pollinators!** If the flowers do not get pollinated, their seeded payload cannot come to fruition. I realized I must plant **MANY more flowers** in and near my garden to attract the Bees, Birds, and Butterflies! This past Summer I had flowers sprinkled all through the garden and had wonderful (and beautiful) results. A little further into this chapter, in the Gardening section, are some secrets I learned about **Companion Plants** you can scatter across your garden to bring in the workers to do the pollinating and pest remediation. Here is a list of some of the best Pollinator Plants to buy and grow, but also to discover in your yard and rescue from the weed killers and lawn mower. Dedicate places all over your yard to entice, feed, and offer water to our fabulous flying workforce! Your garden will produce so much more abundantly with better partnership through pollination.

🍇 POLLINATOR PARTNER PLANTS 🍇

Alyssum	Cranberries	Marigolds	Salvia
Anise Hyssop	Dandelion	Milkweed	Scarlet Gilia
Asters	Dill	Morning Glory	Scarlet Globemallow
Bee Balm	Dogwood	Motherwort	
Begonias	Echinacea	Nettle	Scented Geraniums
Berry Bushes	Elderberry	Nicotiana	
Black-Eyed Susans	Evening Primrose	Oregano	Serviceberry
	Fennel	Oregon Grape	Strawberry
Blackberries	Fleabane	Pansies	Sunflower
Blanket Flower	Floss Flower	Parsley	Thistles
Blueberries	Fruit Trees	Penstemon	Thyme
Buttercups	Goldenrod	Peppers	Tomatoes
Celosia	Grindelia	Rabbit Brush	Trumpet Vine
Chives	Hibiscus	Raspberries	Uva Ursi
Chokecherry	Hollyhock	Red Clover	Violets
Clarkia	Honeysuckle	& all the Clovers	Wild Bergamot
Columbine	Lavender	Rosemary	Willow
Cosmos	Lemon Balm	Roses	Yarrow
Cottonwood	Lupine	Sage	Yellow Buckwheat

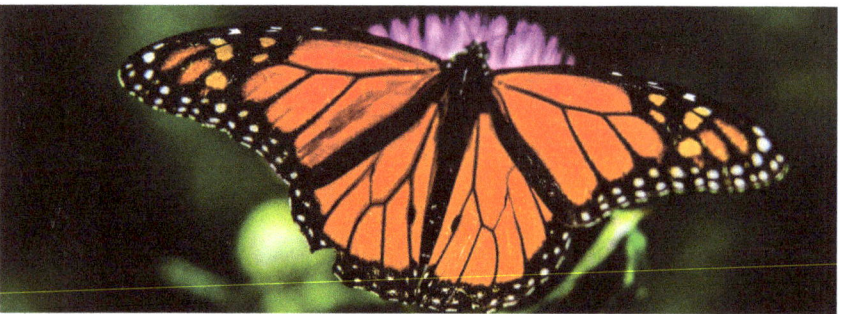

BUTTERFLY HIGHWAYS

Watching people create a living, loving Partnership with Nature is one of my *most* favorite things. In Canada, a group has begun making life more beautiful for their Bees & Butterflies - and it is brightening up the whole community!

> "The Butterflyway Project began in five Canadian cities in 2017. We recruited a team of volunteer Butterflyway Rangers in each. Their mission was to plant native wildflowers in yards, schoolyards, streets and parks to support Bees and Butterflies. The goal was to establish local "Butterflyways" by planting at least a dozen Pollinator Patches in each neighborhood or community."[5]

Now it is years later, and this organization has recruited more than **400 communities** to participate. They have built an *entire habitat*, in a long and beautiful Butterflyway that stretches across the whole country of Canada! They have thousands of volunteers who plant and dedicate habitats as "Pollinator Patches" in their yard and neighborhoods. The intended and spectacular results are magnificent rainbow gardens that benefit everybody! What a beautiful and mutually beneficial action - for the Butterflies, the Bees, EVERYTHING THEY POLLINATE along the way - and the lucky People who get to watch them in wonder.

North Carolina has instituted a similar practice, and their entire state is blooming with Flowers, and filled with Butterflies! There is also a successful **Monarch Highway** program that currently traces the Monarch Butterfly's path across the United States. *"The I-35 corridor, or the "Monarch Highway," runs along the central flyway of the Monarch migration in the states of Minnesota, Iowa, Missouri, Kansas, Oklahoma, & Texas."*[5] The Monarchs can sense or smell flowers two miles away!

I am pleased to report that the Winter of 2022 saw a **resurgence of the Monarch Butterflies** in California. Where they had counted 2000 in the previous year, they counted 100,000 that year! I believe efforts like these are finally impacting these important pollinating partners in the most supportive way.

THEY SEE YOU

Bees and Wasps utilize **FACIAL RECOGNITION**. They actually *know* your face if they have seen it once. They don't want to bother you, they are getting to know you! When we lived in Stagecoach, Dave Allen and I were able to coexist peacefully with every Bee and Wasp on the land. There might be a few on the screen door to the mudroom in the morning and we would peacefully let them out. For seven years we **allowed** them their nests

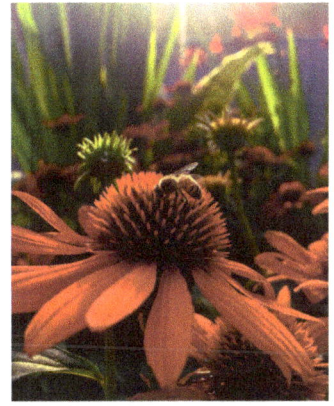

and never had a problem. We never had any fear and they never had any aggression. They have **zero desire to hurt** you so please don't fear the Bees! Learn ways to support them as dear friends, for they are all working so hard for us and for the Planet.

Did you know that many **Beekeepers TRAVEL all across the country with their hives**, *following the flowers*, bringing pollination assistance for what is no longer there? As soon as Beekeepers discovered you could move Beehive colonies by train in the 1860's, **Migrant Beekeepers** have been the Heroes of abundant yields and assured food supply for this whole country, influencing and ensuring everything we grow and that we export. **Andy Card**, one of the legendary Bee Wranglers featured in the book *Following the Bloom*, says it this way:

> "We're the last real cowboys, the last people moving livestock across the United States."
>
> ~ Andy Card

Yeah, BEES. More than a *thousand* commercial pollinating operators wrangle their Bees on Bee Drives, traveling late nights down long highways with pallets of Beehives in semi trailers. They go from flowering to flowering, north in the Summer and south in the Winter. Some of them loan their colonies out to fruit orchards, then blueberry barrens & cranberry bogs, then almond groves, then clover, then wildflower. **About half of the Bee Colonies in the United States are on National Tour!**

Some of the Beekeepers are famed "Bee Wizards" - magic-makers and hive-fixers who are in touch with the colony and able to breed Queen Bees, split hives to double output, or attract more Bees to join and grow the hives. Some of them place colonies with a Queen in "packages" to sell for Beekeepers to start or increase their hives. Some of them rent out their hives in emergencies and travel sleepless nights to fill in when other Beekeepers can't make a route. The flowers don't stop, no harvest can be delayed and **the Bees must *be* there**. Some of them lobby the government for new laws and protections for Beekeepers everywhere. ALL of them are completely worn out from the immense amount of contributory work they perform with and for their amazing, Heroic Bees. **We owe the Beekeepers our GRATITUDE** for caring so much for the Bees who are pollinating the Flowers that produce all our Food and Honey! Thanks to you, **Bees and Beekeepers**, it all keeps working.

TAKE THE HONEY AND RUN

Besides the Pollination market, it is a "run for the Honey" literally. And the money. The world's annual production of **Honey** is worth currently $7.9 Billion US dollars. Every country uses Honey, with India and China the greatest producers. But many, many small-farm, personal Beekeepers exist who are learning and passing down this fine art. Since the statistics show the average person in the US consumes about **one and a half pounds of honey yearly**, even small home Beekeepers can have a piece of that pie! Farmer's Markets, natural food stores, restaurants, coffee shops and bakeries are all great places to sell homemade honey. If you can't *be* one, support hard-working local Beekeepers by buying their delicious Honey.

This means you are consuming *Local Honey*, which is rich with the pollen from your local and indigenous plants. Locally-produced Honey will desensitize your allergic irritation to the local flowers. This primes your immune system to be less reactive to the nearby pollens in hay fever season, so your allergies will lessen & maybe even go away. Honey is antimicrobial so it preserves itself, and protects the health of every creature who consumes it. Everybody wins.

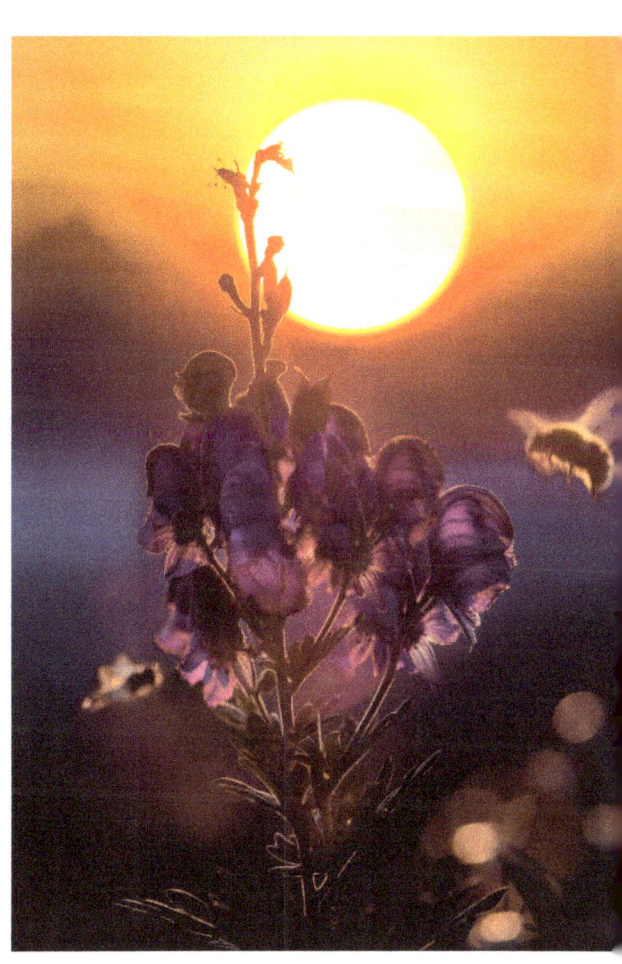

CORRECTION

**Last night I dreamt
that I had a beehive
here inside my heart.
And the Golden Bees ~**

**were making
white combs
and Sweet Honey
from all my old
failures.**

~ Antonio Machado
translated by
Robert Bly

HONEY

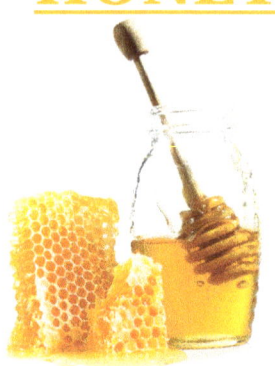

is a **completely wild, LIVING, Miraculous, Medicinal Healing Food.** Bees make it for feeding their hive, and they store the extra, so we (and many other creatures) are able to collect it and enjoy it. Honey has helped humans survive in times of great hardship, and on its own can prevent starvation. Honey is a major food supply miracle for us - as long as *we save the Bees who make it!* Honey will preserve food and last forever. An explorer found a 3000 year-old jar of Egyptian Honey (they called it the "tears of Ra") and it still tasted delicious! Because our ancestors subsisted on Honey, *their* relationships with Honey and the Bees are **written into our DNA**. Honey has one of the largest **energy fields** under Kirlian photography, offering Divine Frequency support for our energetic field as well. It is made from Liquid Light - a high vibrational, levitational, golden nectar created by the Sunshine and Flowers - transformed by the brilliant Bees.

Our lives as well as the lives of **all Flowering Plants**, and animals of all sizes, are intimately connected with these special flyers. Honeybees have to collect the nectar from **two million flowers** to produce one single pound of Honey. Luckily they work in large hives! Worker Bees (all female) cover many miles in search of the perfect flower and can collect from 50-100 flowers during each gathering trip - it's a full-time job. The **taste, medicinal action, color and scent of each different flower is collected in the Honey**, producing a wide range of healing effects and flavors from each flower's particular pollen contribution.

Honey on its own is a **soothing demulcent syrup**, great for sore throats, to stop a tickle, moisturize vocal dryness, soothe asthma, and reduce coughing. You can make a great, all-purpose *Herbal Lung Syrup* with Honey, early Spring Spruce tips & Violets (recipe pg. 226). I love to make *Garlic Honey* each Fall to ward off colds and flus all Winter long. Honey is full of living **Enzymes, Vitamins, Pollens, Minerals, Antioxidants, Amino Acids and Flavonoids**. Honey is a low-glycemic nutritive sweetener, with fast-absorbing natural sugars that provide the body with lasting physical **energy** that has no blood sugar crash. The "Honeymoon" is named for an ancient rite where just-married lovers eat honey for fertility and sensual bonding.

Eat a big spoonful of Honey the next time you need fast energy! Make a "HoneyBall' or "Honey Spoon" with Honey and your favorite powdered herb, like Clove Powder for flu and sneezing. Honey makes herbs easy to give to kids (over 3 years of age) and adults who hate pills. Honey and Turmeric make a crazy strong antibiotic syrup, and Honey with Cinnamon balances blood sugar.

Honey is widely used by premiere athletes and performers who rely on its **levitational ability to lift** their performance. This **miracle nectar** contains over 200,000 still-being-discovered phytochemicals that perform many miracles for Human bodies, including healing DNA and shutting down the growth of cancer. Honey is produced from **Teamwork**, inherently coded with worthy advice and cooperation energy from the Bees. From them we also receive spiritual **insight** for understanding **Community, Levitation** and **Flight**. A teaspoon of Honey will also enhance **Meditation, Visions** and **Dreaming**!

Use this miracle healer internally to add extra ENERGY and LIGHT to any system. Honey **stimulates libido**, heals digestive ulcers, calms inflammation, promotes gut health, dries post-nasal drip, soothes laryngitis, eases joint pain, helps **memory & brain issues** and all neurological problems, encourages sleep, **boosts immunity and fertility**, fights staph and bacterial infections, and also heals respiratory infections, gingivitis, hot flashes, dementia, stomach aches, headaches, **adrenal fatigue**, bronchitis, cancer, parasites, and diabetes. Honey is super helpful for many of the "abbreviation disorders" like **ADHD, MRSA, SIBO,** and **PTSD**. Sayer Ji suggests that Honey has ancestrally fed & healed our gut microbiome with its "80 million-year-old, time-traveling probiotic microbes."

Honey is a natural **topical antibiotic & wound-healer**, useful for burns and scrapes, acne, and eczema, is helpful for healing scars, and can be life-saving for dressing wounds in emergencies. **Manuka Honey** is an herbally-enhanced, especially healing Honey, which receives its particularly strong anti-microbial properties from the pollen of the Manuka bush, a relative of Tea Tree. This **Myrtaceae Family** member has potent essential oils that transfer to the pollen, which kill bacteria and miraculously heal wounds. Coconut Oil with Manuka Honey, and a little Castor Oil makes a healing salve beyond compare. Manuka Honey has extensive *internal* medicinal benefits, and is graded for its healing potency.

Many years ago, Gaia told me that because Bees were affected by weather changes, Humans, chemtrails and toxic pesticides, many of them had MOVED to regions of the Planet where it had **now become more hospitable for growing food**. She suggested that we would be wise to find and *follow* the Bees! Since seasons are shifting a bit and weather conditions are creating new water in places where it simply wasn't before, she said the **Bees already know** that it is now possible to grow a variety of plants in *places* you'd never expect. And that they sense and **predict weather,** seasons ahead of time.

This is why the Essential Pollinators are already there! Growing new crops in new places at new times for a new climate is something we all need to consider. It is time to experiment and adapt, to harmonize with all of the changes we are going through environmentally. We can debate *who*, or exactly *what* is to blame for climactic changes, but regardless - we must pay attention to the way conditions are NOW, not the way they always used to be. We must take what is happening to our systems into account and alter our ways. We can always look for clues from Nature about what to do next. Dave Allen tells a story about an old rancher who offered him this wise adage: *"Farm according to the Weather, not the Calendar."*

Later in this chapter, I have compiled a list of similarly old-fashioned, absolutely fantastic folkloric sayings. These still provide valuable advice, regardless of when they were first used, because they preserve so many helpful signals and clues from Nature!

THE BEAUTIFUL SOUTH

The second motivating factor for writing about Food is that we moved to the Deep South, after living most of our lives in Colorado. I had personally only experienced the South from childhood roadtrips and holidays with my Father's family in Texas. I spent a summer in Kentucky after high school, but that was about as far as I had ventured. Just like many of us, I grew up thinking the stereotypical Southern diet was fried chicken, casseroles, collard greens and okra! It has been exciting to discover the true cuisine here and to experience some amazing, unrivaled Southern home-cooking. To be clear - we LOVE it here, and think the People, the Food, the Plants are truly special. I've been totally sidetracked by the Trees in this area, I am researching and will feature the many uses of different kinds of Trees in the upcoming *Volume Four*.

There are *outstanding features* of every regional cuisine, and each one has its characteristic foods and spices. Now that I actually live here I can say: food in this part of the World seems to be based on **indulgent home-cooking and deep comfort**! In the South, there are a lot of fried foods, almost everything is sweet, even the meat is rich with caramelized, sugary barbecue sauce. Most of the vegetables are heavily cooked and served with sauces or gravy, people don't eat a lot of fruit or raw veggies. Many Southerners love their biscuits, bacon, fried chicken, BBQ, sweet rolls, cornbread and pies, and love to drink Cokes and Sweet Tea. This is, of course, a **VERY** gross generalization, but a revealing one (and I do apologize if I have offended any of my Southern friends in proving my point).

Living in the South simply helped me to realize **we did not all grow up eating the same stuff. We have not all learned the same things!** In this region - and all across the Planet - many people have simply *not been taught* to make the connection that **Food influences their Health.** They are simply too busy enjoying it! People of the South love the way they eat and don't feel much need to change. As the late, brilliant Wandering Herbalist **Frank Cook** said, *"Most Americans only eat 25 species of Plant foods a year."* He would teach about this, while he served an outdoor meal made with 25 wild species he had gathered on a hike just that day!**[6]**

Many people stick to the *handful* of foods they know and love. We *are* creatures of habit - we just need to alter them, add to them now and then! People are very in touch with the Pleasure of Food and many simply eat what their families have always eaten. Most were never taught the *consequences* of eating that way. Or else they live in a culture where they have come to believe heart disease and dying early are natural.

It is a little harder to convince the older generation of the value of **organic food**, because they did not *have* as many pesticides in their food when they were growing up, it wasn't necessary. Even fast food USED TO BE more nutritious than it is today, with "chicken" nuggets made of pink goo, burgers made of dubious "beef," and the like. So it's important to go the extra mile to help everyone understand what is different NOW, in this recent age of engineered, pesticided, over-processed, artificial Food.

The South boasts abundant health care, hospitals, and cancer centers, **because they need them!** I am astonished at the many compromised people I see everyday with all the same health problems, and the laundry list of medications they take. Nearly every single one of them is severely **inflamed, dehydrated, and truly sick** with the side effects of their medicines - and the food (and sodas) - they regularly eat. I join the growing rally of experts exclaiming, *"You can eat differently to make your body well!"*

BETTER FOOD GETS IT DONE

You do not have to be unhealthy, I promise you. Your body can heal itself if you offer it the very best nourishment.

Food Is The Key That Unlocks And Creates Your Health.

Another reason many people don't know enough about the Healing Power of Food, is because they have had to equate food with **money** alone. Not knowing any better, and many times out of necessity, they tried to buy the least expensive food possible. I've been there - I, too, ate a lot of ramen noodles and popcorn for dinner in grad school!

Even recently I have debated which is more important this week, the cat's food or our food? Economic hardship is very hard to live within. With grocery prices these last few years we can all relate to the quandary we feel when deciding what food to buy.

People always complain, "*It takes money to be healthy, to buy health food.*" Yes, that is true. But I like to tell them that they **deserve food that makes them well** and prevents them from **spending so much money** on doctors and medicines! The trade off is worth it - more good food, less pharmaceuticals. It's just important to examine the *quality of nutrition* implicit in anything you can buy at "20 for $2.00!" Belly-filling, wallet-saving, yes, but nutritionally bankrupt, dead food (not even Food). **For your health**, I promise you the extra money will be worth it, until you can learn to provide better Food at a better price for yourself.

S*aving money on health food* is very easy because you can actually **GROW YOUR OWN**, at a fraction of the cost of store-bought. And you can make inexpensive home remedies with your bounty that serve you and your Family well in times of need, saving so much money on medications.

I know many people did not grow up with a **local health food store**, or have access to *health pioneers* who supported alternative diets. They were never taught about raw food or herbs or food combining. Possibly no one even spoke to them about the consequences of taking so many pharmaceutical medicines at the same time - which they think are their only hope to fix their failing bodies. They have never had the *resources* or the *education* to know how to eat any better to resolve their health issues.

It is a plain fact that the Southern region is ALSO a rapidly **growing** area for *new* health food store development, as the educational tide changes. I know people in the South *want* to be more healthy and they need support. Young people would come up to me in the health food store and say, "I don't know about any of this food, I only eat the same way my Grandparents always have. How can you help me learn?" This boosted my inspiration to answer this call, to help **create Food Change**. And to provide evidence and support for not just the people of the South, but to *everyone* who simply **may not**

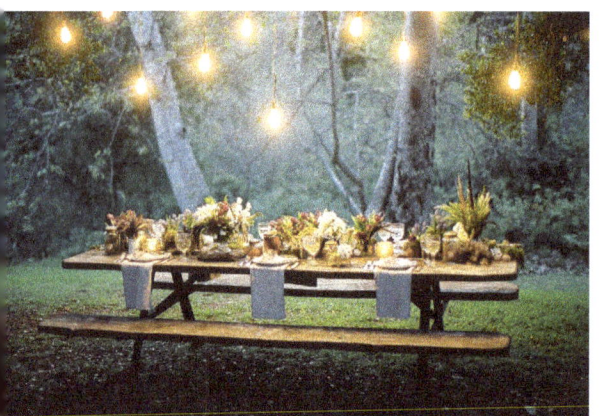

know how to utilize the good food of the Garden in this way.

The REAL healing is done *everyday* at MEALTIME. Everyday you have a chance to USE FOOD WISELY, adding in Superfoods, changing the variety of your diet, adding your blessings, and eating with Joy.

I don't believe the answer will ever be found in overusing a bunch of

UNNATURAL, symptom-creating, poison pharmaceuticals which only mask the problems! Let's learn more about how *eating better food* works. Every one of us, even the nutrition and survival experts, need to keep learning all the time about how to **nourish ourselves and help others to do so.** We must all make strides to discover and preserve Real Natural Health. In Chapter 3, we will explore **Vital Nutrients and Food Medicines** from specific plants that can change your attitude and energy, divert the course of disease, radically change your health, maybe even save your life!

There's so much we can do with healthy Organic Food. AND - *growing it yourself* adds a special energy just for your benefit. Many experts even believe your Plants will grow specifically to suit your particular biological needs! Whether you grow your own or just seek out Organic Food at the stores, I can assure you, you will find your best way to real health through enhancing and improving your diet.

DO THE VEGANS KNOW SOMETHING?

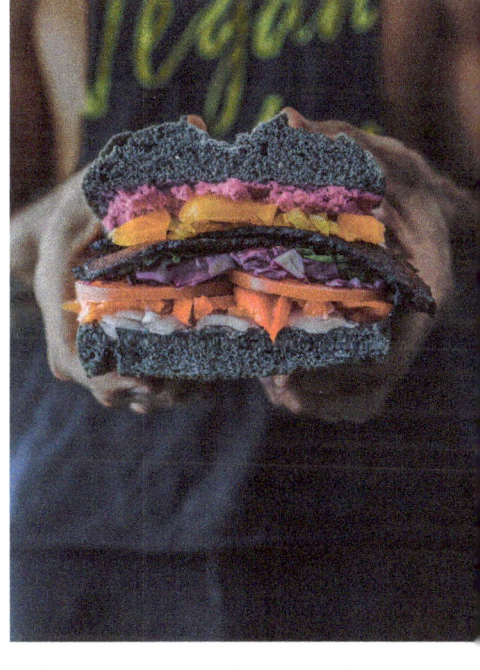

Eating "Red Meat" at all three meals a day is unhealthy, both physically and spiritually. Maybe it is something you have always done, or learned from your parents. But it is not really an example of eating "all things in moderation." Eating anything that much is more like a habit (or an obsession)! Focusing on the nutrient profile alone, Red Meat **does not** provide cell-protective Antioxidants, nor enough essential Vitamins, nor a variety of Phenolic compounds that aid its digestion, the way Plants do. Excess Red Meat intake causes inflammatory and acid overproduction diseases. Because of this, Meat can actually remain undigested in the gut for years, clogging and stopping up the system, adding weight and eventually an unnatural girth to the belly. With such a focus on Meat, there is little room for Fruits and Vegetables which should be the **mainstay of the diet.** *This habit compromises the body's health more every day.* Our bodies *depend* on the essential nutrients and vital force found in **Living Food**, grown from the **Living Ground.**

Plant-based diets are not just promoting a current fad, they are a **necessity, a lifeline for health, another Divine connection to the Planet.** Vegetarians and Vegans have realized for centuries that there is also a *spiritual potency* to Living Plant Foods, harvested lovingly and without the karma that cruelty to animals creates. AND, the **youth-preserving, age-reversing nutrition** inherent in a Living Food diet shows right on your Vegan friends' faces - their healthy glow simply radiates. Plant Foods are high in Minerals necessary for *every bodily function* and Vitamins that can remediate deficiency-based illnesses. Many diseases (including diabetes) have been *reversed* with a Raw/Vegan diet and its health-improving benefits are well documented. Recent food experiments have scientifically proven the healing value of eating high-quality, **homegrown, Vegan garden produce.**

The cuisines of most cultures offer **complete protein Vegan dishes** (like Red Beans and Rice) that equal the protein of full-Meat meals. It is a potent motivation to know we could reverse diseases and poverty and food shortages (and possibly even slow down AGING) if we would rely more on what we can **GROW**.

> "If we gave up eating beef we would have roughly 20-30 times more land for food than we have now."
>
> ~ *James Lovelock*

Just Saying. Maybe you don't have to *give up* Meat, but focus on it a little less? Use some of the land for other vegetable crops? I am obviously a strong supporter of **reducing our *reliance* on Meat**, and helping more people utilize the varied **gifts of the Plant Kingdom**. You only need to watch one video about overcrowding chicken sheds or inhumane animal treatment of milking cows, or take a trip to a slaughterhouse to agree with me. Our meat production and *consumption* has become out-of-balance with what is natural. It has become INDUSTRIALIZED and gluttonized, and consequently the increasing demand has pushed already unnatural practices into overdrive. Overcrowding creates more disease and smaller animals, who are then fed growth hormones and antibiotics to counter this, and wind up unable to walk. The meat actually retains the antibiotics, hormones, adrenaline, poisons, chemicals and FEELINGS from such horrible practices, and then people eat it! Imagine the physical impact and hormonal disruption this causes us, not to mention the emotional impact incurred from eating such unhappy animals full of stress chemicals and growth enhancers.

> **"The cow's in the kitchen. it'll be cooking soon -**
> **Feeding all the people,**
> **Eating Red 'til they're blue....**
> **Turn off the tele - stop watching the News**
> **Start filling your belly**
> **With some Home-Grown Food."**
>
> ~ *"All in the Numbers" by Dave Allen*

There are *many alternatives* to combat the unnatural evolution of this way of eating. **We *have* solutions to this problem**: kinder, more humane ways of raising Meat, as well as alternative foods on which to focus. We can turn to better Food Combining for complete proteins and optimum digestion. Mushrooms and Mycoprotein are a wonderful Meat substitute, as well as Texturized Vegetable Protein and all the many Vegan protein sources listed below. At this moment, Chefs and Scientists alike are working on ways to reduce our dependence on animal proteins.

This is where the old saying, "Careful what you wish for," becomes appropriate. An **overly-engineered** Vegan alternative may not be the answer either. I am definitely not an advocate of laboratory-created, flat slab, fake meat that bleeds with artificially engineered heme-molecule blood, sprayed with preservatives and antifungal poisons for shelf life! Or cricket and insect proteins which are over-refined to hide all the legs!! YUK! So much processing, refining and meddling does not make "engineered plant-based" food any better, it takes the "Natural Food" right out of the equation.

The real answer is in utilizing all of the many **Living Whole Plant Foods** we can get. Most people would find radical **better health** if they'd eat less meat, or maybe only eat it once a day, or even only a few times a week. Others might want to experiment with replacing it altogether. There are options to learn about, regardless of your commitment, ways to get back to **Superfoods, Herbs, Mushrooms, Sprouts** and all the vivid colors and *medicine foods* of the Plant Kingdom.

VEGAN PROTEIN SOURCES

Almonds	**Flax Seeds**	**Oats/Oatmeal**	**Sesame Seeds**
Amaranth	**Hazelnuts**	**Peanut Butter**	**Soybeans**
Avocado	**Hemp Seeds**	**Peas**	**Spelt**
Black Beans	**Hummus**	**Pecans**	**Spinach**
Blue-Green Algae	**Kale**	**Pistachios**	**Spirulina**
Broccoli	**Lamb's Quarters**	**Poppy Seeds**	**Sprouted Whole Grain Breads**
Buckwheat	**Lentil Flour**	**Potato**	
Cannellini Beans	**Lentils**	**Pumpkin Seeds**	**Sunflower Seeds**
Cashews	**Lima Beans**	**Quinoa**	**Sunflower Shoots**
Chia Seeds	**Macadamia Nuts**	**Radish Sprouts**	**Tahini**
Chickpeas	**Mung Beans**	**Red Kidney Beans**	**Teff**
Chlorella	**Mushrooms**		**Tempeh & Tofu**
Edamame	**Nutritional Yeast**	**Seitan**	**Wild Rice**

HOMEGROWN SOLUTIONS

Recently, there were more than a few times when I could say I was glad we had so much food stored. The supermarkets were out of organic Raspberries for weeks this

Spring, but I had plenty in my freezer. When cyberattacks on the food chain began happening, there was no organic chicken available for weeks, but we thankfully had more than we needed. Just watching the hardship our friends in Texas endured in the "Deep Freeze of Winter 2021" and some of our families in the recent "Hurricane/Flood in North Carolina of 2024" opened our eyes even wider. Witnessing many people living without power for more than two weeks, or with no grocery store trips possible because the road simply wasn't THERE anymore, reminded us how wise it is to have emergency food on hand. While I was writing this, another hurricane just hit New Orleans and they "can't say when" power will be restored or any store will reopen. It makes me feel so grateful for the Real Food I have set aside and preserved, as well as the many Sprouting seeds and trays I have on hand for Fresh Food I can *grow* for us in any season, for any reason. It is wise to have our gardens and pantries prepared for what may become a changing *new normal* with our access to Food.

What we will most likely experience is that our food supply could become more **local** and **seasonal** again, and may be interrupted and compromised occasionally. We all unknowingly got in the *habit* of eating grapes in midwinter, without thinking how difficult they were to obtain from South America, simply because our stores always provided them! Some people do not even realize food production is (by the nature of our weather) **seasonal and regionally specific**, simply because we have had such *easy access* to an international supply chain and millions of trains and trucks and drivers moving it around easily in every month of the year. Our access to food and supplies has never been greater, as long as the workers, trucks, planes and trains are all still *moving*! And the electricity and technology that runs such enormous food conglomerates stays secure and unhacked.

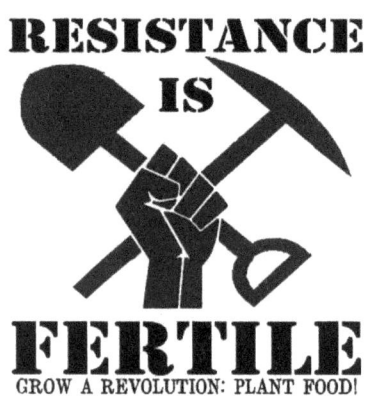

Because challenges could at any time confront us, we need to actively seek and create **Food Solutions**. If you notice that your easy public access to the "Abundant Food Supply" you count on has become affected, or if you just want **better quality, less expensive, guaranteed Organic Food** straight out of the Garden, you will find possibility and inspiration here! This is one of Humankind's most special skills, that we possess a drive for solution and a creative ability for problem-solving that is unrivaled. We can apply this to the changing food situation. **JUST LIKE NATURE**, our Universal Design provides ways we can adjust to changing circumstances. Now is the perfect time to have some adaptive plans in place for growing and providing for yourself in a sustainable way. Gardens are a *living gift* for your Family, and the entire Ecosystem - benefiting everyone including the Wildlife, Birds and Pollinators! Let's all learn to be **Plant Partners** at Home. Let's return to GROWING MORE FOOD FOR OURSELVES.

~ the garden of earth ~

🌿 GARDENING 🌿
growing for your table, pantry, & medicine cabinet

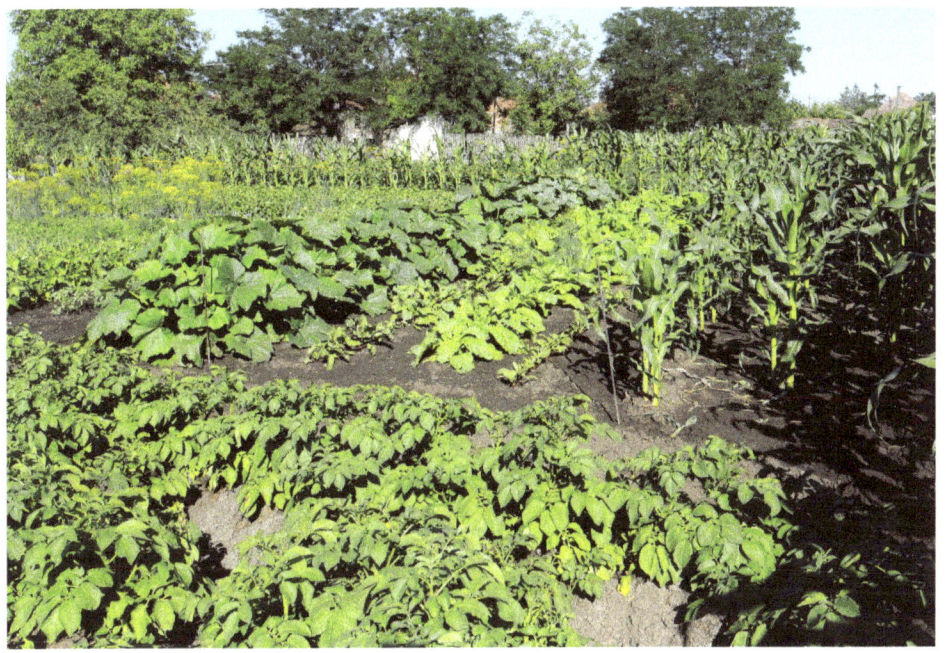

> "Maybe a person's time
> would be as well spent raising food
> as raising money to buy food.
>
> ~Frank A. Clark

Growing your own Food is a great MONETARY value and saves trips to the store. It offers you more personal choice, the adventure of exploring what is possible, and the joy of watching it grow! It gives you time in Nature to reset and be healed. It is a sacred communion you make with the Plants, Elementals, Nature Spirits, Birds, Animals, Soil, Air, Water - deep in the Elements of Nature - *and you both grow*. The Food you harvest will also provide you with Seeds, so you can grow it again or spread it to others. Gardening is a **remarkably healing, sharing, RENEWING practice** with the fruits of your labor providing many essential gifts for your Family, Friends, Neighbors and Wildlife. In Chapter 5, you will find lots of awesome ways to **preserve and share** all the many Gifts the Garden offers.

For now and the future, let's teach ourselves to grow Personal and Community Gardens! YOU can be the one to bring medicinal herbs and food plants into your yard, your home, and your neighborhood. Think of the items you regularly purchase at the store and try growing them for yourself. It may be a challenge to grow different things in some climates, but I always think you should try. Nature is an amazing adaptor. Lots of food can be grown INSIDE in all seasons as well. Search the seed catalogs and websites early to prepare your plans for growing what you need, and consider planting a Medicinal Garden and a Kitchen Herb Garden, as well as Food and Flower Gardens.

EDIBLE YARDS

My dear friend **Brigitte Mars** has a **Garden like no other**, wrapped all around her house in Boulder, Colorado. It is abundantly overflowing with *what grows there naturally*. She cherishes and nourishes her many Weeds the way most people care for their cultivated, store-bought perennials! This is simply because she realizes what potent food and medicine plants she has been given: **Nettles, Peppermint, Rosemary, Motherwort, Purslane, Lamb's Quarter, Dandelion, Chicory, Roses** - the list goes on. She harvests Wild Weeds *everyday* to make juices and raw meals, teas and medicines. Brigitte to this day does not have a driver's license and has never driven a car, in dedication to the environment - but believe me, she still gets around! And she needs fewer rides to the store because her Garden provides wild fresh food for her DAILY. And she feeds everyone who comes over! As I mention in the following chapter about Weeds, when you tend your special Wild Plants and harvest them and work with them, they grow like any other garden - abundantly!

Check your yard for what dear Mother Nature has already planted, just for you. In the Springtime in Jackson, our entire backyard is filled with Violets in a purple carpet that I know grows denser each year, just for me. I have made many medicines with my remarkable Violets, and their generous, giving spirit lives on in the bounty I am able to enjoy and share year round. Find space in your yard to set aside *wild gardens* that honor and are in support of the Weeds, Nature Spirits and Medicinal Plants that may be already there to please you.

Brigitte is a brilliant proponent of **The Edible Lawn**. She'll prove the value of **sustaining the wild world** to you. WATCH this awesome video to see her in action in the Weeds. She puts forward the plan that we need to start creating EDIBLE LAWNS: www.brigittemars.com/other/eat-the-weeds/

This is actually a growing trend right now: **FOODSCAPING**, they are calling it (what a brilliant and obvious idea). Think of the green, green lawns in front of nearly every house and apartment building. All this real estate used to tend a lawn of *grass*, from a likely foreign species, that has to be regularly watered constantly (*think* of all the precious water required with no food resulting!). Note all the grass-seed, the mowing, the maintenance of these plants that produce *nothing of value* but a green carpet, and worse, the many weed killers and pesticides required to keep it pristine. Nowhere in Nature does only one Plant grow anywhere at a time. All the space we have dedicated to unproductive lawns could be rededicated to **feed entire neighborhoods**. *Water your Food, not your carpet!* Start planting Sustainable Backyards, at least. I have seen many self-sufficiency books and posts about people who are learning how to be completely self-reliant with the food they produce in their own **yards**, regardless of geographical location. Here is a beautiful, full backyard garden from my friend Meredith Kaye-Clark. Don't you wish we all had this?!

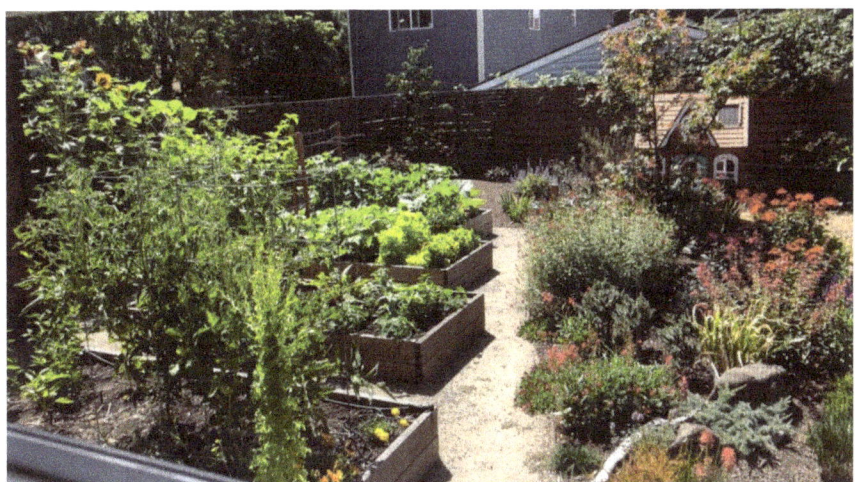

I wrote about **Kin's Domains** in *Volume One*, the idea from the Vladimir Megre's *Anastasia* books, that every household should be provided (by the government) with a 2.5 acre farm from which they could grow everything necessary to feed a large family. This land would produce food to spare for neighbors, or for sale or barter. Instead of billionaires hoarding our farmland, **I believe the government should reclaim the precious land and spread it around to all people.** In Russia they practice this, and whole communities have sprouted up around the Kin's Domains, feeding their neighbors solely with their locally grown food. It's working, living proof of this genius and humanitarian Gardening idea in action. In some places they even use gardens to remediate prisoners, and give them something of which they can be proud.

PLANT GARDENS WITH YOUR CHILDREN

We need to teach our children to grow gardens. They LOVE watching plants sprout and will be MUCH more interested in eating their vegetables if they grow them! My surrogate grandchild Rowan is constantly informing me about what they are growing and how many plants and of what types. The Garden is nurturing him and providing him a lifelong passion! His scientist/father Sean Ballard Bruce teaches him all the botanical names for the plants they are growing. Who doesn't love hearing a 4 year-old exclaiming plant names in

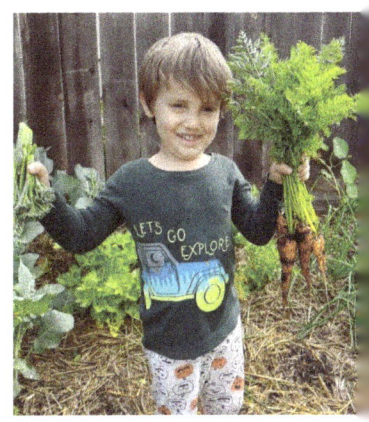

Latin! Rowan grows like a weed, he is great at sports and loves to go to Farm Camp, too.

Another truly inspiring Gardener of Change is my dear old theatre friend, and long-running KKFI Radio Personality **Mark Manning**, who is involved with the Kansas City, Kansas School System. He actively teaches thousands of schoolchildren each year how to grow Food and fall in love with Gardening. This picture makes me cry - look at all those raised beds, the food potential, and the happy children outside!

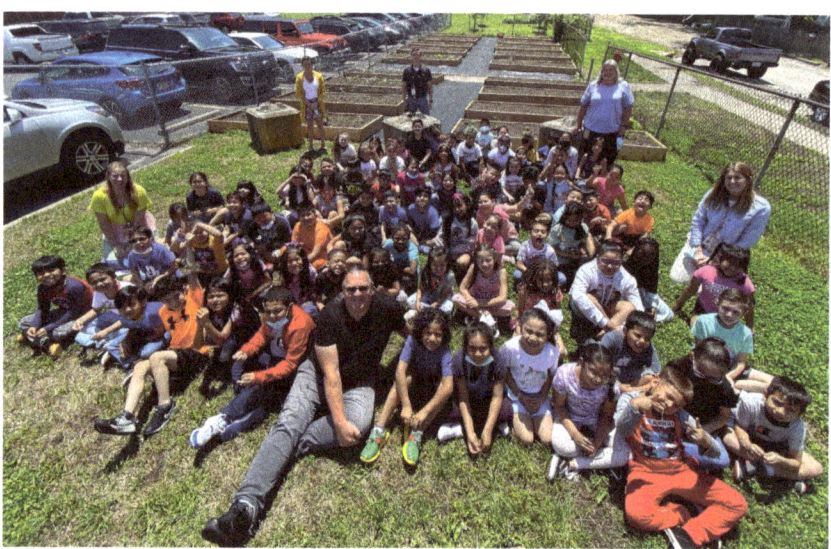

"Located at seven schools, the KCK Organic Teaching Gardens have built organic, "raised bed" gardens directly on the school grounds of three Middle Schools and four Elementary Schools in the inner city of Kansas City, Kansas. Each year 1000 to 2000 students, between K-8th grades, participate in nine months of workshops that include: *Planting and Harvesting Fall, Spring and Summer Gardens, Learning about the Parts of a Seed and the Parts of a Plant, Composting and Worms, The Multiculturalism of the Garden, George Washington Carver and the History of Sweet Potatoes, Trees and Tree Planting, Bees, Insects and Spiders.* Workshops involve preparing Food harvested from the garden for students to eat, reading from garden literature, and connecting students to their own classroom curriculum benchmarks. Garden Coordinator, Mark Manning conducts over 300 workshops annually in classrooms at these schools."[7]

Now THIS is progress with the younger generations, Gardens growing right on their playgrounds! Thank-you to the schools who believe in the *importance* of the education a Garden can provide. I am so proud of you Mark, my friend, think how many souls you touched! May your inspiration continue through generations.

I salute **Michelle Obama** and all the heart-warming, Gaia-loving good work she did planting new White House Gardens. In her book entitled *American Grown,* she writes all about the Kitchen Garden she planted on the South Lawn! She tells about her many experiences as a novice gardener there, as well as fascinating tales about gardens all over the US. She invited school children to help build and maintain the White House Gardens, and Mother Nature herself taught them all together. Everybody learned more than they expected from the Garden - in her words:

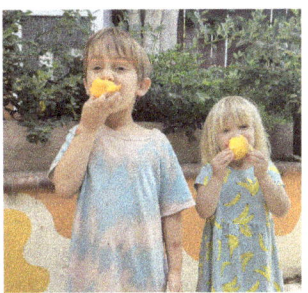

> **"People from all walks of life and every sector of our society are coming together and using Gardens - and the food they grow and the lessons they teach - to build a healthier future for our children."**
> *~ First Lady Michelle Obama*

She writes about Thomas Jefferson who grew more than 100 species of flowers and 330 varieties of herbs and vegetables; about Victory Gardens planted during World War II which produced about 40% of America's food; inspiring stories of many other wild-growing Gardens and do-good Gardeners from New Jersey to Seattle. This is a beautiful book full of heart-warming success stories of Family Farms and Community Gardens, Farmer's Markets and Soup Kitchens, all inspired by Nature, feeding the World with homegrown food.

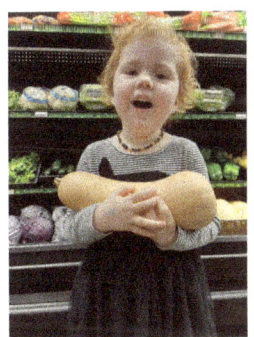

> **"Why try to explain Miracles to your kids when you can just have them plant a Garden?"**
> *~ Robert Brault*

FUN WITH FRIENDS AND NEIGHBORS

I love the energy generated from Community Gardening, and the way it brings neighbors and families together. It encourages sharing of the crops, as well as seeds, stories, and plant wisdom throughout the tribe. Everybody learns and works in cooperation for the literal "fruits" that all of the labor will bring. One of the most joyous results of gardening is the abundant **return on investment** - usually armloads of more food than you could personally consume. It is as if **each plant wants to provide a plenty that extends beyond just your Family**. Give your extra food to those in need, to your friends and neighbors, to homeless shelters, soup kitchens, or even sell it as homegrown produce to your local restaurants and stores! I know many hobby Gardeners who soon became Farmers because they discovered another revenue stream growing right outside! Here is the perfect example of the Plant Kingdom teaching us to grow and share, then richly rewarding *all of us* for it. Mutually Beneficial - that's a great system.

You may have no space of your own for growing outdoors. But most of you have a **spare table, windowsill, small deck or balcony, or a sweet rooftop** you could commandeer for the purpose! Maybe there are people in your building who would want to grow a garden together on the roof? Stretch your imagination about what is possible and how you could find spaces in which to allow the Plants to flourish. Lettuces and Tomatoes grow great in small pots on a kitchen windowsill or countertop. Herbs are perfect to raise in containers, and cookie sheet pans can be used for an Indoor Microgreen Garden. You, and Nature, can find a way to make sure you can have Fresh Food.

SEEDS OF CHANGE

These days I take my **Seed Collection** a lot more seriously! The demand for seeds has skyrocketed in the last few years. I decided I want seeds as gifts from now on for any occasion. And I have made plans to specifically **gather and share** seeds from my garden after the harvest each year. In order to keep seeds viable for years they should be stored in airtight glass containers like mason jars, in their packets. Some people suggest **freezing** seeds for long-term storage, but do at least keep them very cool and dry, 32-41 degrees, in a refrigerator or a cool dark basement. Real gardeners will tell you even ancient seeds can still germinate, so don't be overly worried about dates and having new seeds, just make sure you have a back-up if they don't sprout. Saving seeds each growing season is a ritual we should all practice - there are so many free food seeds that go to waste each year! When you begin to pay more attention to seeds you will realize they are everywhere.

Get together with your friends and do a "Seed Swap." Many of us have purchased more seeds than we can grow, or have open packets we may never use. It is fun to gather with your buddies and some little jars to share seeds and garden success stories. I envision someday we could have **Little Seed Banks** the way we have the Little Lending Libraries, where you could drop off the spare seeds you have and pick up some seeds that another gardener may have left. What a cool way to spread the literal seeds of change! A year after I wrote this, I found this image posted on social media by John Forti. He has written a brilliant book called *The Heirloom Gardener*. His book is incredibly helpful, and his invention of a Seed Library is exactly what I am talking about! Let's all share our seeds, and any other overabundance we have in this unique way. I have seen a box like this near my vet's office for spare animal food and supplies, and read about some Free Food 'Fridges in New York City where you can put your extra food to share.

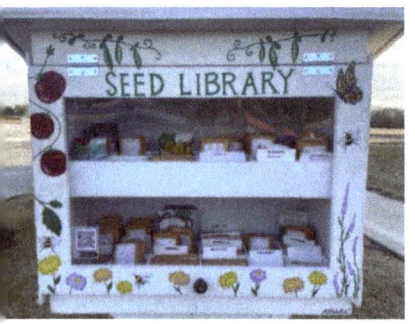

FRUIT TREES EVERYWHERE

A perfect new trend is to save your Peach, Plum, Apricot or Cherry pits, Avocado seeds and other large seeds to throw out the window on road trips, or for rooting and planting in your own garden. Apparently the *government* of Thailand recently suggested a plan for all their people to save their fruit pits and plant them, or toss them out onto the roadways and into fields. The country is now boasting its largest share of food-providing fruit trees ever, thanks to a simple act of saving seeds and releasing them into Nature instead of landfills. With this one campaign, Northern Thailand and Malaysia have been able to provide a SUSTAINABLE, generational food source for their people, for many years to come. Streets should be lined with Fruit Trees to feed the People.

Or you could be a Plant Champion like **David Avocado Wolfe** and start a **Fruit Tree Planting Foundation,** and plant over **1 million fruit trees**! His amazing team, TreeEO Cem Akin, and all the Arborists and all of the volunteers at the organization are vital to this mission. In November of 2020, the Fruit Tree Project & FTPF accomplished the mind-blowing goal of planting their 200,000th fruit tree in the Los Angeles area *during a pandemic*! I guess they used their "downtime" well! They figure this amounts to roughly **28 million pieces of fruit, 33 million pounds of breathable oxygen, and the elimination of 40 million pounds of carbon dioxide** from the atmosphere *each year*. FTPF wants to plant 18 billion trees - close to three trees for every person alive on Earth - to demonstrate organic and organizational standards and encourage food freedom and self-sufficiency for all cultures.

> "***The Fruit Tree Planting Foundation*** is dedicated to planting fruit, nut and medicinal trees to alleviate world hunger, combat global pollution, strengthen communities, and improve the surrounding air, soil, and water. Our programs strategically donate where the harvest will best serve communities for generations - including public schools, city parks, community gardens, food banks, low-income neighborhoods, Native American reservations, international hunger relief sites, and animal sanctuaries." ~ *www.ftpf.org*

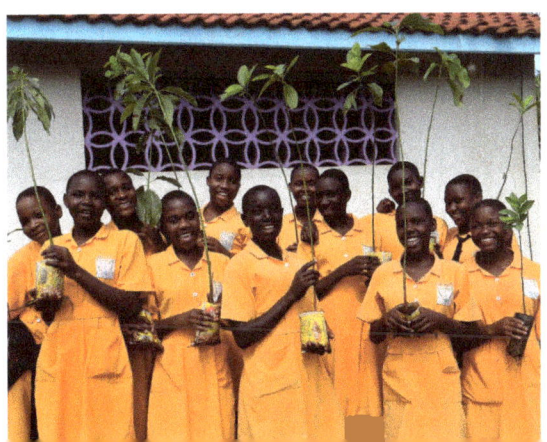

~ the garden of earth ~

GARDEN SECRETS

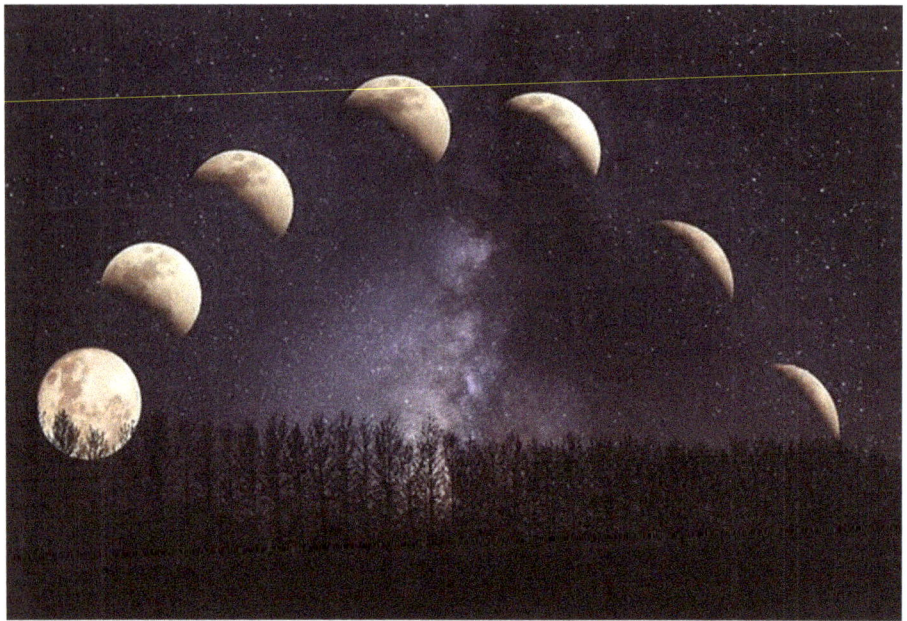

PLANTING BY THE MOON

Utilizing the **Moon Phases** is an ancient planting practice that is super effective and oddly supportive for your Garden. The Moon creates repeating natural cycles that influence the water in our bodies, the ocean tides, and also the growth of our garden plants by pulling on the water in their bodies and in the soil. When the Moon is Full, water gravitationally ascends to the surface to nourish seeds, causing them to swell and germinate faster. When the Moon is New (dark) everything descends, as the gravitational pull lessens and water returns to nourish the roots. For superior results, choose your planting times in harmony with the Moon cycles below and you will be rewarded with healthier, more vigorous plants, and much better harvests.

- NEW MOON to FULL MOON ~ WAXING PHASE: Best for planting and sowing seeds of **Annual Flowers, Fruits and Veggies - above ground crops** like Corn, Tomatoes, Melons, Lettuce, Beans, Cucumbers and Squash. The building, waxing, Bright Moon energy encourages expansive growth of leaves and stems. Transplanting or splitting plants is most favorably done during this phase as well.

- FULL MOON to NEW MOON ~ WANING PHASE: Best for planting **Flowering Bulbs, Biennial and Perennial Flowers, and Veggies - underground root crops** like Potatoes, Beets, Carrots, and Peanuts. Dark and below ground items like roots, tubers and bulbs are encouraged to grow downward as the energy of the waning

Moon is darkening and contracting, and the gravitational pull upwards decreases. The **completely dark New Moon** is a *resting time* for plants, so do not plant anything during those few days. However, this is the perfect time to weed, and tend the soil. Transplanting seedlings right at the **Full Moon** helps with root shock.

More detailed celestial assistance will be found when the **Moon is in particular Zodiac Signs**. The Moon stays in each sign for about 3 days, and you can determine what sign/when by searching online at astrological sites like **www.astro.com**. You can also find the Moon dates and signs in the Farmer's Almanac, you can check it when in line at the grocery store, or read online at **www.almanac.com**. I have found it is a wonderful reference for timing guidance, Moon details, weather predictions, awesome stories, planting suggestions, old timer advice and planning tools for your gardening adventures.

⭘ Advanced Moon Gardening ⭘

WHEN THE MOON IS IN:	TAKE THIS ACTION:
Cancer, Scorpio, Pisces, Taurus	Plant, transplant, graft, water
Aries, Leo, Sagittarius, Gemini, Aquarius	Harvest, plow, weed, control pests
Capricorn	Build garden beds, plant roots, fix & build fences, structures
Aries, Leo, Sagittarius	Prune & deadhead

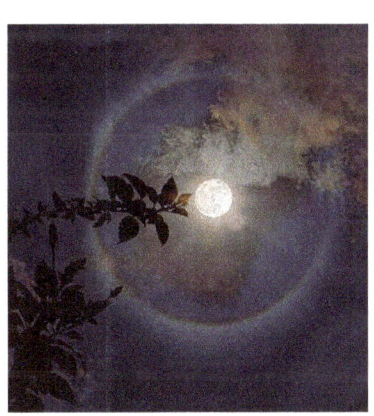

"Learn to do common things
uncommonly well;
we must always
keep in mind that anything that
helps fill the dinner
pail is VALUABLE."

~ *George Washington Carver*

AT THE GARDEN'S DIRECTION

A deeply spiritual way to connect with Nature is to **ask advice of the Garden itself** - the Angels of the Landscape, the Nature Spirits, and the Devas of the Plants you grow. Consulting them, connecting to an Elemental Realm, is very educational and surprisingly beautiful. They are responsible for guiding you and love to assist with your acknowledgement. Here are some very exceptional **Gardens Who Became Teachers!**

~ the garden of earth ~

FINDHORN GARDEN

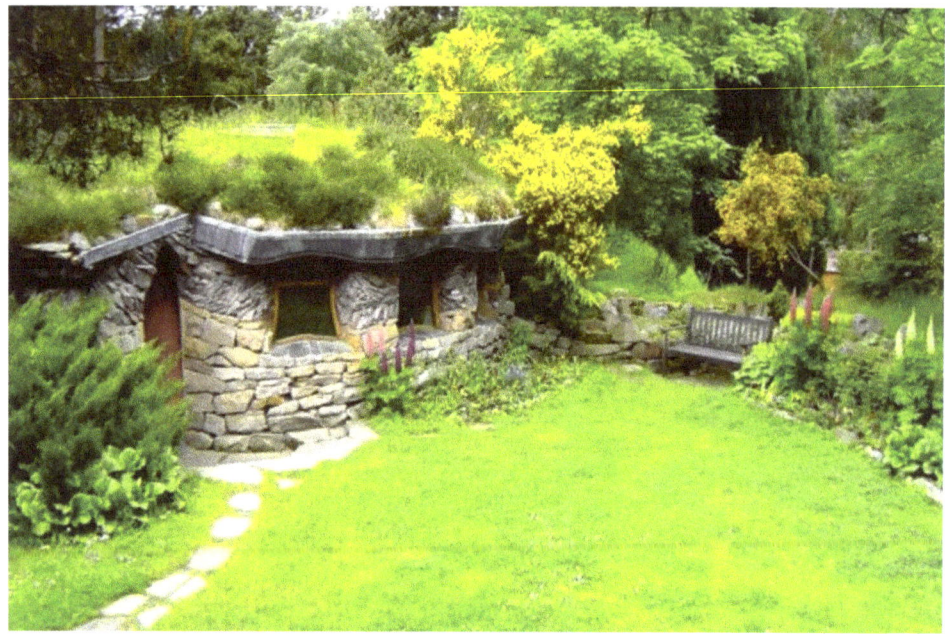

The most famous Spiritual Gardening Experiment *ever* still flourishes today in Scotland. More than sixty years ago, dear friends **Dorothy Maclean and Peter & Eileen Caddy** built and nurtured a small, humble garden that would one day become the world-renowned *Findhorn Foundation Garden and Spiritual Eco-Community*.

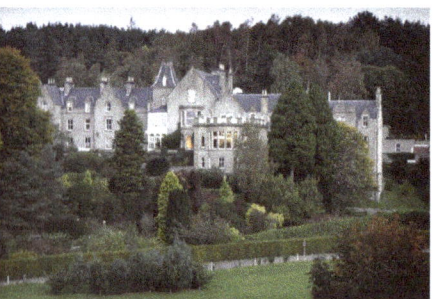

In 1962, after a successful run of five years as management team for the gorgeous castle-like Cluny Hill Hotel in Northern Scotland, Dorothy, Peter and Eileen were unexpectedly released from their employment. They received Innate Guidance that they were to all stay together, and so they moved nearby into a small "caravan" (like an RV trailer) in a park near the coast. Since they couldn't actually feed themselves suitably on their shared government unemployment benefits, they quickly realized they *needed* to grow food to survive.

Initially they really struggled, until one day Dorothy was contacted in meditation by the **"Overlighting Intelligence of Plants"** which she would eventually call the Plant's Angels, or Devas. They answered questions, made suggestions, and would give her detailed instructions to help remediate the sandy, coastal soil in which they were trying to grow. Eileen also received visions and spiritual guidance. Her messages would instruct her husband Peter to build specific kinds of garden beds and fences to suit the particular needs of the growing Garden. Every morning, they would all make time for querying Nature and *"Attuning to the God Within."* They prepared questions and sought a most unique and organized, business-like approach with which to receive guidance. They got their answers. Tuning-in to the Voice of Nature gifted them with revelations they could not have imagined, and offered them a quality of Divine answers they could find nowhere else. A real partnership (with real instructions) was established between the Humans, the Land, The Plants and the Beings. They asked for Angelic Guidance and abundantly received it, and with it the Garden revealed its very own intelligent and magical plan.

The Angels ultimately gave them three Founding Principles for success in the Findhorn Garden and Community:

1. **"Inner Listening"** ~ listen to the Voice inside seeking to support you

2. **"Work Is Love In Action"** ~ give your whole self & highest Love to each and every task you do

3. **"Co-Create with the Intelligence of Nature"** ~ be fully, lovingly engaged, asking and wondering about everything outside

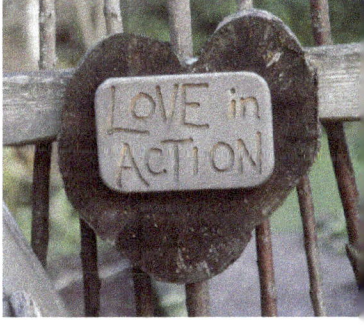

What *unexpected motto* were they given by the Angels, for trying to live on what Nature alone could provide? They were told to **"Expect a Miracle."** They did, and it happened! In 1969, their Garden would attain world-wide recognition for its **40-pound Cabbages**, in addition to Flowers and Herbs and Food no one expected could ever grow there! Suddenly everyone wanted to know just what they were doing in this little corner of wind-torn Scotland. Horticulturists came from all corners of the World to study their stunning successes. They were on the Evening News! People came from many countries.

Upon visiting the Gardens, many were drawn to the mystery and magic of Findhorn's land and its unconventional ways. They wanted to live there, settle into the community to learn, and many people did. Eventually, the trio would *buy* that brilliant castle hotel they were *fired* from, to add to their seaside caravan park, providing much more land and housing with which to expand their budding gardens and growing community.

Ironically, the enormous Cabbages might have made them famous, but they were not the whole story at all! **An entirely new way of Gardening** was co-created by these dear people who simply took the time to listen to Mother Earth. Teaching people to work WITH Nature, communicating with the Angels of the Plants and the Place, creating strong intentions and asking for help from Spirit became their true legacy. They have since taught millions of people to tune in and receive helpful guidance from Mother Earth in all her forms. The beauty that continues to grow in the hearts of the many people they touched is an **unexpected second flowering**.

Dorothy advises that you seek to **communicate with EVERYTHING!** Everything in Nature is connected to the Whole. Notice how each creation has its own unique **spiritual energy, frequency** and **personality**. *Everything* is available to communicate

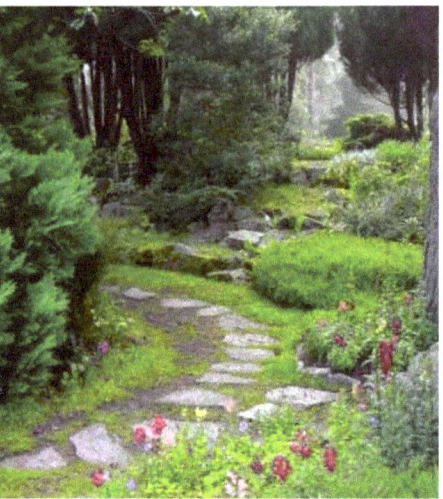

with you if you will just ask, and Everyone can do this if you just believe. We are all equipped with the internal senses and abilities to connect with energy around us, but we use the skills so infrequently. You will be astonished how much more there is to living when you begin to connect to EVERYTHING!

When you go to a new place connect with the Angel of that City or Forest or Beach. When you see a plant you do not know, seek to meet its Deva and ask about it. When you are in a particularly beautiful garden, thank the Landscape Angel for the design. When you have trouble in your yard or garden, connect with its Land or Garden Angel for assistance.

What wonders could happen if we all started communicating with every being and thing more? We don't feel odd about communicating with our pets, and we love it when they "talk back" in their own way. How enriching will it be, for both parties, when the Angels, and Spirits of Nature, and the PLANTS THEMSELVES communicate back to you, expressing what they really want you to hear?!

> **"There is nothing fey about consulting the Intelligence of Nature. It is, as I see it, entirely practical: an efficient method of finding solutions to problems that otherwise would have humanity stumped."**
>
> ~ *Dorothy Maclean*

Read Dorothy Maclean's amazing books to discover more about the Angelic Guidance she was able to cultivate. They are truly special. You can explore the many innovations of the Findhorn Gardening process, watch live Garden demonstrations, peruse articles, and learn more about their brilliant and successful philosophy at **www.findhorn.org**

> **"Talking to plants is one way of talking directly to Spirit."**
>
> ~ *Rosemary Gladstar*

~ the garden of earth ~

~⚘ PERELANDRA GARDENS ⚘~

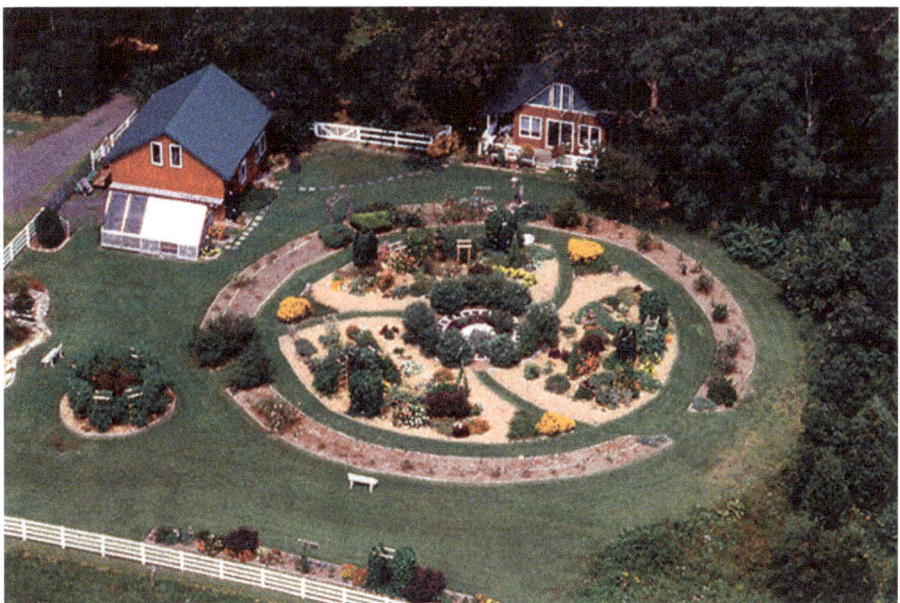

Another radical Gardener is **Machaelle Small Wright** of **Perelandra Gardens**, and her revelatory partnership with the Nature Spirits, in her neck of the woods in Virginia. She knew of the Findhorn Garden and had studied their ways of connecting to Nature and using intention. Through experimentation and communication, *she* discovered her own way to work directly in co-creation with Nature. She pioneered a method where Nature advised HER what to do, what to plant, and how to improve the Garden!

> "The Perelandra Garden thrives because of a new approach taught to me by Nature. What I'm going to describe to you does not fit comfortably into the recognized notions of tradition, logic or even sanity. In fact, it tends to thumb its nose at all three, especially sanity."
>
> ~Machaelle Small Wright

Her approach to "Co-Creative Gardening" will not only change your Gardens, but will also change your Life! She uses fail-proof muscle testing and meditation to access the **Intelligence of Nature** for answers. She teaches that Gardens are a purely Human construct, and as we are building something somewhat *unnatural*, the Plants need us to define our **Intention, Purpose** and **Direction**. If you were working with people, you would tell them what you expect, or hope for from them for the project - do the same with your Plants. Give them a mission, goals, your vision, and hearty encouragement.

Her Research Garden is a sanctuary where Machaelle and her staff all study and listen. In direct response to the guidance Nature has provided they have built a Nature Spirit Area and an Insect Sanctuary, a Wildflowers Only Garden, and an Elemental Annex

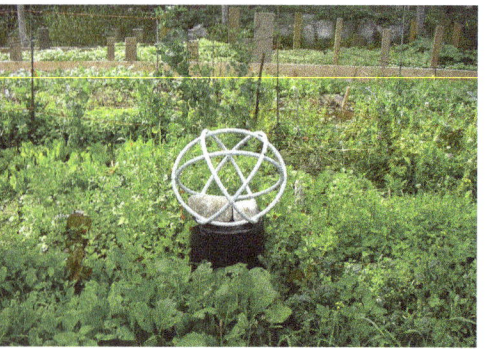

especially for the Elementals. In the center of everything, Machaelle has placed what she calls the *"Engine of the Garden."* It is a beautiful quartz crystal cluster on a slab of slate, inside a Genesa Crystal made of copper tubing that concentrates the Life Force of the surrounding area, to be utilized for the Garden. It is surrounded by quartz, shells and other minerals, with cacao shell alkalizing mulch for nourishing the first ring of Herb Gardens.

It was from her Garden, and her books, that I learned to **ask the Land** and the **Plant Devas** what *they* wanted to grow. After all, they are the Universal level *architects* and keepers of Nature Intelligence for the Garden! I learned to work *with* the **Nature Spirits** (which she defines as the specific plant's focus within my specific environment). I learned to make the Nature Spirits a special wild place on the land that was all theirs, and to mark it off for them. This is a very *deep* level of Gardening that works in a harmonious dance with all the energy there, physical and spiritual, seen and unseen - and it will blow you away.

Machaelle also speaks of "Gut Gardening" in which you simply trust yourself and your gut feelings after making a few specific connections with your Garden. Define clearly your Intent and Purpose for the garden, then specifically **ask for Nature to partner with you** as you go out to plant and tend. Express thanks and release its energy when you are finished. It's kind of like turning on and off a button that connects you to a shared focus. She counsels us to seek Nature as a **partner** and listen to anything your gut feelings reveal about your process. You may feel nervous at first, but eventually you find that your questions are answered by your magnificent partner before you even finish asking them!

Machaelle was originally inspired by Findhorn, and now we are inspired by her Gardens. You will find there are many people who believe in the Spiritual approach to Gardening and working with Nature, one in which you let Her do the teaching. The defining element of this kind of work is the level of LOVE and devotion that it requires. But it is not like work; true connection with Nature *liberates and creates* this cooperative and connective energy that makes it easy and exciting. You feel compelled to do the right thing because it feels best to you and the Plant and the Land and the Angels. It just feels like Love.

Take a video tour of Perelandra Gardens, plus discover many fabulous resources, research, books and products, on her website at **www.perelandra-ltd.com**.

Just ask **Luther Burbank**, one of America's most prolific and innovative horticulturists. He developed more than 800 new varieties of plants by *attuning to Nature*. Luther was even able to convince a Desert Cactus that it was **safe and loved** enough that it *no longer needed thorns*. He did indeed produce a smooth cactus variety and it grew to be enormous! He is remembered for his incredible communications, his devotion to and protection for the Plant Kingdom. He is pictured here with his remarkable Thornless Cactus, a revolutionary partnership in our midst.

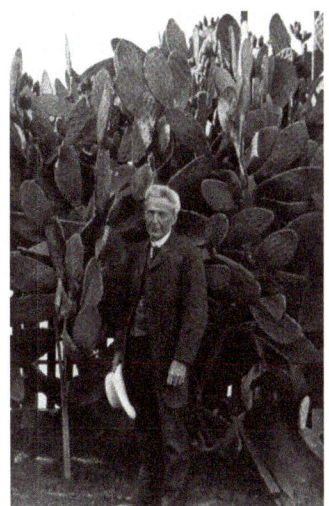

> **"The Secret of improved plant breeding, apart from scientific knowledge, is LOVE."**
> ~ Luther Burbank

NATURE TO THE RESCUE

Everyone experiences Gardening **challenges** at times. The mistakes are part of the journey, with Nature just teaching you how to do better. Don't think of them as failures but as real lessons in the School of Gardening. Like the *one night* I leave the Garden buckets outside and everything freezes. UGGGGH! Here are a few more "trade secrets" of the Garden that might be helpful to know (in addition to suggesting you *always* consult the overnight temperatures!).

PROTECTIVE PLANT PARTNERS
Naturally Repellent

Sometimes it becomes necessary to change the balance of insects and pests around you. If the bugs or animals become a problem, here are some great things to plant or to use to discourage them. You could plant a border of these plants around your garden, near your patio or next to your house entrances. Plant these aromatic helpers in pots that you can move around to repel pests where needed - while they enhance your space with their beauty.

REPEL MOSQUITOES: **Aromatic plants** - Geraniums, Mosquito Plant, Basil (all scents but Lemon Basil especially), Citronella, Lemon Balm, Catnip, Oregano, Tansy, Eucalyptus, Lavender, Marigolds, Rosemary, Bee Balm, Thyme, Lemongrass, Feverfew, Patchouli, Rosemary, Mints, Sage, Floss Flower, Garlic, Onions, Pennyroyal, Lantana, Decorative Alliums.

REPEL FLIES: **Perfect for kitchen window boxes** - Basil, Citronella, Sweet Woodruff, Lavender, Lemongrass, Pennyroyal, Coriander, Pitcher Plant, Leeks, Marigold, Rosemary, Bay Laurel, Mint, Petunias, Nasturtiums, Lemon Thyme, Clove

Essential Oil on fabric strips. Pennies in a ziploc bag of water hanging from the eaves or sitting on tables are said to repel flies and freak other pests out.

REPEL WILDLIFE: **Aromatic plants overwhelm the senses of garden pests & predators**: Garlic, Lavender, Daffodils, Catnip, Chives, Scented Geraniums, Mints, Oregano, Onions, Salvias, Rosemary, Tansy, Cinnamon. **Additional pro tips:** Use Garlic & Chili Powder combined with Vinegar sprinkled around garden entrance, Vinegar-soaked used Corn Cobs on garden corners, Coffee Grounds, Grass Clippings, Moth or Camphor Balls, Scented Soap shavings, and Smashed Eggshells. Plastic Forks buried tine-side up between plants discourage animals walking through rows.

REPEL POISONOUS PLANTS: **White Vinegar mixed with Liquid Soap and Water** makes a spray-on solution that is effective for removing plants that are unsafe to keep around, like Poison Ivy. I always do this as a last resort. I verbally warn the plants and tell them to relocate away from people before I apply it. But if they persist, I apologize while I am covering them with this mixture, which is very effective. You may need to apply to young plants each Spring to keep them from recurring.

PLEASING PLANT COMPANIONS
Helpful Garden Friends

One of the more interesting techniques in Gardening is **Companion Planting**. In a stunning example of **service to others**, plants fix nutrients into the soil that other plants need, ward off pests, boost food harvests, and help establish better environments for each other. Certain pairings produce remarkable results, and these are listed under plants they "like." While the plant does not "dislike" other plants *per se*, it shows clear preferences with its yield and size. This year the Eggplant I planted near the Peppers is twice the size of the one I planted near the Fennel. In fact, it is suggested that you **don't plant Fennel in your garden at all** (now I know)! Fennel is what is known as an ***Allelopathic Plant,*** because it contains a growth-inhibitor that affects nearly every other plant nearby. It uses its chemicals to assure its own growth success and water supply, so.... Fennel doesn't make a lot of friends. But it is a beautiful ferny wonder planted in a bed of its own, and its bulb, stalk, fronds, flower and pollen are all edible, licoricey delicacies that are quite expensive in the gourmet stores.

Instead of using poisonous insecticides that will alter your food, water supply, and the genetics of your Garden forever, **plant natural partners that will do the work for you.** Keep in mind that some plants in the **same Family** will *attract* the same pests, so it is better to plant them with other plants that would *repel* predators. Herbs make great companion plants because their powerful essential oils deter damaging insects. Many people plant Flowers right in smaller rows between their Veggies, with fabulous results for pest remediation as well as better pollination. I used this technique the last two Summers and it stunned me with its beauty, simplicity and effectiveness.

TOMATOES
- **Like:** Basil, Marigolds, Carrots, Asparagus, Celery, Onions, Lettuce, Parsley, Spinach
- **Dislike:** Broccoli, Cabbage, Corn, Kohlrabi, Beets, Potatoes, Peas, Fennel, Dill, Rosemary

LETTUCE
- **Like:** Mint, Chives, Onions, Garlic, Beans, Beets, Broccoli, Carrots, Corn, Peas, Radishes, Marigolds, Asparagus, Eggplant, Cilantro, Chervil, Strawberries, Spinach, Cucumbers, Squash, Zucchini, Cabbage
- **Dislike:** Celery, Parsley, Potatoes, Broccoli, Brussels Sprouts, Kale, Kohlrabi, Cabbage, Cauliflower

CARROTS
- **Like:** Tomatoes, Leeks, Rosemary, Sage, Chives, Onions, Amaranth, Radishes, All Beans, Peas
- **Dislike:** Coriander, Dill, Parsnips, Fennel

CUCUMBERS
- **Like:** Nasturtiums, Marigolds, Beans, Celery, Corn, Lettuce, Dill, Peas, Radishes, Oregano, Peanuts, Onions
- **Dislike:** Melons, Potatoes, Sage and other highly aromatic plants can stunt growth

BEANS & GREEN BEANS
- **Like:** Corn, Eggplant, Nasturtium, Summer Savory, Broccoli, Brussels Sprouts, Lettuce, Peas, Squash, Strawberries, Cucumbers, Potatoes, Radishes, Cabbage, Celery, Kale, Spinach
- **Dislike:** Beets, Onions (whole Family) impair growth, Peppers, Tomatoes, Marigolds

CORN
- **Like:** Beans, Cucumbers, Purslane, Melons, Peas, Pumpkin, Zucchini, Basil, Dill, Radishes
- **Dislike:** Tomatoes, Cabbages, Broccoli, Kale

ONIONS
- **Like:** Carrots, Beets, Cabbage, Chamomile, Lettuce, Parsnips, Tomatoes, Marjoram, Savory, Rosemary, Strawberries, Radishes
- **Dislike:** Asparagus, Beans, Peas

SQUASH & ZUCCHINI
- **Like:** Corn, Beans, Peas, Dill, Radishes, Marigolds, Borage, Peanuts, Mint,

Nasturtiums, Garlic, Oregano, Lettuce, Onion, Melons, Lemon Balm

- **Dislike:** Potatoes, Cucumbers, Cabbage Family (Brassicaceae)

MELONS

- **Like:** Onions, Oregano, Chives, Catnip, Leeks, Cabbage, Broccoli, Carrots, Sunflowers, Lettuce, Peas, Kale, Okra, Brussels Sprouts, Squash
- **Dislike:** Cucumbers, Squash, Zucchini, Pumpkins

PEPPERS

- **Like:** Basil, Onions, Spinach, Tomatoes, Carrots, Cucumbers, Radishes, Squash, Eggplant, Lettuce, Beans, Peas, Chard, Parsley, Dill, Oregano, Garlic, Nasturtiums, Potatoes
- **Dislike:** Beans, Cabbage Family (Brassicaceae), Fennel, Apricots

NATURE'S MANY SIGNALS
Fun & Functional Folklore

There is a great amount of valuable, age-old wisdom to be found in the "Old Sayings." Folklore, old wive's tales, and stories about Nature's ancient signs provide a wealth of information that is fading and in danger of being forgotten. Our ancestors searched the Natural World for clues about how to survive and prosper. They often used *rhymes* to remember the conditions and features of Nature's seasonal cycles. Their "folk-lore" stories would preserve advice passed down from many years of living WITH Nature, and observing the patterns in Plants and Weather. They repeated the adages to every generation - ask your Grandparents what they used to say. **Accurate guidance** is actually encoded within this folklore that people counted on for their livelihoods. I remind you of these wise words from your wise ancestors in an effort to preserve this fount of INFORMATION. Let's keep our Earth Family's knowledge intact. Please email me if you have heard any other good old sayings (littlelauralamun@gmail.com) so I can add them to future printings of this book!

"Start your Garden beds when the dirt clods don't stick to your boots anymore."

"If you can sit on the ground with your trousers down, it's time to sow the seed."

"The moon, her face be red, of water she speaks."

"Clear Moon, Frost soon."

"Give the slugs a dish of beer, and you'll both be happy all the year."

"What you love and nurture will one day love and nurture you."

"Who weeds in May throws all away."

"Nothing will grow under a Walnut tree."

"When dew is on the grass, rain will never come to pass."

"A wet Spring, a dry harvest."

"Rain before seven, clear by eleven."

"The sharper the blast, the sooner 'tis past."

"Red sky at night, sailor's delight; red sky in morning, sailors take warning."

"Mackerel sky, mackerel sky – never long wet, never long dry."

"Trout jump high, when rain is nigh."

"When leaves show their undersides, be certain that rain betides."

"A warm January makes a cold May."

"If the first week in August be warm, then the winter will be white and long."

"When Dandelions are blooming, plant Beets, Carrots, Spinach and Lettuce."

"Plant Chives in orchards to prevent lightning strikes."

"Peppers grow spicier if you plant them when you are angry."

"Plant Cabbage when the Dogwood is in bloom."

"Twelfth of May, Stow Fair Day, Sow your kidney beans today."

"Plant a cucumber on 6th July, you'll have cucumbers, wet or dry."

"Plant Corn when the Oak leaves are the size of a squirrel's ear."

"Put Potatoes in the ground when the Forsythia blooms, or on Good Friday."

"Never plant vegetables that sound alike together."
    (separate Tomatoes & Potatoes, Beans & Greens)

"Always plant something in the yard when someone dies."

"Hold an empty wallet to the Full Moon and soon it will be full."

"Plant old rusty nails around your hydrangeas – iron for more vivid color."

"Tell your Bees everything going on in the house, and their honey gets sweeter."

"When the ass begins to bray, surely rain will come that day."

"If the new moon holds the old moon in her lap, fair weather."

"If you don't treat your Scarecrow with respect your crops will suffer.
    Give him a hat."

"Birds fly low when the rain is set to go."

"Birds fly away from water in the morning, and toward water at evening."

"Rain on Easter Sunday, and it will rain the next seven Sundays."

"When woodpeckers share a tree, it's a cold winter for thee."

"A ring around the Sun or Moon, means that rain or snow is coming soon."

"If the goose honks high, fair weather. If the goose honks low, foul weather."

" If spiders are many and spinning their webs, the spell will soon be very dry."

"Doors and drawers stick before a rain."

"When clouds appear like rocks and towers, the Earth's refreshed with frequent showers."

"Three snows after the Forsythia bloom."

"Walnuts and pears, you plant for your heirs."

"Frogs will look through ice, twice."

"February fog means a frost in May."

"Cut a thistle in May and it'll be there the next day.

    Cut a thistle in June, it'll come again soon.

        Cut it in July and it's sure to die."

"Pennies in a bag of water, the flies will leave you to laughter."

"Use a cucumber end on a squeaky door, silent hinges evermore."

"Note on your calendar the first day you hear thunder, or see lightning in spring. Count exactly six months ahead and you can predict the first frost or snow."

"When the final Fireweed flower blooms, snow is just days away."

"A straw best shows how the wind blows."

"Ringing in the ears at night indicates a change of wind."

"The higher the clouds, the better the weather."

"When the wind is in the East, it's good for neither man nor beast.
When the wind is in the North, the old folk should not venture forth.
When the wind is in the South, it blows the bait in the fishes' mouth.
When the wind is in the West, it is of all the winds the best."

CARE FOR THE WHOLE HABITAT

> "Just as the Bee takes the nectar, and leaves,
> without damaging the color or scent of the Flowers,
> so should the Sage act in a village."
>
> *- Dhammapada, Sayings of the Buddha*

When you are digging in new places to make your gardens, take great care not to disturb the many native inhabitants. Disrupt their home environment in the least destructive way you can. That way, the natural system in place will continue to work with your minor alteration. There is a whole world going on underground with the interconnecting mycelium, and insect pathways that create ideal growing conditions. Don't mess with it! Remember that **leaf blowers, lawn mowers and weed eaters use electricity and gas to create noise and death**. They disturb the peaceful habitats, blowing away and destroying the nesting grounds for many insects and small animals, butterflies, bees, and other helpful pollinators. INSTEAD - you could simply allow the peaceful, quiet yard to *nourish* and provide everything you and the indigenous species need. Leaves that fall are Nature's fertilizer, provide shelter for many, and can be mulched with the lawn mower in the Spring instead of bagged in plastic in landfills. The weeds that grow abundantly early in the seasonal cycle can be harvested for food, but always leave plenty for incoming Pollinators and Wildlife.

I love the scene in the movie *Seven Years In Tibet,* in which the Buddhist Monks must dig up all the worms in the ground, chant to them, and carefully and lovingly remove them before they can construct a new building. Picture a whole line of monks, bowing and praying, as they each carry a single earthworm to a new spot they established, and over which they prayed intently. The Buddhists treat *all* creatures like they *could* be the reincarnation of their Mother. They lovingly provide for *All Beings,* no matter what, knowing the good returns to them.

In Co-Creating all your wondrous gardens, always notice and care for the Native Beings and the habitat they have built for themselves. They are a blessing with which your yard is gifted. They are a crucial part of the natural ecosystem and will act as your Partners. They are required for a healthy balance of the natural food chain, and will assure your soil is aerated, your plants are pollinated, and the ongoing abundant harvest of your Garden is exceptional. Thank-you, Mother Earth, for ALL of the Helpful Beings, great and small!

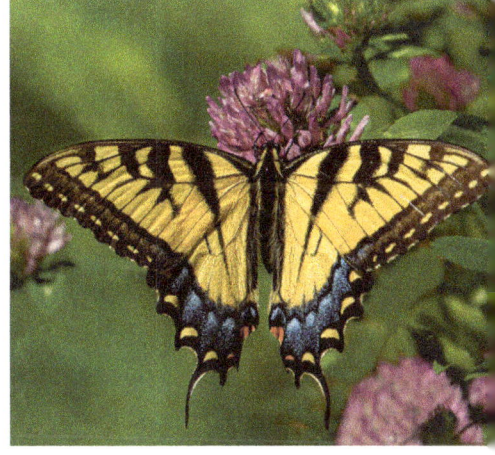

~ the garden of earth ~

~ SPROUTING ~

living food that grows anywhere

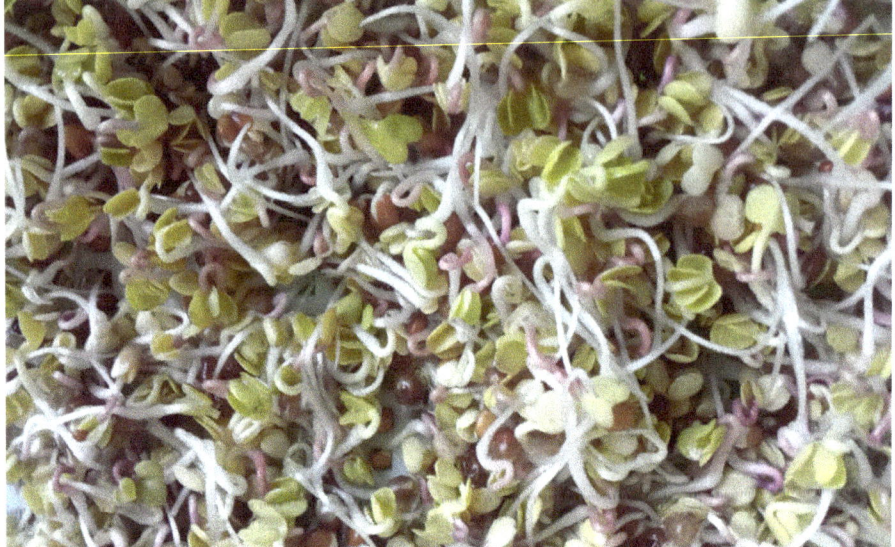

Consider **Sprouting** as an amazing way to **grow Fresh Food in ANY Season, especially** if you have some challenges with Gardening, or don't have the right kind of space for it. Maybe you got caught unawares by a storm, experienced a drought, or had a tough growing season? *Sprouting* can provide fresh, protein-rich food in just a *few days*. You might have some great preserved food in your pantry, but what is missing is anything fresh, green, living, that is filling and nutritionally dense to eat in the Winter. **SPROUTING OFFERS IT ALL.** Get yourself some basic supplies and Sprouting Seeds, and you will always have great, *nutritious* LIVE food at your fingertips, and be able to grow it anywhere, in any season.

THE INDOOR GARDEN

What I love so much about Sprouting is that you get to **enjoy the Plants inside**! Watching food grow for you is a wondrous sight. Seed-to-harvest goes super quickly with Sprouts, so it makes it extra fun (and great for kids) to see such fast progress. You reap your delicious harvest within days instead of months! Sprouting is one of the best ways to keep **Living Food** available anywhere - even in a **hotel room or on the road in a suitcase** - I have done it! It takes hardly any space at all to grow Sprouts and Microgreens, just a jar and a lid and some water. Once you begin, you may likely become obsessed with growing such ridiculously **vital food**. The trays and Mason jars of growing, precious baby plants infuse your space with Living Light Energy and vital Oxygen! It's a pretty beautiful process. Sprouting makes a great **family or**

home-schooling project that not only teaches many concepts about growing, but creates a massive amount of truly delicious Superfood plant material for early brain nourishment. **Imagine what kinds of adults we could grow if we taught all children how to Sprout!**

My favorite book on Sprouting is from long-time raw fooder **Doug Evans**, and is simply called *The Sprout Book*. Doug was an early juicing maven, who co-founded *Organic Avenue* in New York City in 2002, the country's *very first* organic cold-pressed juices and raw food retailer, which grew to 12 stores in Manhattan alone. Later he produced *Juicero* juicing machines for cold-pressed juice at home. After those successes - he realized his next product was sitting on his shelves right front of him, as he had been obsessively **Sprouting** for 20 years! His book is an amazing story of his life, as well as a great reference source, filled with interviews from leading doctors and nutrition specialists, real Science. **He tells you how to Sprout just about ANYTHING.** *His* energy is as inspiring, uplifting, and infectious as the Food itself! You want to get his book, hunt down some of his videos and watch this guy in action in his Sprout Laboratory. He's a wizard - the scale of his operation is mind-blowing. Here's one of my favorites with Avocado - **www.youtube.com/watch?v=lTysT1-BpY4.**

Because the only thing you need is Seeds, pure water and care, and *no electricity* is required for Sprouting, it makes it an **ideal Survival Food process**. If you have no outdoor space (or time) for Gardening, Sprouting helps you quickly garden in small spaces, anywhere indoors. But the best reason for beginning a Sprouting habit is the **Exceptional Nutrition found in the brave baby plants!** The *germinative energy,* and all the nutrients for new growth act like stem cells in our bodies, creating new cells, enhancing the environment, **preventing and healing many diseases**.

> "Sprouts are the most efficient delivery system for the heroic amounts of veggies we need to eat and maintain our health. In fact, there is no food on Earth more nutritious than Sprouts."
>
> ~ Doug Evans

- Sprouts contain bioavailable sources of **Protein** and **Amino Acids**, full of absorbable **Minerals, Antioxidants**, and many cancer-fighting compounds. Sprouts are rich in **Folate, Magnesium, Phosphorus, Vitamins C, B's, and K**.
- Sprouts are low in calories, are low glycemic, and suited to many diets including **Keto, Paleo, Atkins**, and **Bulletproof** diet protocols. They are actually considered a "zero points" food in **Weight Watchers** - but are packed with nutrients.
- Sprouts are the perfect food for people with diabetes because they are so high in Fiber, Protein, and other vital

nutrients, *without* any sugar, and can be eaten plentifully.

- **Sprouting a food increases its Protein content by 20%! Vitamins and other nutrients are increased by up to 500%!!** This is a real Life hack.
- Sprouts contain the *information* that will build the entire mature plant and its offspring, and the *nutrition* it needs to make it so. They are full of living potential.

One of the greatest health challenges to the body is cancer. **Sprouts** of all kinds carry such cell protective nutrients and antioxidants that they are literally *cancer-repelling!* They would be vital to any anti-cancer protocol diet, and of incredible assistance for prevention in the future. Studies done at Johns Hopkins University found many cancer-preventive chemicals in **Broccoli Sprouts,** at astounding levels. These chemicals, called ISOTHIOCYANATES, are the Superstars of Sprouts, and the real reason Broccoli

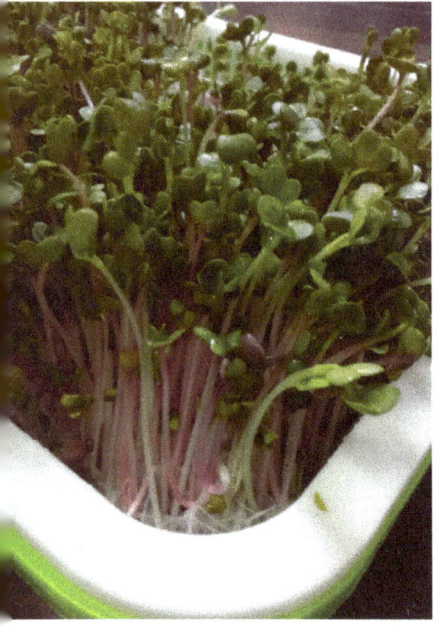

and other cruciferous veggies are famous as tumor-shrinkers and cancer-destroyers. If you need to eat a lot of Sprouts, grow different varieties so you can eat them at every meal.

Even *one serving* a day of these preventative Sprout nutrients will reduce the likelihood of breast cancer by 50%.[8]

Radish Sprouts have *even more* nutrition than Broccoli Sprouts. Doug Evans says they are really the "top dog" in Sprouting, with the greatest amount of nutrients as well as truly superior cancer-killing support. I feel like you can taste their power.

Sprouts make a wonderful snack! They are quite filling, and provide **instant Sunshine energy that lights up your cells,** providing a major energy lift, with **Protein** to keep you going. Because they have a mild flavor, you can pair them with flavorful condiments (like mustard, hummus, soy or hot sauce - or even sweet toppings like peanut butter or chocolate spread) for a flavor and texture burst that relieves food cravings. Add them to every juice or smoothie you make, and juice Sprouts by themselves or with other herbs to add to sauces, and preserve as frozen flavor cubes. When they are blended, your Family will never know the secret radical nutrition lurking within their innocent shake! Sprouts can help you substitute good foods for your least healthy habits or food cravings. Sprouts absolutely assure good health, good fun, and taste good, too!

∽ SPROUTING: Basic Steps for Jars ∽

1. **Inspect your Sprouting Seeds while dry,** remove foreign objects and pebbles, discard any seeds that are damaged or discolored. Measure out ¼ cup of seeds and place them in your **clean Mason Jar.**

2. **Rinse** your seeds and wash thoroughly, right in the jar. Strain water out.

3. **Soak** seeds with fresh, cool, good water and let stand for 2-3 minutes. Here you can add a **Sanitizing Agent** if you choose like Grapefruit Seed Extract (2 drops per quart) or 35% Food-Grade Hydrogen Peroxide (5 Tablespoons per quart), or Apple Cider Vinegar (2 Tablespoons per quart) but this is not necessary. I have personally never used any, you decide.

4. **Cover** the jar with a special screen **Sprouting Lid**, or place some cheesecloth or a piece of screen under the Mason lid ring.

5. **Drain** out the liquid (and sanitizing agent if you used one), rinse again, add more fresh water & soak again for 2-3 minutes. Drain one more time.

6. **Cover and soak** seeds with about ¾-1 cup of water (about 3:1 ratio water to seeds) so they are all submerged. Swirl the jar and make sure all seeds are soaking underwater. **Let sit for 4-12 hours.** Check TIPS under each Sprouting Seed for specific times and suggestions.

7. **Drain and tilt the jar** just off upside down into sink or tray or shelf (at about a 70 degree angle) so any water can run out. Keep out of direct sunshine and send good vibes for growing!

8. **Rinse and drain** the seeds in the jar a **few times a day** if you can. **Taste** them at every rinse and decide at what point in their growth you like them the best. Use this time to love and sweet-talk your seeds into growing! They are sensitive Plants after all! Enjoy the sacred act of engaging them.

9. **Sprouting Tails** that are close to an inch long, with leaves that have begun to form and split mean your Harvest is nearly ready! Green them up a bit by placing the jar in a bright location for a few hours (but never in direct sunlight), so they can photosynthesize and produce more vital phytochemicals for you. Then, they are ready!

10. **Store** Sprouts in the same Jar, or pour out and rinse if you want fewer seed capsules. You can store them in glass containers, ceramic bowls or ziploc bags. **Refrigerate and consume them within a week.** It's helpful to rinse Sprouts every few days to refresh.

Once you master the basic process with jars you can move on to *trays* of **Microgreens** and **Grasses**. Keep in mind the **quality of the Water** is quite important - the seeds and seedlings won't like chlorine any more than you do! Use Spring Water, Filtered Water, Gem Water, even Distilled Water if necessary. If you have to use tap water, let it sit uncovered overnight so the chlorine will evaporate. Or soak Shungite pieces in it to restructure the water and absorb the toxins.

Now is the time to stock up on Organic Sprouting Seeds, jars and trays. You can usually buy seeds very cheaply in bulk from organic growers or supply houses. Store some along with Mason jars and cheesecloth in your **emergency food supplies**, as well. Any lettuce, herb or salad green seeds can be grown in dirt or in water trays as **Microgreens**. These are all-the-rage as fancy salad decorations, and can even be found in upscale restaurants perched in little haystacks on juicy prized steaks!

For doing it yourself, nearly any **bean, vegetable, grain or nut** will work for Sprouting in jars and sheet pans. Source your seeds from collections that are actually called **"Organic Seeds for Sprouting"** so you make sure not to get irradiated, conventionally sprayed or contaminated raw material. *Only the best seeds are what we need.* But in a pinch, remember that almost any old, edible plant seeds in packets can be sprouted for superior survival nutrition.

CAUTION: Store-bought and restaurant sprouts (particularly Alfalfa Sprouts) can become contaminated through many people handling them, or exposure out on salad bars for long hours. Bacterial infections that may have serious complications can result. These are highly unlikely with Home Sprouting, but do take extra care to sterilize jars, rinse sprouts well, and always store them in clean containers. To be quite certain, take the extra **Sanitizing Step** (#3 above) at the beginning of the Sprouting process and you will have no trouble at all.

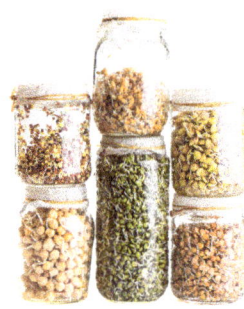

Sprouts can get **moldy** quickly, so make sure they are always slightly damp but not wet. When storing them, discard any slimy portions and rinse well every few days. Always use your nose to make sure the smell is fresh and green, and not sour (indicating advanced decay or culture).

If you are **SENSITIVE TO SEEDS**, and have to avoid them, **you can still eat Sprouts.** Simply rinse the seed capsule away, or trim them from the bottoms of your Sprouts and Microgreens.

Consider assembling a **Sprouting Gift Basket** with Seeds and supplies, and add Doug Evans' Sprouting book (or this one) for anyone you know who has cancer.

Animals LOVE Sprouts! They can be a vital way to deliver nutrients to Pets, especially any animal challenged by illness or cancer. Feed them Broccoli Sprouts and see what they think! Give your animals sprout choices and see which ones are their favorites. They tend to like the crunchy Bean Sprouts, Sunflower and Soybean. Chickens LOVE sprouts! Grow some extra batches of sprouts for your animals in the Winter, when fresh food is not available, and watch their health soar and digestion improve.

~ the garden of earth ~

◎ THE BEST SEEDS TO SPROUT ◎
Powerfully Cool Sprout Facts

<u>ADZUKI BEAN</u> Sweet-tasting, small but protein-rich, loves to sprout, filling snack, keeps blood sugar balanced, great for the heart & cholesterol, high in Protein, Iron, Magnesium, B$_6$ and antioxidants. *TIP: soak for 12 hours first*

<u>ALFALFA</u> Called "the Father of all Foods" - this is the quintessential sandwich sprout you see everywhere, reduces risk of breast cancer, full of Vitamin A, Niacin, Calcium. Avoid in lupus, use sanitizing agent first, and rinse more often for safety. *TIP: best to eat at days 7-10 of growth*

<u>AMARANTH</u> My favorite is "Red Garnet" - this one grows the most glorious, magenta red sprouts full of Antioxidants which lower inflammation, assist weight loss, are antihypertensive, high in Selenium, Manganese, Phosphorus, Vitamins A. B, C, E. *TIP: run cool water through seeds for 1-2 minutes, soak in cool water for 30 minutes*

<u>BARLEY</u> Look for "Purple Barley," grow it to inches tall barley grass & juice for great nutrition, reduces hunger, helpful for weight loss, sprout Barley before grinding into flour, make into porridge, source of Manganese, B$_1$, Selenium, Molybdenum, Niacin. *TIP: soak for 12 hours first*

<u>BASIL MICROGREENS</u> My other favorite - best grown on sheet pans, harvest day 14-21 when sprouts have grown greener and tall into shoots. Dark-colored varieties do well, juice microgreens for shots and flavor blast, source of Vitamin, A, B$_6$, C, E, K$_1$, Calcium, Iron, Zinc. *TIP: do not soak, Basil is a light germinator, do not cover*

<u>BROCCOLI</u> One of the finest anti-cancer remedies in the world, sulfur compounds (sulforaphane) are anti-tumor, lower inflammation, prove great treatment for autism, increase glutathione, prevents heart disease, protects nerves. Strongly antioxidant and detoxifying, source of Vitamin A, C, Calcium, Iron, Potassium. *TIP: sprouts may have tiny fuzzy hairs, this is normal*

<u>BUCKWHEAT</u> Make sure you get "Sproutable Raw Buckwheat Groats." After Sprouting, dry groats in a super low oven and grind into flour for pancakes or pasta great for blood pressure, blood sugar balance, source of Rutin, CoQ$_{10}$, Magnesium. *TIP: very starchy, rinse often & until water clears*

<u>CABBAGE</u> Green or red both work, but red is especially antioxidant (4-5x green cabbage), can be fermented for a sprouted kimchi, lower cholesterol, prevent heart disease, helpful for weight loss, delicious mild taste, source of Vitamins A, C, K$_1$. *TIP: Day 3 move to bright area, not direct sunlight, harvest day 5-6, rinse to remove hulls*

<u>CHIA</u> Superfood for supernatural strength, long-lasting energy, and stamina, high in Calcium and Essential Fatty Acids (the good fats) and Protein. Makes the gelatinous goo for Chia Pets, grows anywhere, no rinsing needed, easily transferable to any

porous ceramic surface or tray. *TIP: don't soak, keep moist by misting*

FENUGREEK Nutty and bitter, actually a legume, high in Protein, Iron & Fiber, great for menstrual cramps, breastfeeding, to relieve constipation, aid digestion, heal the respiratory system. Helps diabetes & improves sex drive, antibacterial, boosts immune system, hulls are edible, but chewy. **NEVER EAT IN PREGNANCY.** *TIP: soak for 8-12 hours first*

HEMP SEEDS Look for "Whole, Organic Unhulled Raw Hemp Seeds," they have a nutty flavor and are very crunchy. Anti-inflammatory, helpful for the heart, menstrual cramps & PMS, skin problems, 35% complete Vegan Protein, hugely nutritious, high in Essential Fatty Acids, Vitamin E, Potassium, Phosphorus, Calcium, Iron, Sulfur. Grow in trays, harvest anytime after short tail to 6 days, eat or grind. *TIP: soak 4-12 hours*

GARBANZO BEANS (Chickpeas) Lectins are neutralized by sprouting, which assists bean digestion (less gas), perfect protein to fat ratio for building muscle mass & weight loss, same quantity of Protein per serving as in steak, high in Iron & Fiber. Sprouted hummus is excellent! *TIP: soak for 8-12 hours first*

LENTILS Easy, fast & fun sprouters, ready to eat in 2-3 days, full of Protein, Zinc, Iron, Folate, Vitamin C which increases 400% with Sprouting. Balances blood sugar for hours, reduces osteoporosis & colon cancer, one of the most nutritious sprouts. Great simply soaked in Overnight Oats. *TIP: soak for 8 hours first*

MUNG BEAN Super fast & easy, full of Iron, Folate, Fiber, Manganese, Vitamin K_1 and loads of Vitamin C, half the carbohydrates when sprouted. Harvest day 2-6, make great smoothie additions, super hydrating, full of electrolytes. *TIP: soak for 12 hours*

MUSTARD One of the spiciest sprouts, grind in mortar to a paste & use like wasabi, contains helpful Sulfur compounds like Broccoli, cancer-preventative, full of Copper, Magnesium, Iron, Selenium, Vitamins A, B_6, C, may prevent asthma attacks, can regulate blood pressure. Harvest in 5-6 days, microgreens in 11-14 days. *TIP: turns gelatinous like chia, no need to soak, mist to water*

PEAS Super high in Protein, sweet & tender, best as a shoot or mature microgreen in salads. Good source of B Vitamins (especially Folate & Niacin), Vitamin C, Iron, Magnesium, highly antioxidant & cell protective, anti-cancer, good for anemia, brain food. *TIP: soak for 8 hours first*

RADISH Spicy, similar to mild wasabi, thermogenic & great for weight loss (16 calories/cup). Has the highest anticancer action, assists cardiovascular health, breaks down atherosclerosis, lowers risk of all diseases, epicly full of Vitamins A, B (especially Folate), C, E, K_1, and most minerals especially Calcium, Magnesium, Iron, Potassium, Phosphorus & Zinc. Gets creamy when blended for Vegan dips. *TIP: soak for 8 hours first*

RED CLOVER Highly medicinal sprout, contains anti-tumor Genistein (stops blood flow to tumors which starves them), high in Phytoestrogens for PMS, menopause, hot flashes, fibrocystic disease. Helps anemia, is a powerful source of Vitamin C, Folate, K_1, Calcium, Iron, Zinc. *TIP: soak for 8 hours*

SUNFLOWER (BLACK) Use "Raw Organic Whole Unhulled Seeds." A great staple survival food (complete Vegan protein), amazing wildlife food, small amount contains over 100 enzymes. Great immunity food, high in Iron, Potassium, Magnesium, Calcium, Zinc, Vitamins A, B's, D and E, Chlorophyll. Hearty/good travel food, harvest at 10-12 days for tall shoots. *TIP: soak for 8 hours first, grow in trays for large shoots that can be moved into sunlight to green & grow taller for salads, jars for smaller sprouts*

WHEAT BERRIES High in Chlorophyll, Flavonoids, B Vitamins, C, E and Antioxidants. Lower cholesterol, anti-cancer, reduce inflammation, detoxifying, balance blood sugar, helps weight loss. Grow into 3-5 inch tall Wheatgrass in trays for Juicing, or for your pets to eat. Chewing Fresh Wheatgrass makes an instant remedy for nausea, blood sugar crashes, or anxiety, and will bolster energy quickly. Wheat Grass Juice and Sprouts are **GLUTEN-FREE.** Juice is sweet but liver stimulating and too much too soon can cause temporary nausea. *TIP: soak for 12 hours first. Freeze extra Wheatgrass juice into ice cubes for use in smoothies and shots*

- **CAUTION:** Do Not sprout and eat raw Kidney Beans (still too high in lectins after Sprouting, can make you nauseous and ill, even when boiled out for 10 minutes) or Quinoa (they have many saponins which make them more allergy-inducing).

The miraculous Sprouting process breaks down the *anti-nutrients* which coat and protect the seeds, known as **lectins** and **phytic acid**, as well as **amylase and protease enzyme inhibitors**. These plant defense chemicals disarm your body's ability to break down and absorb nutrients from food. For predatory animals, this signals it is not a good food. For Humans, the lectins and all are not *that* challenging for most people, but are highly allergenic, taste bad and cause digestive distress. On the bright side, since Sprouting the seeds *destroys the anti-nutrients*, many people find that if they are sensitive to a particular grain or legume (like Wheat/gluten), they can tolerate the sprout of the same plant with no trouble at all.

SEEDS EVERYWHERE

Become more aware of all the seeds contained in your food. What if you saved every single seed you came upon? Think of the food seeds you would quickly acquire, and the wondrous SPROUTING YOU COULD DO! It is mind-blowing the number of perfectly good seeds we spit out and throw in the trash every day. Start saving them.

Also, you can use the Sprouting techniques to grow old packet-seeds instead of throwing them away. You will have less time invested in growing them in case they do not sprout, and if they do, you can eat them! I have so many old half-used packets of Basil because I love growing it so much. This spring I sorted through them, and began Sprouting all my old Basil seeds into MicroBasil for salads. What a feast!

REGROWING FOOD SCRAPS

With very little effort, some of the food we would send right to the Compost Pile can live to grow and produce food again. I have seen some interesting articles and videos lately about regrowing food from the unused ends of fruits and vegetables. Check out the books and videos of long-hair dude **Armen Adamjen**, **@creative_explained**. His fact-paced videos and wildly educational content is really catching on - as in he already has 9 million followers on Instagram, and that many millions more on other platforms. Armen was even featured on *The Today Show*, demonstrating his super sustainable and innovative food-growing and house-cleaning hacks. What started for him as a "nerdy lockdown hobby" turned into an Information Empire. He has since collaborated with Jennifer Garner and Bryan Adams and won an award for Sustainability Influencer of the Year.

- Cut the top off of your trimmed ORGANIC **Beet**, or **Carrot**, or the bottom inch off of **Lettuce, Celery** or **Potato**. Surround your vegetable top (or bottom) halfway up with water in a small bowl or dish. The end of Celery will grow an entire celery plant, many veggies will send up sprouting leaves. I have been trying this with real success, the top of my Golden Beet is growing like crazy! I can eat the young greens that sprout, or plant it in dirt, in a small pot or the garden.

- **Pineapples** are quite easy to re-grow this way. Just make sure to offer your re-growers plenty of fresh water, start with high quality organic produce to begin with, and keep an eye on it! Once it has matured enough to be a real plant of its own, transfer it to the dirt for further growing. This is another great homeschool project that provides real nourishment on many levels for kids and adults alike.

- I use this technique to root fresh **Mint** or **Basil** stems from friends. When someone shares their amazing harvest with me, I save one or two sprigs to grow roots in a glass of water. When the roots look nice and frilly I plant them in my Garden!

- Neglected, sprouting **Potatoes** or **Garlic** can be placed in the garden and grown. Quarter the Potato, or cut a large piece around a sprouting Potato eye, and plant. Plant Garlic as is, green tips up. If it sprouts, get it OUT - into the Garden!

- **CAUTION: Do NOT eat raw sprouts that grow out of the plants of the Solanaceae (Nightshade) Family** which include **Potatoes, Tomatoes, Hot & Sweet Peppers** and **Eggplant.** But do plant them in your garden for great success. See more cool information about the Nightshades in the Plant Families section.

~ the garden of earth ~

FERMENTING
culture your own probiotic garden

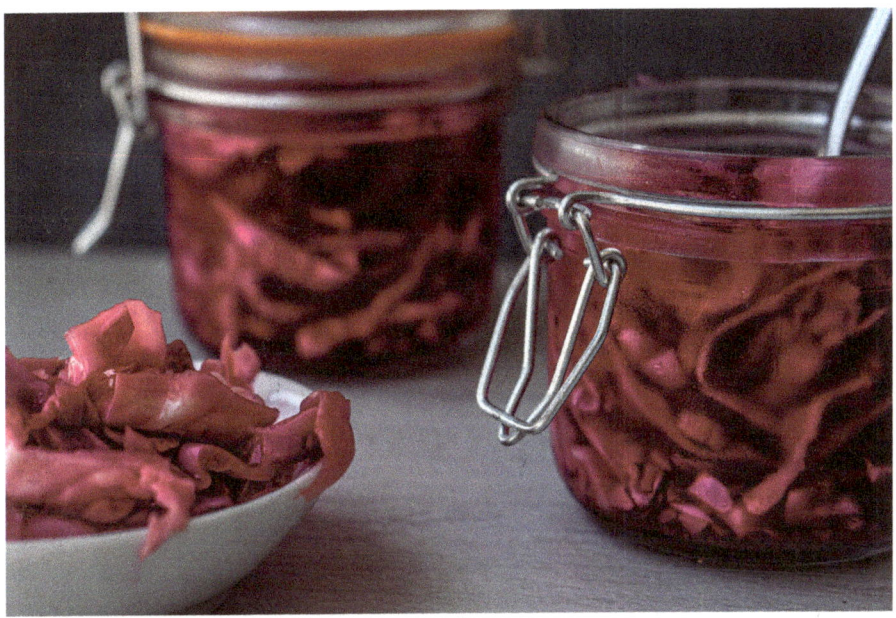

> "For me, Fermentation is part health regimen, part gourmet art, part practical food preservation, part multicultural adventure, part activism, even part spiritual path as it affirms again and again the underlying interconnectedness of All."
>
> ~Sandor Ellix Katz, Fermentation Pioneer

Sandor Katz is, in many ways, the "Father of Fermenting" in this country. He wrote the brilliant book that started a whole fermentation revolution, called *Wild Fermentation*. He had some serious health challenges and he says Fermenting probably saved his life! Plus, his entire life changed because he wrote that one book! As a result of his efforts to educate people about culturing foods, he got to travel the World lecturing, demonstrating, teaching, writing, sharing and LIVING the Magic of Fermentation.

Many of the foods you enjoy are **Cultured or Fermented** first, before you eat them: **Coffee, Chocolate, Vanilla, Tea, Cheese, Beer, Wine, Sauerkraut, Pickles, Vinegar, Yogurt, Kefir & Kvass, Sourdough Bread, Preserved Lemons, Pickled Herring, Tofu & Tempeh, Miso, Kombucha, Soy Sauce, Seitan, Natto, Kimchi**, and many more.

Alcohol was most likely discovered by ancient people who found Honey and Water bubbling in a tree stump, drank it and realized how refreshing a fermented, sparkling beverage could be. And how silly the alcohol and bubbles made you feel! That was most likely the original Mead, and we can see in the historical record that many cultures, all over the World, sought the conditions it took to replicate it.

ALL indigenous people used some form of Fermentation to preserve food, from the North Pole to the South Pole. Fermentation provided our ancestors the ability to produce **probiotic beverages** to enhance their digestion, and **yeasts** to leaven bread. Eventually, they would discover how to ferment malted grains into raw whiskey, create cheese from cultured milk, produce alcohol from potatoes, and turn fruit juices into vinegar with which to pickle vegetables and meat. Food Preservation (and alcohol abuse!) was forever changed with these discoveries.

The Magic of Fermentation is found in the helpful *microscopic communities,* naturally-occurring bacterial cultures and yeasts from the air that **transform the nutritional value of Food, in a kind of** *pre-digestion* **that actually increases nutrient absorption.** It is a partnership of Food with Microbial Life, in which the Food magically alters into something even better! Fermentation also *preserves* the food in a liquid bio-preservative that it generates as a natural byproduct of the culture (acetic acid, lactic acid as well as alcohol). These cultured liquids help the Ferments retain all their nutrients and prevent spoilage.

But they also enhance your Food with essential, active **Probiotics,** helpful flora and new *transformed nutrients* that offer powerful support for better gut health. Fermented foods are different than they were before - altered by Nature - and are encoded with that transformative power, a life-altering energy. Fermented Foods included regularly in your diet will change your Life and make it sparkle! Top your salads and entrees with a scoop of fermented vegetables for righteous nutrition, tang, and color.

Fermenting is a great way to save and store perishable fruits and vegetables. You can even Ferment and store milk (as kefir & yogurt), fish, and meat. This is how you can provide YOURSELF a living and constantly growing, sustainable source of Probiotics - no more expensive trips to the health food store. Once you get into it, you will LOVE Fermenting. It is so easy to ferment and store or pickle your extra produce in a flash. Your gut will thank you for giving it natural support and your digestion and immunity will improve dramatically.

> "How ironic that the road to Culture in our germophobic technological society requires, first and foremost, that we enter into an alchemical relationship with Bacteria and Fungi, and that we bring to our tables foods & beverages prepared by the Magicians, not machines."
>
> ~ *Sally Fallon Morell*

Simple Sauerkraut

(or Beet Kraut, Turnip Kraut, Carrot Kraut, Rainbow Kraut, Wild Weed Kraut, Seaweed Kraut, and so on)

1. **Scrub clean all the vegetables really well, but do not peel.** Grate or chop your cabbage, weeds or veggies into a big bowl - eyeball your jars or crocks to see roughly how much you need to prepare. Grating is great because it liberates the **Ennobled Water** in the vegetables which we are using as our fermenting liquid, and creates surface area for better culture growth.

2. **Sprinkle liberally with Salt** as you go, and other seasonings & spices if you like. Traditionally, **Caraway Seeds** are used in Sauerkraut, but **Fresh Ginger, Turmeric, Cumin, Dill, Garlic, Juniper Berries, Chili Peppers** or any herb you can imagine can be used to impart flavor and add considerable medicinal value. Some people add **Beer**, or some **Brown Sugar** to sweeten the sourness. Taste it to see what it needs, don't oversalt.

3. **Squeeze, pound and bruise the veggies** for a few minutes to break down cell walls to release more juices. Use clean hands, a potato masher or wooden spoons & mallets.

4. **Pack into a clean jar or crock**, and really cram it in there with your fingers and blunt utensils, so the air bubbles are released and the liquid completely covers your kraut. Fill the jar nearly, but not totally to the top with your brining veggies.

5. **Keep the kraut under the liquid with a weight.** It can be a specially-designed ceramic insert, a cabbage leaf, or some hand-cut veggie (or other invention you design) to keep the veggies covered and the liquid on top.

6. **Check everyday and release any off-gassing** from the jar by cracking the lid, and after a few days taste your product. You can eat it at any time, but the flavors will continue to grow & alter into the Umami-filled yumminess of Fermentation the longer you leave it! **Refrigerate** when you want it to stop processing based on flavor. Enjoy your Living Probiotic Food and remember to drink the leftover Juice as a gut tonic.

- **Don't be afraid of the helpful bacteria, microorganisms and yeasts!** The USDA has ZERO cases of incidence of food poisoning occurring with fermented vegetables and fruits. Stick with those until you learn your basic skills and you will be safe. Later when you get a good handle on growing this kind of a culture garden, you can advance to preserving dairy and meat if you have a need, seeking specific guidance for safety

SOURDOUGH ADVENTURES

Do you love the unmistakable tang of Sourdough Bread and Pancakes? They begin with the simplest Fermentation - a culture made with water and flour, that is activated by the many airborne wild yeasts in our atmosphere and on the grain. This kind of leavening raises bread and baked goods without baker's yeast, utilizing just the sprinkled-in, magical Fermentation of Nature! A good sourdough starter is a prized possession, can last indefinitely, and can be passed down to the next generation. It is a living culture that requires weekly maintenance but offers a wonderful texture in baked goods, a distinct bubbly quality, and a sour taste like nothing else on Earth.

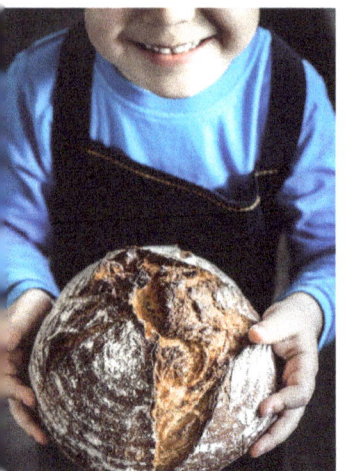

Sourdough starters could be found in the covered wagons that blazed a trail across to the Western US in the 1800's. Tales are told of gold-miners sleeping with their Sourdough starters to keep them warm during the cold nights on the way to the Gold Rush. Ancient Egyptians most likely used Sourdough as their first form of unleavened bread. One of the oldest relics of Sourdough use was found in Switzerland and dates to 3700 BC! **San Francisco Sourdough** became so famous because the taste could not be duplicated out of the area. Researchers later established there was a particularly sour bacterium in the culture found only within 50 miles of the city, so they named the strain *Lactobacillus sanfranciscensis* in tribute.

Lucille Dumbrill of Newcastle, Wyoming may just have the *oldest* living Sourdough Starter recorded in recent history. Her culture is currently **136 years-old**, and it was given to her husband by a student of his from the University of Wyoming. The student's family traced the starter back to a **shepherd's wagon from 1889**, and Lucille maintained this gift for her entire life! For this feat of food preservation, Lucille Dumbrill won a Wyoming State Historical Society Award. She liberally shared this remarkable age-old starter with her family and friends from all over the country, so this original 1889 culture is still bubbling and regenerating, creating Sourdough delicacies nationwide. And will be for years to come.

Start with *sterilized, super clean utensils* and a fairly large, widemouth glass jar. Use filtered or spring water (or even distilled) to start with, most tap water has chlorine that will kill the living culture. For a **gluten-free Sourdough Starter**, you will have best results with ***Teff, White Sorghum, Brown Rice*** or ***Buckwheat Flour.***

Sourdough Starting is a lesson in Patience as it takes a while (7 days to mature) and requires your effort on a weekly basis to keep it active. But don't be scared away. Sourdough Starter is an AWESOME resource to have! Because a warm environment is needed, some people sit and read or watch TV with the jar in their lap, or by their side, to keep it warm and active!

Sourdough Super Starter

DAY 1 - MAKE INITIAL STARTER: Combine ½ cup flour with ¼ cup warm water in your starter glass jar. Mix with a fork, it will be thick and paste-like. Cover with plastic wrap or lid and let rest in a warm spot (75-80 degrees) for 24 hours. Place it near a heat outlet, in a cold oven with the light on for a few hours, or in the microwave with the light on (do not try to heat or cook).

DAY 2 - LOOK FOR BUBBLES: Check for Fermentation which is indicated by bubbling. No need to do anything else today, let rest in a warm spot for another 24 hours. A liquid (kind of like a fermented liquor) may be forming called "hooch." It can be smelly but is totally normal, usually just means your starter needs to be fed. Don't freak out, drain it off and feed Starter tomorrow.

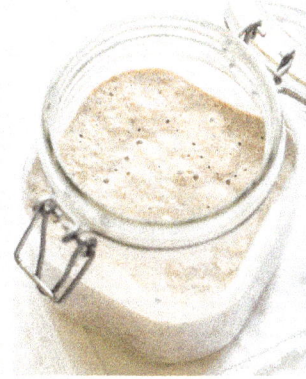

DAY 3 - FEED THE STARTER: Remove and discard half of the Starter, it will be stretchy, use a spoon. ADD ½ cup flour and ¼ cup warm water. Mix until smooth, like pancake batter, cover and let rest in a warm spot for another 24 hours.

DAYS 4, 5 AND 6 - DISCARD & FEED ALL 3 DAYS: Discard half of the Starter (great uses for it below) and feed exactly like Day 3, for each of these days. Place a rubber band around the jar or a small mark at the top of the Starter level to gauge its response, as now it will start to rise and fall. When it falls below the line it is time to feed again.

DAY 7 - DOUBLED IN SIZE: Starter should be very active, bubbly, soft and spongy like a roasted marshmallow. It should smell pleasant. Remove and use or discard half of it. If it doesn't seem active, keep feeding and discarding, it could take up to 2 weeks to get a great culture. Once it seems ready, transfer to a clean jar and refrigerate. Date it, and name it! This is your very own traditional Sourdough Starter to share for years!

<u>**FEED WEEKLY** (if possible, and at the most)</u>**:** Refrigerate, to slow the culture process and maintain. Mature Starter does not need to be split in half and discarded anymore. But it should have weekly feedings. If you get too much, take out what you need and make something with it. ***Don't worry*** if you forget all about your Super Starter for weeks or longer, follow the principles to revive it and it will likely be just fine!

<u>**FLOAT TEST:**</u> Fully active Starter will float in water. Take a small spoonful after Starter has doubled in size, and add to a glass of water. If it floats, it is ready to be used.

<u>**USE INSTEAD OF YEAST:**</u> One cup of Super Sourdough Starter would be about the equivalent of one package of dry baker's yeast in your bread recipes.

<u>**GATHER GOODNESS:**</u> Forage for Wild Weed seeds (like Plantain, Lamb's Quarter, Wild Mustard) to combine with the Starter to capture even more airborne yeasts.

FOR RECIPES: Remove the amount of Starter you need **2 days before you need it** and allow it to warm on the counter overnight. Make sure it is bubbling and active, feed it the second day to get it really ready. Use on the 3rd day.

- **UTILIZE THE DISCARDED STARTER:** While it seems wasteful to remove and discard half the Starter when feeding, it concentrates the cultures and helps the Starter mature faster. **Here are some handy and ingenious ways to USE the discard.** Place in a new clean jar and give it for gifts as a Super Sourdough Starter for friends; add into batter for baked goods, pancakes and brownies; coat fried chicken with it or use for fish batter or tempura batter for veggies; use to thicken sauces or gravy; make dumplings with meat or veggies and a little extra flour; add to matzo balls; make into pizza dough, biscuits, popovers, cornbread or crackers; dehydrate and add to salads; freeze it, or refrigerate it to use later; make flatbreads, pita bread or tortillas; and you can always offer leftover Starter to the compost pile. Wildly enough, the **Lactic Acid** in the Sourdough makes a great anti-aging and **Exfoliating Face Mask!** Mix with some Aloe Vera and 2 drops of Essential Oil and paint on the face.

QUICKIE QUICHE - Make a super easy Quiche that makes it own pie crust. Mix Sourdough Starter with 4 eggs, pour over veggies, meat or cheese, bake until golden.

DRY IT: Super Starter can be dehydrated so it can last nearly indefinitely or be shared over long distances! This is a great solution if it is inconvenient to feed it, or if you are moving or traveling. Spread mature starter on parchment paper and let air dry for 24-48 hours until brittle. Or place in a dehydrator on very low (95-100 degrees) until it snaps. Pulse in a food processor to a dry powder, or store broken pieces in a glass jar. To revive, rehydrate with equal parts Water at room temperature for 3-4 hours, then resume feeding with Water and Flour for 2 days until active.

- **YOUR STARTER IS A ONE AND ONLY ORIGINAL!**
  Since making your own Sourdough Super Starter is done by capturing and culturing *your* local wild yeasts and bacteria at a certain time, your Starter will have its own complex flavors. And it will be **unduplicatable by anyone, anywhere else!** Cultivating your very own Culture gives you the honor of naming the new bacterium for your own area, for its flavor, its inspiration, or with your last name. Indicate on your gift labels that your special Sourdough is called *Lactobacillus* _____.

> "God made yeast, as well as dough, and loves Fermentation just as dearly as he loves vegetation."
>
> ~ *Ralph Waldo Emerson*

❧ MAKE YOUR OWN YEAST ❧

During 2020, many people were home with extra time on their hands, and baking bread became a runaway trend worldwide. The unexpected demand for Yeast was not able to be met, and for several months you could not find dried Yeast in the stores. But as Microbiologist and Yeast Scientist, Sudeep Argawala says, *"There is never a shortage of Yeast. Yeast is EVERYWHERE!"* In yet another natural miracle, helpful organisms and potent yeasts are all out there in the air, and can be gathered in many wild ways! You can use the solvent action of Water to collect them from your fresh organic garden produce. Your harvest has been exposed to many yeasts and probiotics for its entire growing season. These helpful bacteria, elevated biotics and wild yeasts that have blown through the air onto your harvest will begin to colonize in the water. They feed on the sugars and starches you provide them to begin the Fermentation process, creating a new Yeast-producing culture.

Argawala suggests you start your Yeast Ferments with the **washing water from organic produce, unsulphured dried fruit** (which retain yeast especially well), **dregs of your Belgian beer, the last few sips of wine** at the bottom of a bottle (with the sediment), **crusts of bread sourdough bread** from restaurants or artisanal bakeries- your imagination is the limit. As he says, *"We've been doing this for 12,000 years. I think everyone's a little late to get to the party."* He recounts tales of some Paris boulangeries making baguettes with more old bread than yeast during tough times! Brewmasters will tell you that for hundreds of years Belgian Ales have been exposed to the fresh air in wide open collector vats where the same hybrid medieval "super yeasts" will settle into the mash, creating the characteristic lacey foam. Let your yeast starters sit in an open window or in the garden for a few hours to enhance yeast uptake.

Bread is currently the most wasted food in the World, with more than **44% of perfectly good bread discarded** because it may be stale or because people don't like the crusts! In the UK alone that equates to 24 million slices a day that get thrown away. **Roz Bado,** a development baker at **Gail's Bakery** in the UK, discovered a way to repurpose day-old bread by pulverizing it and Fermenting it into a porridge to feed and leaven their famous Sourdough Bread. The resulting loaves are nearly one third **"Rescue Bread"** which costs much less than regular bread and tastes delicious, with a wonderful crumb and texture. Some other cool Brits invented **Toast Ale**, a surplus-bread-based beer that they boast saves and recycles "1 slice per bottle." You have to admit, it is a pretty brilliant and sustainable idea to utilize good food instead of destroying it.[9]

Both of the following Yeast-Gathering recipes follow this same principle of Fermentation, resulting in a truly helpful leavening product made from magic - and literally out of thin air! The process is much less involved than the Starter above, though your Yeast will still need to be refrigerated and maintained. But you will always have a wonderful natural Yeast when you need it!

Wild Yeast Cultivation

Use **Distilled, Filtered** or **Spring Water** to start with, as most tap water has chlorine that will kill the living culture. **For a Sugar-Free Yeast,** experiment with **Honey, Monk Fruit, Molasses, Erythritol** and other nutritive sweeteners. The very best fruits to use are **Organic Raisins, Figs, Dates, Grapes, Blueberries, Apples, Plum,** and **Prunes**.

RAISIN OR DATE YEAST WATER: Add 2 ¼ cups of water to a large clean jar, more than 32 oz. (like an old vinegar bottle). Add ¼ cup of **Raw Sugar** and some **Raisins** or 2-3 **Dates**. Put the cap on and shake really well to dissolve the sugar. Loosen the cap a half turn and place someplace warm, 78.8 degrees is ideal. For the next 4 days shake vigorously twice a day, releasing any built up pressure inside. The fruit will likely rise to the top. You'll see lots of bubbles and foam by Day 5, on which you add 1½ cups **Water** and another few **Dates or Raisins**, 1 ½ Tablespoons **Sugar** and 1 teaspoon **Salt**. Shake vigorously. Place in a warm spot and repeat daily shaking twice for 4 more days. Strain out fruit (bake with it or compost it) and refrigerate Wild Yeast until needed.

TO USE: Bring Yeast Water to room temperature. Take 1 cup **Yeast Water** and add to 2 cups **Flour,** stir well and let rest overnight or 16 hours. It is active when there are bubbles and the texture changes. Use in any recipe as you would Sourdough Starter.

Bread made with this method does seem to have slower rising and doubling compared to regular Starters or dry Yeast, but upon baking it comes out wonderfully, and the taste is more mild. The upside is very LOW maintenance, it does not need to be fed, and refrigerated like Sourdough. Yeast Water will last for months. You use no Flour, and you don't discard, so it is a great thrifty method. If it has been awhile since you used it last, you may need to revive it for a day or two by feeding it with more fruit, water and sugar and keeping it warm.

POTATO YEAST: Boil **Organic Potatoes** in water (set aside and use the potatoes in some awesome dish) and reserve the water to cool. Take 1½ cups of the cooled Potato-boiling water and add to a quart-sized jar. Add 1 cup **Flour** and 1 Tablespoon of **Sugar** or **Honey** and mix thoroughly but gently. Cover with a paper towel or dish towel overnight in a warm place. In the morning it should smell yeasty and be bubbly. Refrigerate and feed weekly just like the Super Starter above, removing and discarding half of it first, before adding 1½ cups **Flour** and 1½ cups **Water** plus 2 Tablespoons of **Sugar**. When you are ready to use, bring to room temperature and feed and keep warm a bit to get activity (bubbles & a distinctive and yummy, yeasty smell).

TO USE: 2 Tablespoons Potato Yeast = 1 Tablespoon regular dry yeast. Experiment a bit to see what works best for your needs.

USING FRESH PRODUCE, BREAD SCRAPS, OR DREGS: Take a small handful of your fresh unwashed garden Produce, or Pine Needles & Wild Weeds, or small Bread scraps, or last dregs of Beer or Wine and add into a wide mouth Mason Jar with 1 cup of water. Swirl around well, and notice the cloudiness develop, that is the Yeast. Leave uncovered in a warm place for a few hours, then strain out any solids and add the yeasty water to an equal amount of **Flour.** Cover and let rest in a warm place (like on the countertop while the dishwasher runs). Within about 12 hours bubbles should start to form. After about 48 hours it should be ready to use or feed. Similarly to the Super Sourdough Starter, take a small amount and add it to equal parts Flour and Water to make a new Yeast Starter. When it doubles in size 12 hours after feeding, you can refrigerate it and use it in any recipes just as you would a Sourdough Starter.

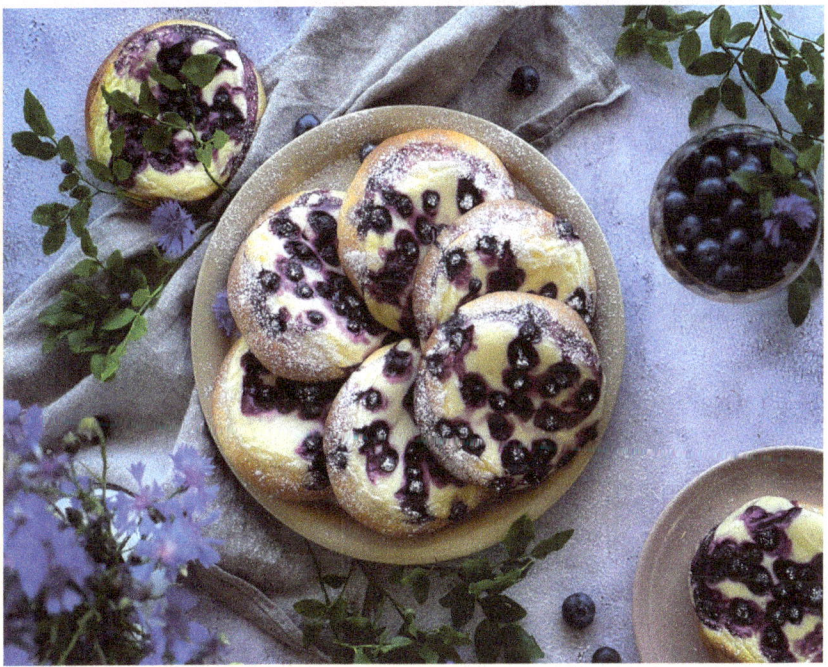

It is all a grand science experiment, so if you don't succeed with one kind of Fermentation, try another. **Be patient and nurturing with the process just like you would with your other Gardens.** With a little effort and practice you will have grown and fermented wonderfully unique, vital, **microbe-enhanced** Super Foods! You will soon have living success stories, a new and wonderful survival skill, and many delicious experiments to share.

~ the garden of earth ~

COMPOSTING

growing something just for the Garden

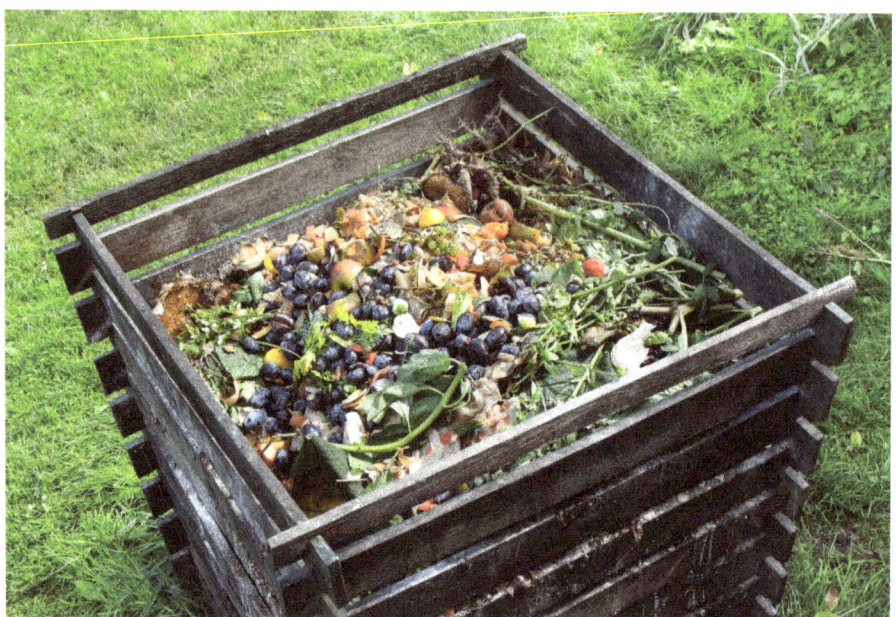

CREATING HOME ENVIRONMENTS

When you build a Compost Pile, you establish a spot in your yard where you **INVITE the Living Elements of Nature** to colonize and perform their *decomposing jobs* in order to break down food material into vital soil. You are building a home - a living, growing environment for a variety of enzymes, bacteria, worms, and insects. These in turn feed other insects, birds and eventually the soil organisms for a much healthier ecosystem altogether. Composting is a little like returning the favor, giving something back to the Garden so it can produce more abundantly.

There are **Community Composts** available in some places if you want to contribute your scraps. Many Zero-Waste initiatives have sprung up around the country and you can find compost bins right next to trash & recycle bins near stores, restaurants and in shopping malls. Some cities like Boulder, Colorado, pick up compost waste curbside! This is yet another AWESOME cog in the wheel of tending the Planet. Start a neighborhood compost pile for your community gardens. See if you can get a composting program established in your town.

Composting creates the most fertile and supportive soil-enricher imaginable. Many farmers call this **"Black Gold"** and its value in gardening is immeasurable. Composting also keeps your vegetable and fruit leavings OUT of plastic garbage bags and landfills, where they may never have the appropriate conditions to decompose as Nature intended. Some households cut their trash in HALF by beginning to compost. Landfills are methane generators, along with producing carbon dioxide, greenhouse gasses which are particularly harmful to the environment. To prevent this, we need to be more careful about what we send to landfills and dumpsites. There is simply no reason at all to throw food scraps into the trash system in plastic bags.

Composting generates the three main minerals we need for soil health and properly growing plants - **Nitrogen, Phosphorus and Potassium**, and a whole host of other nutrients including **Magnesium, Calcium, Zinc** and **Iron**. It seems silly to BUY fertilizers that are often smelly and expensive, when the very scraps we want to throw out can *make it for us*! **Most commercial fertilizers contain hidden harmful chemicals, hormone-mimicing, growth-stimulating poisons and genetic modifiers that we definitely don't want in our food.** Science has also proven that the soil retains the *good* minerals and nutrients many times better when it has been treated with home-grown compost. It also enhances the soil's ability to retain water, which makes for healthier plants while it lowers water usage.

The National Resource Defense Council states that the **average American household throws away about $150-$200 in wasted food PER MONTH**, up over 50% from the 1970's. And the most wasted of all foods were fruits and vegetables. All of us hate that feeling of opening a box of greens just to find they are all slimy, or finding the orange at the bottom of the drawer that has gone soft and moldy. All these less than perfect food items can be recycled right into your compost piles and their advanced stage of decay is perfect for stimulating further processing in the pile. What a joy to know that even if you didn't get to eat it in time, your expensive produce will still have an afterlife by providing vital fertilizer for your next garden.

I have heard some people say they don't want to compost because they think it will smell. Ironically, the worst smells from garbage are ANIMAL proteins decomposing, which you never put into a compost pile. If you keep your composting VEGAN, you should never have a problem with odors. There is a certain balance of nutrients necessary to maintain the best "life" in the pile, and if you ever have odor there is a remedy for that, too, read on.

There are many compost bin systems available in the gardener's supply stores and online/mail-order offerings. Some of them rotate so that your pile gets easy turning and aerating which does help a lot. However - all you really need is a 3 square-foot cube somewhere in the backyard, that you can easily make out of old pallets or chicken wire fencing. This is about the ideal size to assure the organisms stay warm enough in the pile, and for you to be able to turn it easily. The smaller pieces your food waste is in, the faster it will decompose, so it can help to chop up your scraps first, keeping them about finger-sized for best results. A little preparation helps you to create faster-producing compost.

Choose a dry and shady spot, avoid any place with excessive rain run-off, and ideally place your bin or pile *away* from the house. You can make an easy open compost pile, or a bin closed-style system which increases heat and speed of compost maturing, but needs to be monitored more often so it doesn't get wet and moldy. Moisture is important in both cases, as a pile or bin that is too dry may cause the reactions to slow and the composting to take much longer.

There are essentially 2 different methods of Composting - a **COLD** (passive), and a **HOT** (active) method. **Cold Composting** lets Mother Nature do most of the work at lower temperatures and will yield good mature compost in about 1-2 years. This is a great method if you are not in a hurry for your compost, or have less time to devote to turning, correcting levels of nutrients and preserving higher temperatures. This is a slow but sure method and requires patience. It is basically anaerobic in nature at low temperatures, and fairly nonreactive, so the compost does tend to retain bacteria, fungi and viable weed seeds, and could have more of an odor.

Hot Composting requires a bit more attention to detail, but the returns from this style of composting are much faster, with viable mature compost in as little as 4 weeks to 12 months. In this method, a specific kind of closed container or bin is used that will stimulate greater heat and moisture, and the carbon and nitrogen rations are more easily managed. The higher temperatures fostered by the correct balance of conditions (see below) result in a much faster end product. This is more of an aerobic process that reaches higher temperatures to completely destroy all pests, weed seeds, plant disease bacteria, fungi, and insect eggs or larvae. Optimal temperature for Hot Composting is about 130-140 degrees Fahrenheit.

It is crucial to **"turn"** any style of compost often. This term means just what it says - rake and turn and unearth the pile to expose every layer to air. This is typically done about once a week in the Summer months, and about every 3 weeks during the Winter if it is possible. Work to assure that everything is getting air evenly, and that the moisture level of the pile is like that of a wrung-out sponge - not wet, but moist and consistent throughout, for ideal decomposition.

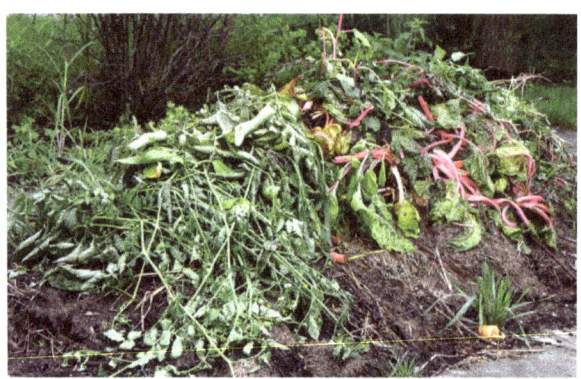

GOOD VS. BAD FOR THE PILE

<u>GOOD:</u> Composting is not just for Food alone, but we want to add only the best ingredients in order to create prime organic material. **It is also safe to compost: GRASS CLIPPINGS, FIREPLACE ASHES, COFFEE GROUNDS, NEWSPAPER, SAWDUST, HAY & STRAW, FUR & HAIR, NUT & EGGSHELLS, CARDBOARD, LEAVES, PAPER TOWELS AND NAPKINS, USED TEABAGS, OLD DRIED-UP GARDEN REMAINS** and many other organic materials from the yard that can be recycled by this process. What a better way to dispose of these things, instead of in plastic bags in a landfill!

<u>BAD:</u> **What should NOT to composted: FATS, GREASE, OILS & LARD, BLACK WALNUT HULLS, LEAVES & TWIGS, COAL OR CHARCOAL ASH, EGGS, DAIRY PRODUCTS, MEAT & FISH SCRAPS & BONES, PET OR HUMAN FECES, CAT LITTER, DISEASED OR INSECT-RIDDEN PLANTS, INORGANIC MATERIAL LIKE PLASTICS,** and **ANYTHING TREATED WITH CHEMICAL FERTILIZERS.** All of these will increase odors, attract pests, and can infect the pile with unwanted bacteria, fat residues, and chemicals.

BALANCING THE GREENS AND BROWNS

Your compost pile needs five main components to thrive: the balance of **Nitrogen** and **Carbon, Air & Water,** and **correct Temperature**. The pile needs to contain more Carbon items than Nitrogen items, preferably in a perfect ratio for the best conditions for the decomposing microorganisms. How can you tell the difference? The Garden yet again provides.

<u>GREEN</u> items are mostly high in **Nitrogen**, which includes most fresh food vegetable scraps, as well as grass clippings, manure, seaweed, alfalfa, garden waste, weeds, and even coffee grounds (once a green bean before roasting). These will all increase the Nitrogen of your pile, making sure the decomposers of the pile grow and reproduce more quickly. Too much Nitrogen and the pile turns cold, slimy, wet and smelly.

<u>BROWN</u> items are mostly higher in **Carbon** and act as the food source for decomposers. You can find more Carbon for your pile in dead leaves, sticks, plain paper, ashes, cornstalks, nut shells, woodchips (untreated), sawdust, fruits, cardboard, pine needles, straw and twigs. Too much Carbon will make the pile dry, slower and lifeless.

Ideally, use **2-4 parts of BROWNS for every 1 part of GREENS**. Have a leaf pile on hand near your compost from which to pull each time you layer new scraps in, and remember to add sticks and twigs and the other additives regularly.

Compost must be mature and complete before you utilize it for the garden, or else it can damage the plants and attract rodents and pests. Look for crumbly and smooth soil texture, with no evidence of food or paper scraps, with a great rainy day, rich earth smell, with no ammonia or sourness, and a dark rich color. The pile should have shrunk in size by about ⅓, and the temperature inside the center of the pile will be within about 10 degrees Fahrenheit of the outside temperature. It's ready! Now you can use this "Black Gold" to add to potting soils, place around your plants, use as a mulch, surround fruit trees, distribute into your lawn, rake nourishment into the garden soil, enhance houseplants, and remediate old flower beds.

TRENCHING

One of the easy Composting techniques is to build a **trench-style compost pile** in your yard. Dig a trench between **12"-24"** deep, as long as you like. When a section is full, simply bury the waste beneath soil and lawn clippings at one end of the trench and continue to the other end. You will want to pick a shady and dry spot away from roots, near a fence is good. This is the *only* style of compost in which you could also bury small amounts of meat, grain and dairy waste as they will be deeply below the ground. Earthworms and soil organisms do all the work. As long as your soil doesn't freeze solid, this method can be used year-round. If the soil gets too dry it is suitable to water it to support the process. This compost is also **invisible and odorless**, might be better if you have neighbors nearby. As this is a Cold Composting method, it will take longer to produce healthy soil, maybe **up to a year or more**. It is a little more effort to harvest the rich soil from the trench, so some people build these adjacent to where they want to garden for years to come. While still actively Composting, do not plant anything on top of the trench, as it could fall in and sink as the matter decomposes. However after a year or two, this would make a perfectly-prepared area for your garden or flower plants. Turning the soil well before planting is best, and is also a great way to check for thorough decomposition and maturity of the new soil. Mark the trench with a flag or rock circle so you can find it in every season, and also so no one steps into it.

WORM COMPOSTING

Vermicompost or Vermiculture is an INDOOR method of composting, utilizing **Worms**. This method is highly effective, odorless and easy to do, and is all-the-rage with some gardeners. Worm compost can work actively year-round, and can be placed in a closet, basement or even in the kitchen under the sink. This method produces organic worm castings in about 3-6 months and takes very little time and effort, only about 30 minutes per week to feed the worms. You have to get over (or perhaps never have had) any **fear or aversion to worms**, as they are the essential workers of this process, and must be purchased initially to create your composting community. The best worms for the job are the "Red Wiggler" species (*Eisenia fetida*) which you can purchase at bait stores or from many online retailers. Make sure to read reviews, check the worm species you are buying, and confirm also that you receive a FULL pound of worms (about 1000) for each bin you start. There are lots of YouTube, Rumble and TikTok videos detailing the finer points of this method.

TROUBLESHOOTING YOUR COMPOST

FOR FRUIT FLIES: Cover your compost pail in the kitchen at all times, and get fruit fly traps from the health food or gardeners store. Increase the amount of Carbon-rich Browns into your pile, and bury your GREENS scraps every time beneath the BROWNS to discourage flies. Add food to your pile only about once a week to encourage them to go elsewhere for food. Make sure the pile is not too wet.

FOR BAD ODOR: This can be a moisture problem, or an imbalance of Nitrogen & Carbon. Add more BROWN items like sticks, leaves, sawdust and paper to your pile and keep the watering down to a lesser amount. If the pile smells like Ammonia, there is too much Nitrogen and you need more Browns. Turn your pile more often as it may have gone anaerobic and lacks oxygen. Work more sticks, wood chips and cardboard into the pile for air channels.

OVERHEATING: Temperatures above 160 degrees Fahrenheit can kill the microbes in the pile and cause it to go sterile. Get a good compost thermometer and keep track. Ideally keep below 155 degrees.

COLD TEMPERATURES: If the pile seems too dry or too cold, consider covering it with a tarp and watering it more often. You can add Blood Meal, Cottonseed Meal, Kelp, or Manure to increase Nitrogen. Add some fresh dirt for more microorganisms. Temperature will go down when the compost is ready, check it with your compost thermometer.

GRASS CLIPPING CLUMPS: Sprinkle grass clippings instead of adding huge amounts into the bin. Use excess clippings instead as mulch around trees and flowers.

IF YOU NEED IT FASTER: You can add Nitrogen boosters and compost boosters to the pile, but MAKE SURE THEY ARE ORGANIC. Chop up clumps and any larger than finger-sized pieces of waste. Turn the entire pile out of the bin and aerate it, add wood chips to the bottom of the bin to create airspace, add fresh Greens and water, Return it to the bin in layers with Browns and small sticks, put a lid on it, and turn often until it is in perfect condition to use.

*****

SPARE THE WEEDS FOR THEY ARE SO USEFUL.

Always plan on *utilizing* whatever Weeds you remove from your yard in your Salads, Sauces, Smoothies, Ferments or Juices. Many Weeds make great main dishes! The entire next chapter will help you learn how to recognize and utilize all the **WILD WEEDS, glorious Free Food** that our beloved Mother Nature *already* provided for us. You will find it hiding in plain sight, in and amongst that which YOU seek to grow!

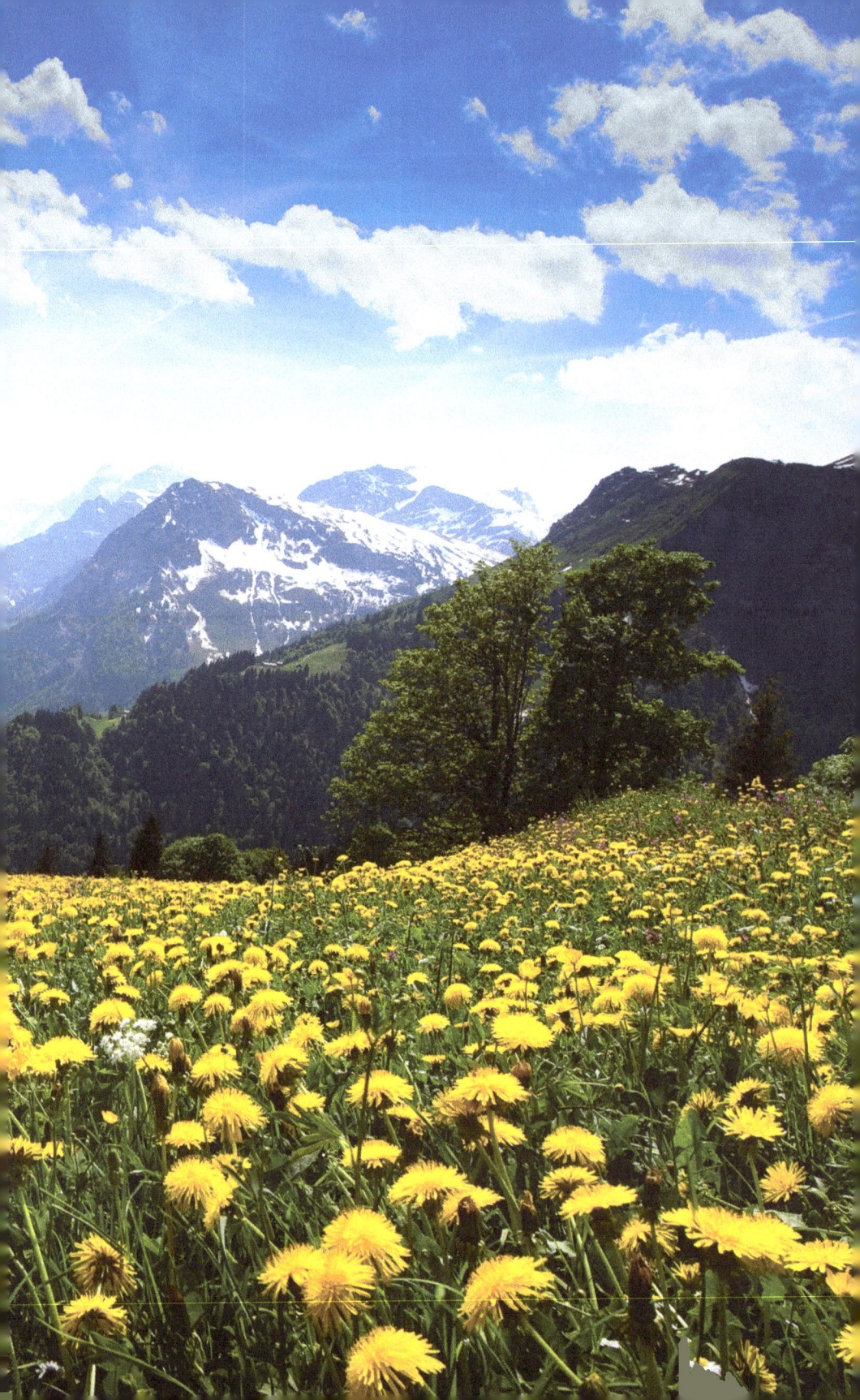

~ the garden of earth ~

~ Chapter 2.15 ~

OUTLAWS OF THE GARDEN

> "The Wild gatecrashes our civilized domains, and the domesticated escapes and runs riot. Weeds vividly demonstrate that Natural Life - and the course of Evolution itself - refuse to be constrained by our cultural concepts."
>
> *~ Richard Mabey*

UNTAMED DEVOTION

This chapter is dedicated to my wildest, free-range, true Outlier friend, **GONZO**, aka **Mark Lemke**. Gonzo was one of my best friends and a river-running buddy. He became Totally Unlimited, left the Earth in 2007, but not before he taught us tons of lessons, cracking us up for many years. His gift was teaching people all about Nature by immersing them in it, making them wiser and more in touch in the process. His legacy includes the often-quoted, completely time-shattering concept: *"It's Always 2:15."*

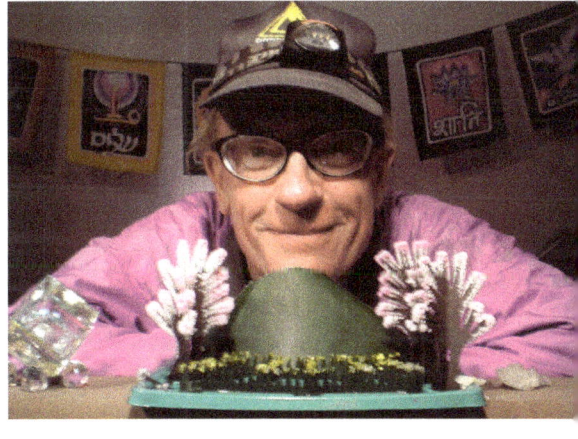

Gonzo and I first met when we were invited (by my Best Friend Kathryn) to join a 22-day, guides-only, Grand Canyon rafting trip. Boating 266 miles of the Colorado River, descending a mile deep into the Earth, is a truly life-changing event. Being away from society, money, hot and running water, shelter and electricity for nearly a month is an exercise in survival and self-examination. Everybody on the trip would face their own personal challenges, all while floating deeply through a major portal vein of Nature. The Land and the River become your companions, and are so supportive you can't help but feel comforted. The minerals, the red rock, the feel of the River every single day, the wonderful plants and birds and animals all play a part in your personal transformation. You come out of the Canyon a whole new person. Plus, the friendships you make on a trip of that kind last a lifetime! You literally put your life in each other's hands daily, and everyone has to bond, pitch in, and constantly watch each other's backs, to make it out alive.

It takes an enormous amount of preparation for a private raft-trip of that nature, even for a group of just nine people. Food, snacks and drinks for 24 days had to be bought and deep-frozen in our coolers. There was so much gear, and so much BEER! My first time down the Grand Canyon, I was kind of nervous about being around all these wild, outdoor-living raft guides. I felt suspiciously like a mountain girl in a big city girl's clothing. But I had one secret weapon: I could really COOK! Kathryn was kind enough to guide and teach me at every turn, and give me jobs at which I could excel.

Gonzo and I were assigned to do the shopping for the travel days prior to the river trip. I had menus and lists and big plans, because it was my job to prepare the road meals. I was all ready to run to the store, when Gonzo said, *"Hey there, the first thing we need to do is stop rushing all around so much! It's only 2:15! Now just calm down. Sit down here and smoke this joint. We have all the time in the World!"*

Needless to say, shopping later was hilarious (and effortless). But I learned a powerful lesson. Slow down, make it more fun, enjoy it all more! That was Gonzo's mantra, proving time does not matter when you are a mile into the Earth - or actually anywhere! Rafters would ask him, *"When is breakfast?"* and he would say, *"2:15."* *"When do we get to the takeout?"* *"2:15."* *"What time will the Sun go down?"* *"2:15."* Eventually you get it, get *off the clock* and realize **"It's always 2:15!"** It's River Time, Vacation Time, I Don't Give a Damn About Time, Time. Let that clock go, toss your watch and phone away.

Gonzo's constant lesson was to stop being ruled by time - or actually ruled by *anything* - BE FREE. Find times when you get to LET GO of worrying. You might enjoy it all more, *and still have plenty of time.* For a few summers, we both lived by the side of the

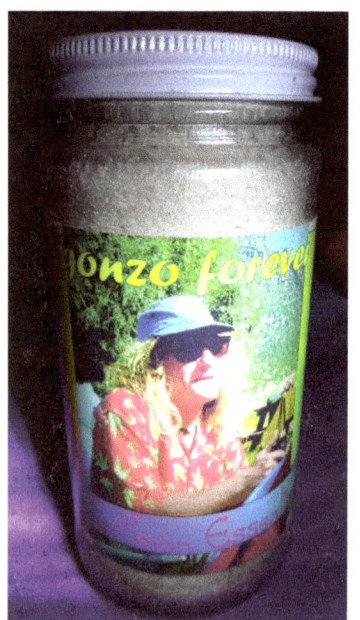

Colorado River working for the same rafting company, and we took many mellow AND wild river trips. We rafted through the Grand Canyon twice together, although the second time he hiked-out early with a 90-pound backpack to leave for Antarctica to work Search and Rescue! His herbal influence will stay with me forever, but it's also this Wild-Free-thing he had that changed me forever. I DO believe the Marijuana Spirit chose him as an ambassador, because his Life was a Stoned Spiritual Service Success Story. He would be as enthusiastic about a "Chapter 2.15" as he would be thrilled that this chapter is about Weed (*Weeds,* Gonzo!).

My Dear Gonzo, the way you lived with **Plants** was a true revelation to me! You were one of the first people I met in Colorado who dug his own Osha and made herbal pantry stores of Wild Plants. I watched you gathering Horsetail by the river, making tea in your teepee with all your baggies of Peppermint, Ginger, and Valerian, chewing long pieces of Licorice root, smudging with Sage you'd gathered, adding herbs to the fire, dancing around madly. I always knew where you were by the smell of Patchouli (and the coughing!). Thanks to you, to this day, *I always know what time it is*. You gave me a whole Free and Natural Life View I would never have acquired any other way, teaching me so much about Plants and People and Playing. It is totally appropriate that this chapter about the craziest, hardiest, most *free* Weeds, be dedicated to YOU.

THE WILDEST FOODS EVER

There is **Free Food** living in your yard, right now, waiting to be utilized. Regardless of season, water shortage, level of neglect, weather or geographical location, there are Food and Medicine plants (some call them Weeds) all over your neighborhood. They grow for you freely. You did not have to plant them or maintain them. Ironically, they prefer to grow with no effort on your part! Once you learn more about them, you won't ever look at Dandelions (or any of the other Plants you may have thought were pests) the same way. Journey a little further to unpopulated areas, and you can discover even more Wild Food. You will begin to recognize that **Food is Everywhere!**

The Weeds are the **UNDOMESTICATED OUTLAWS** of the Plant World - the Outliers, Outlanders, the Outcasts. They naturally contain an **extra drive to survive** and will adapt to do so, growing abundantly in drought and in floods, on forest fire clearings, construction sites, around abandoned properties and in disturbed ground. We find such powerful medicines in the Weeds because they are used to neglect, they *have* to be extra hardy, and they count on nothing! As a result of enduring their particular hardships, Weeds make *much stronger* **vital phytochemicals** than most plants, to ensure their survival. Their potent saps and essential oils rebuke parasites, *increase* their ability to deter pests and fight bacterial, fungal & viral invasion, repel predators, and hyperstimulate their own growth against any and all odds. Their medicinal and adaptogenic content is off the charts, because they are always creating a personal pharmacy within their "body" with which to heal and preserve themselves (much like the biology of Humans)! Their precious ingredients have great worth. Their self-healing design is evident by their natural, resilient and persistent survival.

Weeds create a Living Garden that requires **no watering or maintenance**. Weeds will push up through a crack in asphalt, grow through a fence, or overtake a garden simply for survival's sake. Weeds will grow in the worst soil in the driest conditions and create a beautiful flower. Weeds also wildly and quickly reproduce in radical expansion, so they provide an abundant food supply! In a shocking drive to stay alive, some Weeds even *double* their output when they have been harvested once.

Weeds are by nature not only abundant, they are the **Rebels**, they have the Rebel Gene! They don't behave like our more civilized, cultivated garden plants. They will sprawl through a whole field, climb over every telephone pole, or cling to the edge of the canyons. They'll grow in the crook of a tree or make their home in your whole front yard. They will take over, however and wherever they can, to survive and multiply. They have even been known to *imitate* other plants to keep from being recognized!

I've always thought of the Weeds like secret, less popular friends. They always turn out to be the coolest and most loyal, and when you notice them, they start to call to you more! I believe the Weeds, like all Plants, WANT you to befriend them! To stop a minute and explore them, say hello, and help them to realize their potential. They want you to search for them, spread the good word about them, to eat, and enjoy them. They are so busy just trying to provide for everybody - we must *utilize them*.

#WEEDSTOO

Why were we ever taught to believe that some Plants are "good" and some, like the Weeds, are not? Who decided this? Who proclaims and enforces the labels? **Why make LAWS against certain Plants?!** There is not a single plant on Earth that has no uses, they are ALL here for a reason, made purposely for us. And all of them for a *multitude* of reasons. Gaia says that every single creature has a **Seven-Fold Purpose** for being here on Earth (just as you do). So why not recognize those purposes inherently expressed by *every* plant. Especially all the many Weed-Plants we carelessly discard? It is foolish to overlook and discriminate against these "different" Plants. We need to start a revolution and a social movement - **#WeedsToo!**

The real question is, *why are we being taught* to ignore such an important and abundant FOOD and Medicine supply? And much worse, instructed and neighbor-shamed into using poisonous pesticides to destroy them? **Especially in a time of food and income challenges?** The **pesticide industry** *(brought to you by to the pharmaceutical and oil industries)* is a mega-billion dollar entity with a lot of Power, and the full ability to effectively sell their death-wish for Weeds. Their reach is large and their propaganda is convincing. Simply because many people lack education, money and accurate information, they have been brainwashed by the makers that it is NECESSARY to decimate perfectly wonderful plants right in their own yards. These are the very plants they could be using to feed and heal the whole Family... it seems weirdly intentional.

What slander against the Plant Kingdom, that modern industry has vilified the Weeds. You can see commercials on TV saying "*We have to destroy all the Dandelions, it's war!*" Well - **stop buying it**, literally. This is "fake news" if there ever was! The ORIGINAL fake news, quite possibly, their same story going on for a century. Let's all try to restore some reason. It's time we revive traditional, ancient wisdom and work for a re-education of all people about Weeds, *especially* Dandelions. Everyone needs to understand the fact that Weeds are just **one MORE Garden** our beautiful Earth has made for us. **Stop the Killing!** Stop spraying the poisons that leach into our water supply and ruin our topsoil and contaminate our Organic Gardens and our rivers and impact our children, pets and wildlife! Stop removing our Food and Medicine Plants, stop altering our seeds with pesticide-ready genetics. People have a sovereign right to keep their own Heirloom Seeds and Precious Weeds - and to grow whatever they like. Let's break the artificial control cycle and take our Wild Indigenous Food back.

This is made even easier by simply letting the **WILD FOOD GROW FREE** in your yard. It's exciting to see what comes to feed you, no purchase necessary! "Allow" the *natural growth* as an experiment, even if just for a little while, to see what thrives easily on your land. Try it in the Spring when the Pollinators need the most support. Many of the Plants in the following **"Materia Weedica"** will lovingly show up to greet you, and abundantly beg to be noticed. It will be so much fun to use them! If you don't have a yard, locate some quiet nice fields nearby, and visit them often to see what develops. Keep track of secret spots you can forage for real Wild Foods and visit them like friends.

With some simple tips, you can be harvesting their complementary foods from your very own yard today. It will be exciting to keep track of your natural bounty, when you get to know the plants a little better they will show you things about the condition of your World. You'll also see that Weeds you recognize from home also grow in many places **all around the World**. They are waiting to greet and feed you there, as well. I remember seeing the same Weeds I knew and loved in France, and realizing I had friends already there waiting for me!

BE SURE TO STAY ALIVE

It is MOST IMPORTANT to be CERTAIN of the Wild Foods you eat. Bear in mind the story of the young man named **Chris McCandless**, who went out adventuring in the wilds of Alaska, and decided to live there year-round in an old school bus. In a state of near starvation he wrote in his journal that he had eaten many wild plants, some that may have weakened his body (and would eventually kill him). I read Jon Krakauer's book about him, *Into the Wild*, then watched as it was made into a movie in 2007. I never forgot this potent foraging lesson. Years after publication of the book, Jon added to his story, writing two follow-up articles for *The New Yorker*, the last of which was called, *"How Chris McCandless Died - The Update."* Krakauer had the seeds of *H. alpinum* which Chris ate (he referred to them as "potato seeds") analyzed for toxins. After much research, he discovered new information about the actual cause of poisoning being a neurotoxic amino acid called L-canavanine from an otherwise non-toxic plant. **"The death of Chris McCandless should serve as a caveat to other foragers: even when some parts of a plant are known to be edible, other parts of the same species may contain dangerous concentrations of toxic compounds."**[10] This makes a case for Chris identifying the plant correctly, but the wild food guides being nowhere near explicit enough about which parts NOT to eat, and which food toxins to avoid. In this case, his malnourished and stressed condition created a *extra sensitivity* to the L-canavanine that turned deadly. Many Alaskans took offense at the

"Hollywoodizing" of this story and they worried others would follow. But the advice remains the same: **Be Careful.** When I saw the movie, the *deadly* effect of a simple plant misidentification (or misuse) was tragically and visually impressed upon me. You can never "un-see" that. Consequently, I embraced a whole new level of caution. I received it as a teaching moment, especially important for those of us who feel we "know a lot about plants." **Be Informed. Be Humble. And Be Extremely Cautious.** Your Life and the Lives of those you love depend upon it.

Many Weeds are commonly known, but always CONFIRM to be sure, and check **multiple sources**. Experts suggest finding at least **three photographic references** that match your plant sample. To make sure your identification is sound, ask a Park Ranger, use Wild Food guides, carry Plant books, phone-an-Herbalist, consult agriculture experts in your area, ask botanically-inclined friends, use identification apps and search the internet as well. It is wonderful to have so many tools with which to research and learn the benefits of your food sources. I think it is wise to have some **physical Plant Identification BOOKS and MAPS** on hand for reference as well. We want to be prepared for strange weather, or any Earth changes that may be possible - and the internet on our sometimes fragile electrical grid is not a reliable constant. Having alternative, *non-electrical sources of information* in your home, backpack and car (like good old-fashioned BOOKS) is a smart idea!

WISE FRIENDS GROWING LIKE WEEDS

I write all through the book about another "Free-the-Weeds" influencer, my mentor and dearest friend Brigitte Mars. She encourages the Wild Weed plants to grow freely, all over her entire yard. She constantly has Food and Medicine galore within steps of

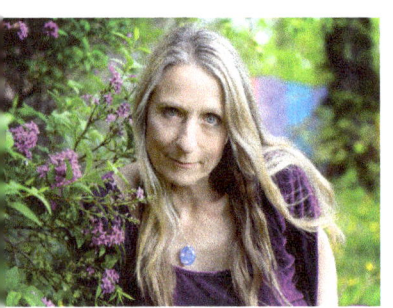

her kitchen door. Brigitte is a Living Psychedelic Legend. She wears colorful, flowing, goddess rockstar clothing, and has an enormous closet room, arranged in spectral rainbow order. Her exotic, trippy Breezy Dream House is filled with fairies and doll houses and mushrooms (oh my!), sacred art and about a million books, many of which she wrote! Her deep purple office has books all over, bottles of magical potions and charts and collages, notes and book ideas, notebooks everywhere - research heaven. Brigitte's kitchen is filled with bottles of natural medicines, all of her Unitea Herbs Tea blends in big gallon jars, dozens of remedies, extracts, ferments and crystals, and the everpresent wild Nettle from the garden for juice. She *always* has a dozen raw dishes in the fridge from which to feed me, and every single time I'd visit, she'd make me a "to-go" plate for my drive back to Steamboat. She'd garnish it with edible flowers and minty aromatic herbs to keep me awake while driving, ALL WEEDS we'd picked together as we walked her Wild Gardens.

Brigitte's **Herb Walks** and **Classes** in Boulder are not to be missed, she has encyclopedic knowledge, spending time with her is a gift, and a true education. Brigitte dedicated her first book entirely to the King of the Weeds, appropriately titled *Dandelion Medicine!* She teaches so many people how to learn and love what comes freely from the land. I am in awe of Brigitte Mars - and I want to serve Earth like her.

Brigitte knows literally Everybody, and the parties at her magical Dream House are LEGENDARY - three floors of the wildest, most rainbow-filled, sparkly, alternative, psychedelic fun anyone could ever have on Earth! With Celebrities, Gurus, World-Famous Poets, Musicians, Herbalists, Yogis and Artists - you never knew who'd you meet next (*"That's Ron, he's an Alien,"* right Jasper?).

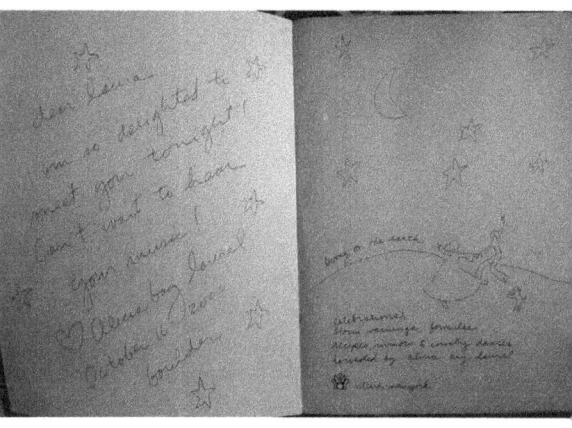

On the night of October 16, 2000, Brigitte was having a particularly festive party with tons of superstar guests, and she introduced me to one of my true Natural Woman Heroes, author/activist/artist **Alicia Bay Laurel**. While I have a nice library of survival manuals and self-sufficiency books, her book, *Living On The Earth*, is my very favorite. You can learn **everything** in her book from how to make soap, clothing, food, shelters, or medicines to how to make sunflower seed yogurt or tan a hide, to how to build a kayak or await rescue if you are stranded in the water! It is a remarkable book, full of great information to have on hand. Her original single-line artwork and hand lettering make this book so unique. It's a helpful handbook for working with Weeds, too, with many awesome Wild Food recipes. What an honor, I got her to sign my well-worn copy! She is transcendent and one of our Inspirational Wise Elders. Recently, she celebrated the 50th Anniversary of the first printing of this remarkable book! DO get yourself (and a friend) a copy here: ***https://indigo-with-stars.myshopify.com/products/living-on-the-earth-5th-english-edition-50th-anniversary-edition***

Allow me to remind you that everywhere you go there are similar **Wise Elders** growing their incredible knowledge like weeds. Seek these people out! Find out who the Plant Pioneers are in your town, and go meet them. I met Brigitte Mars because I sent her a letter, and that one letter changed my life forever! *Write* the Authors you love, connect with them online, become friends with these Legends of the Plant World. Many of them are on social media and have lots of FREE videos and resources with which to educate you. **But meeting the living person is the greatest education of all!** There is something in the vibration of these great thinkers that passes on to you, their drive and desire is infectious (in the very best way). Go to their classes, read their books, watch their videos, listen to their guidance to get out in Nature more, teach yourself all about the Plants. And one day, you may find YOU have become a Wise Medicine-Person yourself! You may be offered a chance to teach *your* children and *your* friends and *your* neighbors all about the Wild World. You will want to share your knowledge. And I tell you, I am going to want to read YOUR book.

PLANTS TEACH YOU

Keep in mind as you forage and study, that especially in Spring and Summer, a plant will most likely be showing you **all of its life stages at once.** In a field you can find the new shoot of a plant, it's growing basal leaves, perhaps the plant in flower, examples of growing fruits nurturing seeds. You will likely even find the same plant from last year in a dry dormant state somewhere nearby, from which to gather seeds. Details you can glean from the field will show you how it reproduces, what it creates, how it is designed perfectly to spread its seeds. This gives you great clues about the life cycle and mission of that plant. All this evidence, when you take time to see it, offers you ways you can identify it in many seasons (which could prove helpful someday). I like to keep notes about where I find certain plants that I want to come back to for harvest and observation, and date them, too. Secret stashes of plants may not come up the next year but might the year after - it can be helpful (and fun) to have records. I read about a woman who kept a calendar of all the plants that came up for her, renaming the days each year by their current blooming Flowers.

I know I have said it before, but let the Plants teach you **caution**, too. Never eat anything of which you are unsure. Take small cuttings or make drawings in your notebook, or take pictures so you can later positively identify any unknown or "new-to-you" plants.

If you look closely and begin to keep track, you will be able to recognize **PATTERNS** in plants that look alike, which indicate they are **related and likely have similar actions**. These *characteristics* teach you who the plants are and what they might do. Botanists noticed patterns like this and agreed to call plants that fit into such identifiable groups a **FAMILY**, noting the characteristic, repeated details that united them.

> "Learning to identify Plants by Families will forever change the way you look at Plants."
>
> ~ *Thomas J. Elpel*

You may have noticed that your **Mint** plants have a *square stem*. **Every member of this Family will always have a square stem**, with alternating and opposing pairs of leaves. Mint flowers grow in circular whorls that ascend to the top of the stem, and almost all have that aromatic minty smell. Just like that, you have learned how to identify plants in the **Mint Family!** You have likely eaten several varieties of Mint in candy flavors, so you probably have a good guess about what they do, and how quickly they help your stomach! *Family Identification* is a super helpful way to figure out the **kind of plant** you have found, what it might do, even when unsure of the *exact specific plant.*

I highly recommend *Botany in A Day* by the above-quoted Thomas J. Elpel, and his website **http://www.wildflowers-and-weeds.com/**. He says that if you could learn just *eight key Families* you would have a great amount of success identifying *most* of what is out in the field. Here are his <u>**Super Eight Plant Families:**</u> **Mint, Parsley, Mustard, Pea, Lily, Grass, Rose** and **Aster** (some of these because there are poisonous plants you need to know in the Pea and Parsley Families). His methods taught me more in one afternoon than I learned in many years of foraging and herb books! Now I can identify plants all over the World by knowing their Family characteristics.

All members of the **Rose Family** have a 5-petaled star flower and produce fruit - like Apples, Peaches, Strawberries, and Almonds. All members of the **Mustard Family** have a 4-petaled flower in a cross, and all make edible Mustard seeds! Knowing the Plant Family gives you clues about identification, medicinal nature, edibility, where to find the seeds, when it will mature, and where it will grow.

Here are some cool highlights and interesting facts about some of the "better-known Families." There are actually **452 Plant Families** classified so far! I have included some of the more likely and popular ones you will encounter out in the World. But don't worry, it is not necessary to grasp all the finer details of each Family. I offer them as a *reference* so you can look them up when you DO want to know more about a certain plant, or a food you are eating, or the other kinds of foods in that particular Family. You'll be able to utilize this information right away in the upcoming section about the Wild Weeds, as the Plant Family is noted at the top of each plant.

PLANT FAMILIES

ANACARDIACEAE ~ Cashew, Mango, & Sumac Family ~ small trees
and shrubs with 3-lobed pinnate, compound leaves, many single-seeded white, pale yellow, red or bright orange berries, flowers 3-5 petals, 5-10 stamens, some have a bracts, or a flower cone above the leaves. Resinous (usually poisonous) milky sap flows through tubular channels in the stems, and most trees in this Family have that characteristic sap also in chambers in the bark. Mostly tropical, but members of this Family grow in Southern states. Family name comes from the Greek meaning *"upward heart"* which describes the outward facing nut that is characteristic of this Family.

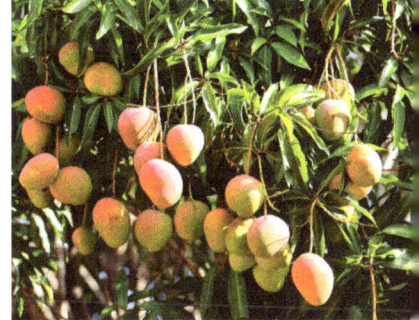

- Mango, Pistachio, Cashew, Staghorn Sumac, Mastic, Peruvian Pepper Tree (Pink Peppercorn), Hogplum, Smoke Tree, Marula, Zebrawood, Cuachalate, Smooth Sumac

NOT ALL HARMLESS, BEWARE - **Poison Oak, Poison Sumac & Poison Ivy** were a part of the Rhus genus in this Family but they have attained their own genus status (see **Toxicodendron**, below). They share many similar characteristics.

Mango, Pistachio, and **Cashew** all contain smaller amounts of **Urushiol**, which is the same key component that makes Poison Ivy and the Toxicodendrons (great band name) so irritating and "poisonous." Some people with bad Ivy reactions, have allergies to *these foods* for that same reason. Several plants of this species produce viscous adhesive fluids, oils, lacquer, resins and mordant for red dye.

- **TOXICODENDRON** - "Poisonous Group" A Subfamily of **Anarcardiaeae** - **Poison Oak, Poison Sumac** and **Poison Ivy** are identified best with the old adages *"Leaves of Three, Leave Them Be" "Longer Middle Stem, Don't Touch Them" "Hairy Vine, No Friend Of Mine."* Poison Ivy leaves are notoriously glossy and droopy (bullies with a bad attitude). White or yellowish berries may or may not be present. Edges may be smooth or toothed, and leaves turn red early in the Fall and so become more visible in the brush. The best way I have found to identify them is the longer stem on the middle of the three-leaf leaflets, and that they only grow one leaflet-of-three from each side of the stem at a time, alternating singly down the stem (which is sometimes red) and they droop a lot and look shiny. Opposite, balanced double three-leaved stems (like a Y) are most likely Box Elder seedlings. Keep in mind *burning* poison toxicodendrons creates toxic smoke - so don't do it. If you need to remove it, use a strong Vinegar and dish soap solution to spray on the plant while asking kindly for it to find a different place to grow. Remember, these too are sacred plants with a multi-fold purpose on the Earth and they still deserve respect and some places to grow.

APIACEAE (formerly Umbelliferae) ~ Parsley, Celery & Carrot Family

~ flat-top, compound umbrella flowers usually white, yellow or pink (not blue) with alternate ferny, complicated pinnate leaves. Stems hollow between the leaf joints, seed capsule is a twin with 2 seeds in each capsule.

- Carrot, Fennel, Osha, Anise, Coriander, Dill, Angelica, Gotu Kola, Parsley, Celery, Dong Quai, Lomatium, Lovage, Cumin, Cilantro, Asafoetida, Bupleurum, Caraway, Chervil, Ajwain, Cow Parsley, Sweet Cicely, Parsnip, Sea Holly, Wild Carrot, Queen Anne's Lace

NOT ALL HARMLESS, BEWARE - There are many deadly Hemlocks and other POISONOUS PLANTS in the Apiaceae Family, but many great Medicines as well. Water Hemlock has an obvious **spotted stem and really stinks**, which in Nature generally means, **"I'm Poisonous, don't touch me."**

MANY of our Culinary Spices come from this Family, and they are full of potent and medicinal essential oils. The greens are very aromatic and make great flavor boosters and digestive aids. The roots of this Family are highly nutritious, vegetable food staples.

ASPARAGACEAE (formerly in Liliaceae) ~ Asparagus Family

~ includes the sub-families of Agave, Beargrass and Brodiaea, which were all formerly classified in the Lily Family. Each of them have characteristic but different appearances.

> ☙ **Asparagus, Shatavari, Agave, Yucca, Butcher's Broom, Lily of the Valley, Solomon's Seal, Queen's Cup, Trillium False Solomon's Seal, Bluebell, Grape Hyacinth, Spider Plant, Beargrasses**

2,900 SPECIES, **NOT ALL EDIBLE** - **Lily of the Valley** is toxic.

Asparagus is a super edible Wild Food, with the youngest feathery shoots in Spring, as well as mature stalks, all deliciously edible. It is also known to be diuretic and an aphrodisiac, with its potent, upward thrusting growth.

Trilliums are endangered so picking them is illegal in most states. They have sets of three - 3 petals, 3 sepals, 3 leaves representing the Holy Trinity. They hide in the forest floor and you should count your blessings when you see them.

ASTERACEAE (formerly Compositae) ~ Daisy & Sunflower Family

~ distinct Daisy flower with many rays, center disc can grow into a tall cone. Flower is actually a composite of many tiny flowers. Milky sap. Multiple layers of bracts below the flower, some grow prickly burrs or thorns. These plants never grow into trees, and are never aquatic, but otherwise grow so abundantly that their relatives can be found worldwide.

> ☙ **Dandelion, Sunflower, Chamomile, Burdock, Chicory, Echinacea, Arnica, Yarrow, Stevia, Calendula, Mugwort, Elecampane, Milk Thistle, Feverfew, Grindelia, Lettuces, Coltsfoot, Salsify, Aster, Tansy, Fleabane, Tarragon, Artichoke, Marigold, Chrysanthemum, Dahlia, Zinnia, Sagebrush, Jerusalem Artichoke, Goldenrod, Prickly Wild Lettuce, Pyrethrum**

32,000 KNOWN SPECIES MOST EDIBLE - One of the BIGGEST families containing many staple foods and herbs. Herbalism students used to complain about the DYC's - *"Damn Yellow Compositaes"*- because there are so many yellow, Daisy-looking flowers to learn in this Family.

Asteraceae is an important Family for the economy, providing many food crops as well as medicinal herbs, tea and coffee substitutes, and cooking oils. **Lettuces, Dandelions,** and many wild edible greens are a part of this Family.

Artemisia, Wormwood, Sagebrush, Mugwort, Sage, White Sage and 51 other Bitter Herbs that are all highly **anti-parasitic** come from this Family. **Echinacea** is a potent immune-building herb. Many of these plants are used as vegetable dyes. Sunflower Family plants are also used as ornamentals in gardens across the World. Their milky white sap is a leading cause of dermatitis in sensitive people, and many experience allergies to **Ragweed** and **Goldenrod**. Some members of this Family contain too many pyrrolizidine alkaloids to be safely eaten (**Golden Ragwort, Tansy & Coltsfoot**). **Cocklebur** is toxic to farmyard animals, and **Yarrow** can cause photosensitivity.

BORAGINACEAE ~ Borage & Forget-Me-Not Family ~

mostly periwinkle blue flowers (but some yellow and red) that are multiple with 5 petals, alternate and sometimes opposite lance-shaped leaves that clasp the stem. Hairy stems & leaves can cause skin irritation. Flowers coil into a curly shape (scorpioid flower) and start out red or magenta, and fade to blue on the same plant. Capsules have 4 seeds, and dry into flat, tear-drop burrs that look like a tiny dog's tongue.

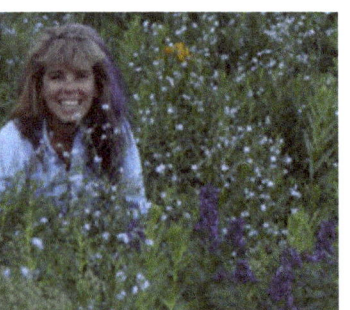

- **Forget-Me-Not (pictured), Comfrey, Borage Hound's-Tongue, Field Gromwell, Bluebell, Lungwort, Heliotrope, Viper's Bugloss, Alkanet, Stoneseed, Stickseed, Miner's Candle**

2000 SPECIES OF SHRUBS, TREES AND PLANTS - many edible, utilized as astringent and mineral-rich herbs, the leaves of many **Borages** edible as well. Their gorgeous periwinkle edible flowers are one of the very few **Blue Foods.**

Comfrey (also called Bone Knit) is a powerful but much maligned member of this Family, due to its high content of pyrrolizidine alkaloids which can irritate the liver when overused excessively. Used in moderate quantities and especially in Tea form, Comfrey provides an amazing mineral matrix remedy for bone healing.

Borage has perfect, blue, shooting star-shaped edible flowers that look awesome in ice cubes, on cakes, and in salads.

BRASSICACEAE (formerly Cruciferae)

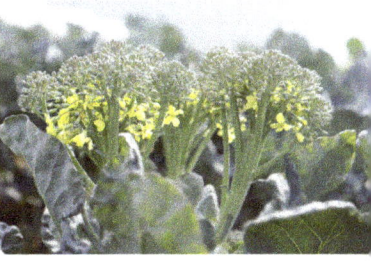

~ **Mustard & Cabbage Family** ~ flower always has 4-petals in a cross, 6 stamens - 4 tall 2 short. These plants grow a tall flower spike that becomes the vegetable and produces seeds, but may also grow below ground like a tuber or rhizome (Turnips & Beets). Seeds (held inside leaf-like pods on the stem after flowering) can be easily found in all seasons.

- Broccoli, Kale, Cauliflower, Cabbage, Brussel Sprouts, Radish, Beets, Horseradish, Wasabi, Maca, Bok Choy, Daikon, Kohlrabi, Rutabaga, Turnips, Wild Mustard, Collard Greens, Napa Cabbage, Watercress, Arugula, Rapeseed, Mustard Seeds & Greens, Shepherd's Purse, Penny Grass

ALL 4000+ SPECIES ARE ALL EDIBLE - it's a long list that includes some of our best staple foods. Cruciferous Vegetables feed the world.

Wild Mustards make perfect trail seasonings, you can literally always find one around with its very obvious seeds. This Family was originally named for its crucifix-like flower. **Mustard** has always been considered a holy seed, mentioned in the Bible five times. There is a spicy element to all Mustards that make them easily identifiable. **Cabbage** of some sort is featured in all major international diets. Most every cuisine makes use of **Mustards, Broccoli** and **Radishes**, as well.

CANNABACEAE ~ Hemp Family

~ coarse, sturdy-stemmed, upright ropey plants or woody vines with palmate or pinnate leaves. No petals on the flowers - just clusters of bracts. Thomas Elpel notes the Hemp Family, *"may not have much in the way of showy flowers but the Family does claim one of the most recognized plants on Earth: MARIJUANA."* Highly aromatic, fast and abundant-growing plants.

- Marijuana (Cannabis), Hemp, Hops, Hackberry, Trema, Qing Tan (Blue Sandalwood), Muku *(Aphananthe aspera)*

170 SPECIES EDIBLE & HIGHLY USEFUL - small Family but super nourishing food plants, providing hundreds of products made from flowers, fiber, juice, oil, and seeds.

Cannabis was one of the earliest-discovered domesticated and farmed plants. There is evidence of its widespread use over 10,000 years ago, and as long as 27,000 years ago in the Czech Republic. **Hops** is famously known for its use in beer, but it is also a sedating, nerve-nourishing **Cannabis Family** member. Hops contain terpenes and terpenoids similar to the Marijuana plant that increase the neurotransmitter GABA in the brain. One subspecies *Humulus yunnanensis* contains CBD and THC and has been bred to contain as much as 18% CBD, for a marijuana-free CBD alternative. Hops can be sewn into Lavender pillows or sachets to promote deeper sleep.

CARYOPHYLLACEAE ~ Carnation & Pink Family ~

spicy edible flowers, usually with ruffled or jagged tips, can be dense with many petals or in a single layer. Flower parts usually in 5's, large sepal clasping the base of the flower, sometimes a large bulb ovary below the flower. Long, stiff and pointy, veined, dark ovoid leaves. Stems are coarse and durable with distinct nodes. Flowers taste like wintergreen or clove and are beautiful in salads.

- **Carnation, Chickweed, Soapwort, Scleranthus, Pinks, Wild Sweet William, Mouse-Ears, Campions, Sandwort, Baby's Breath, Pearlwort, Corncockles, Snow-In-Summer, African Dream Root**

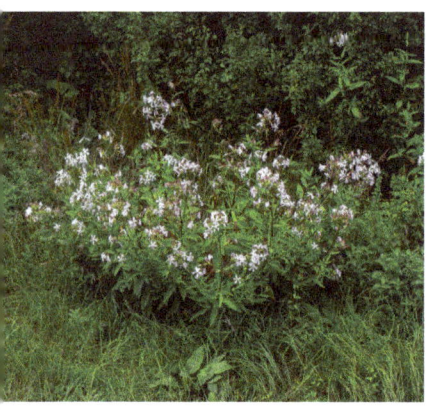

OVER 2000 SPECIES - many grown for the floral industry, but also used as edible garnishes.

Soapwort *(left)* grows near streams and waterways and can be used as sudsy soap for washing hands and clothing, it even works for shaving. Recognize it by its light pink flower and tendency to foam right up when rubbed between your hands with water.

African Dream Root (*Silene capensis*) induces vivid visions and promotes lucid dreaming. Silene is used is used in flying potions for levitation.

CLUSIACEAE (also called Guttiferae) ~ Garcinia Family ~

mostly tropical trees and shrubs, broad-ended oblong leaves, milky or colorful sap, capsule or berry fruit. Tropical fruits **Garcinia** and **Mangosteen** are all the rage in weight loss.

- **Garcinia, Mangosteen, Kokum, Kamani, Caulophyllum, Waika Plum, Bitter Kola**

800 SPECIES — Trees have been cultivated for many years for timber and resins. But now they are grown in many orchards for diet aids.

Some plants in this **Clusiaceae Family** provide not only pollen and nectar, but a kind of resin that Bees and other Pollinators use in building their nests. See also **Hypericaceae**.

ERICACEAE ~ Heath Family ~ think **Rhododendron** with woody stems, alternate thick, leathery & shiny evergreen leaves, clusters of urn-shaped, fused-petal flowers, also tube or trumpet flowers with 4 or 5 petals joined at the bottom, abundant red to deep purple berries. Grow in shrubs or small trees in acidic conditions, sometimes in bogs. Ericaceae are dependent on mycelial masses to live.

- **Blueberry, Cranberry, Huckleberry, Azalea, Heather, Wintergreen, Bilberry, Manzanita, Pipsissewa, Lingonberry, Heath, Rhododendron, Mountain Laurel, Uva Ursi/Bearberry, Indian Pipe**

4250 SPECIES - mostly flowering and dwarf evergreen ground cover, shrubs & climbers which provide food for many animals and humans.

Wintergreen (normally associated with Mints as candy and gum flavoring, although this is their true Family) can be found in small patches in deep woods, berries are edible. You may also be lucky enough to see the mysterious, ghostly white, non-photosynthesizing **Indian Pipe**, (also called Ghost Pipe) pictured above.

FABACEAE (formerly Leguminosae) ~ Pea & Bean Family ~ also called Caesalpiniaceae, Mimosaceae, Papilionaceae. Think Clovers and Lupines, which are all legumes with an irregular flower with banner, 2 wings & a keel, sometimes in a tall stalk or a ball, giving way to long pea like seed pods.

- **Red Clover, Peanut, Alfalfa, Licorice, Astragalus, Fenugreek, Peas, Beans, Crimson Clover, Owl's Clover, Lupine, Mesquite, Locust, Mimosa Tree, Butterfly Pea**

NOT ALL HARMLESS, BEWARE - **Lupines** are poisonous, **Locust** and **Mesquite** have brutal thorns. But there are many helpful food plants in this Fabaceae Family as well. **Beans & Peas** provide vegan protein worldwide.

Astragalus, Red Clover and **Licorice** are some of the Medicinal Herb Superstars of this family. **Peanut** wins the contest as the most useful member of this Family, thanks to George Washington Carver who discovered over 300 uses for it, and with it, subsequently saved the economy of the South (more details in Chapter 4).

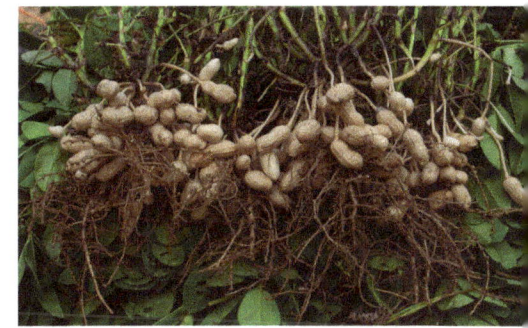

HYPERICACEAE ~ St. John's Wort Family ~ A Subfamily of **Clusiaceae**.

Yellow flowers with 4 or 5 parts with many stamens like a firework, leaves are opposite on the stem and have dark glands or clear dots on them.

👉 **St. John's Wort, Hypericum varietals, Triadenum**

UP TO 700 SPECIES - Hypericum plants make a surprising red-colored extract, oil & dye. Stems, leaves & flowers produce a powerful medicinal oil for nerve support.

St. John's Wort has powerful antidepressant action, and is an effective alternative to Prozac. Some people say it lessens the effect of birth control pills, use with care. Taking extract of St. John's Wort a few times a day can stop a herpes sun blister in its tracks, due to its strong anti-viral nature. Homeopathic **Hypericum** (St. Johns Wort) is specific and helpful for nerve complaints like neuropathy, sciatica, and fibromyalgia.

LAMIACEAE (formerly Labiatae) ~ Mint & Nettle Family ~ always

have square stems, alternate and opposing leaf pairs, and are usually highly aromatic. Mints have whorled flowers which clutch the stem all around like a ball successively up the stem to a crowning flower. Their smell and taste are instantly recognizable, very few do not have scent. Flower matures into a seed capsule with 4 nutlets. This is one of the largest Plant Families containing many of our medicinal herbs, and likely over half of your spice cabinet, as popular savory spices are from the **Mint Family**.

👉 **Peppermint, Spearmint, Basil, Lavender, Oregano, Chia, Lemon Balm, Rosemary, Marjoram, Nettles, Henbit & DeadNettle, Motherwort, Self-Heal, Skullcap, Hyssop, Horehound, Coyote Mint, Bee Balm, Catnip, Bergamot Mint, Thyme, Coleus, Culinary Sage, Pennyroyal, Patchouli**

OVER 7000 MINTS, MOSTLY ALL EDIBLE - Mints are generally harmless but **Nettles** do sting terribly if touched, and **Pennyroyal** can be toxic, so it is best to identify these two in particular, so you can stay away from them. **Rosemary** is an evergreen member of the Mint Family.

Patchouli is not usually thought of as a member of the Mint Family, but it does show many of the characteristics, as it is insect-repelling, strongly aromatic, anti-microbial. It is highly prized for perfumes, incense and to flavor chewing tobacco. Patchouli has been associated with the hippie movement, because it was used to mask the smell of Marijuana. Very recognizeable, Patchouli is also one of the most *disliked* and triggering smells, while simultaneously being one of the best loved! Patchouli Oil was **embedded in the plastic** of the Masters of the Universe toy, **Stinkor** (made by Mattel in 1985) making it true to its name.

LAURACEAE ~ Laurel Family ~ aromatic leaves & bark, flowering shrubs & trees, sometimes evergreen, with alternate shiny, leathery leaves. Most of the flowers are small, yellow and strong-scented, and the fruits are berries or drupes.

☙ Avocado, Cinnamon, Bay Laurel (Bay Leaf), Sassafras, Camphor Tree, Litsea Cubeba, Spicebush, Lindera, Ocotea

2850 SPECIES PROVIDE MANY ESSENTIAL OILS - highly valued for medicinal herbs, spices & perfumes, and wood for timber and furniture.

Avocado (also known as **Alligator Pear**) is considered a large *berry* with a single seed, and its aromatic leaves can be ground into a spice that tastes like Anise. Wood from **Lauraceae** trees has a high essential oil content, so it repels pests and thus is found unmarred and of high quality. **Bay Leaf** is an evergreen aromatic herb usually added to sauces and soups for flavor, but it makes a lovely fragrant tea and is supportive for the heart, may lower blood pressure, and is helpful for migraine prevention. The Oracles at Delphi used the smoke of **Bay** to inspire their visions and hallucinations.

LEGUMINOSAE ~ Pea & Bean Family ~ renamed, see FABACEAE

LILIACEAE ~ Lily Family ~ showy flower with parts of three, flower actually made of 3 sepals and 3 petals usually identical in size and color so they look 6-petaled, deeply lobed and funnel shaped, with landing strip color changes guiding pollinators toward the center, 6 stamens (sometimes only 3 with very polleny heads), one large showy pistil. Parallel veins in the leaves like stripes. Flower matures into a 3-parted seed capsule. Lilies grow from starchy bulbs or corms rich in inulin polysaccharides.

☙ Day Lily, Tiger Lily, Glacier Lily, Sego Lily, Tulip, Mariposa Lily, Fritillaria, Toad Lily, Stargazer Lily

610 SPECIES - NEARLY ALL LILY FLOWERS ARE EDIBLE* Originally 3700 species, currently Botanists disagree about categorizing this Family, and have tried to split it into as many as 70 subfamilies!

Lily flowers make amazing fritters stuffed with goat cheese and quick-fried in a light batter, or as dramatic salad garnishes. Lily buds can be sauteed or steamed like vegetables. **Tulip** bulbs are edible when cooked, be sure to use those you have grown yourself for more than one year, or from an organic source, as commercially they are usually sprayed with fungicides.

> *This edibility does not include **Lily of the Valley** which is poisonous (and **not** actually a true Lily at all, but in the new **Asparagaceae** Family), or **Death Camas** (very poisonous).

ALLIUMS ~ Onion Family ~ a sub-Family of Liliaceae, bulb-ended on a firm stalk, ending in long green leaves, with compound BALL flowers. Have a paper-thin bract wrapped around the flower in simple umbels or advanced full spheres. The onion-scented sulfur glycoside compounds in this Family are notorious - **if it smells like an Onion, it is one, and it is edible**. Alliums are digestive helpers, powerful expectorants.

❧ **Onion, Garlic, Chives, Leeks, Ramps, Wild Onions, Ramsons**

925 SPECIES ALL EDIBLE — like the Lilies to which they are related.

Garlic is especially medicinal and helpful as a strong antiviral, cough reliever for colds, to lower cholesterol and blood pressure, and for remediating candida and resistant infections. Make **Garlic Honey** - simply add cleaned and peeled Garlic cloves into Honey and take liberally after a month or two. It is one of the best remedies ever! **Onions** are fascinating in that they absorb airborne bacteria, so try to eat them freshly cut only, completely avoid on salad bars. Onions can be used to clean and clear the air of bacteria in sickrooms and make great poultices on the feet if you can stand them!

MALVACEAE ~ Mallow & Cacao Family ~ Hibiscus-style flower with 5 separate petals fused at the base in a funnel, around a main large & showy pistil with many striking stamen. Leaves look like a ruffled fan and are slippery. All parts of the plant are mucilaginous when crushed and can be used like Aloe. Flowers and later large fruits with many seeds grow right out of the limbs of trees in this Cacao Family.

❧ **Cacao, Cotton, Okra, Macambo, Hollyhock, Durian, Linden Tree, Marshmallow, Hibiscus, Mallow, Rose of Sharon, Baobab, Blue Malva, Kola Nut**

MORE THAN 4200 SPECIES ALL EDIBLE - Many of Earth's most important food, textile & commerce plants come from this Family. **Cotton** is used worldwide in clothing and is probably on your body right now. Cotton does have medicinal properties, though it is highly pesticided, poisonous and abortifacient at high doses, so it is technically considered the only *inedible* Mallow.

Cacao is the Most Delicious of the Malvaceae! Here is her glorious Hibiscus-like flower. You will usually find **Vanilla** (Orchid Family) as a vine growing right on Cacao Trees, as they love to grow together. Cacao is the true name for the plant from which we make **Chocolate**. We have mistakenly called it **"Cocoa"** all of our lives because of a spelling error that was made in merchant transactions in England in the 18th Century! Cacao is more accurate, and usually indicates the RAW, sugar-free, and original form of "chocolate" which we enjoy today as Cacao Nibs, Beans, Fruit, and Powder. I add Nibs to my oatmeal, cookies, salads, chia cereal - everything.

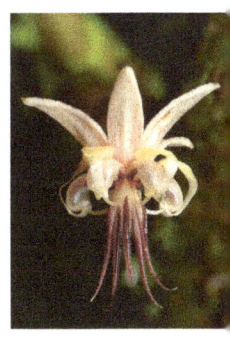

Okra is actually an edible fruit and a kind of **Hibiscus,** and it is slimy and gooey like they all are! The mucilaginous leaves of the **Mallow Family** are great for burns and sunburn. All members of this Family can be made more texturally edible when used in pesto, sauces, or smoothie additives, and most are quite good as pot greens.

MYRTACEAE ~ Myrtle & Tea Tree Family ~
are ancient woody trees and shrubs characterized by oval leathery evergreen leaves. They have shiny oil glands, which account for the many aromatic oils and strong spices that come from this potent Family. Flower parts in multiples of four or five, often star-shaped with many stamens.

- Tea Tree, Clove, Guava, Allspice, Eucalyptus, Manuka, Bay Rum Tree, CamuCamu, Paperbark, Surinam Cherry, Ohi'a Lehua, Bottlebrush, Java Plum, Feijoa, Rose-Apple, Lemon Myrtle, Syzygium

OVER 5900 SPECIES MANY EDIBLE - some of our great Food, Essential Oil and Medicine Plants come from this Family.

Tea Tree, Clove and **Eucalyptus** essential oils are veritable first aid kits in a jar, and can be used to treat nearly any body ailment. Botany experts believe this Family dates back to 56-60 million years ago.

ORCHIDACEAE ~ Orchid Family ~
evergreen, bilateral symmetrical flowers, usually 5 petals and a cone, fused stamens, very small seeds. These are perennial plants that lack any real woody, permanent framework and may exist on air alone. Orchids are cosmopolitan, they can grow in all Earthly locales except for glaciers. Orchids are cultivated and hybridized, prized and collected for their beauty.

- Vanilla, Dendrobium, Coral Root, Dragon's Mouth, Venus Slipper, Early Purple Orchid, Cattleyas, Fairy Slipper, Spider Orchid, Ladies Tresses

28,000 SPECIES - BLOOMS OF ALL ORCHIDS EDIBLE - the 2nd largest Plant Family.

The Karma Orchid is a deep magenta & white beauty grown for leis, but you would also recognize it from garnishes on plates all over the World. It is completely edible.

Vanilla is the most famous and only edible fruit-bearing Orchid in the World. We utilize most the extract of its fermented fruit pod. **Dendrobiums** have a long history of use in Chinese and Japanese Medicine for cancer, indigestion, headaches, eye disorders, and fertility treatments.

OXALIDACEAE ~ **Oxalis or Wood Sorrel Family** ~ small plants, shrubs and even some trees, with sour-flavored, heart-shaped shamrock leaves, full of Vitamin C, and flower parts in 5's. Plants display "sleep movements" spreading open in full light and closing in the dark. Grow all over the World except for polar areas.

⬥ Wood Sorrels, Purple Shamrock, Iron Cross, Oca, Carambola (StarFruit), Redwood Sorrel, Bilimbi, Candy Cane Sorrel, Sourgrass

900 SPECIES - MANY WITH EDIBLE PARTS

Small Family that gets its **Oxalidaceae** name from the presence of Oxalic Acid which is sour-tasting, and should be avoided in people who are prone to kidney stones.

Wood Sorrel is a great source of Vitamin C and minerals when hiking, and can be used as a survival food in the wild. To make a great hangover remedy, steep a handful of leaves in boiled water for 10 minutes. Drink hot or cold for a soothing and sour, liver-friendly remedy that will ease nausea and headache.

PASSIFLORACEAE ~ **Passion Flower Family** ~ circular and symmetrical, wildly ornate flower with multiple sepals and fringe, with a climbing vine and 3-lobed leaves, and curly-cue tendrils for grasping as it climbs. The fruit is a delicacy. Passion Flower is also associated with Jesus and the crucifix with its large cross-shaped pistil.

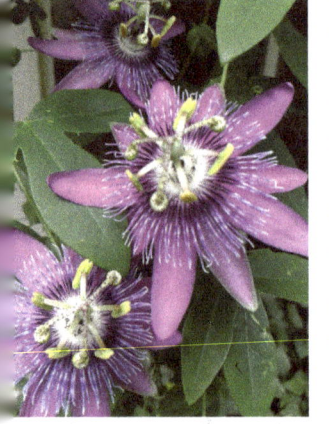

⬥Clematis, Passion Flower, Maypop, Turnera Granadilla, Adenia, Astrophea,

750 SPECIES - USUALLY EDIBLE FRUIT, grown as ornamentals and found in the wild as well.

Passion Flowers are all very nervine (soothing to the nerves), and make wonderful tea additions. These abundant vines and flowers are great companions, indoors in pots they will grow freely all over your windows and doorways. I had one that grew two stories up into the staircase of my log cabin, and even in Colorado it thrived indoors!

POACEAE ~ Grass Family ~

hollow stemmed, tall sturdy grasses, rows of seed capsules at top of long stalks are the flowers. They are wind-pollinated, so they don't need to invest energy in dramatic or showy flowers to attract pollinators. Grasses generally have knees or nodes in stems, and they are designed to withstand frequent cutting, to produce harvests often and abundantly.

- Rice, Corn, Wheat, Barley, Rye, Millet, Oats, Vetiver, Bamboo, Lemongrass, Teff, Spelt, Hay, Thatch, Straw, Cereal Grasses, Pampas Grass, Lawn Grass, Kentucky Bluegrass

ALL 12,000 SPECIES EDIBLE - *The most economical Food Family,* feeding the World inexpensively for generations. Eaten in moderation, Grasses are great survival foods.

Grasses are the dominant vegetation in most areas. They feed large as well as small animals, and in emergency food crises can feed people. Grasses provide Grains which make up more than 51% of the dietary energy available worldwide, generally consumed in some form at every meal. There is much controversy about whether or not Grains are healthy, but many of the accompanying health problems arise from pesticide contamination in non-organic Grains. Every body is different and some cannot tolerate what other cultures live on, but most live on Grasses of some kind.

Lemongrass is the most fragrant of the grasses. It is a potent medicinal herb and essential oil that kills *E.coli* and *Staph*, and has been used to treat parasites, herpes, cholera and cancer, as well as colds, fever, flatulence and insomnia! Topically it is helpful for arthritis and painful inflammations, and a bath with Lemongrass can relieve aching muscles.

POLYGONACEAE ~ Buckwheat Family ~

has an interesting flower, but is characteristically named for swollen knees or nodes on stems. The Latin name means "*many knees*" and also relates to the many seeds they produce. Curly or ruffled (but toothless) leaves are common, simple and alternating leaves, all clasp the stems at their base. Lots of small flowers with no actual petals in clusters & spikes. Triangular-shaped seeds, sometimes lens-shaped, many in a tall cone, sometimes with wings.

- **Rhubarb, Buckwheat, Fo-Ti, Yellow Dock, Knotweed, Bistort, Curly Dock, Sea Grape, Wild Buckwheat** *(Erigonum),* **Mountain Sorrel, Japanese Knotweed**

1200 SPECIES MANY EDIBLE - Buckwheat Family plants grow all over the World and include some of the most prolific weeds, like Knotweed. But there are strong food crops in this Family as well.

Buckwheat is not a wheat and not in the Grass Family so it is known as a **pseudocereal**. Its grain is a distinctly different kind of *triangular* groat that is gluten-free and high in Protein, Fiber, Vitamins and Minerals. Many cultures make Buckwheat noodles, known as Soba in Japan, and Buckwheat is used in the production of gluten-free beer.

Fo-Ti is a medicinal herb that is known to prevent and repair grey hair. It is a full body tonic and one of the tastiest herbs to snack on, as its root is dried and cut into large, thin chips that taste sweet.

ROSACEAE ~ **Rose Family** ~ trees and bushes with abundant 5-petaled, 5-sepaled, cup-shaped flowers, lots of stamens radiating from the center, alternate oval, serrated leaves. Flowers are showy and fill the entire tree or bush in Spring.

- **Apple, Apricot, Peach, Strawberries, Quince Plum, Pear, Cherry, Almond, Rosehips & Wild Rose, Nectarine, Loquat, Serviceberry, Blackberries, Raspberries, Crabapple, Hawthorn, Rowan, Chokecherry, Blackthorn, Medlar, Prairie Smoke, Silverweed, Cinquefoil, Potentilla, Mountain Ash, Meadowsweet, Yellow Avens,**

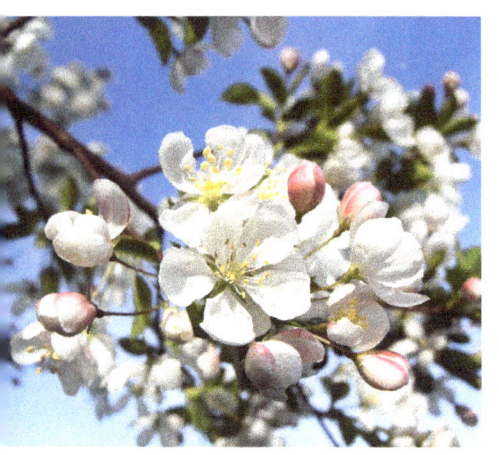

OVER 4800 SPECIES - MOST OF THE EDIBLE FRUITS. One of the **six most important food crop Families**, fruits of the **Rosaceae** are eaten everyday, by people and animals worldwide.

Leaves of the plants in this Family are astringent with tannins that tighten tissues, like **Raspberry Leaf which** helps tighten, tone and prepare the Uterus for Motherhood, and also helpful for soothing swellings, wounds, and easing diarrhea. **Rose Family** plants provide forage food for wildlife, as well as nectar & pollen for pollinators, and then fruit and medicine for all! Cyanide and amygdalin compounds are found in the leaves, seeds and pits.

RUBIACEAE ~ **Coffee, Madder or Bedstraw Family** ~ simple opposite leaves, "interpetiolar stipules" (little hooks or straws coming off the stem), tubular

flowers which produce nectar for pollinators, sometimes multiple in a ball shape, with inferior ovary. Grows as shrubs, trees and flowers all over the World.

- **Coffee, Cat's Claw, Gardenia, Cleavers, Woodruff, Cinchona, Kratom, Noni, African Medlar Fruit, African Peach, Breonadia, Ipecacuanha, Rose Madder, Gallium, Morinda, Yohimbe, Chacruna**

13,500 SPECIES - 4th LARGEST FLOWERING FAMILY - Super medicinal plants in this Family, some very **psychoactive**.

Coffee is one of the most economically important plants on Earth, as it does *power* the World. It alters the mental as well as the physical state. **Rose Madder** makes a beautiful red dye that was used to dye textiles by the Egyptians, and was found in the tomb of King Tutankamen. It was used in cave and tomb painting when mixed with minerals including gypsum. **Cinchona Bark** is a natural source of Quinine.

Chacruna *(Psychotria viridis)* contains natural DMT, and is one of the two plants used to brew ***Ayahuasca***. It is considered a supreme Plant Teacher in the Amazon rainforest. The second partner plant is *Banisteriopsis caapi*, (also called **Caapi**, **Jagube**, or **Yage**) and it is also a Teacher Plant from the Malpighiaceae Family.

SOLANACEAE ~ Nightshade Family ~

have alternate leaves, flower parts in 5's with united petals often in trumpet or star shapes, and fruit is double-celled with colorless juice. Solanaceae refers to the *sleep-inducing* properties of many Nightshades, and the fact that many plants in this family are **narcotic, addictive and deadly**.

- **Tomatoes, Potatoes, Bell & Chili Peppers, Eggplant, Sacred Datura, Cayenne Pepper, Ashwagandha, Pimentos, Tobacco, Jalapeno, Petunia, Goji Berry, Tabasco, Paprika, Tomatillo, Cape Gooseberry, Chinese Lantern, Goldenberry, Henbane, Deadly Nightshade** (also known as **Belladonna** *Atropa belladonna)*, **Mandrake, Groundcherry**

2700 SPECIES - 4th LARGEST FLOWERING FAMILY. Nightshades are one of the biggest food families as well, packed with super nutrition.

Some people are sensitive to the alkaloids in the **Solanaceae**. But many sensitivities occur because of the way they are *prepared* and the things we pair them with (eaten before ripe, deep-fried, or slathered with heavy dairy, like baked potatoes). **Potatoes** provide courage, are strongly antiviral, full of the amino acid lysine, and should be *added* to the diet, not subtracted.

Hot Peppers are full of Vitamin C, and they stimulate the release of pleasure-chemical endorphins, so they are consequently mood-altering, as well.

Goji Berry is one of the most healing, antioxidant foods on the Planet. It raises low testosterone levels, strengthens the immune system, and supports hormone production. It is helpful for many ailments including eye problems, vertigo, senility, tinnitus, hypoglycemia, hair loss, high blood pressure, menopause and more, and is a longevity tonic for the liver and kidneys.

URTICACEAE ~ The Nettle Family ~ a sub-Family of Lamiaceae (Mints)

❦ Stinging Nettle, Wood Nettle, Clearweed *(stingless)*

Hidden hairs sting and release formic acid into the skin causing painful rashes. The remedy for **Stinging Nettle** usually grows right next to the plant. Look for **Jewelweed** or a ruffly-leaved **Dock**. Crush and rub on the Nettle rash for relief.

VIOLACEAE ~ Violet Family ~ heart-shaped, deeply veined, simple alternate or basal leaves, with low-growing ground flowers on single long stem. Can be ruffly lobed flower with 5 petals, 2 on top, 2 on the sides and one more on the bottom, narrow and usually striped.

❦ Violet, Viola, Pansies, Johnny-Jump-Up, Hybanthus

1000 SPECIES - ALL EDIBLE - Some people get digestive distress from the Yellow flowers in particular. It is necessary to keep the edible flowers organic (no pesticides).

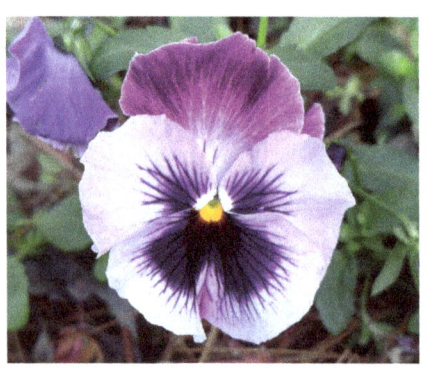

Violet Leaves are heart-shaped and tasty salad greens, high in Vitamin C, and the flowers are perfect for decorating desserts, cookies and salads. **Violet Leaf & Flower** are soothing, cooling and helpful for lung ailments, and clear heat and swellings from the body. Violet-scented liqueurs, flavored candies and desserts were popular during the Victorian era, before World War I. Look under Violet in the **Weeds** section for recipes and details. **Pansies** are my very favorite edible flower. They are SOOO gorgeous in a salad, on chicken, over veggies - and people always ooh and ahh that they can eat them! They come in every color imaginable, so this year I am going to plant a Rainbow Pansy Garden *just* for eating.

ZINGIBERACEAE ~ Ginger Family ~ creeping, rhizome-producing tropical plants with mouth-like, long tube, or beehive-like compound flowers, with long thin basal leaves that overlap to form the pseudostem.

- **Ginger, Turmeric, Black Turmeric, Cardamom, Galangal, Myoga, Grains of Paradise** *(Melegueta)*, **Shell Ginger, Thai Ginger, Korarima**

1600 SPECIES OF POTENT MEDICINE - some of our finest analgesic and anti-inflammatory medicinal herbs (used for milennia) are in this Family.

Turmeric is one of the Earth's strongest anti-inflammatory healing herbs, with uses from arthritis to cancer, eczema to yeast overgrowth. It has powerful staining dye principles and can be used instead of yellow food-coloring. Do not use it in the tub or you (and the tub) will be yellow for weeks! I found out the hard way, and spent lots of time explaining my yellow feet and hands.

Ginger is a "Wonder Spice" as Paul Shulick, who founded New Chapter Vitamins, wrote in his Ginger book. It can literally heal just about anything. My very first product for my company Little Moon was *Letting Go*, a potent Ginger Detox Bath I formulated because of his book and research. An organic Ginger Bath works wonders for every ailment from pain to chills to hangover relief! **Banana** is in a related family (Musaceae).

ZYGOPHYLLACEAE ~ Caltrop Family ~ trees, shrubs, or herbs of the desert, parts in 5's with alternate and pinnate leaves. Like many desert dwellers, they have thorns, stipules, spines and burrs. Stemhave swollen nodes for storing water.

- **Chaparral, Creosote Bush, Tribulus Terrestris** *(Puncture Vine or Goat-Head)*, **Syrian Rue, Lignum Vitae, Orange Caltrop** *(Arizona Poppy)*

285 SPECIES ALL VERY POTENT - highly aromatic and oily.

These survivors of the Desert are actually ***ancient plants*** that protect themselves with thorns and bristles and turpentine-like medicines. They make great fire starters.

Lignum Vitae (Guaiacum) is now an endangered member of this Family as it was over harvested for its many medicinal properties, known for healing arthritis to syphilis. It is also called "the Tree of Life" and is the hardest wood in the world, reported to be so dense it does not float.

"King Clone" *(Larrea tridentata)* is an **11,700 year-old Creosote Bush** ring in the Mojave Desert that is a whopping **67 feet wide!** It has been designated and definitively

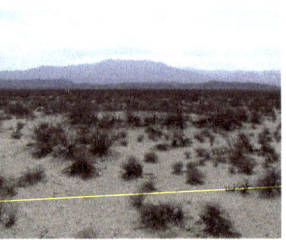

named by botanists to be the world's oldest living organism. King Clone is a true *"champion of survival,"* scientists believe it was one of the first Plants to take hold after the last glacier of the Ice Age retreated (about 12,000 years ago). It is so hardy that it has fought off every other plant for water in the desert, and has won. The wind moves all around the individual pods of plants, whose roots have created mounds of sand in protection. So they now grow on their own hills, providing some small shade for desert creatures. There are directions for visiting this stunning work of Nature in the Footnotes.[11]

FORAGING BY THE RULES

Before I take anything in the Wild, I first **greet the Plant**, and the Plant Spirit, with my Heart wide open, and say *"Hello."* I **ask for permission** from any Plant I seek to harvest, and take the time to await an answer. Usually it is yes, so I continue, explaining *"it's just a little haircut"* or something like that, while I harvest or prune. **I speak right to the Plant while I collect,** explaining all the many wonderful Medicines and Meals I plan to make with their contribution. I say *"Thank-you,"* and offer my great appreciation love, and respect. Make your own connection and you will know exactly what to do. Here are some other tips to Forage the *right way*, respecting each Plant and Creature.

1. **Search for the best and most abundant locations for harvesting that will make the least impact** on the Ecosystem. Remember you are harvesting Food that many other creatures eat. Never harvest more than ⅓ of what you find.

2. **Choose some Plants to look for, and identify positively through at least 3 sources** *before* you go into the field, and especially before you touch it or eat it. Bring a pillow case, glass jar, or organic muslin to gather your harvests - and a notebook for revelations, communications, and field notes.

3. **TAKE VERY FEW ROOTS**, and only a small percentage of what you find. Harvest roots infrequently and very sparingly (**as you are removing a plant forever**).

4. **Never forage for Plants closer than 100 feet to a road or parking lot,** to spare your body the intake of a harvest exposed to traffic exhaust chemicals, oil residue, rubber and microplastics. **Never collect Plants near any pesticide-sprayed fields** or questionable industrial locales.

5. **Keep your "wits on" in the wilderness** and listen for animals and other creatures at all times. Make sure to have a big stick at your side just in case!

6. **Identify possible dangerous Plants** before you go, know the poisonous ones to avoid. Keep an eye on the kids and make sure they stay away.

7. **Choose healthy and abundant Plants to take**, the ones that seem to call out to you. But **Leave the Big Grandmothers**, the biggest, oldest generations, alone. Sit with them instead, and listen to their stories, they are the sacred Elders.

8. **Always Double-Check First, Eat Later!** If you are not certain, don't eat it, *"when in doubt, leave it out,"* don't let the kids touch it, save it for later. Bring home a leaf cutting or a fruit or a flower to aid in your later identification.

FORAGING for Wild Foods that grow nearby helps you to discover a gift that was always there. Teach this skill to your children.

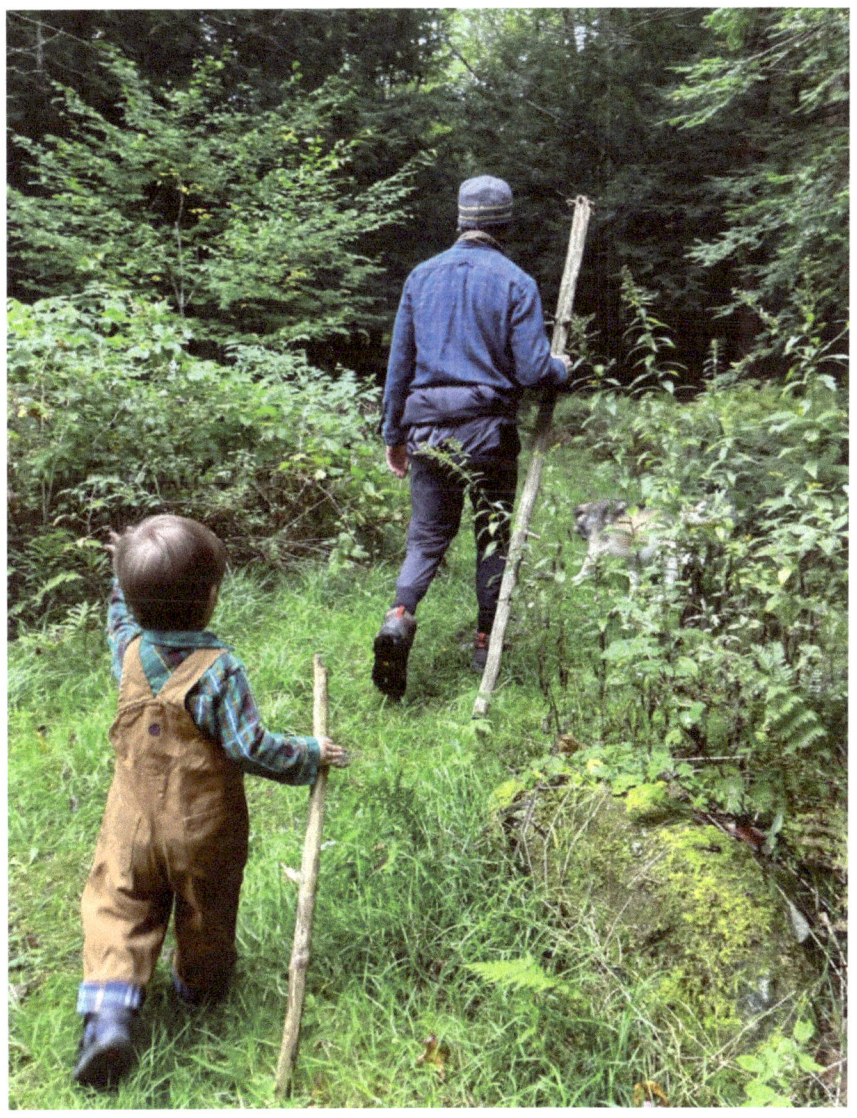

~ the garden of earth ~

MATERIA WEEDICA
The Mind-Blowing Secrets of 25 Wild EDIBLE Weeds

How do you choose *which* **Weeds to write about, from all the many wild and wonderful Outlaws?** I designed this book with *self-sufficiency and food preservation* in mind, so I chose the most obvious and most suitable for **EATING**. Most of these Wild Weed Foods grow right in your neighborhood and are generally considered the **easiest to identify correctly**. These are the plants that will come to your aid if you need them, can provide you with more than you can imagine, and will grow with no effort on your part! And, *Weeds look the same all over the world,* so they can provide you with convenient options anywhere you go - whether you are looking for Food to prepare, seasoning for your dinner, a trail snack, or Plants on which to literally survive.

Don't be put off by the **Latin botanical names**, learn from them. Common names are helpful, but the Latin is plant-specific and helps with exact identification. It is essential in communications between Herbalists and Experts, and when creating recipes. Plus the Latin names are absolutely guaranteed to impress your friends! If you pay close attention to these botanical names (as well as the many folk names for each Weed), they give clues about the Plant's traditional usage or something about its look, and may help you remember what the plant does. To learn more, notice and remind yourself of the characteristics of the **Plant Family** noted for each Wild Weed - then go meet them in the wild. You will begin to see the natural patterns being revealed to you about each one, until you finally feel you know WHO exactly each PLANT really is.

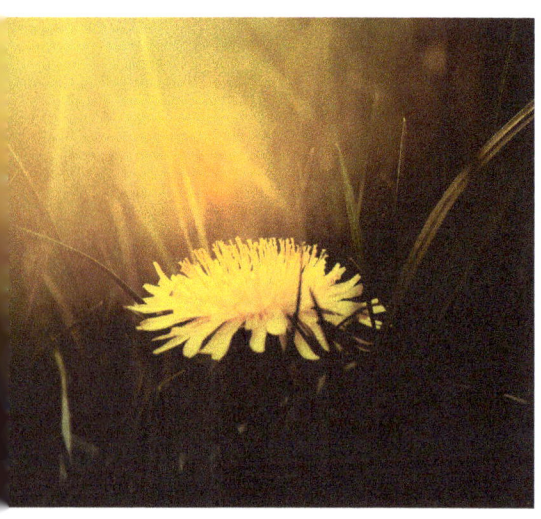

"If you see a Dandelion as a weed, you'll spray it. If you see it as a Flower, you'll draw it close, turn it this way and that, and become lost in the colossal burst of slender golden petals that spew sunshine into the darkest of souls. And so, how many things have we *sprayed* that could have illuminated our souls if we would have LET them be more than what we let them be?"

~ *Craig D. Lounsbrough*

NOW GO FIND THESE PLANTS, USE THEM & PROTECT THEM.

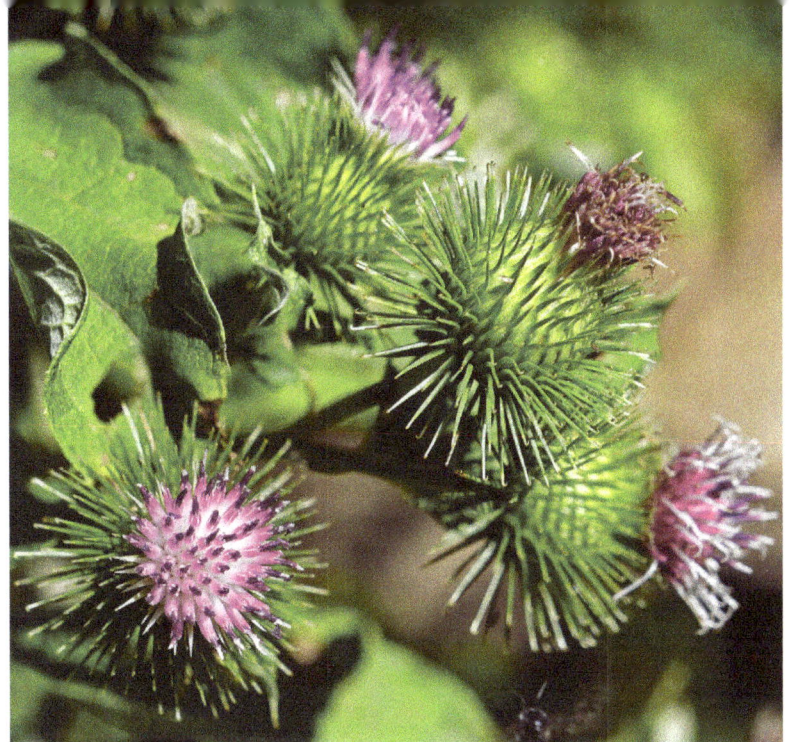

BURDOCK

Arctium lappa, Arctium minus   Sunflower Family/ **ASTERACEAE**

FOUND: In every state in the US except Alaska, Burdock covers disturbed ground in most Western states - Idaho, Wyoming, Colorado, Montana, Utah, New Mexico, Arizona, Nevada, and some In southern California, where it grows in middle altitudes of 5,000-8,000 feet. A native to Europe and Asia. Grows next to roads and paths where animals and humans drop the burrs, in damp areas near creeks and in empty lots.

IDENTIFYING FEATURES: THE BIG ROUND BURRS ON YOUR CLOTHES! Burdock makes lots of big, hairy prickly burrs from thistle-like purple flowers, assuring its seed is spread far and wide. The plant starts with already very big leaves as a seedling, in a low rosette the first year much like Mullein. Then it puts up a tall branched stalk, with hairy, wavy-edged large leaves and extensive veins, all with sandpapery texture. Stalk is somewhat striped and fibrous and NOT red like Rhubarb which it is confused with sometimes (Rhubarb has poisonous shiny and smooth leaves). Long carrot-like yellowy white root has dark brown skin, aromatic and fibrous, and can be 1-2 feet long. Seed capsule is inside the protection of the burr, with a bunch of shiny black seeds loose inside. Burdock seedlings sprout before most other green plants, so that makes them easy to spot and keep track of as an early food source.

FOOD: Burdock can provide food for a large portion of the year as the root can be harvested nearly all year. Young leaves can be eaten raw in salads. Older leaves must be boiled in several changes of water to be able to be eaten - and are not that great.

Better to use them as wrappings for cooking and storing food. Young stalks make a great celery substitute, harvest them before the plant sets flowerheads and the stalk gets hollow, and peel through 2 layers to the center meat which tastes reminiscent of artichoke hearts. The seeds will literally sprout anywhere you pull them off your clothes, so be constructive and make a place for dropping burdock burrs in your yard so you can have reliable food and medicine at the ready. Root is sweet, starchy and slightly bitter, should be peeled before cooking and can be roasted like a potato, cut up for stir fries, dried and pickled. Fresh juice of the root is soothing, cooling and particularly healing.

CONTAINS: Vitamin C, Calcium, Iron, Magnesium, Potassium, Zinc, Mucilage, Tannins, Flavonoids, Polyacetylenes, Inulin, Chlorogenic Acid, Lactone, Essential Oils. Seeds Contain Essential Fatty Acids, Arctigenin, and Actiin.

BODY BENEFITS: Blood Purifier and alterative, supports LIVER & SKIN - great for psoriasis, eczema, acne, and liver ailments. Root contains desmutagens which neutralize cancer-causing waste products and reduce fevers. Detoxifies the blood and supports the body during fasting. Burdock is a hitchhiker by Nature - it wants to be spread far and wide. It can be used to release that which hangs around too much, or to encourage healing expansion.

QUALITIES: Leaf is bitter, seed is pungent, stalk is similar to celery. The root is sweet, demulcent and soothing, calms and clears heat. Seeds are astringent, and leaves are anti-inflammatory. Burdock is adaptogenic, alterative, antibacterial, antifungal, antiinflammatory, antitussive, aphrodisiac, demulcent, diaphoretic, diuretic, expectorant, galactagogue, mild laxative, nutritive, and rejuvenative.

FOLKLORE: Folk names Beggar's Buttons, Gypsy Rhubarb, Bardana, Clotburr, Cocklebuttons, Hareburr, Burr Seed, Happy Major, Hardock. An Asian delicacy, you can find it on menus and in Asian markets as Gobo. French women wrapped their butter in the leaves of Burdock to take to market, which is one of the origins of the common name reflecting the French "*beurre*" for butter. The botanical name references the Latin words for "*bear*" and "*to seize*" - which refer to the hairy burrs that cling to everything!

FIRST AID USES: Leaves on soles of feet apparently cure gout, blisters or sprains, and you can use the tincture for lymph drainage when the throat feels constricted by swollen glands. Utilize fresh juice for inflammations and rashes.

SPIRITUAL PROPERTIES: Ruled by Venus and the Water Element, protective in Nature when burned, said to ward off negativity when scattered around the house. Feminine and flowing, the energy of the plant is known to be healing and loving.

MAGICAL USES: Scott Cunningham suggests digging the root in the waning moon, cutting it into small disks for beads, and threading onto red string while still fresh.

When dry, wear the necklace for protection against evil and negativity. Add Burdock root to protection sachets.

FLOWER ESSENCE: Cleansing and soothing, helps you break through obstacles and clear them away. Can remove anger or memories that feel "stuck on you." Helpful for children going on sleepovers or camp adventures where they may have a little trepidation. Has a protective, easing, and healing effect like a fairy grandmother.

PREPARATIONS: Michael Moore recommends digging the root SPARINGLY during the Spring of the plant's second year before it puts up its big stalk. Burdock is best dug with a long thin spade: dig a deep hole about 2-3 inches out from around base and about a foot down, loosen dirt and pull the root into it sideways, cut off the tough lowest end. Loosen seeds from their capsule with a rolling pin, by whacking the seeds in a cotton towel with a wooden spoon, or a quick pulse in the blender. Tinctures of the seeds are remedies for joint pain and are known to be diuretic and astringent.

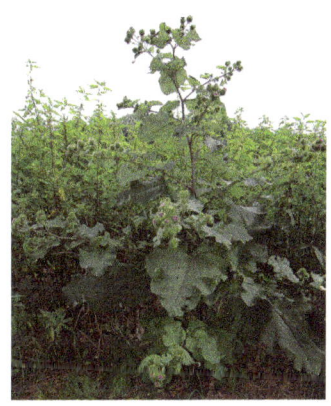

Extracts of the root are supportive for any inflammation. Teas are made with one rounded teaspoon of the dried root per cup of water, brought to a boil and then simmered for 20 minutes at least. MM recommends twice daily for at least 2 weeks, for skin disorders. Burdock makes a perfectly nutritious and soothing tea during fasting and can help with sore throats, mouth ulcers, abscesses, indigestion, unproductive coughs, . Use in small frequent doses. Fresh roots can be juiced and also pickled and preserved for winter. Brigitte Mars recommends burdock as a Bath herb for sore joints and gout. Leaves can be made into a poultice for ringworm. Compresses can be made from root and leaf for swellings, boils, sprains, swollen glands and tumors. Stalk must be peeled twice, then can be eaten raw like celery, made into spiralized noodles, cooked and split open and eaten with the teeth like artichokes, or chopped and cooked in stir-fries & stews. Leaves can be used like aluminum foil for cooking in campfires, or for wrapping leftovers or found trail food. Burdock Vinegar can be made with a whole root and used for digestive upsets and for washing wounds, or rinsing the hair for dandruff. Flower stalks can be sliced and cooked in maple syrup or honey to make a kind of candy.

INVENTION: Velcro was invented in 1948 by Swiss engineer George de Mestral after a particularly burr-y walk with his dog. He examined the tiny curved hooks on the end of the Burdock burrs and how they clung to loops of nearly any fabric, as well as hair on his dog regardless of motion, and even the skin of his fingers. He realized there might be an application for a similar technology in the clothing business. He devised a loop and hook closure that became a standard in the industry based on his observations of Burdock. His trade name Velcro comes from a description of each side of the closure - "vel"vet on one side, "cro"chet hooks on the other.

LAURA: When I moved to Colorado in 1988, I had a bit of a time adjusting to the altitude, new water and climactic dryness. I had a big flare-up of skin inflammation, eczema that was wildly flushing and itching all over my face and body. Burdock tea, and juicing the fresh root, is one of the few things that helped put out the fire. I started to think of Burdock's cooling touch like a sweet, ancient Indian grandmother who would heal me with her soothing medicines. Twenty years later, I used Burdock when I was battling some histamine intolerance during menopause, experiencing Liver Fire Rising heat in the face. Again, Burdock cooled and sedated the Fire, soothed me right out, and seemed to also help the hot flashes! Recently, I have had dreams about Burdock, and have been using it as an antiviral and anti-inflammatory when it calls.

Upon researching, I discovered all the many more things this "simple" plant could do. Its disease-fighting effects are profound and its medicine is far from simple, as it has been used effectively for staph infections, PMS, mumps & measles, cancer, gonorrhea & syphilis, tonsillitis, urinary inflammation, rheumatism, jaundice, diabetes, smallpox, HIV, candida and prostate inflammation...the list goes on. In noticing the many viral conditions it treats, I thought I'd point out how much the flower looks like a virus molecule. Another great clue (and wink) from the Plant Kingdom. I imagine that Burdock could be soothing much of the current viral panic, symptoms, & problems of "the latest viruses" - if we'd just befriend and use it.

If you can't find it growing nearby, this precious "WEED" can now be purchased as seed and grown as a medicinal food plant. Now that's a positive improvement in stature for a once-discarded weed! As I get older, I realize I lived through a generation who lost their love for plants and began eradicating them. Thanks to Herbalists (like Richo Cech below) who sell the seeds and techniques for growing Burdock yourself. And great gratitude is given to all the Weed Enthusiasts everywhere for helping us reclaim these special plants.

> **"If digging is not your thing, take an old bale of wet hay and knock together four 1 x 4 boards to create an empty-bottomed flat, to fit right on top of the hay bale. Then fill this with garden soil and plant your Burdock seeds in there. They will germinate and send their roots down into the hay. To harvest, remove the boards and pull apart the hay to reveal perfectly formed and tender Burdock roots."**
>
> *~Richo Cech*

https://strictlymedicinalseeds.com/product/burdock-gobo-arctium-lappa-packet-of-100-seeds-organic

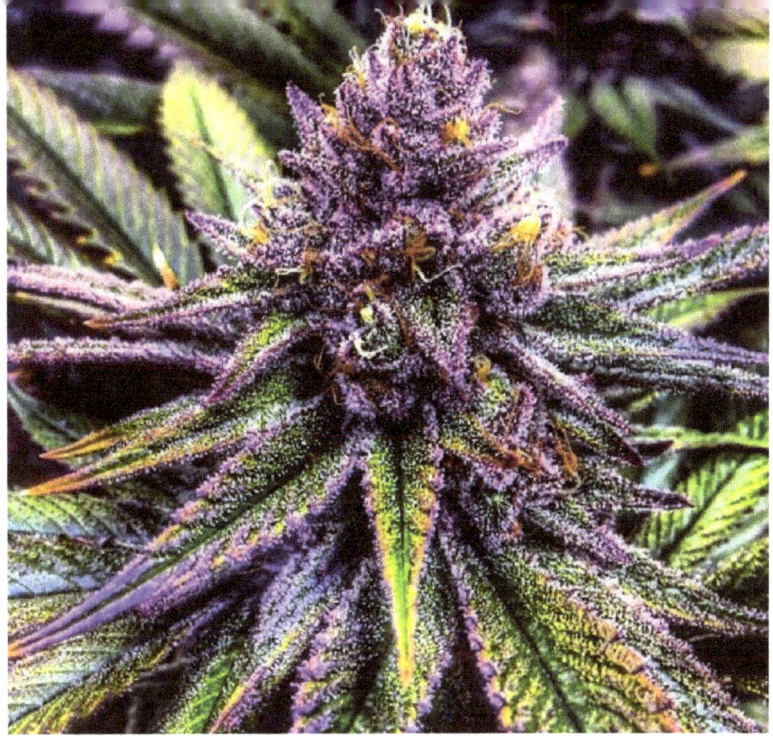

CANNABIS

Cannabis sativa, Cannabis indica Hemp Family/ **CANNABCEAE**

FOUND: Depending on variety, Cannabis grows all over the world, wild, farmed and cultivated for Food and Medicine.

IDENTIFYING FEATURES: Serrated edge, compound leaf with odd number of leaflets in a fan shape, growing on sturdy stalks, with cone-shaped, compound bud flowers rising above the plant with no petals, but 5 stamen, including many hairs and a tantalizing, sparkly dust. These are called the "trichomes" - which on closer observation look like crystal droplets growing out of the leaves, but which are actually the essential oil factories that produce a resin so strong-smelling and tasting it is repellent to animals and pests. This combination of chemicals also protects the flower from wind, cold, fungus and parasites, and produces the medicinal cannabinoids and terpenes. Members of the Hemp Family are characteristically dioecious, meaning there are male plants and female plants with different features. The Female plant provides the medicinal flowers and nutritious seeds.

FOOD: This one plant can provide nearly every single nutrient the body needs from its leaves, seeds, stems, and stalk. Hemp Seed is one of the most nutritious foods on the Planet, full of protein and essential fatty acids. And it has NO psychoactive properties so you can add it to every salad and smoothie you make. Bhang (a juiced-leaf drink very popular around the world) is an incredible way to derive nutrition from spare leaves. Many different foods can be made with the seed, flower and leaves including dairy-free milk and cheese, soy-free tofu and vegan protein meat alternatives as well as side dishes and desserts galore. With the emergence of legal recreational Marijuana, some states now boast entire restaurants dedicated to food that is paired with the plant as it is smoked, or utilizing its many flavor compounds in fascinating new infused cocktails and gourmet dishes.

CONTAINS More than 150 Phytocannabinoids, Magnesium, Calcium, Phosphorus, Essential Fatty Acids (perfect 3:1 ratio of Omega 3 to Omega 6), Fiber, Polyphenols, Sterols, Protein, Trace Minerals, Essential Oils, Flavonoids, Amino Acids including Lysine & Arginine, Terpenes, Choline, Inositol, Enzymes & Lipids. Low in Carbohydrates.

BODY BENEFITS: Extensive and highly medicinal. Your body's Endocannabinoid System is a balancing, full-body system that not only works with cannabinoids from this plant and others, but also makes its own cannabinoids internally. Childbirth is an event a Mother needs to "forget" in order to repeat it with more children, and her body releases endocannabinoids into the bloodstream to ease the anxiety and lessen the painful memory. *Because it does slow thinking, reflex and reaction time down it is wise not to drive, operate machinery, or engage in activities that require swift focus when using this plant.

QUALITIES: Feminine in energy, nurturing and soothing but in a strong and potent way when necessary. Cannabis is psychoactive, aromatic, expansive and renewing, and balancing, regulating for all body systems. Analgesic, anesthetic, anticonvulsant, antidepressant, antiemetic, anti inflammatory, antispasmodic, aphrodisiac, appetite stimulant, bronchodilator, cerebral sedative, euphoric, hallucinogenic, hypnotic, hypotensive, vasodilator.

FOLKLORE: Folk names Hemp, Weed, Pot, Ganja, Pakalolo, Kaya, Spleef, Wacky Weed, Chanvre, Gallowgrass, Neckweede, Tekrouri, Kif, Hanf, Hippie Lettuce, Nodge. Used for millennia as a food crop, dispersed around the globe through trade and travel. Early ritual use from 3000 years ago was confirmed in China and the Pamir mountains of Tajikistan in Central Asia, and in Israel in the 8th century BC. "Bhang" is served at wedding banquets to spread an immense amount of happiness to all participants.

FIRST AID USES: Stress and Anxiety relief: use CBD oil for anxiety attacks, tremors, and nerve disorders, hold liquid in mouth under tongue for immediate results. CBD is also effective for remedying overindulgence in THC (feeling "too high"). Cannabis smoke is a **bronchodilator** and expectorant (traditionally used for asthma), and in a Harvard study has been proven to actually be **good for the lungs** in moderation.[12]

SPIRITUAL PROPERTIES: Ruled by Saturn and the Water Element which is an odd pairing - I guess Saturn builds the foundational vessel for the emotional work of Water. Spiritual revelation and self-actualization are the spiritual actions of this plant as it opens the fabric of the known matrix and expands awareness. Cannabis aids in meditation, bringing the brainwave to the Alpha level very quickly (the slower state found in deep meditation). Many people find it helpful for inner journeying and relaxation. Shamanic indigenous rituals all over the World are accompanied by the smoking of the Peace Pipe or the use of Cannabis in incense and drinks. Rastafarians smoke the herb in their Bible-based religion to bring them closer to Jah (God). They hold sacred ceremonies called "Reasonings" to meditate deeply, pray, ponder and discuss all the latest issues.

MAGICAL USES: Cannabis has a long history of magical and shamanic use that was stunted in the US by the still-on-the-books laws of the 1930's laws restricting its use and sale. Recent generations only know it as a restricted plant and many may have missed its many abilities. Love spells and smoke-scrying divinations were made more potent with Cannabis, and it was used as an additive to meditation incense. Useful for visions and divining when burned with Mugwort, sometimes utilizing a mirror, candle, water bowl or crystal ball. "Hemp" is actually the old Witch's name for Marijuana. Cannabis allows one to slip in between realities to view the future and aids clairvoyance.

FLOWER ESSENCE: It helps you lighten up, removes the heavy load, unburdens and opens the heart, and adjusts the attitude. Cannabis Flower Essence helps to clarify your will and in mental freedom, spiritual liberation and enhances the ability to stand tall. This is a great way to experience the mood-altering Spirit of the plant without smoking.

PRACTICAL USES: Avocado used to say you could build, run, fuel, and feed an entire airline all with the Hemp Plant - planes, runways, seats, food, pilots and all. Hemp can be used to make a plastic, wood or concrete substitute that is stronger and more weather- and pest-resistant for building. Hemp oil can be made into fuel, a fact Big Gasoline never wanted us to discover. You can make rope, textiles, upholstery, clothing, shoes, seatbelts, paper and newspaper, insulation, tea bags, packaging and food from Hemp fiber. Other parts of the plant can be used in the production of cosmetics, internal and external body remedies, ink, wood preservatives, detergent, soaps, lamp oil, carpet, shopping bags, surfboards and batteries. Medicines and anxiety-soothers are widely made with Cannabis these days, powered by THC, CBD, CBG and its many other cannabinoids. Let's face it - you would be hard-pressed to find a more worthy and useful plant.

LAURA: In his book *Botany of Desire*, **Michael Pollan** describes Cannabis as a plant that has domesticated us! It has convinced us to cultivate it and grow it abundantly, use it, sell it, make things with it, use it for recreation as well as for medicine. It has convinced us to farm it widely both indoors and outdoors until it has become the MOST DESIRED plant on the Planet. But is it a Weed?

Seeds of Cannabis germinate in one week, while most other seeds take 10-14 days. It grows voraciously, sometimes more than 2 inches in one day. It completely renews itself every 3 months and creates abundant seeds and will propagate and root by clones. It is wind-pollinated for ease, and some plants can reach up to 20 feet. Before a sanitation department worker (who will not be named) eradicated them in 1951, there were more than **41,000 pounds of Cannabis plants growing wild in New York City**. After the things you have learned about Weeds so far, what do you think? I think it definitively qualifies as a Weed, as well as one of the greatest food, fiber and medicine plants of all time! And I think some people qualify as murdering exterminators for trying to eradicate it, criminalise it and spread harmful disinformation about this God-given miracle plant.

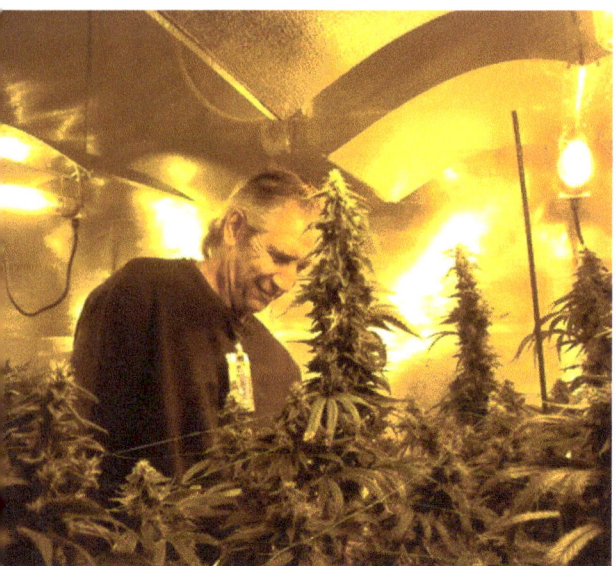

But there is hope for Humanity yet. **Dave Allen** worked in a commercial Medical Marijuana grow operation in Steamboat Springs, Colorado, running his own 500-plant warehouse for Rocky Mountain Remedies. During that time I got to visit a lot, and witness all the stages of the plants while he lovingly tended them (you'd be lucky to have a person look at you the way he looks at those plants!). I learned more with every visit to these beautiful and abundant creatures, and definitely developed a kinship with the Cannabis Spirit. One way to change your attitude about this plant is to watch it grow and feel its genuine positive energy. Seeing so many strains growing in one warehouse also taught me their differences. Here are some of my own research observations, and some anecdotal data I gathered on the major types of Cannabis, so you can understand their effects and definitively tell them apart!

SATIVA Nicknamed "sun-tea-va" ~ euphoric, energizing and mentally stimulating. Sativa helps you get up and keeps you going for tedious work or mental effort, way better than caffeine! It is the taller lanky species, **higher in THC and lower in CBD**, with long and narrow leaves, loose spear-like flower clusters. The entire plant has less chlorophyll so can exhibit other colors of orange and gold. These plants are more wild, tall and leggy and can grow more than 12 feet tall, and have thin, sword-like leaves. Sativas grow better in hotter climates near the Equator, Central America,

Africa and Western Asia. They also take longer to grow than Indicas and have smaller medicinal harvests. Sativas are cerebral, bring inspiration and a brighter awareness to the mind, they are uplifting like brain candy, physically energizing and can make one giggly. They heighten all sensation, and sensationalize all input, increasing serotonin uptake, which is the positive mood, "happiness" brain chemical. These are the best strains to use for migraine and other headaches and can be good for nausea without being heavy. Sativa is the perfect plant for focus, learning and creativity. It raises the appetite and lowers the awareness of pain. There are some Sativa strains that are higher in CBD like Charlotte's Web and many hybrids.

GREAT FOR daytime, more alert use - WORK, FOCUS, STUDYING, CREATING, HIKING, SHOPPING or HOUSEWORK.

FAMOUS CHEMOVARS / SATIVA STRAINS: MAUI WOWIE, ACAPULCO GOLD, SOUR DIESEL, CHARLOTTE'S WEB, HEADBAND, JUICY FRUIT, AGENT ORANGE, LIME GREEN SKUNK, SUPERNATURAL, TRAINWRECK, PURPLE HAZE, GRAPEFRUIT, PANAMA RED, LEMON HAZE, JACK THE RIPPER, STRAWBERRY COUGH, AC/DC, STRAWBERRY BANANA, PANAMA RED, JACK HERER, MOBY DICK, HAWAIIAN SNOW, AMNESIA HAZE, DURBAN POISON, GODFATHER, SUPER GLUE, SUPER SILVER HAZE, GREEN CRACK, CANDYLAND

INDICA
Nicknamed "in-da-couch" ~ heavy, euphoric and sedative, higher in CBD but not always lower in THC. With short and broad, extra dense leaves and chunky solid flower clusters, this type of plant is short and stocky and wide. These plants have more chlorophyll and the buds are fatter and broader, tending toward darker colors of deep green and purple. Indicas tend to have their ancestral roots in the Himalayas, Turkey, India, Afghanistan, Pakistan and SE Asia. Their energy is more downward motion action, and they act mainly on the physical body, and are generally higher in CBD. This makes Indicas the choice for chronic pain relief, insomnia, anxiety, tremors, nausea and inflammation, and nerve damage of fibromyalgia and MS. A good Indica will make people feel better emotionally, and promote a deep relaxation that makes their physical bodies respond with better healing. There is a noticeable body buzz with Indicas, as it increases dopamine, the "pleasure" brain chemical. Indicas slow the brain way down, sedate the body, and can make it hard to think and remember things. This is the reason for the quintessential stoner attribute: "no term" memory! These are the strains that are famous for relieving eye pressure for Glaucoma relief. These are also the strains that assist with "forgetting" - a crucial component to healing PTSD in veterans. Indicas are mostly used for major pain-relief and can replace opioid addictions. Used for preventing seizures, spasms, and convulsions in Epilepsy, Parkinson's and other nerve disorders. Indicas are helpful for nausea and increasing appetite in chemotherapy. May be very helpful for autism and social disorders.

GREAT FOR nighttime, sedated use **- for SLEEP, PAIN, TENSION, UNWINDING AFTER WORK, SPACING OUT, DAYDREAM CREATING.**

FAMOUS CHEMOVARS / INDICA STRAINS: NORTHERN LIGHTS, PURPLE KUSH, PURPLE URKLE, BUBBA KUSH, GRAPE APE, HINDU KUSH, PENNYWISE, GRANDADDY PURPS, AFGHANI, G-13 (*US government's own research strain from the 70's*), **AURORA INDICA, L.A. CONFIDENTIAL, BLUEBERRY, PAKISTAN VALLEY, BLACK D.O.G., SUGAR BREATH, HASH PLANT, CHOCOLATE MINT OG, KOSHER KUSH, AFGHAN KUSH, WHITE RHINO, BLUE CHEESE**

HELPFUL HYBRIDS

A combined hybrid strain has a more cultivated, balanced action can be useful at night as well as in the daytime - all-purpose. These were created to balance the effects of two kinds of strains, to get the best of both. Many cultivators experiment with breeding Cannabis plants for different effects, flavors, aromas, and percentages of THC and CBD. Some wonderful examples are the Chemovars below which are combined strains that exhibit the best of both worlds.

FAMOUS CHEMOVARS / HYBRID COMBINATION STRAINS: BLUE DREAM, WHITE WIDOW, GIRL SCOUT COOKIES, GOLDEN GOAT, PINEAPPLE EXPRESS, WEDDING CAKE, GELATO, SHERBET, OG KUSH, JACK HERER, AK-47, GORILLA GLUE, CHEMDAWG, CHERRY PIE, GG4, CANNATONIC, SOUR TSUNAMI

{**CANNABIS** cross section at high magnification reveals microscopic hilarity!}

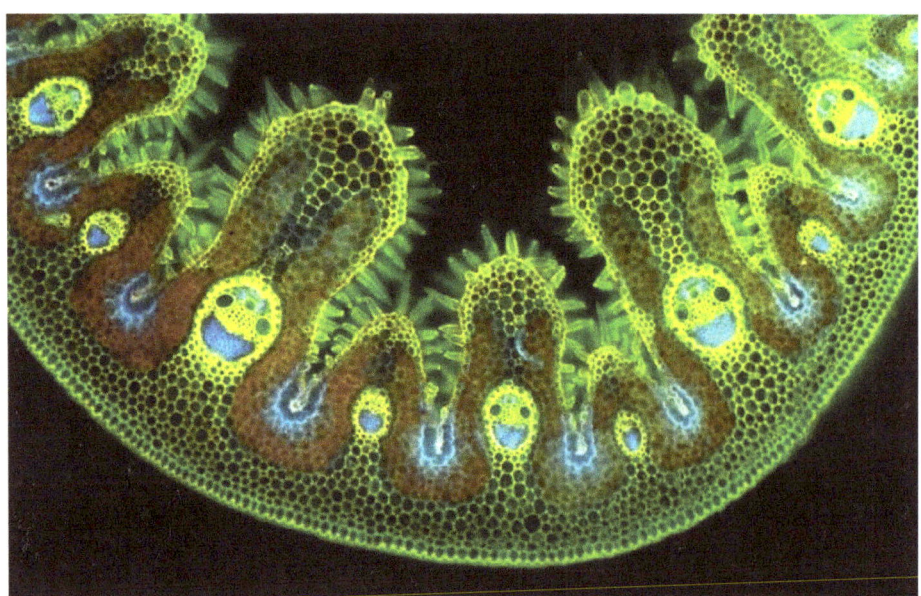

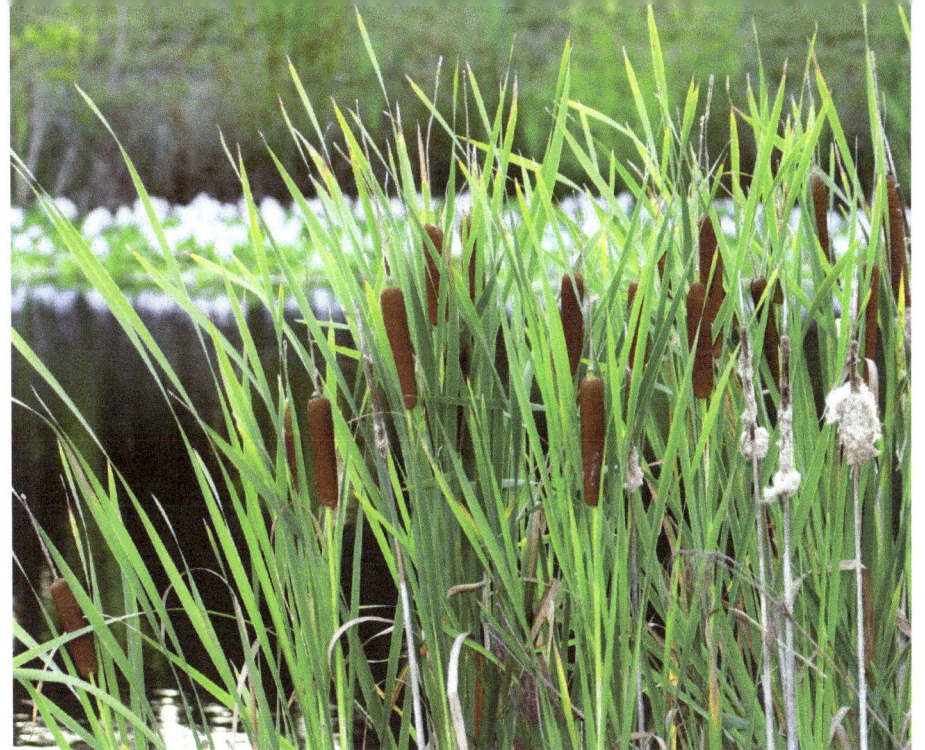

CATTAIL

Typha latifolia   Cattail or Bulrush Family / **TYPHACEAE**

FOUND: In swamps, wetlands and ditches, edges of ponds and rivers, Cattail is native in all 49 continental US states and Canada (and was introduced into Hawaii) — plus, it grows all over the World. This spreading plant usually prefers to overtake ditches and shallow, flooded areas that are an average of 1-1½ feet deep.

IDENTIFYING FEATURES: Tall panicle flower that looks like a brown hotdog on a stick or a fat cigar. Usually found growing in water, in a stand of tall leaves that sheath the stem and are pointy, long, flat, bright green and sword-shaped. Cattails form colonies that grow from 5-10 feet tall. Wild Iris (Yellow or Blue Flag) are poisonous look-alikes, but have distinctly different colored Iris flowers.

FOOD: All parts of the plant and Pollen are edible. This is one of our most accessible survival foods and it can be prepared in dozens of ways. Choose Cattails where you can see many old brown seed heads for best identification. Harvest the plants that are in the cleanest water you can find, as it can absorb toxins from stagnant or pesticide-laden water.

CONTAINS: New shoots contain Vitamins A, B's and C, Potassium, Phosphorus. Pollen is a great source of Protein, Antioxidants and Beta-Carotene. Whole plant is high in Fiber as well as Calcium, Iron, Magnesium, Manganese, Phosphorus, Potassium, Sodium, Vitamin K, Choline, Carbohydrates, Starch, and Bioflavonoids.

BODY BENEFITS: Fully nourishing to the body, Cattails are a wonderful food source that immeasurably increase your chance of survival in the wilderness. This awesome food plant is so rich in carbohydrates that it will also support healthy weight gain when needed (think Cattail Pollen Pancakes!). Cattail is useful for anemia, cancer, to benefit the kidneys, for malnutrition, high blood pressure, excessive menstruation, diabetes, atherosclerosis, and as a cardiac tonic — and it helps heal boils, sores, and scars of the skin. While Cattail is not normally gathered and used as a medicinal herb in the West, the Chinese have always studied the many positive effects of this helpful plant, and use it with great success. In their Traditional Chinese Medicine, the Cattail Pollen is gathered and encapsulated for a remedy called Pu Huang that is used for nosebleeds, uterine bleeding, shrinking tumors, and blood in the urine. Cattails can also reduce lipid deposits in the arteries.

QUALITIES: Masculine, cooling, astringent, diuretic, analgesic, styptic, and healing to the skin. Cattail provides highly nutritive, bowel-supportive, metabolism-boosting, wonderful food.

FOLKLORE: Folk names Cat-O-Nine-Tails, Bulrush, Corn Dog Grass, Swamp Sausage, Water Torch, Copper's Reed, Punk, Reedmace, Cumbungo, Raupo, Balca. Excavated grinding stones with Cattail residue prove it was eaten over 30,000 years ago in Europe. Depictions of Jesus in ancient art show him holding a Cattail as a scepter. Pan's flute was said to be made of the hollowed out stalks of this plant cut to different sizes. Stalks were also used for arrows. The downy fluff from the mature flower was used as down-free bedding, to stuff pillows, create insulation (stuff large plastic bags with it), and to line diapers, cradles and menstrual pads. Leaves can be woven for mats, hats, shoes, baskets and shelter. The long basal leaves of Cattail were originally dried and stripped to form Rushes, which were used to weave chair seats and make super strong and long-lasting lashing.

FIRST AID/SURVIVAL USES: In the Spring, the young leaves make a gel that can be used for relieving pain and the stopping itch of bug bites, and will coat a wound like a bandage. This small drop of honey-like nectar at the base of the plant between the leaves can also be used for spider bites and toothaches. Leaves can be burned to create a styptic powder that stops bleeding and is antiseptic and astringent for wounds. A poultice from the pounded root will relieve inflammation, pain and infection. The Cattail stem will make tea to relieve dysentery and fevers. Browning and roasting the pollen increases its ability to staunch blood flow as a styptic powder, and it can be mixed with honey to apply. The flower fluff can line a shoe for blisters, pad a splint, and be used as tinder to feed fires — and the dried stalks can be used as a hand drill to start a fire. Dried seed heads on the stalk can be dipped in oil or wax and used as torches, and to repel mosquitoes. Boil the leaves with Sesame Oil to make a wonderful pain-relieving massage oil. Stuff the down of the old flowers into your sleeping bag and arrange into a mat under you for warmth when cold camping.

SPIRITUAL PROPERTIES: Ruled by Mars, and the Fire Element, Cattail has the power to inspire Emotional Fire, Passion and Lust. Cattail has a very upward motion of energy and supports reaching, strength and striving. This is an aggressive, spiritual warrior force that can be used for drawing in courage, offering you the ability to stand tall in the Spirit Realm as well.

MAGICAL USES: Carrying Cattail is said to increase a woman's sexual desire and enjoyment of sex. Use Cattail on an altar for Virility, as a symbol of erect strength and potency. Cattail carries the power of Lust and can be used in Love Spells. This is a potent warrior plant that can be placed on altars, and called on in meditations for standing your ground and protecting yourself.

FLOWER ESSENCE: Made most often with the Pollen, the Cattail Flower Essence is for connecting with Inner Truth. It holds a lantern up to illuminate your personal path, helping you to validate your deep knowing and be able to stand up for it.

PREPARATIONS: This plant is the gold mine of Wild Foods. Euell Gibbons, one of my heroes, calls Cattail the "Supermarket of the Swamps." He says "no plant, wild or domesticated tops the common Cattail for it tastes best when prepared hot, but in the raw Cattails have many delicious uses. In early Spring, harvest 2 foot tall young shoots and eat the inner core (heart) of the stalk raw, or prepare like Asparagus, grill, or slice for salads like Hearts of Palm. The young corms (which are small shoots growing out of the rhizome) can be eaten raw after peeling, sliced into salads, cooked like a vegetable or pickled for a Winter surprise. In May and early June, before the flower spikes erupt into a cloud of pollen, the green bloom spikes can be eaten like corn on the cob, roasted or boiled or cooked over a fire — and shucked for a corn substitute for porridge, sauces or cornbread. The rhizomes can be dug, peeled, pounded and placed into a jar of water to separate the good starchy sediment from the fibrous root. Drained, collected, and washed in fresh water, this starch makes a great white flour (containing gluten for better rising in bread-making) that can be used even without drying first. For best eating, harvest the full rhizome after the flowering in Fall, Winter and through to Spring and prepare like a root vegetable. The remarkable bright yellow, antioxidant-rich pollen usually shows in the month of June. Watch your Cattail patch, plan ahead so you can be ready to roll when the flowers are perfectly fluffy and ready for gathering.

LAURA: I vividly remember gathering Cattails at the side of the road with my Mother, knee deep in water in a ditch, laughing and shouting for joy. In the 1970's, they were very popular for floral arrangements, and she trimmed them down and used them for beautiful Fall decorations in the house. I remember thinking my Mom was so cool, she used Nature as an interior decorator! This experience opened my eyes a bit more to what was naturally growing nearby, and widened my interest in how and what you could gather for yourself.

Cattail Pollen Pancakes

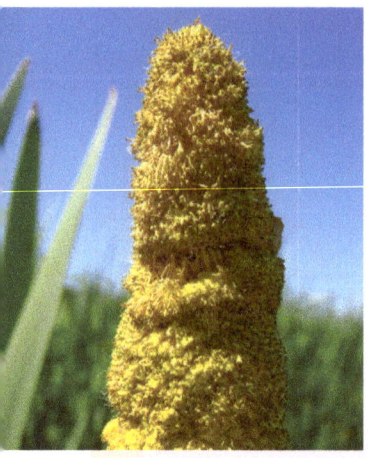

- **GATHER and REST DAY: A day ahead of time**, go out to a Cattail patch with scissors and a big ziploc bag. Find the yellowest, fattest flowers that have exploded with pollen and bend their heads over into the bag and snip off. Take them home and let them sit for 24 hours or so. Then shake the heads into the bag until all the pollen seems spent. It WILL STAIN - so be careful handling it and where you wipe your hands. Snip a corner of the bag to pour out the magical golden powder.

Store it in a glass jar, and compost the rest of the flower.

BRIGHT YELLOW FLAPJACKS: Measure your **Cattail Pollen** and use ½ and ½ with your favorite biscuit or pancake mix* or favorite scratch pancake recipe for the best, richest, most golden pancakes you have ever tried! There is a sweet pollen taste to these pancakes that is flowery and exotic - but it's the color that will blow your mind! The Pollen adds considerable nutrition and potent antioxidants, making these SuperFood Pancakes, that also happen to be perfectly sweet without syrup. *I love *Birch Benders Pancake Mixes* from Vermont. You make them with water alone, and they come in resealable pouches, perfect for camping, rafting and hiking - and Sunday breakfast.

OTHER USES FOR CATTAIL POLLEN: It is great in savory dishes as well as sweet, perfect for curries and paella, fish and fowl, golden rice dishes and Golden Milk. It can be used the way you would Bee Pollen or Turmeric, sprinkled on yogurt, oatmeal, salads, smoothies and in cookies, cakes and desserts.

Cattails fix Nitrogen into the soil to actually feed all the other plants, as nourishing to the whole ecosystem as they are to our bodies! Cattails help the environment by absorbing and removing toxins from wild and contaminated water sources. Studies show Cattails can remediate a tainted water supply within a few months when grown specifically for this purpose. So Cattails care for EVERYONE.

We all need to know where this plant grows, and learn about harvesting from it. BETTER YET - go get some plants from your favorite secret and pristine location to plant in your own yard! Cattails will handle transplantation well and will grow in soil or in water, in the ground, or in pots! Ask first, then take only a few plants from an abundant stand. Dig down *at least a foot* to liberate them by their rhizome, which is white and spreading and looks like Ginger. Keep the rhizome covered and moist in a bag until planting. Ideally, replant them next to water sources or ditches or low areas that receive lots of rain. Water them abundantly to the flood stage — they like to have "wet feet" for most of the year. Care for them like a garden plant, and you will have a wonderful new friend and a YEAR-ROUND food source.

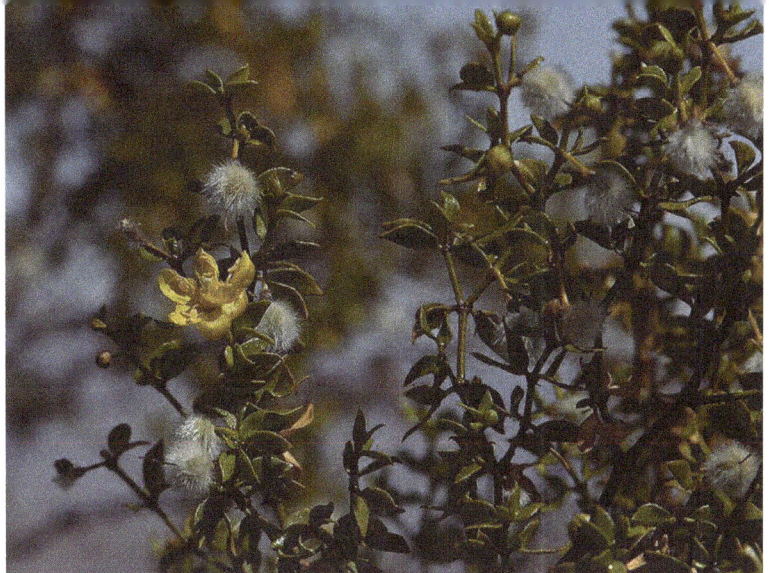

CHAPARRAL

Larrea divaricata, Larrea tridentata   *Caltrop Family/* **ZYGOPHYLLACEAE**

FOUND: In 5 Southwestern US states: Texas, Arizona, New Mexico, California and Nevada, also in Europe in the Mediterranean Basin, Australia, and South Africa. Chaparral grows in biomes like Aspens do, as a member of a fully functional community of plants and animals, all connected. This is characteristic of the Family.

IDENTIFYING FEATURES: Super strong-scented, shiny, leathery and pointed, small oval nibs of leaves on a wide and leggy evergreen bush, or small tree growing 2-10 feet tall. Has small pinwheel yellow flowers, and expired flowers explode into a powder puff. When you find one, look around, they often cover the landscape (in California they cover 5% of the terrain). One squeeze of the leaves and your nose will tell you it is turpentine-y Chaparral! It is a perennial evergreen, so the plant can be identified and harvested in all seasons. Leaves are considered sclerophyll, which means "hard-leaved" in Greek, and their waxy coating keeps in moisture, so the plant can grow in desert climates. Bushes are oddly flammable in late Summer and Fall, due to their high essential oil content, so they are good firestarters for emergency fires.

FOOD: A medicinal herb much more than a food plant, Chaparral is to be used with care as a tea, made with the fresh or dried leaves and stems. Some herbs are simply too strong for regular food usage, and this is one of them. But it comes in handy as a potent medicine comes and anytime you find some you should harvest a jar of it to take home.

CONTAINS: Vitamin A (Beta-carotene), Calcium, Chromium, Potassium, Magnesium, Molybdenum, Quercetin, Resins, Lignans, Saponins, Essential Oils, and NDGA (see my comments below).

BODY BENEFITS: The ultimate blood & lymph cleanser and purifier, Chaparral is thought by Native Americans to be a cure-all plant. It is a real killer with antibacterial, antiviral, antitoxic, antiparasitic, antifungal and antiseptic properties. It increases the body's stores of Vitamin C in the adrenal glands. It is highly antioxidant and free radical scavenging. Great as an external remedy as well, Chaparral is effective as an antiseptic wash or poultice, in a salve or as an extract applied to wounds, abscesses, boils & growths, ringworm, rashes, herpes, impetigo, scalp and body sores, as a douche for yeast infections, and as a foot soak for athlete's foot and gout. It can support treatment of urinary tract infections, shorten the duration of colds and flu, reduce anemia, and flush out swollen glands with lymphatic drainage. Its cleansing action can aid in symptoms of alcohol withdrawal.

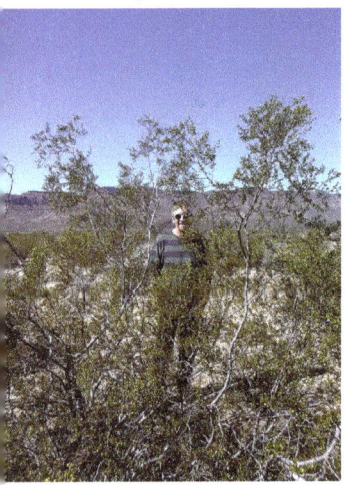

QUALITIES: Chaparral, with its high saponin content, is like a detergent for the blood, and can be very effective for atherosclerosis and removing plaque. It is considered to be cooling, yin, salty, drawing, drying and very bitter. Chaparral is alkalizing, alterative, antiarthritic, antibacterial, antifungal, antiinflammatory, antioxidant, anti parasitic, antiseptic, antitumor, antiviral, diuretic, emetic, expectorant, immune-boosting, laxative, lymphatic flushing, and tonic.

FOLKLORE: Folk names Creosote Bush, Black Bush, Greasewood, Chapparro, Hediondilla ("little stinker"), Jarilla, Dwarf Evergreen Oak, Gobernadora, Goma de Sonora. Many of the folk names refer to the very turpentine-y scent of this bush and its many volatile compounds that cause it to burn well. The resin from Chaparral has a glue-like consistency and was traditionally used to mend pottery and make baskets waterproof. This same strong resin makes it difficult for other plants to grow nearby, assuring "home security." Traditionally used by the Native Americans in protection rituals for the home.

FIRST AID USES: Tea used topically, cooled in the refrigerator first (or frozen in an ice cube) is soothing and cooling for sunburns, Poison Ivy, bug bites and rashes. Tea can be used as a rinse to prevent dandruff, clean wounds, and to cover Poison Ivy so it doesn't spread. Drink when cool to bring down a fever.

SPIRITUAL PROPERTIES: Ruled by Saturn, and focusing the Element of Earth, Chaparral is a Protector plant, an upholder of the natural matrix, and a banisher of evil. It is grounding and cleansing, while it helps the unnecessary and unwanted to move on. Chaparral clears the way for the new, helps it to first crystallize in the Ethers.

MAGICAL USES: Chaparral makes a great home or workplace smudge. It is cleansing when burned by itself, or with other potent herbs like Sage or Palo Santo. Chaparral protects the home, and small dishes of the herb can be placed strategically at the corners of the house to create a field of protection. It is considered a banishing herb for removing negative influences and energies. Chaparral can be worn in a medicine bag when entering into controversial communications.

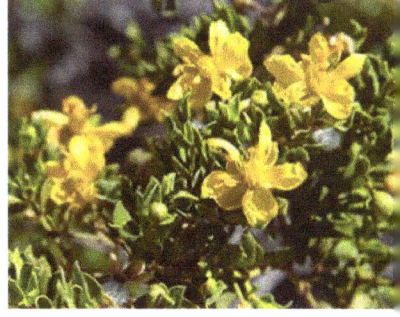

FLOWER ESSENCE: Chaparral is very cleansing and cathartic, as a flower essence on a deep spiritual level. It can be super helpful for psychic toxicity, nightmares, psychic or dream invasions, hallucinations, and drug detoxification. It can be especially soothing for the fear and paranoia surrounding current events, and for ridding the psyche of violent images and storylines from the news, television and movies. I read about a case where someone's Father was nearly permanently drugged and institutionalized with violent dementia and hallucinations. Using Chaparral and St. Johnswort flower essences, which helped rid him of the "ghouls" and haunting images that had been plaguing him, he recovered completely.

PREPARATIONS: Chaparral is so strong that it is best in small doses. You only need 1 teaspoon of herb to make tea, and use water that has just been boiled. One of the coolest things about this herb is that it gives and gives. You can, and ought to, re-use the same herb for many more infusions when making tea. Chaparral should be drunk on an empty stomach for the most potent cleansing effect. Avoid Chaparral in pregnancy and while breast-feeding, as it does have very strong constituents. ***Do not take if using methotrexate (rheumatrex, trexall).

LAURA: I had just discovered the herb Chaparral through Lalitha Thomas' book *10 Essential Herbs*. I had been doing her 21-day Chapparal Cleanse, in which you essentially use the same teaspoon of Chaparral in hot (not boiling) water, for morning tea for three days, then repeat with fresh herb, drinking the tea everyday for 3 weeks. It had markedly improved my skin due to its special actions for the liver (in moderation), and the blood cleansing action which helped remove the toxins and accumulated wastes which lead to my skin problems. I was impressed with anything that helped my skin, and the results with Chaparral were significant. I reveled in the strength of even the 4th or 5th infusion, the herb was so potent. I had really come to love Chaparral (even the strong turpentiney taste) after a long herbal dieta of daily use. I was so grateful for my health improvements and the mysteries of the plant that we became fast friends.

I was there in 1992, working at the original Alfalfa's Market in Boulder, Colorado when "they" came and seized all the Chaparral. Men in Suits from the FDA bullied into our herb department and took all the bottles and bags of dried herb and extracts and capsules we had on the shelves, violently putting them into trash bags, in a real RAID with law enforcement support. In Colorado! And in hundreds of other stores ALL over the country that week. They acted as if we were harboring a secret stash of heroin (instead of a very abundant Medicinal Weed). They very, very seriously inquired if we had "any Chaparral hidden in any other part of the store?!" They made us feel like criminals for selling this mighty herb, and made us *promise to destroy* any further orders that came in for this "banned substance." Within a few days, there was simply no more supply of Chaparral in any of the stores, to be bought at any price, in any form. Sweeping herbal assassination.

At the time, the Herbalists' gossip was that the FDA was releasing a new brain cancer chemotherapy drug, and wanted every other remedy to be "off the shelves." Because Chaparral contains a super powerful anti-tumor agent called Nordihydroguaiaretic Acid, it was a target. This phytochemical NDGA has a rich history of effective treatment for brain cancer and leukemia, so they quite possibly banned this plant for the medicine it contained. As potent as Chaparral is, I find it not at all surprising that Big Pharma felt threatened, and forced a literal coup with the FDA to remove it from public sale and use.

The public excuse for the FDA raids, like the one at Alfalfa's, was that Chaparral alkaloids were harmful to the liver (hepatotoxic) in large quantities. *Two people* allegedly developed non-viral hepatitis from using enormous quantities of the herb and that was enough for the FDA to take direct action. Lab mice were given hundreds of times the normal dose and developed liver anomalies (which would be expected in any animal, with irresponsible use of any plant remedy) to back up their findings. This is one of the reasons Herbalists teach us to use the same herb many times and in tea, to spread the action out and dilute it for easier assimilation without side effects. As is usually the case, the bad publicity highlighted only some remotely dangerous isolate of the plant, with no mention of the 10,000 other amazing things Chaparral CAN do in its natural form! After more thorough research Chaparral was found to be safe, there was no evidence of hepatotoxicity, and the ban was lifted in 1995. However, by then so much harm had been done to the reputation of the plant that many people were afraid to use it simply because of the bad press.

From that moment on, I made sure to travel to the West regularly, stopping every time to hike and forage for my own personal supply of my beloved Chaparral. Take empty glass jars with you on roadtrips. KNOW and note as you travel where your favorite medicinal herbs grow. Someday the information could prove vital and necessary for your sourcing it, as was true for me. I keep a nice full half gallon jar full of Chaparral now and love to travel to replenish it!

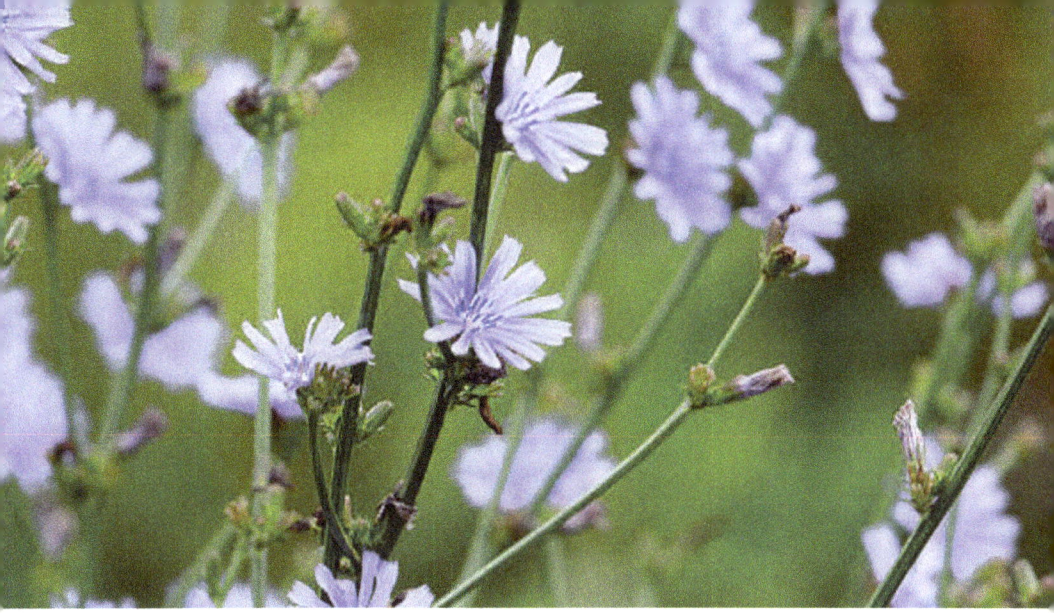

CHICORY

Cichorium intybus   Daisy Family / **ASTERACEAE/COMPOSITAE**

FOUND: Originally from Eurasia, and Egypt, now grows along roadsides, against poles, and by mailboxes in all 50 states in the US, and worldwide. Chicory is PERFECT for young homeschoolers & new foragers to find, as this plant is so abundant and recognizable with its unusual blue flower, and it has no known poisonous look-alikes.

IDENTIFYING FEATURES: Perennial. Bright periwinkle-blue daisy flowers grow right on the long woody naked stem, and petals are fringed, square-tipped, and somewhat irregular. Blooms regularly close at noon in the Sun. Leaves grow in radiant circles like Dandelion, mostly in dry soil in disturbed areas like ditches and building sites. The plant ultimately grows to 1-3 feet tall. It has alternate leaves on the stem which are lobed and irregularly-toothy with a purple midrib. Stem produces a milky latex sap. The root is most commonly used, dug the second year before the plant flowers, and looks like a white carrot or parsnip.

FOOD: The very first leaves of Chicory resemble Dandelion greens nearly identically, and it can be harvested mistakenly with it in the early Spring. However, that's a good thing, as they taste the same, are perfect when young and tender and both have great body benefits! Chicory has become a cultivated delicacy, especially in Europe, for its leaves for salads and as Winter greens, though the older greens are very bitter. The root is roasted and ground, used as a coffee additive or substitute, especially in the South US for New Orleans style reduced-acid coffee. The flower buds are blanched and called chicons (used like capers). It is widely used as a forage drop food for livestock as a substitute for oats. Chicory is one of the traditional "bitter herbs" of Passover. The Flowers are edible and look gorgeous on the plate or in salads. The root or whole plant can be juiced for a nutritious, cooling beverage.

CONTAINS: Chicory contains Beta-carotene, Vitamin B, C, K, Flavonoids, Zinc, Folic Acid, Manganese, Iron, Potassium, Choline, Sesquiterpene Lactones, Oligofructose, Coumarins & Latex. The root contains the highest amount of Inulin of any known food. Inulin is a fiber ingredient of the moment because of its Prebiotic capability for feeding our healthy gut flora & supporting your Probiotics. Chicory is used as a source of dietary fiber and a sweetener that enhances sugar or its sweet substitutes.

BODY BENEFITS: Its bitter greens are stimulating to the Liver (increasing bile for better digestion) and also help clear heat and toxins from the blood. The root can help with acid reflux and oligofructose sugars from the Inulin can reduce appetite by lowering the "hunger hormone" Ghrelin. Inulin, like all good fiber sources, has also been found to reduce cholesterol and stimulate bowel regularity. Chicory can ease the angry emotions of the Liver, helping to dispel irritability, ease jaundice, control temper tantrums, & cool rage. Helpful for gout, UTI's, depression, diabetes, gallstones, and constipation.

QUALITIES: Bitter, sweet and salty, yang but cooling and moist, Chicory is alterative, antibacterial, antiinflammatory, antiseptic, cardiotonic, diuretic, digestive, astringent, mild laxative, and stimulant.

FOLKLORE: Folk names Succory, Blue Sailors, Ragged Sailors, Watcher of the Road, Coffee Weed, Horseweed, Wild Endive, Belgian Endive, Whitloof, Blue Daisy, Cicoria, Achicoria, Barbe a Capucin. The flowers will yield a yellow dye, and the leaves will make a blue dye. Chicory grew all along the banks of the Nile, and the 18th century Dutch brought it home to use in coffee.

FIRST AID USES: Use tea as an anti-bacterial, anti-inflammatory and cooling wash for wounds, bug bites, eczema, and acne. Crush the fresh leaves to rub on, and use as a poultice for swellings. Use as a tea for rapid heartbeat,

SPIRITUAL PROPERTIES: Chicory is generally ruled by the Sun, but also has been associated with Mercury, Venus, Jupiter & Uranus, and the Element of Air. Has a masculine energy of clearing the way, building strength both physically and spiritually, and putting down deep roots.

MAGICAL USES: Removes obstacles like a Garden Ganesh! Chicory was traditionally carried in an amulet to remove life's obstacles and help maintain one's frugality. Once upon a time the herb was considered to make people invisible, and to open locked doors and boxes when prepared correctly. Old texts support anointing your body with the chicory latex to obtain favors from great people. I say, try a small patch on your skin first to make sure you don't have any side effects before you go slathering it on in the hopes of favor! Carry Chicory flower to bring good luck, and remove curses.

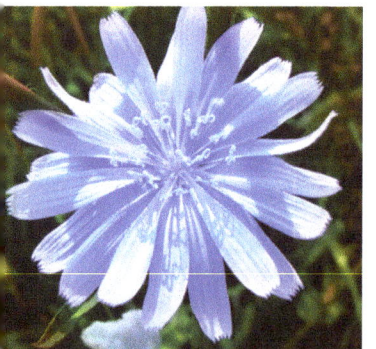

FLOWER ESSENCE: Supports a relief from "emotional congestion" and "misdirected love forces," and can open the flow of Love. Good for people who can't separate the trials of the World from their own. Great for self-pity, martyrdom, possessiveness and rejection. Great for children (or the childish adults) who "act-out" and get fussy, selfish, and throw tantrums to get negative attention. Chicory balances this inner neediness and helps rewire the heart and solar plexus so they can feel easy-flowing energy and personal harmony.

PREPARATIONS: Euell Gibbons suggests "digging" instead of picking this as a salad herb. He recommends digging below the dirt to the place where the root attaches to the leaves, and with a sharp knife cutting through that white top-root to harvest. This less-bitter white portion can be simply chopped & dressed as you would beets along with the leaves. And the tops will grow back! The entire plant can be juiced for supreme, soothing nutrition. Smaller, young leaves are delicious in salads or used like spinach, older leaves can be boiled for 5-10 minutes to reduce bitterness. You can put a flower pot over Chicory and grow it Endive-style in the dark for less bitter greens. Euell also recommends that if you have unwanted chicory plants in your yard, you dig them up carefully, trim off the leaves and put the roots in wet sand or sawdust in your root cellar, from which you can grow several rounds of delicious greens (the Endive). Now *this* is a weed that keeps on giving! The roots are not quite worth the effort of preparing them for a regular food product, but would work great in a survival situation, chopped or thrown whole into the fire to roast. For making a coffee substitute, dry the roots fully and roast in the oven at 200-350 degrees until medium dark brown inside, watch them closely. Chicory can then be pulverized like you would coffee beans. For a powdered beverage additive, use in a ratio of ⅓ of the herbs in the blend while brewing coffee or tea, or about 1 ½ teaspoon per cup of water by itself.

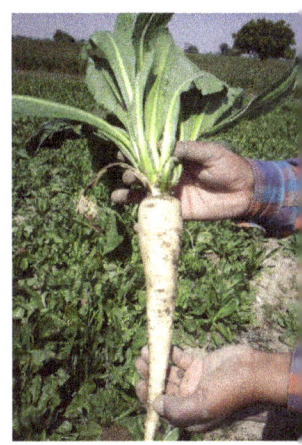

LAURA: When I was growing up, my Mother made the most delicious European dish called *Endive au Jambon,* which she learned to make while living in Switzerland. Belgian Endive is layered with Gruyere Cheese and Ham, baked into hot, cheesy, bitter heaven - stunning, French, and soooo delicious! While researching I discovered that Endive is the small oval cabbage-like green, REGROWN from the mature root of Chicory! It is so expensive because of the process of having to grow twice - first as a lovely Chicory plant (*Cichorium endivia*) from which the whole root is harvested, replanted and then tended to in the dark (to decrease the bitterness) and sometimes underground conditions, to re-grow a dense upright oval cluster of light-colored greens out of the top. This is what we have come to know as Endive. This is a similar process to the techniques described in Chapter 2, growing a new product from an existing stub of the plant. The flavor is bitter, complex and delicious. Radicchio (*Cichorium intybus var. foliosum*) is a bright red-leaved Chicory, and bitter salad green.

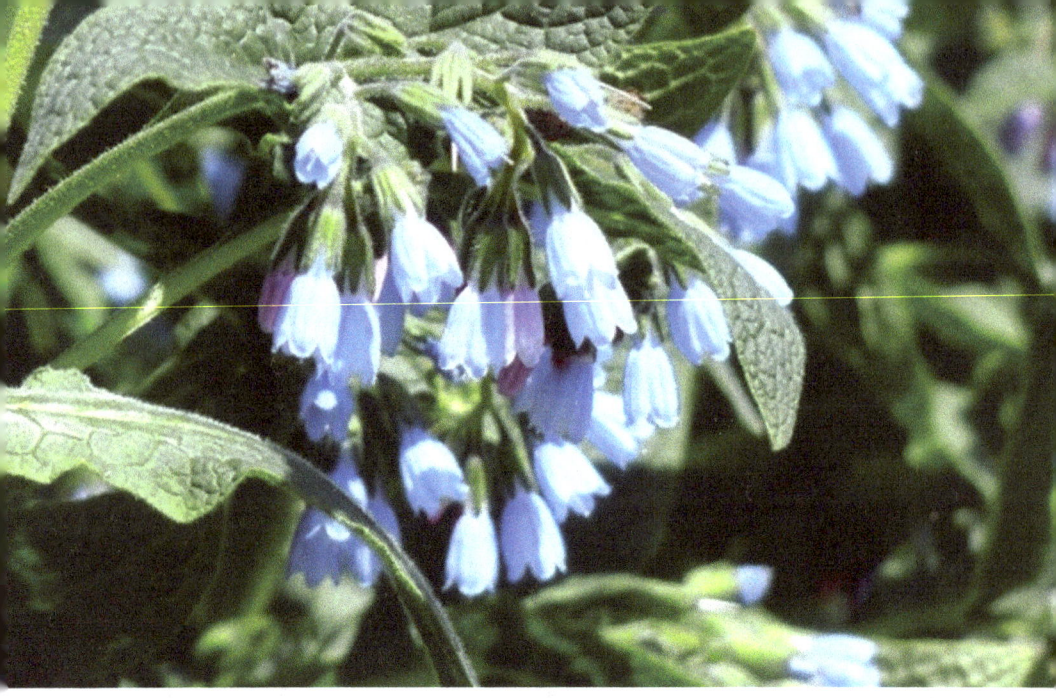

COMFREY

Symphytum officinale   Borage Family / **BORAGINACEAE**

FOUND: A native of Northern Asia and Europe, Comfrey has spread worldwide through forests, along streams, in meadows, and fence edges. It loves to grow in cooler climates, and damp, grassy soils with lots of sunshine.

IDENTIFYING FEATURES: Central, very **hairy** stem grows 1-4 feet tall, with long, lance-shaped or oval leaves, heavily veined and hairy. Comfrey has bell-shaped, scorpioid flowers that curl inward in a spiral and are blue, magenta, pinkish, white or purple. The root is black on the outside, white inside, looks somewhat like a turnip.

FOOD: Young leaves (before flowering especially) are perfect for raw salad greens, and can be cooked or juiced for superior nutrition. Root can be chopped and dried for tea, or candied. There are not a lot of food uses for this plant because it contains such very strong alkaloids, but small amounts are highly effective as a medicinal tea.

CONTAINS: Protein, Vitamin B12, Calcium, Iron, Potassium, Inulin, Germanium, Amino Acids (Tryptophan, Lysine, Isoleucine, Methionine), Inulin, Mucilage, Allantoin, Alkaloids, Saponins, Triterpenoids, Phenolic Acids, Rosmarinic Acids, Sterols, Tannins

BODY BENEFITS: The botanical name *Symphytum* means "grown together." Comfrey accelerates healing to repair broken bones, heal ulcers, and knit wounds back together. It is healing for so many parts of the body including the mucous membranes and skin, and it reduces pain while it renews bones, tendons, and the lungs. Its repairing action is due to its ability to regenerate cells very quickly. It is good for digestive issues, for all complaints of the lungs, as well as being helpful for laryngitis, burns, gallstones, tonsillitis, dysentery, heartburn, low body weight, and hemorrhoids.

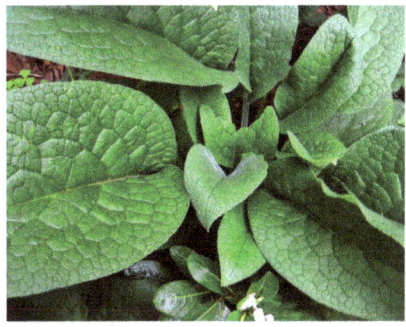

QUALITIES: Comfrey is a fractal multiplier, increasing and expanding what it touches. It is yin, moistening, cooling, soothing, and feminine. Comfrey is alterative, anti-inflammatory, antiseptic, astringent, demulcent, emollient, expectorant, hemostatic, immune stimulant, lung tonic, nutritive, refrigerant, and styptic.

FOLKLORE: Folk names BoneKnit, Boneset, Blackwort, Slippery Root, Bruisewort, KnitBack, Consolida, Healing Herb, Wallwort, Yalluc, Gum Plant, Ass's Ear, Healing Blade, Suelda, Langue-de-Vache, Oreille d'Âne, Consoude, Okopnik. Comfrey has been used as a healing herb for as long as we have written records. Alexander the Great carried this herb into battle for treating wounds, and it has been used as a fracture remedy since at least the Middle Ages. Boiling the root will yield a thick paste that can be used as glue and for waterproofing.

FIRST AID USES: Tea, salve or poultice applied topically for broken bones, gout, rheumatoid arthritis, burns, skin issues, bruises, sprains and strains, back pain, hemorrhoids, varicose veins, scars, wounds and wrinkles. Poultice can be made by pulverizing 6 leaves with a little water to which you add a binding agent like flour, cornmeal or flax seeds. Wrap in place with a cloth bandage. Tea can soothe coughs, congestion and asthma and is a great remedy for ulcers. Comfrey is also helpful as a drawing salve for easing out splinters or infected lymph. Add tea to a bath for broken bones and skin inflammations. Gargle tea for sore throat and swish as a mouthwash for gum disease.

SPIRITUAL PROPERTIES: Ruled by Saturn (planet of foundation and crystalline structure, which rules bones) and the Water Element, is a sacred herb of Hecate. Comfrey leaves can be burned with Mugwort and Bay Leaves for an intoxicating incense for divination purposes. Since it multiplies cells, it also multiplies energy and can be used to take dreams and manifestations to the next level.

MAGICAL USES: For personal protection and protection against theft, especially while traveling, carry Comfrey leaves or flowers, and place in your luggage to keep it safe as well. Make a sachet with Comfrey and hang in your car for constant protection on the road. Comfrey Root is used in money spells and worn for protection and frugality while handling money. Wrap your money in a Comfrey leaf for a few days before going out gambling, and it will return to you multiplied.

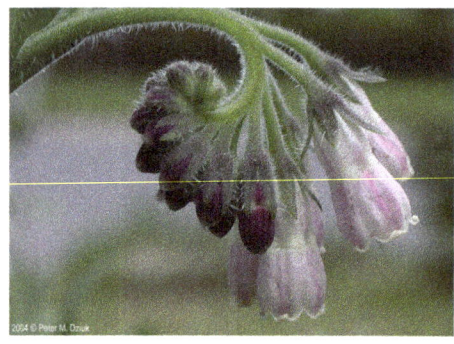

FLOWER ESSENCE: Comfrey is the Super Healer. She helps you sort through old emotional wounds and build a better way. This a the flower for healing from trauma and abuse, especially karmic traumas that may even be remnants of past life experiences that still manifest now. Comfrey can assist with clarifying hazy memories or supporting past life regression. It supports healing on all levels, and can be useful for energy loss, low self-image or negative body image. It assists with recovery from major accidents and emotional incidents in life. Helpful for PTSD & "soldier syndrome." The flower looks like it is giving you a much-needed hug.

<u>Heals It All
Comfrey & Goldenseal Salve</u>

Heals It All Salve is great for healing wounds, removing the itch and sting of bug bites, easing the pain of sprains and bruises, shrinking scars, soothing skin irritations and so much more. Smelling it will stop an anxiety attack and elevate your mood. It is gently antimicrobial as well, like an herbal Neosporin, and will greatly accelerate healing.

Gather **Comfrey Root** (super sparingly, take one only) and half a dozen large **Leaves,** and allow to dry, or dehydrate in a very low oven. Chop dried plant material to increase surface area and immediately add to a large Mason Jar with a tight lid (16 oz or more).

Purchase some **Goldenseal Powder** from a health food store, or open 6 capsules, and place 1 teaspoon of Goldenseal Powder with Comfrey in the infusing jar.

> ★ **Plantain Leaf, Ginger Powder, Calendula Flower,** or **Slippery Elm Powder** would make very healing additions to this salve if available.

At the New Moon, warm 2 cups of **Organic Sesame Oil** (or **Organic Olive Oil, Coconut Oil**, or your preference of Base Oil) in a clean sterilized pot. Monitor the heat until the oil is quite hot, but not bubbling, and pour into the jar with the herbs. Tighten the lid and shake 100 times. Place in a dark warm place to infuse for at least two weeks, shaking daily if you can. Set your intention with the New Moon for this medicine to create a powerful remedy that truly will **Heal All**. Give thanks, as you shake it, for the assistance of the Plant Kingdom.

Prepare enough clean sterilized 1-2 oz. Jars, or Tiny Tins, or old cosmetic containers to hold 16-20 oz. of completed salve.

After the Full Moon, strain the herbs out of the oil and into a pot. Warm very slowly and add 4 oz. of **Beeswax Beads**. Remove from the heat when there are very few beads left, but make sure it is hot enough to melt everything completely. This is a great time to move the salve to a glass measuring cup with a pouring-spout. Cool the mixture for 10 minutes or until it starts to set up just a bit. Add ½ teaspoon (50 drops) **Lavender** and ¼ teaspoon, (25 drops) **Frankincense** Essential Oils, and 10 drops of **Spearmint Essential Oil**. Add any other Essential Oils you like, 5-10 drops each. Stir quickly until oils are well combined, and stir again each time you pour into the prepared salve jars. If it sets up before you are done, rewarm in double boiler on super low heat to preserve the essential oils. Allow filled jars to cool just a bit and then put lids on. Make a pretty label with a clever name for your version of this salve, and give to friends and family members! As some people are sensitive, I think it is nice to include an ingredient list.

- ★ **PRO TIPS:** If you need it sooner than in 2 weeks, you can *"force"* the extraction process with heat. Place the Herbs right into the Base Oil in a pan on the stove, and let the mixture sit covered, on very, very low heat, for at least a few hours. You could also put the whole infusing jar into a pan of water in a low oven for a few hours, and let sit overnight. Strain and proceed to the next step.

- ★ **LIP BALM BASE:** Without the Goldenseal, and with half the Essential Oils, this would make a wonderful **Lip Balm** base. Add a little **Castor Oil** for shine, some **Vanilla Extract** for flavor and a little extra **Beeswax** for optimal hardness in warm weather, or pockets.

LAURA: Comfrey's healing powers are so amazing, and it works so FAST, that a wound treated with it must be carefully cleaned, or the Comfrey will cause it to heal over any debris! The **Allantoin** (the same constituent responsible for the healing powers of Aloe Vera) stimulates cell growth, while it is soothing and protective. Allantoin is coincidentally found in the milk of nursing Mothers.

Comfrey can be propagated by root cuttings and grown in your yard. Plant 2-4 inches into the soil, in full Sun and keep it well watered. It is recommended to cut the flowers the first year so the plant can concentrate on hardy roots and stems. Comfrey is a Weed, so don't be surprised if it wants to spread around. Clip the flowerheads before they release their seeds to control its expansion.

Comfrey can enhance your garden as a companion plant and even support your compost pile! **Comfrey causes compost to break down more quickly**, enriching it with vital nutrients. Comfrey leaves can be spread in the garden for nourishing Nitrogen, and used as mulch around fruit trees. A strong fermented tea can be made of the Comfrey leaves, and used to water plants. This will provide nutrients far better than conventional, poisonous fertilizers.

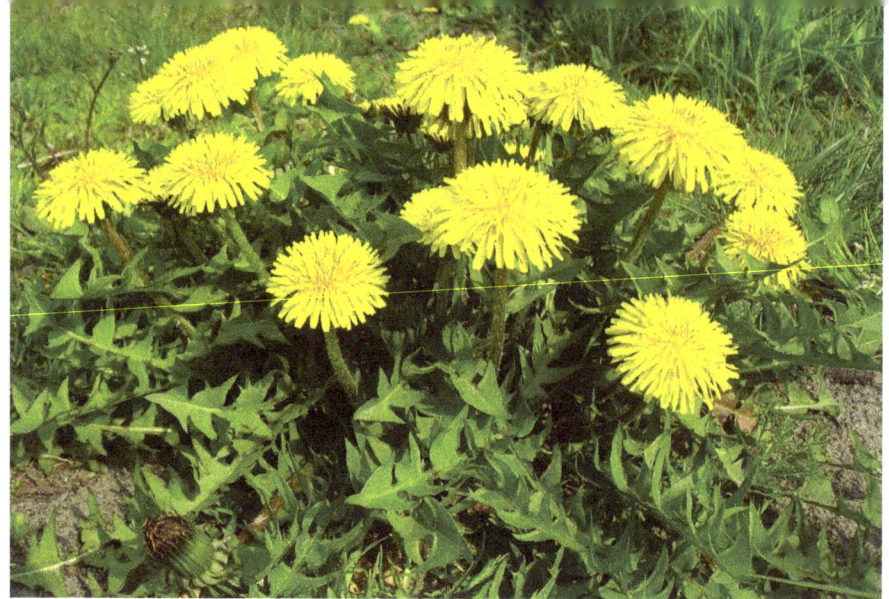

DANDELION

Taraxacum officinale   Daisy Family / **ASTERACEAE**

FOUND: In front and backyards, growing happily in grass worldwide. Dandelion loves Sun and frequents vacant lots, disturbed ground, driveways and cracks in the sidewalk. It will adjust to every kind of soil to grow abundantly.

IDENTIFYING FEATURES: Dandelion leaves grow from a basal rosette, are jagged, dark green, and pointed like arrows, and have no stems. There is just one single stem for each bright yellow, compound Sun-like flower, which later goes to seed as a full grey sphere. Sap is milky white. Dandelion is one of the easiest plants to identify by people of ALL ages, because it grows everywhere, has a bright, sunny recognizable flower which opens in the daytime and closes in the evening (and maintains its starring role in television pesticide advertising). Another amazing Weed, Prickly Wild Lettuce, has a similar appearance to Dandelion early in the season before it flowers. To distinguish them, check the underside of the leaves, the Prickly Lettuce has little spiky prongs all along the rib and Dandelion does not. Dandelion has a long taproot that may penetrate as deep as 15 feet if it is an old plant.

FOOD: ALL PARTS USEFUL. Dandelion is entirely edible, but should be gathered from wild areas away from vehicles and air pollution. Young leaves, before flowering, are delicious eaten raw in salads and added to sandwiches. Older leaves are much more bitter, but can be boiled to lessen their bitterness (water your plants with the Nitrogen-rich water). Buds can be pickled or chopped and sauteed. Roots are dried and roasted for tea/coffee substitute. Flowers make great fritters and brighten anyone's day in pancakes, salads and as tea. Dandelion has one of the longest flowering seasons and in some climates can be found in all months of the year. Roots can be foraged even in Wintertime, as the basal rosette of leaves is an all-season giveaway.

CONTAINS: *Leaf:* Vitamin A, Beta-Carotene, Vitamin B1 and B2, Vitamin K, Choline, Inositol, Folic Acid, Vitamin C, Calcium, Iron, Lutein, Manganese, Phosphorus, Potassium, Fiber, Bitter Glycosides, Terpenoids. *Root:* Calcium, Iron, Phosphorus, Choline, Zinc, Pectin, Inulin, Fiber, Tannins, Gallic Acid, Phenolic Acids including Quinic Acid, Lutein and other Flavonoids, Triterpenes, Fatty Acids & Essential Oils. *Flowers:* Lecithin, Polyphenols, Flavonoids (Apigenin, Isoquercitrin (a Quercetin-like compound, Luteolin), Caffeic Acid, Terpenoids, Triterpenes, and Sesquiterpenes.

BODY BENEFITS: Dandelion is regarded as safe, even in pregnancy (for which it is very helpful for preventing edema and hypertension), for children, and even in large amounts. It cleanses and cools the blood, clears infection and obstructions, supports the liver and its detoxification, benefits blood circulation, and lowers blood pressure. It treats many issues of the liver, skin, kidneys, veins, bladder, spleen and stomach and may even help prevent baldness. It stimulates lactation (which is funny because it makes a milky sap). The leaf tea is a remedy for hangovers as it helps flush the toxins away. The whole plant is useful for liver cleansing and support for recovering alcoholics. The Fiber in Dandelion helps the digestion, reduces cholesterol and helps fight diabetes. Dandelion encourages weight loss and detoxification, enabling the body to feel nourished enough to be able to shed excess weight. Romanian scientists, Elizabeth and Gabriel Racz-Kotilla found that Dandelion Extract, along with a minimum-weight maintaining diet, enabled mice and rats in their study to **lose 30% of their body weight over 30 days**, due to the cleansing and mineral support.[13] Dandelion flower is richer in Lecithin than Soybeans, which helps prevent cirrhosis of the liver, helps the body metabolize fats, feeds the brain, and nourishes the myelin sheath of the nerves. Because it is diuretic, it can be effective for swellings, water retention and promoting urinary flow. The blood cleansing action of Dandelion helps prevent metastasis and is very effective for breast cancer, and other cancerous tumors.

QUALITIES: Its nature is masculine, cooling, salty and bitter, the leaves are diuretic, and roots are blood cleansing, nourishing, and filled with minerals. Dandelion is also considered to be alterative, antacid, antitumor, antiviral, antioxidant, astringent, decongestant, digestive, galactagogue, hypotensive, immune-stimulant, laxative, nutritive, restorative, tonic, and vulnerary.

FOLKLORE: folk names Blowball, Amarga, Lion's Tooth, Cankerwort, Clock Flower, Irish Daisy, Dent de Lion, Fortune Teller, Bitterwort, Sun-in-the-Grass, Priest's Crown, Radiki, Wet-the-Bed, Butter Flower, Yellow Gowan, Chiccoria, Devil's Milkpail, Peasant's Cloak, Consuelda. Blow on the seed head flower 3 times and the number of seeds left should tell the time, or be the number of kids you'll have, or the number of times you'll get married! Dandelion is an old traditional remedy for the eyes. This was confirmed scientifically when it was proven what a great amount of Beta-Carotene that Dandelion provides, as well as the discovery of Lutein in the root. Beta-Carotene is the best Vitamin A source for healing vision, and Dandelion is 30% richer in this nutrient than Carrots.

FIRST AID USES: A healing poultice of flowers works great for wounds or bug bites, chew some up and apply. Put milky sap on warts to remove them. Eat the young leaves if thirsty, the minerals will replace lost electrolytes. If you are uncomfortable from an especially fatty meal, Dandelion Root caps or tea will ease your digestion and help the liver process the fat more quickly so you feel better.

SPIRITUAL PROPERTIES: Ruled by expansive Jupiter and Sun, representing the Element of Air, Dandelion's contribution to the Spirit world comes as if out of thin air; it is believed to call the Spirits. Dandelions shine a bright light on situations that need altering and offer expansive solutions. I believe they are here to teach us on many levels. The Dandelion Flower reflects all the celestial bodies: the Yellow Sun - Flower, the Silvery Moon - Seedhead, and the many, many Stars - millions of Winged Seeds.

MAGICAL USES: Used for centuries for divination, wishing and calling spirits. Some believe Dandelion root tea promotes psychic powers. Leave a cup of tea by the bed to promote dreams with spirit visitations. Children have always used the seed heads for making wishes. Make a garland of the closed flower heads that have bloomed and closed, with tufts of cotton on top - space well on a string, and the next day they bloom! If you bury Dandelion in the northwest corner of the house, it will bring favorable winds of change your way. To send a message to a loved one, blow your intention out with your breath as you blow the seed heads away.

FLOWER ESSENCE: Yellow, Sun-like, joyful, Dandelion is helpful for the *over-doers* of the world (my hand is up)! Great for chronic fatigue, muscle tension, low stamina, and exhaustion. Dandelion Flower Essence provides dynamic physical energy, but also helps one to listen and slow down. It is helpful for grief, over-striving, perfectionism,

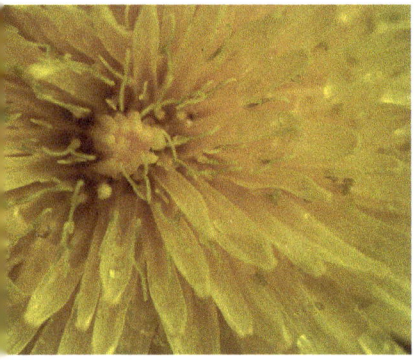

resistance, and tension from exhaustion. This is an essence that brings calm and effortless flow. Helpful for issues of the Solar Plexus or Personal Power chakra. Useful for clearing old anger and other emotions out of the body. Great for picky eaters, people with low self-confidence and those who are indecisive (lacking in personal guidance). The glorious Dandelion has a special affinity for helping to balance the energy of children. A simple fresh Flower Essence can be made with your kids, right in the yard. Place clean Dandelion flowers in a glass bowl or jar of spring water, and allow it to sit for a few minutes to a few hours in the Sun to release the magic. Dandelion Water can be sipped right away, or preserved with a bit of brandy for the big kids.

PREPARATIONS: Fresh, young greens make a very nourishing daily salad, especially for pregnant Moms and kids alike. A juice of the roots will cure what ails you - many symptoms can be relieved this way. Dried root can be gently boiled to make Dandelion Root tea. Fresh flowers make an outstanding Dandelion Wine, Dandy flower fritters, pancakes, bread, jelly, syrup, marshmallows, ice cream and so much more. Capers can be made from the very tiniest young flower buds by pickling them in a vinegar brine (find them deep in the center of the basal rosette before the stem of the flower shoots up tall). Roots can be peeled and eaten fresh or cooked as you would carrots, or pickled and canned. Make a Dandelion pizza - heap the greens onto any frozen pizza or freshly sauced dough, cover with cheese and bake until the cheese is nice and brown. Italians love their Dandy greens and they dress them with lemon, vinegar, garlic and olive oil. You can blanch the young greens for less than a minute and store in the freezer for exceptional Winter nutrition.

Dandelion Root Coffee

Harvest, wash and slice or chop **Dandelion Roots**, place on a baking sheet and spread them out as much as possible for best airflow. Dry in a 250 degree (F) oven for 1 to 2 hours, checking, turning and stirring every 15 minutes or so.

Once they feel fully dry, raise the temperature and roast the roots at 325 degrees (F) for another 35 to 45 minutes, checking & tossing every 15 minutes, taking great care not to burn. Cool and seal in a Mason jar.

TO USE: Grind 1 Tablespoonful Roasted Pieces (the way you would whole beans). Boil 1 Cup Water in a small pot, add ground Dandelion. Simmer for about 2-5 minutes, tasting so it doesn't get too bitter. Add other herbs for taste, like Chicory or Spearmint. Strain, and flavor as you like with cream, nut milk creamers, or sweetener if you desire.

Or you can add ground Dandelion Root to Coffee grounds when you make Coffee. Roasted it is perfect for adding to other teas, enhancing soups and for adding to medicinal extracts and bitters.

If Roasted Dandelion Root Coffee is more than you want to prepare, I have a wonderful product to share with you made from Dandelion Root, called *Dandy-Blend*. Its popularity increases with every cup made - it is delicious, easy, and PACKED with Dandelion's unparalleled nutrition. Dandy-Blend is an instant powder, formulated to resemble coffee in flavor and body, and it is delicious both hot and cold. Dave Allen and I take our liver-loving Dandelion remedy every night, we call it a "Jim Dandy!" For a coffee substitute, this is the best-tasting, caffeine-free, sweet-craving-satisfying beverage I have ever tried, and it is nutritious and so good for your Liver.

RECENT HISTORY OF ABUSE: Dandelion is allegedly the most Ubiquitous Weed, with the worst reputation ever — and if you believe everything you see on the TV, everybody hates it and wants to kill it. I get livid when I see this. Dandelion is a Chief Medicinal Plant, playing a vital role in medicine and health and survival. Its hundreds of uses have not only been forgotten but the poor plant has been demonized, banned and shunned from any "good yard." The same chemical companies who make the pesticides also make the medicines with which this vital plant competes. Their message could not BE more wrong or more opportunistic. I think it is ironic that one of our greatest medicinal plants has been "taken out" by the pharmaceutical competition. Believe me, they are only interested in their own job security and industry domination, not in protecting you from the dangerous Dandelion. And remember, a war on Dandelions kills BEES — our most important food supply Heroes. And that it is estimated that more than 7 million wild birds die annually because of lawn pesticides and herbicides.

In other countries, millions of dollars are made **selling Dandelion**. It is cultivated in Europe as a gourmet food and a vitally important medicine plant. And yet, especially in the US, so many more millions of dollars are spent trying to ERADICATE it! A valuable food plant under siege simply because it likes to grow in the grass? Dandelion is trying to provide, just look at the abundance of them. Doesn't that strike any chord within you? The fact that Dandelion can *grow everywhere*, and is *good for everyone*, is a sure clue from the Creator that it is meant to be utilized.

<u>**LAURA:**</u> Some people say **Dandelion is the most successful plant on Earth**, mastering survival against all odds. And boy, have modern Humans stacked the odds against it! In the old days, the gardeners actually weeded out the *grass* so the Dandelions and other beneficial Weeds could grow better! Dandelions feed your lawn and aerate the soil for helpful insects, so the grass and garden only benefit if you leave them. When you mow them, they grow back with much shorter stalks to stay in line with your cut grass. Dandelion is a perfect food plant that has dozens of benefits and so many more nutrients than most of the garden plants we try to grow! It was only in the mid 1900's that chemical companies decreed that Dandelions had lost their luster and become a nuisance, paving the way for them to offer their toxic solutions.

Likewise, in the early 1900's nobody paid any attention to the "noxious weed" Peanut until George Washington Carver brought it to the attention of the whole World. Suddenly a "useless pest" became a lifesaver for farmers, chefs, oil and food providers alike. The same thing can happen with Dandelion if enough of us continue to educate people and stand up in support. We can all save it, use it and serve it by example! Go out in the yard with your kids and have a talk about this amazing plant. Then gather some, prepare and eat it together - you will see their eyes light up with the joy of making a new friend!

Euell Gibbons called Dandelion *"The Official Remedy for Disorders"* which is the literal translation of its botanical name in Latin. James Beard (famous chef and culinary awarder) uses it, and many of the countries in Europe and Asia prize this remarkable plant as a gourmet food. The Chinese count it as one of the **Six Primary Plants** in their extensive pharmacopeia of thousands of medicinal herbs. Brigitte Mars calls Dandelion one of the *"**five most nutritious vegetables on Earth**.*" Even the

US Department of Agriculture ranks Dandelion above both Broccoli and Spinach for highest nutritional content. Many people believe the "bitter herbs" referred to in the Bible are Dandelions. They grow on every continent (except Antarctica in this modern age). Before salad greens were readily available in the grocery stores Dandelion greens saved millions of lives. People learned how to make everything from coffee to wine to flour with all the parts of this amazing plant, and they counted on it as a fresh, nutritious vegetable that would grow anywhere. Dandelion seeds can spread as far as five miles from their original flower! They also reveal their independence - the flower does not need to be pollinated to produce seed, so it has a fail-safe to survive.

Dandelions have their roots in history as they were thought to have evolved more than 30 million years ago somewhere in Eurasia. Their worldwide use is documented in the writings and pharmacology of Ancient Greece, Egypt, Lebanon, Germany, Switzerland, Portugal, Korea, China and Rome (Italy). Some smart herbalists actually brought stores of Dandelion plants on the Mayflower over to the New World, although the Native Americans likely had already been using it for hundreds of years.

In Bulgaria, scientists have proven that Dandelion leaves can be used to monitor air pollution, as they retain pollutants in direct proportion to their concentration in the environment. In Japan, they honor Dandelions and devote entire gardens to them, with horticultural societies dedicated to studying and developing new varieties.

In Tennessee, Dandelions can be found blooming year-round. Nothing makes me feel quite as good as going to the mailbox in January and seeing a new Dandelion. Hope returns with Dandelions. The flower is a personal Sun growing just for you, and its beautiful yellow flag marks a vital resource plant growing abundantly below. I feel a deeply rooted kinship with it, and the need to protect the Dandelion is strong in me. ALL people should understand the truth about this incredibly useful plant. If you want to remove it from your lawn, do not spray your precious land with poisons, just harvest it, eat it and make good use of it as Nature intended!

Become a Dandelion Champion, spread Dandelion's Good-Weed Gospel to everyone you know. Let Dandelion be a Gateway Weed for you, one that convinces you of the need to forage for many more wonderful, Wild Weed Foods.

> **And the Dandelion does not stop growing because it is told it is a Weed. The Dandelion does not care what others see. It says,**
> **"One day they will be making wishes upon me."**
> ~ B. Atkinson

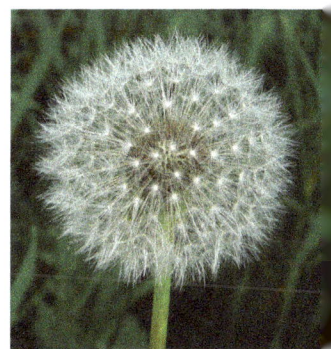

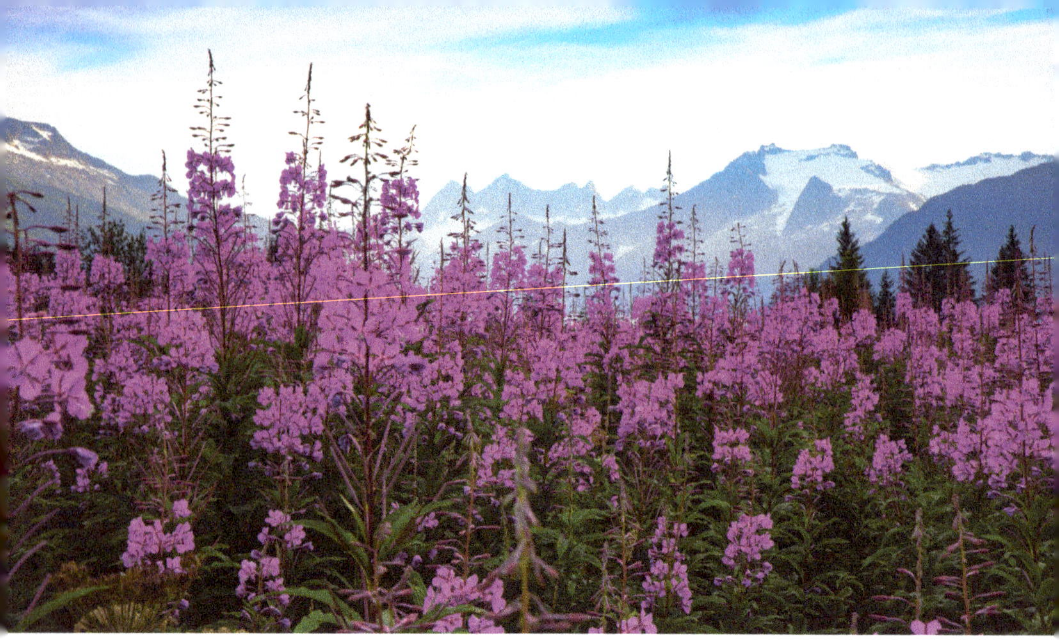

FIREWEED

Chamerion, Epilobium ungustifolium   Evening Primrose Family / **ONAGRACEAE**

FOUND: Widespread in North America, Europe, the Himalayas, and Asia. I always thought of Fireweed as a mountain plant, but it grows in 38 of the 50 US states in varied conditions, altitudes, and climates, in open fields, along roadsides, railroads, in gravel, streams, mountain meadows and at the forest's edge, mainly in full sun.

IDENTIFYING FEATURES: Glorious hot pink compound flowers (up to 50 blooms on one stalk) atop sturdy stalks with an abundance of long, pinnate, narrow, middle-ribbed leaves. The leaf veins are unique and will identify this plant positively (in all seasons and before & after the flowering) as they are rounded and do not reach the edges of the leaf. The stalks reach 4-6 feet high, but have been known to grow as high as 9 feet. Flowers have 4 petals and 4 sepals, and leave behind a long pink capsule which contains fluffy down and tens of thousands of seeds in long thin pink seedpods. Leaves turn red in the Fall.

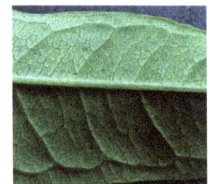

FOOD: Whole plant is edible. Flowers make a beautiful pink jelly, syrup, candy or ice cream and are amazing in salads for decorating cakes. Bees make a delicious and spicy honey with the nectar. The flower buds can be pickled like capers. Stalks are great fresh or cooked, and taste best before flowers bloom. Because leaves can be identified in all seasons by the circular veins, they can be harvested year round for tea. Root can be boiled or roasted like most root veggies or dried and powdered for flour. Cook the early Fireweed shoots as you would asparagus. The green parts of the plant and root become bitter when the flower is in bloom, while the plant is sending all the nectar and sweetness upward to the showy flowers to attract the Pollinators. Use this time to gather the blossoms for their plant sugar and nutritional value. Watch out for the Moose, Bear Deer and Elk when gathering - they all love Fireweed!

CONTAINS: Beta-Carotene, Vitamins A, B3, and C, Potassium, Sodium, Calcium, Magnesium, Lithium, 16 Amino Acids, Trace Minerals, Poly-Phenolic (Ellagitannins), Oenothein B, Glucuronic Acid, Phenolic Acids, Flavonoids (Quercetin, Kaempferol), Sterols, Triterpenes, Beta-sitosterol, Essential Oils, Mucilage, Tannins and Fatty Acids, Pectin, Plant Sugars.

BODY BENEFITS: Fireweed is a great food source, with a readily digestible protein that brings energy and vitality, and is supportive for digestive issues, skin complaints and liver conditions. It normalizes blood pressure, enhances the mood, relieves impotence and stimulates circulation. Fireweed can balance hormones especially in men and is useful for many male health issues. Surthrivalist **Daniel Vitalis** says,"*Fireweed acts as a 5-alpha reductase inhibitor, helping reduce the conversion of testosterone to dihydrotestosterone (DHT) which has been linked to hair loss, benign prostate hyperplasia (BPH), and may play a role in prostate cancer. Preliminary research indicates Fireweed is an excellent herbal candidate for men aged 40 and over, both in the treatment of andropause and BPH, and prophylactically against prostate cancer.*"[14] In Siberia, they make a traditional fermented tea from the flowers that tastes like rich, fruity red wine, called Ivan Chai. This tea can replace caffeinated beverages and provide the body with a nutritive energy that restores (instead of exhausts) the adrenal glands. Fireweed has a soothing, gentle laxative effect and coats the tissues to heal intestinal distress for leaky gut syndrome, colitis, IBS and Crohn's. It is helpful for sore throats and lung complaints as well, and has an antimicrobial effect on staph, strep and candida.

QUALITIES: It is alterative, anti-aging (possible Fountain of Youth?), antimicrobial, anti-inflammatory, antioxidant power rivaling Vitamin C, antiparasitic, anti-proliferative, antispasmodic, astringent, calmative, cytotoxic (acts against cancer cells), demulcent, emollient, photoprotective (sunscreen action), and modulating for the immune system. Fireweed is joyful, feminine, loving, and abundant.

FOLKLORE: folk names Rose Bay, Blooming Sally, Firetop, Willow Weed (the leaves look like Willow leaves and have similar action), Great Willow Herb, Ivan-Tea, Ivan Chai, Koporye Tea, Persian Willow, Bomb Weed, Feuerkraut, Indian Wickup, Burnt Weed, French Willow, and Herb Wickopy. The French eat the young shoots like Asparagus and call it Asperge. Fireweed is the floral emblem of the Yukon, and also the National Flower of Greenland. Native American tribes used it for gastrointestinal problems, constipation, parasites, headaches, insomnia and first aid for wounds and bruises. They also used the fluff of the seed capsules with animal hair and feathers for weaving yarn, and for felting into a kind of fabric for mats.

FIRST AID & SURVIVAL USES: Tea or extract for migraines, insomnia, anemia, the DT's, infections, and colds. Gargle juice or tea for laryngitis and sore throat. Tea can also be used as a sunscreen, spritz yourself with a spray bottle of it regularly while in the Sun. Fluff released after flowering is great fire-making tinder, and also very cushioning under bedding, and to add to pillows or sleeping bags for warmth. The inside of the stem can be cut thinly, soaked in water, braided, and made into nets, twine and lashing.

SPIRITUAL PROPERTIES: Fireweed is ruled by Mercury as a traveler, Venus as a beauty, and the Sun for its love of its light, and represents the Fire Element. Some people believe each Fireweed plant replaces the Soul of a burned down tree. This beautiful plant helps heal and align the Sacred Feminine, repairing damage done by religion or negative male-dominant behaviors. It heals the Heart Chakra and helps release abuse. Fireweed steps you up, and raises your vibration to a higher level.

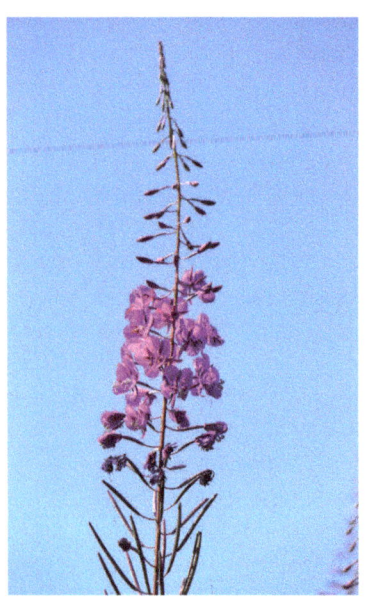

MAGICAL USES: For redemption from trauma, make beads out of the crushed flower blossoms and a pinch of sugar. Put a toothpick through each for a hole. Dry, and then thread flower beads on a string to wear next to the Heart. Know that the Fireweed will transmute and burn away any old wounds creating a receptive space for new growth.

FLOWER ESSENCE: Fireweed brings back beauty and heals the heart. It is like a hot blanket for the Spirit. It dissolves old energy patterns and the negative emotions around trauma, shock and abuse. It frees you of victim mentality and self-pity. Can be especially great for war veterans with PTSD. It burns away the old, creating a safe space for the new, helping all beings shift into higher consciousness. Fireweed is healing and can ease you back to Nature and the loving, nurturing harmony of balance.

A single Fireweed plant can release up to 80,000 seeds each season, which accounts for their ability to reclaim large swaths of burned land so quickly. Fireweed will also help rehabilitate clear cuts and encourage the forest to recover from overharvesting. It fixes nutrients into the soil to build a matrix that prevents soil erosion. Fireweed encourages fresh colonizing growth upon which a new forest can eventually grow back. It will remediate and recolonize oil spill areas, as well. Fireweed can also be an indicator of toxic radiation sites. **When Uranium is present in the soil it causes the Fireweed flowers to mutate and become white,** as they absorb the radioactivity and renew the soil. Needless to say - don't eat the white ones! But know they are purifying the Earth.

Fireweed Jelly

- 6-8 cups of **Fireweed Blossoms & Buds** (no stems, lightly packed & rinsed)
- 5 cups **Water**
- ¼ cup **Lemon Juice**
- 1 teaspoon of **Butter or Coconut Oil** (to eliminate foaming)
- 2 oz. (57 g) of **Powdered Pectin**
- 5 cups **Raw Sugar**

- Pour boiling water over the Fireweed Blossoms and let infuse for 30 minutes to an hour or more (some Alaskan die-hards leave it to infuse for 24 hours, I would). Squeeze flowers with your clean hands, strain this juice and add to a large pot for the jelly, composting the old flowers. Add Lemon Juice, Butter and Sugar. Bring to a boil, and then hard boil for 1 minute. Remove from heat. Stir in Pectin, and stir for 5 minutes. Skim the foam off, if any forms. Pour into sterilized Mason jars, wipe off the lids and jars and tightly screw on lids. It's so beautiful and pink! Process in a hot water bath (details in Canning section). Allow jelly to sit undisturbed for an hour or more, so it can set up fully, then refrigerate and consume within 1 month.

<u>LAURA:</u> While I have never used it in this fashion, Fireweed's constituents have been scientifically proven to be stronger than cortisone creams for healing eczema and skin inflammation (I wish I knew this sooner!). The Glucuronic acid makes Fireweed an amazing remedy for arthritis and rheumatism. Its benefits for men are many, and this overlooked Weed may contain the secret for keeping men virile and healthy. We really should seek this beauty out every year and make MANY medicines from it.

This plant is relatively unknown to some people, but it was used for ages in traditional medicine all around the world. It was named for its ability to be one of the first plants to recolonize in burned out areas, blanketing the land, healing the soil and priming it for life again. Fireweed was the first plant to appear after the Mount St. Helens eruption in 1980, which destroyed all flora and wildlife. In London after WW II, Fireweed was the first to bring color back to the bombed-out grey landscape. The hopeful pink paints a fresh start on the landscape and brings back hope, color and life.

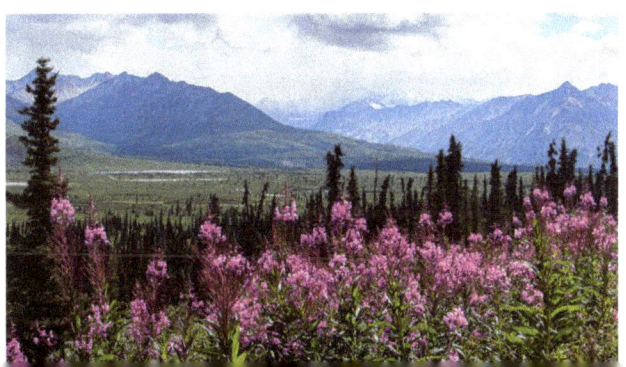

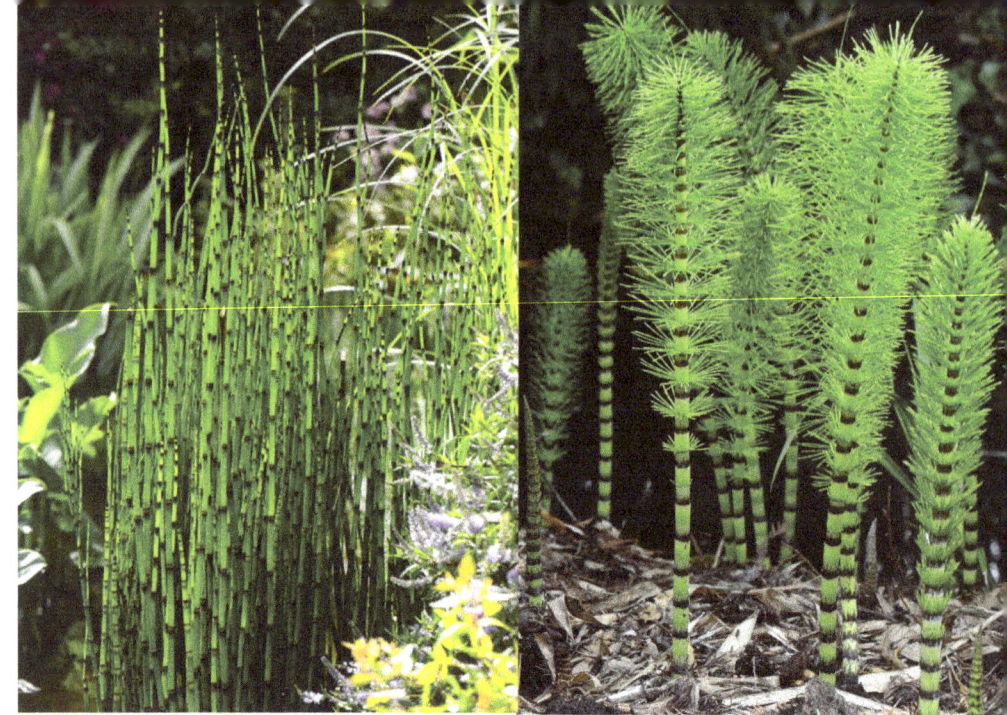

HORSETAIL

Equisetum arvense, et al   Horsetail Family / **EQUISETACEAE**

FOUND: In moist habitats all over the World in woods, along streams, ditches, roadsides and rivers. Horsetail is native to Eurasia, Africa and North America.

IDENTIFYING FEATURES: One tall stalk, like a miniature jointed bamboo, that can reach 2-3 feet tall. Young plants are very needled and hairy, resembling a horse's tail. Mature stalks are bare, black- jointed, tall and hollow. This crazy ancient plant has scales instead of leaves. The cone-like flower on top is called a "strobile," and opens in bands to spread spores into the wind.

FOOD: Young shoots are a wonderful trail food and vegetable staple for Native American and Japanese cultures. Tea is made from the dried stalks. Gather in the Spring and early Summer (to avoid excessive nitrate and selenium content). Do not gather plants with brown spots (not the brown and black joints of the horsetail but actual brown spots in the green stalk) which could be a fungus. Small stalks can be peeled and the heart can be eaten. The tuber-like roots can be eaten raw or prepared like a root vegetable.

CONTAINS: Silicon (a soluble source of Silica), Beta-Carotene, Vitamin C, Calcium, Magnesium, Potassium, Selenium, Sulfur, Manganese, Luteolin, Saponins, Phytosterols, Phenolic Acids, Caffeic Acids, Alkaloids (Nicotine is one), Rutin, Phytosterols, Acontic Acid, Tannins, and 15 types Of Bioflavonoids.

BODY BENEFITS: The Silica that Horsetail absorbs from the soil is a hair and nail strengthening mineral that is also exceptional for strengthening bones in osteoporosis and fusing fractures. It creates a crystalline matrix for bones to recalcify upon and the raw material for tissues to build collagen. It is mineral-packed and acts as a full-body tonic. It will also strengthen and heal ligaments and tendons, prevent kidney stones & and other kidney problems, urinary tract infections, heal ulcers, help heal tuberculosis, and help skin regenerate. It is an antioxidant, shown to protect cells and inhibit cancer-cell growth. Helpful for the eyes, for gout, coughs and asthma, balances blood sugar in diabetes, and is supportive for the Liver. Horsetail is a good source of Quercetin and can be helpful for Springtime allergies. It has been used to remedy incontinence and other bladder maladies. There are encouraging reports of Horsetail as a treatment for Senility (which can be an imbalance of Silicon and Aluminum which this herb can rebalance). Horsetail is able to extract Gold from the water and soil it grows in, and any remedy with inherent Gold is useful for rheumatoid arthritis and joint pain. It clears heat and toxins from the blood and dampness from the body.

QUALITIES: Horsetail is alterative, antimicrobial, antifungal, anti-inflammatory, antiseptic, astringent, diaphoretic, diuretic, healing and restructuring for the connective tissue, hemostatic, mineralizing, nutritive, rejuvenative, styptic, and vulnerary. It has a sweet minerally flavor that is slightly bitter, and it is cooling, dry, yin, and grounding.

FOLKLORE: Folk names Horse Pipes, Bottle Brush, Shave Brush, Scouring Rush, Snake Grass, Bull Pipes, Devil's Guts, Jointed Monkey's Grass, Dutch Rushes, Paddock Pipes, Pewterwort, Joint Grass, Candock, Mare's Tail, Eyes of Fire, Corncob Plant, Canutillo del Llano, Equiseto, Asprella, Equisette. Horsetail was originally used to polish metal (especially pewter) and arrowheads, due to its scratchy action.

FIRST AID USES: It stops bleeding - chew in the mouth and apply as a poultice. Use the tea for nosebleeds, soothing wounds and burns, stomachaches, colds, menstrual cramps, joint pain. Soak feet in Horsetail tea for blisters and infections. Use small joints of Horsetail for brushing your teeth. Gather Horsetail to dry and powder to use as a styptic. Tea can be used as an eyewash for pinkeye or styes. When trying to grow out the hair, rinsing the hair and massaging the scalp with Horsetail tea is super supportive for strengthening hair that breaks easily, and can be helpful for dandruff.

SPIRITUAL PROPERTIES: It is ruled by Saturn and the Earth Element, so Horsetail influences structure, the crystalline matrix, the framework - and offers foundational Earthly Energy as well as ancestral support. Horsetail is an **Ancient**, a true wizard of a Plant and should be worked with in meditation and journeying.

MAGICAL USES: Place in the bedroom for fertility support, use in pouches & amulet mixtures to be worn on the body, place on a fertility altar, or hang by the bed. According to legend, a whistle made of the hollow stem will charm snakes to the player. The stalks make great magic wands or all-natural pick-up sticks.

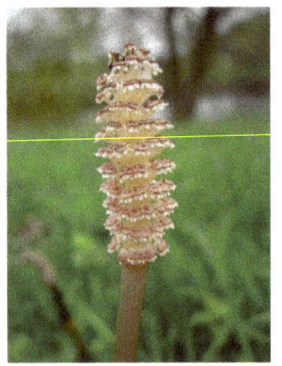

FLOWER ESSENCE: Horsetail embodies stand-up-tall energy, foundational support and the momentum to strive upward. It supports communication at all levels. It enhances interspecies communication (great for work with animals), and connects you with your generational ancestors. Helps open the channel to your Higher Self and Superconscious. Enables you to build step-by-step new foundational structures, crystallize your desires, and strive for your highest potential.

PREPARATIONS: Use 2 teaspoons of herb per one cup water for tea. Also, Horsetail can be juiced, or made into a flower essence or alcohol extract (which, with Coconut oil, can be applied to hair and scalp as a hair mask for better growth). Horsetail contains some nicotine, and can be used in a smoking blend to reduce cravings for tobacco (short-term use up to 3 weeks, do not use it with a nicotine patch, could be too much). Horsetail is a natural gritty abrasive - use a small handful of stalks to scour & clean dishes when camping, use it to polish wood, or to scrape off gum! Horsetail is great as one of the herbs for sitz baths after childbirth. Chew the stalks while hiking for nourishing minerals and to look extra cool.

LAURA: Horsetail was truly here first! The plant we see growing today has been **carbon-dated back to millions of years ago**. Really?! This plant is **PREHISTORIC**. It has been found on Earth for over 300 million years (yes, this is accurate).[15] That's the equivalent of living BEFORE the Dinosaurs or Mammoths! Horsetail is a living fossil. *Can you imagine the intelligence and experience in that Family line?* They are ancient, they have seen it all and survived it all. They must be one of the smartest plants alive today! No wonder Horsetail may help connect you to your ancestors, because your ancestors probably USED THE PLANT. Amazing. This made me fall in love with it all over again. Now when I see Horsetail I realize I am in the presence of Historical Figures, as the rest of this Family are now extinct.

Horsetail plays an important part in the recycling and removal of nutrients in wetlands, and can be found growing on the edges of water in all forms. Ironically, its scaly exterior makes it immune to most herbicides, so spraying it won't kill it. Anything that has lived for so long has developed defensive mechanisms for just about everything! The adaptive Nature is on full display with this ancient one. It grows in communities much like Bamboo. If you have some, be grateful! Harvest it, use it, split and share it and store it. This is a super healing herb that deserves ultimate protection and respect. Through many Ages, Horsetail has earned it.

Instead of filling our bellies with the "all-the-rage" powdered collagen remedies made from bovine tracheas (ughh), let's look to Horsetail with its *natural* Silica that gives the body the raw materials to produce its OWN collagen.

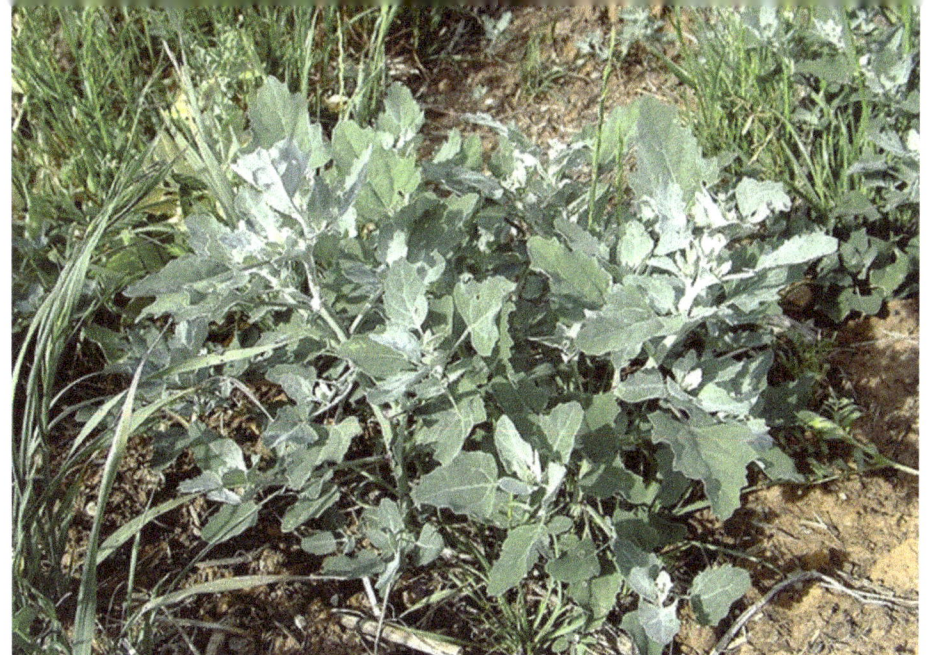

LAMB'S QUARTERS

Chenopodium album   *Goosefoot Family/* **CHENOPODIACEAE**

FOUND: At the sides of buildings, along fence lines, in vacant lots in all 50 states, even in Hawaii, Lamb's Quarters love nitrogen-rich soil and will be found growing near other nitrogen-fixing plants. Originally found in Europe & Asia and used traditionally in many cultures, even farmed in India. Susun Weed says it is *"one of the most widely distributed plants in the World."* For a reason! Along with relatives Quinoa, Amaranth and Spinach, Lamb's Quarters are a powerful wild plant made for feeding the World.

IDENTIFYING FEATURES: Leaves look like a goose's foot, grey-green with white fur-like dust (especially the stem and underside of leaf), and the plant is unwettable (repels water) when fresh. It has a stalk of tiny green and grey seed panicles at the crown when in flower. Can grow to 18 inches high, and in ideal conditions even up to six feet. Lamb's Quarters does NOT smell bad, which is a tip for identifying this plant correctly. The young sprouts have opposite leaves and are somewhat diamond-shaped with the characteristic white dusting (note the botanical name *album* means white in Latin). This dust is made up of mineral salts the plant has processed and created from the soil, indicating its high value as a mineral-rich plant.

FOOD: Naturalists agree this plant is one of the best examples of an abundant, nutritious and forgotten food source that happens to grow as a humble weed. Every part of the plant can be consumed. Lamb's Quarters is the very best wild green, tastes even better than Spinach. Eat raw or steam, boil or saute. Seed panicles can be sprouted, dried and ground for flour, dried and used as a spice, or made into an oatmeal like porridge.

CONTAINS: Vitamin A, B1 B2 and B6, C and K, Folate, Niacin, Calcium, Copper, Iron, Magnesium, Manganese, Phosphorus, Potassium, Sodium, Zinc, Trace Minerals, Tryptophan, Silica, Omega 3 and 6 Fatty Acids, FIber, Protein, Oxalates.

BODY BENEFITS: Lamb's Quarters remineralizes the body (so it is great for anemia), nourishes adrenal function and the ability to process emotions better. It provides Protein for strength and blood sugar stability, and Essential Fatty Acids for cardiovascular and brain health. It can be helpful for liver disorders, spleen enlargement, ulcers, and bilious stomach. Cook in a small amount of water or stock to make a "**vegetable bone-broth**" for healing broken bones and connective tissue. Seeds are especially high in protein. Prevents scurvy and treats worms, intestinal distress and stomach aches. It increases circulation and decreases inflammation.

QUALITIES: This plant is feminine, salty, bitter, mineral-filled, antianemic, antidiarrheal, anthelmintic, antiphlogistic, antirheumatic, astringent, mildly laxative, and odontalgic (helps a toothache!).

FOLKLORE: Folk names Goose Foot, Pig Weed, Wild Spinach, Bacon Weed, Fat Hen, Frost Blight, White Goosefoot, Dirty Dick, Huauzontle, Melde, Bathua, Krouvida, Quelite, Superman. Green dye can be made from the young shoots. There are fossil records indicating this plant has been used as a food source since at least 6500 BC. **Lamb's Quarters received its name because the gathered plants have the same amount of Protein per pound as a quarter of a Lamb.**

FIRST AID USES: Use a tea of the leaves for sunstroke, and to replace electrolytes from exercise. Tea can be used in a footbath for aching or swollen feet, as a wash for itchy bug bites, and a mouthwash for canker sores or bad breath. Use tea for muscle-cramps, stomach aches, diarrhea, to expel worms, and for relieving sore limbs. Chew the seeds for urinary discomfort. The crushed root makes a mild trail soap.

SPIRITUAL PROPERTIES: Ruled by Saturn and the Earth Element, Lamb's Quarters represents the abundant mineral legacy of Earth. Use this plant for connecting the realms, and discovering the connections that are supporting you from the beyond.

MAGICAL USES: Wear a crown of the flowers to speed healing of any ailment. A wreath of Lamb's Quarters and Amaranth is said to confer invisibility.

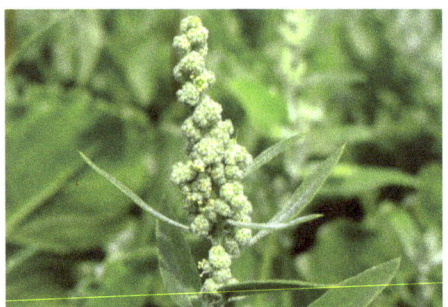

FLOWER ESSENCE: It encourages a heartfelt approach to all things, and helps bridge the gap between what the head wants and the heart counsels. Effective for overthinkers and people who block communication from their Higher Selves by analyzing data instead of just receiving. Helps you soften and hear the voice of intuition. This is a very abundant plant, and the essence reflects its ability to provide great balance and support when in emotional need.

PREPARATIONS: Lamb's Quarters come up early in the Spring and are one of the first edible greens. They are great paired with cheeses and sauces and lots of people add bacon! Cook with your pots of beans to reduce gas upon eating them. You can blanch them and store in the freezer for winter greens, you can dry the leaves for use later, and they are also great for canning. Saute leaves in butter and garlic for a better-than-Spinach side dish. Collect the seed panicles and grind into flour which can be used half and half with other grains for bread and pancakes. Seeds can be dried and cooked with any grain, or added to soups and oatmeal. Add seeds to tomato sauces to mimic the taste of meat sauce. Simmer or steam as a potherb like you would Spinach. Euell Gibbons says *"Pigweeds are too good for Pigs."* He recommends you seek out plants that are young and tender and less than one foot high, and he reminds us we can find this abundant food plant from mid-Spring until frost. Gather tons of it in Midsummer when it is abundant to put up for Winter greens. Frozen or canned Lamb's Quarters that you preserve will provide high-quality Vitamin C and a potent Multi-Mineral source for the whole year. Add the leaves to smoothies and juices for electrolytes. You can make a *Bathua* paste, used in Indian cuisine, by steaming the leaves until well wilted and then pulverizing the herb in the food processor or blender to add to sauces and breads. Dry the leaves, and pulse quickly with Dulse or Kelp (seaweed) and other herbs for an herbal salt alternative. *Eat raw in moderation, and cook the plant to remove the Oxalic Acid if you are prone to kidney stones.

LAURA: On the air during one of my talk radio shows, **Bull**, one of my favorite callers and a farmer himself, was explaining why farmers have to spray so many herbicides. He said it was to keep up with "Superman." When I inquired what plant he meant, he replied, *"Pigweed! It's like Superman! It is always finding ways to resist the chemicals we spray it with - that thing is relentless."* YES, because it is a **major food crop wanting to be grown and utilized**! Stop trying to kill it, to unnaturally grow other stuff, and let the *Pigweed* feed you! When will the people AND the farmers get the message that their same humble SuperMan weed (Pigweed, Lamb's Quarters, Amaranth) **can feed the WORLD?!** And would save millions of dollars on chemicals and their impact.

Lamb's Quarters make the list of my personal *favorite* weeds. This plant gave me my first successful foray into eating and preparing Weeds for others. Back in the old days, I lived in a rustic log cabin at 9,000 feet in **Wondervu, Colorado**, a half an hour from the closest store. One weekend we had unexpected company and were running low on groceries. I wanted to make a Vegetarian Biscuits & Gravy but I was mostly out of fresh ingredients. I decided to go looking for something wild to saute, and then turn into a creamy gravy with some goat cheese I had on hand. I walked out of the cabin door, and just a few paces into the forest's edge I found a beautiful patch of Lamb's Quarters. I greeted it and requested to pick some, and permission was granted. I picked a great large bowl-full, knowing it would shrink when cooked like spinach does.

Once I had the greens, the recipe built itself. I thought the Lamb's Quarters would be good, but I didn't realize they'd be so perfect! The leaves held up (high in silica) and didn't turn soggy or stringy, the flavor was delicious, salty, and they took to the sauce perfectly. I have included the recipe below because it was one of my most satisfying wild meals ever. For many years in Colorado I would make this regularly for company, engaging them in foraging for the plant, watching it cook, and then proving to their taste buds and tummies the delicious benefits of one of our most precious Weeds.

Wondervu Rosemary Biscuits & Lamb's Quarters Gravy

Wondervu Rosemary Biscuits (makes 8-9) - *make these first*

- 2 1/2 cups **Regular or Gluten-free Baking Flour** + a little extra for rolling out dough
- 1 tablespoon **Baking Powder**
- 1 teaspoon **Baking Soda**
- 1/2 teaspoon **Salt**
- 1 stick cold **Butter or Vegan Butter**, cut into small pieces
- 1 cup plain **Yogurt, Buttermilk, Sour Cream, or Coconut Milk Cream**
- 6-8 Fresh **Rosemary Sprigs** (or **Fresh Yarrow Leaves**)

Preheat the oven to 400 degrees F, with a middle rack in place. Line a rimmed baking sheet with parchment paper. Sometimes I butter it, because - butter is medicinal!

Whisk together dry ingredients in a large bowl. Make sure they are thoroughly combined and without lumps.

Using your hands, a steel spatula, or a pastry cutter, cut Butter into the flour mixture until the butter pieces are pea-sized. Make a well in the center of the mixture and add the Yogurt (or substitute). Stir together with a wooden spoon and knead gently in the bowl with your hands to bring dough all together. If too much dry flour remains in the bottom of the bowl, add an additional tablespoon of Yogurt until it becomes a nice dough that holds its shape.

Pull the leaves off half of the Rosemary sprigs, and finely chop, (you can compost the stems). Fold into the dough and knead until well incorporated.

Dust your cutting board or counter with some of the extra Flour. Turn dough out onto the cutting board and press gently into a rectangle until dough is flat and even, and roughly 1-1¼ inches thick. Cut into three or four rounds using a 1-½ inch biscuit cutter or large drinking glass. Place on the prepared baking sheet. Add a sprig of Rosemary or Yarrow or some edible flower like Pansy on top.

Gather any remaining dough together, kneading and repeating the process to cut out all of the biscuits. If the dough seems too soft or unmanageable, chill for 15 minutes.

Bake for 13-15 minutes until the beautiful biscuits are deep, golden brown on top. **This is the perfect amount of time needed to prepare the Gravy below.**

Let biscuits cool for 5 minutes on the pan. Split in half right before serving.

Lamb's Quarters Saute & Gravy

- A Bowl-full of large sprigs of **Lamb's Quarters** (or other sturdy wild greens)
- 2 Tablespoons **Butter or Olive Oil,** more if needed
- 3 cloves of **Fresh Garlic**, minced
- 1 small log of **Goat Cheese** (or Feta cheese), crumbled
- 1-2 teaspoons **Balsamic Glaze** or **White Wine** (or both)
- **Basil Leaves, Lemon Pepper, Cholula, Salt & Pepper** or other condiments to taste

In a hot pan, heat Olive Oil or Butter with Garlic. Watch carefully so you don't burn the Garlic, but heat it thoroughly to release the flavor. Add the Goat Cheese crumbles and Balsamic, and work into a thick sauce. Add a little White Wine, Veggie Stock or Water if you need to thin it up a bit. Season to taste preference with your preferred spices and condiments. I like to add a few glugs of Cholula and Mrs. Dash Lemon Pepper.

Add Greens and stir to coat with sauce. Cook just until Greens are sufficiently warmed, stirring often, and don't overcook.

Heap liberally over split-open hot Biscuits, just as you would a regular Biscuits & Gravy. Garnish with finishing salt, edible flowers, nuts, or the fresh flowertops of the Lamb's Quarters.

- You may by all means substitute regular Wheat Flour for some or all of the Gluten-Free Flour, or add different Whole Grain Flours, or combine them for effect.

- Leftover dry biscuits will taste freshest the first day. After that they can be crumbled into soup or sauces to add body and flavor. However, we never seem to have any left, what with Honey being so nutritious and all (and soooo good on a leftover biscuit).

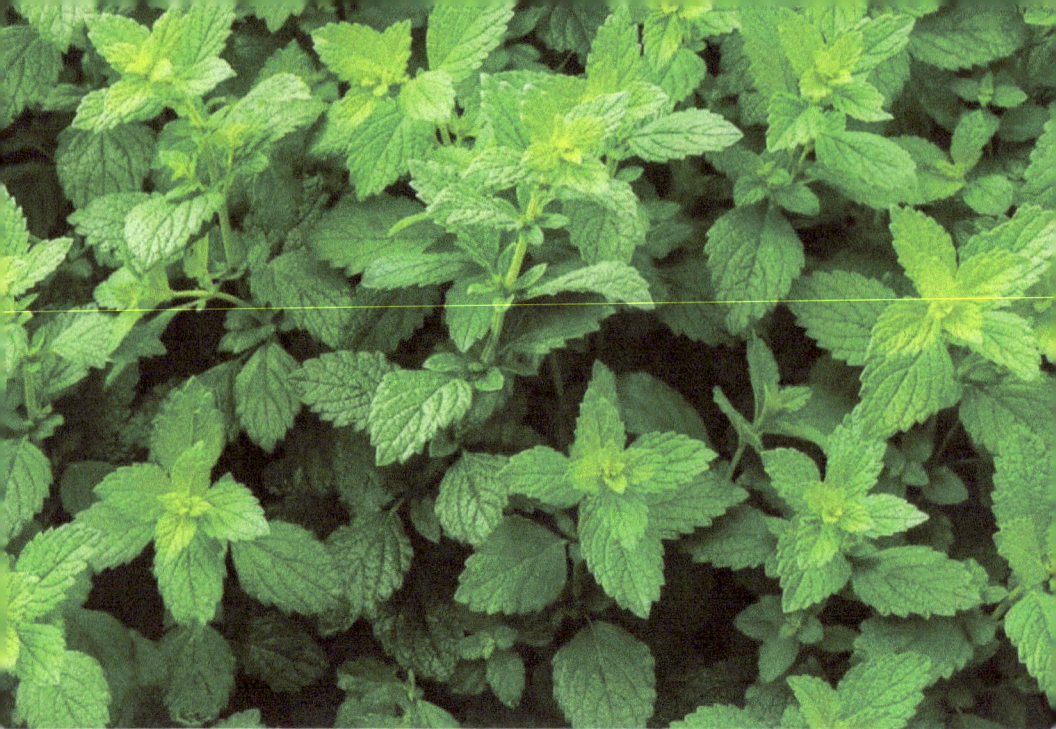

LEMON BALM

Melissa officianalis   Mint Family / **LAMIACEAE**

FOUND: Growing in disturbed ground and open woods, in well-drained soil, Lemon Balm loves the Sun and loves to spread. Originally found in the Mediterranean Basin of Europe, Iran and Central Asia, this impressive and expansive Mint now grows all over the World.

IDENTIFYING FEATURES: Lemon Balm has strongly lemon-scented, bright green, toothed and veined, very abundant heart-shaped leaves. It is a Mint Family member, and has the characteristic square stem, opposing and alternating leaves with the whorled flower which is white to lavender. Flower is in the middle of the stem amongst the leaves, and not at the crown like most Mints. Lemon Balm can reach 2 feet tall and 3 feet wide in one season.

FOOD: Since it is so abundant, you may need to invent many uses for it yourself! I have found the leaves have a divinely lemony taste that pairs well with poultry - but is equally stunning in desserts and for flavoring cordials and syrups. Leaves are a daring addition to salads and soups, adding intense flavor. Use them to decorate cakes, and as a radical flavor for ice cream, similar to Lemongrass.

CONTAINS: Vitamin C, Calcium, Magnesium, Tannins, Bitter Principles, Flavonoids, Hesperidin, Caffeic Acid, Monoterpene Glycosides, Polyphenols, Resins and Essential Oils, Succinic Acid, Rosmarinic Acid.

BODY BENEFITS: The famous Herbalist Nun, St. Hildegard of Bingen, born in 1098 AD, said, *"Lemon Balm contains within it the virtues of a dozen other plants."* It is calming, while being uplifting for the mood and joyfully supportive for the emotions. It soothes the nerves and promotes better sleep. Brigitte Mars says, *"Lemon Balm is generally considered very safe and is a favorite herb for children."* It makes a great bedtime soothing tea to ward off nightmares. Great for all ages, it is also useful for dementia and alzheimer's as it reduces brain damage from plaque-forming proteins, and will increase cognition and soothe agitation. It is heart protective, lowering blood pressure and easing heart palpitations, and with regular use can lower cholesterol. It is a wonderful digestive tonic, treating colic, gastric ulcers, and upset stomach, and is also very helpful for PMS. Lemon Balm increases perspiration and can be helpful in clearing heat, reducing fevers and, for sweating toxins away in detoxes. It improves concentration and focus, and is helpful for ADHD and test anxiety. Lemon Balm is also good for allergies, homesickness, migraines, shingles, teething, flatulence, hyperactivity, nervousness, depression, and anxiety.

QUALITIES: It is sour and citrusy, cooling, dry, yin and feminine. It is anti-aging, antibacterial, anticancer, antidepressant, antioxidant, anti-inflammatory, antispasmodic, antiviral, analgesic, carminative, diaphoretic, digestive, nerve-nourishing, relaxant, rejuvenative, sedative, and a vasodilator.

FOLKLORE: Folk names Lemon Balm, Bee Balm, Sweet Melissa, Dropsy Plant, Heart's Delight, Melissophyllon, Balsamita Maior, Limonnik, Xieng Feng Cao. *Melissa* was the ancient Greek word for Honey Bee. It has been cultivated for farms and gardens since the 16th century, and is an essential ingredient in medicines and perfumes. In the 1st Century, Dioscorides made a liniment with Wine and Lemon Balm for the nerves and sore muscles - I am on it! Carmelite Nuns in 14th century France made a distilled herbal liquor called Carmelite Water or Eau de Carmes, as a panacea for all ills, and digestive tonic. It was so successful for treating the conditions of the day it became known as **"aqua mirabilis" - miracle water**. It was made with a closely guarded secret recipe of 14 herbs that included Lemon Balm, Lemon Peel, Nutmeg, and Angelica root, and it can still be found today. Although, why not make your own? See below. 17th century Botanist Nicholas Culpepper was enchanted by Lemon Balm and wrote in his *Culpepper's Herbal,* in 1652, *"Melissa causeth the mind and heart to become merry... and drives away all troublesome cares and thoughts."*

FIRST AID USES: Extract taken at the first sign of a cold sore may prevent one from flaring. Use the tea for nausea, nervousness, nightmares, to calm hyperactive kids, and for constipation. Make a compress of the leaves for eczema, boils, gout, headache, bug bites, sunburn, tumors and wounds. Use extract for anxiety and depression, and for treating viral conditions.

SPIRITUAL PROPERTIES: Ruled by Jupiter (and quite possibly also the Moon & Venus) and the emotional Water Element. Lemon Balm was sacred to Artemis,

Persephone and Demeter. It used to be grown outside temples to attract Bees which were thought to bring messages from the Divine. Lemon Balm helps the brainwaves to slow into the alpha state of meditation. It inspires dreams and revelations and expansion into the higher realms.

MAGICAL USES: Useful in spells for attracting Love, and also for healing a broken heart (worn in a medicine bag over the heart). It is wonderful for rituals seeking Success, Love and Healing. Just as Lemon Balm has many uses physically, it can be used for nearly any magical intention. Use it to banish dark and evil energies.

FLOWER ESSENCE: Lemon Balm brings deep emotional relaxation & relieves fear. It is perfect for kids who just can't slow down. It helps us to realize our multifaceted nature, inspiring flexibility and versatility. It is useful for releasing emotional trauma and helping you to return to a sunny outlook. Balance is achieved with this essence, and it is perfect for shock, releasing old patterns, soothing the nerves, stimulating emotional renewal and full-body rejuvenation.

PREPARATIONS: Place some Lemon Balm stalks with leaves on top of your chicken while on the barbecue. Crush the leaves and add to drinks or seltzer water. Float some of the fragrant branches in the bathtub to nourish the nerves and the skin. Use it as a seasoning to balance heavy flavors if you don't have Lemon or another acid on hand. Make a Nicholas Culpepper-style "electuary" by infusing dried Lemon Balm leaves in Honey. But the recipe that follows is my favorite - whether you choose Tea or the Wine. It's dazzling, delicious, and actually quite a Cure-All.

LAURA: The famous alchemist Paracelsus called Lemon Balm the "Elixir of Life" and said, "*What is Melissa but a power which exists in the astral light and finds its material expression in the herb Melissa, which grows in our gardens?*" Lemon Balm was his favorite herb, and he believed it contained more healing, **Vital Life Force** (he called it Ens) than any other medicinal plant. Every time we pass it in the garden, we eat a few leaves to enhance our life force, boost our energy and uplift our mood. It makes a great welcome plant in containers, for front porches or patios (and will also repel bugs).

This year, my Lemon Balm was the first green herb to return to my garden in Tennessee about mid-March. Its fresh taste is a harbinger of Spring. Just watch it grow for one season, and you will witness Lemon Balm's zest for Life and understand its ability to expand. Last Summer, I gathered Lemon Balm almost every day for drying, and still had more than I could use or harvest! Since it is a great Pollinator-Attractor for your garden, consider keeping it in pots so it doesn't spread all over the ground - or give Lemon Balm its own garden to take over. The Bees just love it, and its amazing scent also repels pests to keep your garden in balance. Gather it often, and if you need to, before it seeds to minimize the spread. There are so many FREE and wondrous remedies you can make with it, no wonder it grows so abundantly.

Carmelite Water / *Eau de Carmes*

(makes about 3 cups - 24 oz.)

As a New Moon approaches, gather your herbal ingredients for wildcrafting. Sterilize a half gallon jar as well as its airtight lid with rubbing alcohol or vodka.

Purchase an inexpensive bottle of **White Wine (like Pinot Grigio).**

On or near the New Moon, add the following Herbs and Spices to the clean, prepared jar, and cover with **Wine**.

- 1 cup fresh **Lemon Balm** leaves (or 1/2 cup dried organic Lemon Balm)
- 1/4 cup dried organic **Angelica Root**
- 2 Tablespoons dried organic **Coriander Seed**
- 1 Tablespoon organic **Chamomile**
- 1-2 Tablespoons fresh **Lemon Zest** (about 1 small organic lemon)
- 2 teaspoons organic **Mugwort**
- 1 teaspoon organic **Fennel Seed**
- 1 teaspoon organic **Cinnamon Chips**
- ½ teaspoon organic **Sage**
- ½ teaspoon freshly grated organic **Nutmeg**
- ¼ teaspoon organic **Gentian** *(optional, quite bitter, but traditional and very good for you!)*
- 5 organic **Whole Cloves**

Stir the herbs together well, place the lid on, and tighten. Shake 100 times. Place in a cool dark place and shake daily. You may want to taste after a few hours or several days, but the strongest extract will take two weeks. Adjust timing to your taste. I love a long infusion because I love the strong herbal flavors.

After the Full Moon, strain out and wring the herbs well. Or use an herb press or hydraulic press to get out all the good liquid, and bottle into sterilized cordial bottles.

<u>**TO USE:**</u> Take a small amount daily in a fancy spoon, sip in a cordial glass, add to seltzer water, or mix with hot water and Honey for tea. Use medicinally as needed.

Refrigerate the Carmelite Water to preserve it for longer than a few weeks, or add 1 cup **Vodka** or **Brandy** after straining the herbs out for long shelf life and a stronger kick.

- <u>**ALCOHOL-FREE**</u>: add the herbs to 3 cups of Vinegar, Honey or Vegetable Glycerin and process the same way to make a strong remedy with no alcohol.

Recipe can also be made with any Alcoholic Spirit (instead of the Wine) to make a strong **Herbal Extract**. You can add Honey, Maple Syrup or Sugar until thick and rich to make a powerfully tonic and herbal- flavored **Liqueur.**

Carmelite Sister's Tea Blend

You could combine just the herbs into a **Carmelite Sister's Tea Blend** which would be great for soothing frazzled nerves, to remedy stomach aches and headaches, as a powerful anti-viral, and to calm hyperactive children. Use 1 teaspoon of tea blend per cup of just boiled water, and allow to infuse for 5-10 minutes. Use a handful of the herbs (placed in cheesecloth or cloth bag) in water in a Gallon Jar, place in the Sunshine all day, for a delicious. Lemon-Balm-infused **Carmelite Sister's Sun Tea.**

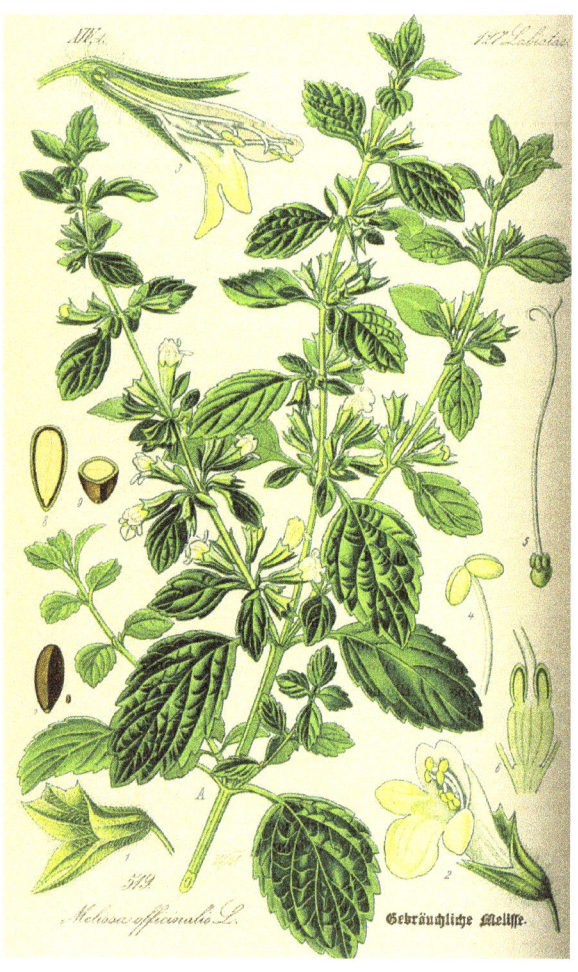

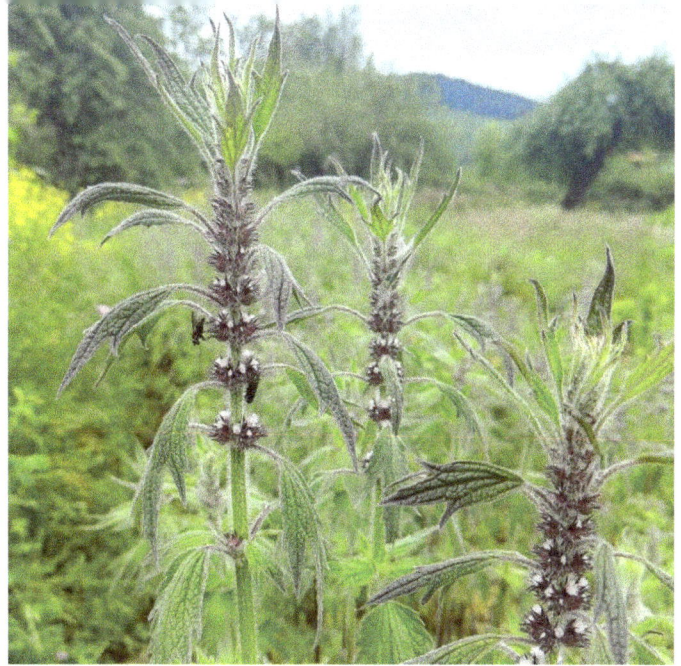

MOTHERWORT

Leonurus cardiaca   *Mint Family* / **LAMIACEAE**

FOUND: Originally cultivated in Europe and Central Asia, introduced to the Americas to attract the HoneyBee. Now misclassified as an "invasive weed," Motherwort can be found in roadsides, yards, gardens, streambeds, and in disturbed ground worldwide.

IDENTIFYING FEATURES: Grows tall on a single square-stemmed stalk 2-5 feet high that is spiky with hairs. Leaves are 3-pronged and deeply veined. Flowers are pink, white or purple-colored, and with the leaves, grow from the center in whorls to a pinnacle on top. Motherwort has the mint Family's characteristic square-shaped stem, and whorled flower calyx and nodes may have purple accents. Like all Mints, leaves are opposite and alternate but on this plant erupt right from a single main stem. It is perennial, and will take over an area over the years, sometimes smothering other plants - so give it a place of its own in honor. Seeds grow in a triangular casing.

FOOD: Young shoots can be steamed and sauteed. Gather the entire plant and dry upside down for use in teas and extracts. Seeds can be dried and used like sesame seeds. The fresh flowers make beautiful edible garnishes for salads, bean dishes, soups, and for decorating plates, and the seeds and flowers have been used to flavor certain types of beer. Motherwort makes a great nutritious addition to Bitters recipes.

CONTAINS: Beta-carotene, Vitamin C, Calcium, Potassium, Flavonoids Quercetin & Rutin, Citric & Malic Acid, Alkaloids (Stachydrine) , Bitter Glycosides (Leonurine), Caffeic Acid, Oleic Acid, Essential Oils, Iridoid, Phytosterols, Tannins, Terpenes, Flavones.

One of the particular Motherwort Alkaloids, Stachydrine, has *"demonstrated various bioactivities for the treatment of fibrosis, cardiovascular diseases, cancers, uterine diseases, brain injuries, and inflammation."*[16]

BODY BENEFITS: Motherwort is a supremely helpful tonic for female hormonal issues from menstruation and PMS mood swings, to menopause and beyond. It is a nervine herb that "gladdens and strengthens the heart," and is supportive for anemia and nervous issues. Famous as a heart tonic (note the "cardiaca" in the Latin name) Motherwort strengthens the heart and boosts endocrine functioning. It is a wonderfully sedating herb for soothing anxiety, tension and stress. Ironically, Motherwort got its name from its use by midwives and doctors in ancient Greece, though some believe it is not safe during the term. But the tea/water infusion of the leaves is definitely helpful for anxiety and muscle relaxation during labor. Motherwort is calming for most "hyper" conditions like hypertension, hyperthyroidism, hyperactivity, hysterics, heart palpitations, hyper hot flashes, night sweats, headaches, restlessness, muscle cramps, fibromyalgia, convulsions, troublesome sleep, spastic colon, irritability, postpartum stress and depression. In the early 1600's, English Herbalist Nicholas Culpepper used it to relieve "melancholy vapors of the heart." He called Motherwort a "loosening medicine" for relaxing muscles, tendons, ligaments, and the membrane covering of organs, as well as loosening phlegm in the lungs and sinuses, for draining water retention and stimulating sluggish digestion. Like a good Mother, Motherwort seems to calm everything that is over the top. Great for use in family meetings or for deep talks. May be of great use in remedying anorexia and eating disorders. Due to its relaxing properties it can cause drowsiness.

CAUTION: Not for use in pregnancy *until* birthing, and Motherwort is best avoided by people with thyroid conditions.

QUALITIES: Motherwort is antibacterial and antifungal, antispasmodic, analgesic, diaphoretic, immune stimulant, uterine stimulant, vasodilator, nervine, circulatory stimulant, laxative. It is warming, drying, astringent, bitter but soothing, mood-enhancing, relaxing, nurturing, sedating and feminine.

FOLKLORE: Folk names Heartwort, Lion's Tail, Throw-Wort, Lion's Ear, Agripaume Cardiaque, Herbe Battudo, Agripalma, Benefit Mother Plant, Gerzgold, Guma, the Lion-Hearted. You can make a wonderful olive green dye with the leaves. .

FIRST AID USES: Serve Motherwort Tea in times of crisis or stress, to quickly calm everybody. It is helpful for heart palpitations and anxiety attacks. Use a small dose of extract for menstrual cramps, headaches or pain, or heart palpitations, every 15 minutes until relieved. Take tea, extract or flower essence for anxiety and fear, or when you feel you need your Mother and need a hug.

SPIRITUAL PROPERTIES: Ruled by Venus, Leo and the Water and Fire Elements. Motherwort is a Sacred Big Sister for all Women, and a Guardian Mother for Men. I have heard it called the "Mama Bear of the Plant World." She is comforting, grounding, protective and magically healing.

MAGICAL USES: Motherwort repels evil spirits, counters hexes and curses, protects babies in the womb like a Mama lioness, and guards against the dark arts. Wear it to dispel bad luck and envy. May be of assistance with clearing spaces (and in exorcism rituals) when calling on the Divine Mother for support. Brings good luck and makes you cheerful! Use to SHIFT things, get them moving again. The Victorians used Motherwort to symbolize "secret love." Burn as an incense to promote astral projection.

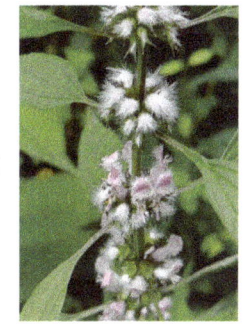

FLOWER ESSENCE: Reverses the feeling of being attacked, or not-at-home in your own skin. Helpful for family issues, resolving childhood trauma & abuse. Benefits those who suffer from food anxiety, eating disorders, overworry about ingredients and allergies, rigid dieters. Use for "Empty Nest" syndrome and other cases of being unable to Mother. Helps you stand tall with authority and trust in benevolent outcomes. Helps with all kinds of transitions in parenting. Helps relieve fear and worry on sleepovers.

LAURA: Motherwort has long been known as a longevity herb. There is a story told about a beautiful mountain spring that ran through many Motherwort plants. All the people in the village who drank from the spring lived to be over 100 years of age.

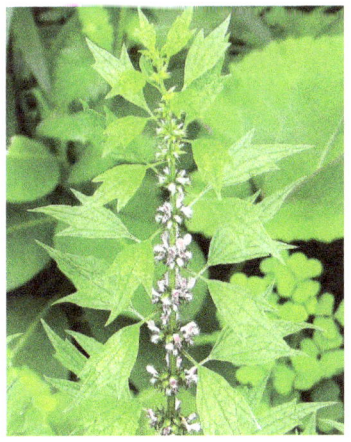

I met this plant in Brigitte's front yard for the first time - and I remember saying, "What is that glorious thing?" Motherwort can be a little shocking in its beauty, you HAVE to notice it towering over a field of grass, or standing regally by a stream. It looks like another one of those ancient plants that *intends* to be noticed and utilized. Motherwort is the Queen Mother, the Lioness, the Mama Bear, who wants to support and comfort you. Her energy supports you and lifts you up above the rest, beautifying and harmonizing your nature.

And the Mothering aspect of this plant is no joke. Try taking some in tea when you need the support of a long-gone Mother, and then get ready to feel loved and nurtured. Your Mom is calling, you better answer.

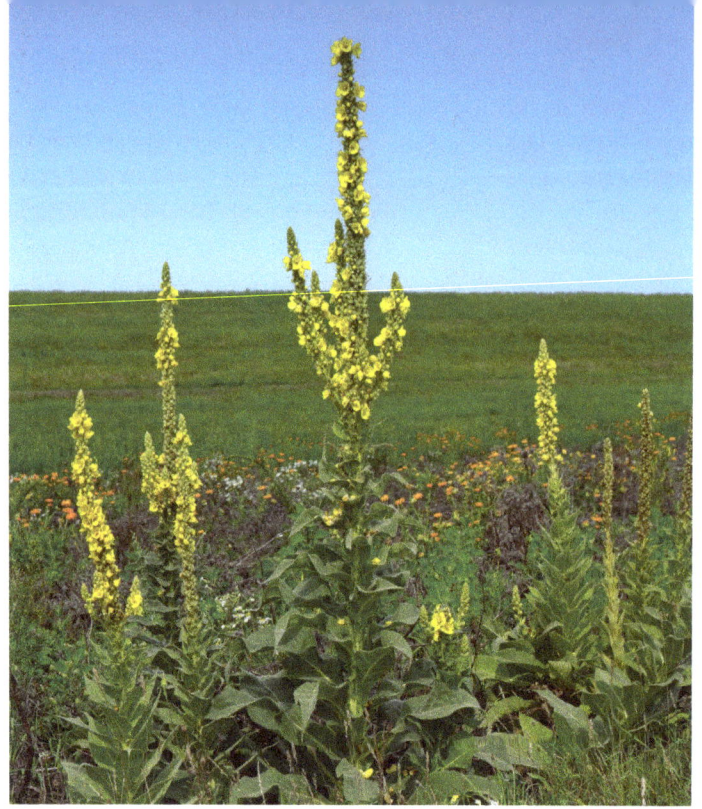

MULLEIN

Verbascum thapsus   *Figwort Family* / **SCROPHULARIACEAE**

FOUND: Originally found in Central Europe and Western Asia, it grows in temperate climates the World over, Found in disturbed ground, compacted soil and wild fields, by railroad tracks and roadsides. This majestic plant can soar to 8 feet tall and grows in communities.

IDENTIFYING FEATURES: Light silvery green, soft, velvety oval leaves are deeply-veined and very hairy. Mullein grows as a low basal rosette of leaves early in the first year, then sends a wide, tall flower stalk up the second year that blooms with many individual yellow flowers clustered and circling the entire top of the stem like a cola. The flowers only open for one day, but stagger their opening, so some can be harvested when closed as well.

FOOD: Mullein is not a food plant per se, but is a very potent medicinal herb for tea, medicinal oil preparations, ear oils, smoking blends and compresses.

CAUTION: Seeds should not be eaten, they are toxic.

CONTAINS: Calcium, Magnesium, Carotene, Choline, Sulfur, Saponins, Glycoside (Aucubin), Flavonoids (Hesperidin, Verbascoside), Polysaccharides, Sterols, Mucilage, Tannins

BODY BENEFITS: Cleanses and nourishes the lungs, liquefies phlegm, moves lymph, soothes swellings, relaxes spasms, prevents infection, relaxes the bronchial pathways, soothes intense spasmodic cough, and is soothing for the digestion. Can be helpful for shortness of breath, asthma, allergies, bronchitis, colds, dysentery, kidney infections, laryngitis, tuberculosis, and whooping cough. Softens tumors and catarrh, inflammations of skin and hardened deposits. The root has been used to treat incontinence.

QUALITIES: Mullein is alterative, antibacterial, antihistamine, anti-inflammatory, antiseptic, antispasmodic, antiviral, astringent, demulcent, diuretic, emollient, expectorant, vulnerary. It is nourishing and tonic for yin, and feminine, moist and cool. This herb tastes sweet with some bitterness. As Brigitte Mars says, *"The flower is more demulcent than the leaf, and the leaf is more astringent than the flower."* The plant has softening qualities.

FOLKLORE: Folk names Jupiter's Staff, Velvet Dock, Feltwort, Velvetback, Beggar's Blanket, Flannel Plant, Candlewick, Hag's Tapers, Aaron's Rod, Adam's Flannel, Blanket Leaf, Doffle, Torches, Hedge Taper, Peter's Staff, Fluma, Shepherd's Herb, Old Man's Club, Barbasito, Gordolobo, Molene, Lady's Foxglove, Graveyard Dust and Wild Tobacco. In the Ozarks men would bend a stalk of Mullein toward the direction of their true love's house. If she loved another it would die, but if it grew straight again her love was true. Mullein leaves can be wound and wrapped in string for candle wicks. Magicians and witches used oil lamps made with the stems and leaves, and the whole stalk was dipped in tallow for a torch that would last a long while (at least until another stalk could be found). The root can be sliced, dried and made into a teething necklace like it was by the Abenaki Indians. The Navajo smoked it to banish negative thoughts and prevent mental disorders. Yellow dye can be made from the flower.

FIRST AID & SURVIVAL USES: Put a few leaves in your pocket when hiking or camping - the soft leaves make great biodegradable toilet paper. Place a leaf in your shoe for blisters, to keep feet warm, or as a soft cushioning insole. Tea from the leaves can be used for relaxation, pain relief, lung support, nervous tension release and to induce sleep. Smoke dried leaves for asthma and congestion. Last year's dried brown Mullein stalks and leaves can always be found and make amazing firestarters and torches. Leaves can be rolled and tied with string for wicks to use in oil lamps - even a jar with olive oil in it will burn as a lantern with this good wick. Leaves can be fed to animals who have a cough. Tuck a few leaves under the pillow to prevent nightmares.

SPIRITUAL PROPERTIES: Mullein is ruled by Saturn and the Fire Element. It has an overlighting protective Plant Spirit who seeks to heal and keep the positive peace. The Mullein stalk has been traditionally used as a sacred torch representing the Sun god in Midsummer rituals. It is reputed to protect against lightning, and rid the home of demons. Mullein can be blended into an incense with Sandalwood or Myrrh resins and burned for protection and courage.

MAGICAL USES: Carry Mullein in a pocket or medicine pouch to attract Love, confer protection, inspire bravery and courage, stimulate fertility, and to prevent attacks of wild animals while in the wilderness. Leaves were dried and powdered and used as "graveyard dust" in old spells and recipes. In India, Mullein is considered the most potent protection herb, and is hung from the doorways and carried as a talisman to banish evil spirits and negativity.

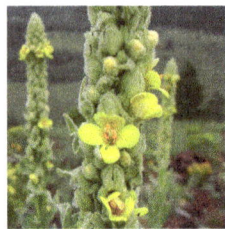

FLOWER ESSENCE: For truthfulness, strong spine, and upright behavior, this essence helps you connect with your conscience, your inner light (Innate) and its true guidance. Use when confused, lacking will, indecisive, or suffering the consequences of being less than truthful. Kindly reconnects you to your perfected, foundational honor structure. This is a great essence for team-building and promoting trust and moral strength.

PREPARATIONS: The plant is not particularly edible as a food, but is a truly healing medicinal herb when prepared as a lung-supporting tea, ear oil, extract or powdered leaf capsule. When making teas with Mullein leaves, use a fine strainer or coffee filter after infusion to strain away the small irritating hairs. Smoking the dried leaves is the preferred method for treating lung issues, this is how the medicine is best delivered. I especially like combining Mullein with Coltsfoot, Lavender and Damiana.

LAURA: Mullein was one of my first Colorado plants, and became a constant companion living there in the West. We had some growing on our land in Wondervu, and during the first season there, at an altitude of 9000 feet, I made Ear Oil from the Flowers and dried the leaves for Tea and Smoking Blends. I found her again in the Grand Canyon and yes, availed myself of her toilet paper prowess. I lovingly met her here in Tennessee showing her yellow-flowered head high above the cotton fields. We found Mullein growing in France and said hello yet again! It is so nice to have Weedy friends you can count on, all over the World.

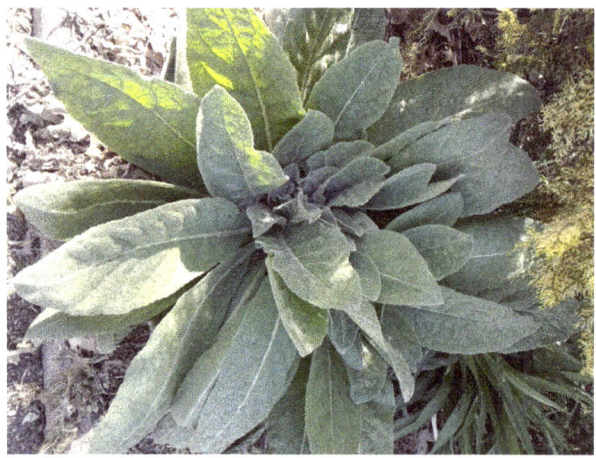

Mullein Flower & Garlic Ear Oil

Designed to be made in small batches so one bottle can be used fresh within a few days and one can be stored. Refrigerate what you don't use right away, or freeze to use the next time.

OIL INFUSION: In a small saucepan, bring 1/4 cup **Olive Oil** to a warm temperature, check it with a drop on your wrist like a baby bottle. Add a small handful of **Mullein Flowers**, and 2 crushed or diced cloves of **Garlic**. Let simmer on very low heat for 20-60 minutes. If you have any growing nearby, or in your herb cupboard, add some **St. John's Wort or Calendula Flowers**, too. Check the mixture often to make sure it doesn't get too hot and the herbs don't burn. Strain. Use when warm but not hot, and bottle the rest in a sterilized dropper bottle. Add Vitamin E Oil from 1 or 2 capsules to the bottle if you are storing or sharing, to preserve it more fully.

TO USE: Warm the dropper bottle of oil in a cup of hot water for a few minutes, test on the wrist to make sure it is not too hot before you use it in the ears. Drop the warm oil into the ears, allow the excess to drain out into a cloth. Put a bit of cotton in the ears to keep in the rest of the oil. A "Warm Salt Sock" can be very comforting for earaches, especially for children. Fill a medium weight sock with salt and warm it in a low oven or microwave until comfortably warm. Place the hot sock or a hot water bottle over the ear, after applying the Ear Oil, move it around neck and shoulders.

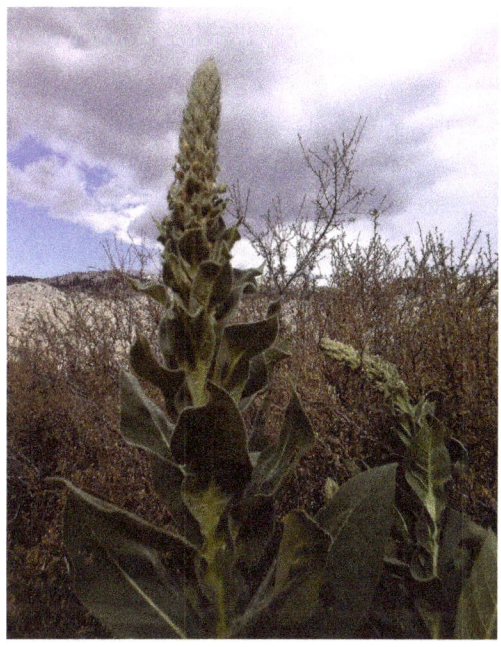

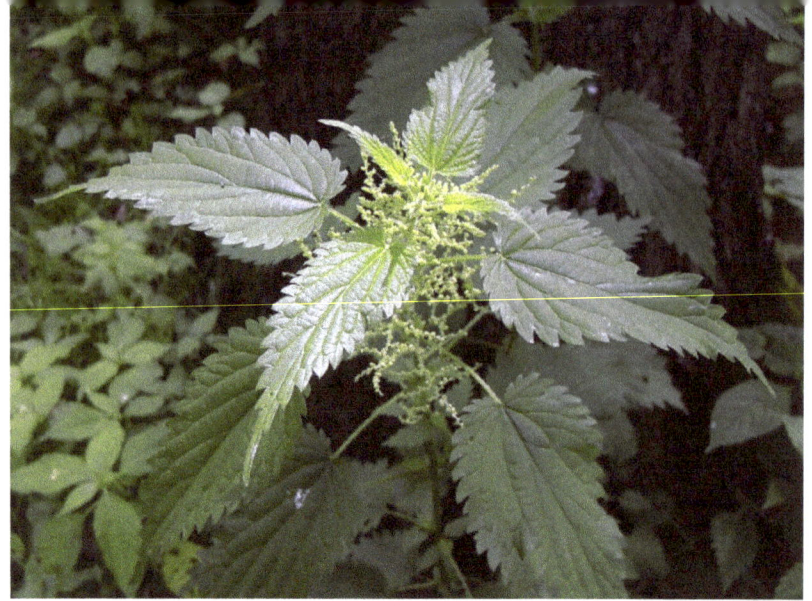

NETTLE (Stinging Nettle)

Urtica dioica Nettle Family / **URTICACEAE**

FOUND: Nettles will grow in nearly any light or soil conditions, in yards, old manure, compost heaps, grasslands, roadsides, woods and wasteland areas. Originally native to Europe, North Africa and temperate Asia, it is now found worldwide.

IDENTIFYING FEATURES: Stinging Nettle STINGS - if you brush against it once you never forget it. This deep green plant can grow from 3-7 feet tall and has alternating opposite, heart-shaped, and deeply toothed leaves, somewhat like a Mint. But this harmless-looking plant is covered with thousands of tiny trichome hairs that are actually hollow silica needles, capable of injecting a stinging irritant right into the skin. Tiny green panicle-like flowers are secondary to the foliage. The root is bright yellow, as are the spreading rhizomes.

FOOD: Avoid eating Nettles fresh and raw for obvious reasons, but the leaves, stalk and flowers can be cooked, juiced, dried or pureed and there is no sting at all. Pick with gloves and scissors. Nettle is a SuperFood for sure, and much more nutritious than Spinach, but it can be prepared much the same way. The root should not be consumed.

CONTAINS: Protein, Beta-Carotene, Vitamins B, C, E and K, Calcium, Chromium, Iron, Magnesium, Potassium, Silica, Silicon, Manganese, Zinc, over 40 Trace Minerals, Betaine, Mucilage, Tannins, Flavonoids (Quercetin, Rutin and more), Xanthophylls, Albuminoids, Agglutinin, Amines (Acetylcholine, Histamine, Serotonin), Glycosides, Saponins, and Tannins

BODY BENEFITS: Nettle is good for everything. As noted British hippie herbalist, David Hoffman says, *"When in doubt, use Nettles."* It has a great affinity for moving stagnant blood - helping to prevent blood clots, building blood with its minerals, and helping it to course around the body freely, improving the blood quality and veinic elasticity. It supports allergy relief by improving resistance to irritating allergens and toxins. Nettle helps curb the appetite and energize the body, and it provides exceptional nourishment that enables the body to lose weight. It clears toxins, speeds recovery after surgery, and restores vital force. Nettles treat inflammatory conditions like gout, arthritis, and rheumatism, relieving pain and reducing heat. The tea as a wash or bath is super helpful for eczema and other skin conditions. Internal use of extract or tea is helpful for anemia, asthma, arteriosclerosis, bronchitis, candida, diabetes, headache, kidney stones, hypoglycemia, bruising, infertility, leukemia, mononucleosis and many viruses including EBV and shingles, nephritis, night sweats, PMS, bloating cold hands and feet, alopecia, PTSD, grey hair, sciatica, sinusitis, and varicose veins, and so much more. Nettle is a remarkable remedy for adrenal fatigue that is many times misdiagnosed as perimenopause. Its nourishment of the adrenals enables them to contribute to the production of all the necessary reproductive hormones for fertility.

QUALITIES: Masculine and warming, Nettle is adaptogenic, acts as an adrenal tonic, is alterative, antiallergenic, antihistamine, anti-inflammatory, antioxidant, anti-radiation, antirheumatic, antiseptic, astringent, blood tonic, carminative, circulatory stimulant, decongestant, diuretic, endocrine tonic, expectorant, kidney tonic, nervine, nutritive, rejuvenative, thyroid and uterine tonic, and vermifuge. In other words, it is a SuperHerb in Weed's clothing.

FOLKLORE: Folk names Common Nettle, Burn Nettle, Devil's Leaf, Bee Sting Nettle, Devil's Plaything, Burn Weed, Burn-Hazel, Hidgy-Pidgy, Hoky-Poky, Indian Spinach, Seven-Minute Itch, Tanging Nettle, Ortie, Ortiga, Krapiva, Kopriva, Wergulu. The common name may be derived from the word for "needle." Makes a great dark green dye. More than 2000 years ago some people practiced Urtication with the Nettle plant, stinging areas of the body on purpose for an antiinflammatory effect. I believe this was also a (very painful) part of religious rites of self-flagellation. The Saxons used Nettle for textiles. Nettles are an important larval food plant for butterflies and moths, so leave it if you find it. After marching for days in cold weather Roman soldiers would strike their legs with Nettle to restore warmth and relieve muscle pain. The fiber of Nettles is strong and has been used for centuries to make rope, textiles, paper, and fiber. In Denmark, clothing and ropes made from Nettle fiber are still intact that were found in tombs from over 5000 years ago.

FIRST AID & SURVIVAL USES: The remedy for Stinging Nettle usually grows right alongside it! **Plantain or Yellow Dock** can be chewed and quickly rubbed on the skin to stop the sting. A sitz bath or mist of the tea will relieve hemorrhoids. Make a double-strong infusion with 2 tablespoons of dried herb per cup of boiling water and when it cools, apply with cotton balls or Mullein leaves for sunburn, bug bites, stings, wounds, and rashes. Fresh Nettle juice can be used in place of Rennet to curdle milk into cheese. Place dried Nettle leaves with your fruit in the root cellar or pantry to deter pests & mold, help preserve freshness and keep the flavor bright. In the wild, pick Nettle with gloves or clothing on your hands, strap onto a backpack for a potherb later, or dry by the fire or on dark rocks in the Sun, and carry with you for a lightweight nutritious snack. Collect stalks and dry them, remove inner fibers, twist and braid into twine for fishing line and nets. For greater strength use 2 or 3 strings braided into rope.

SPIRITUAL PROPERTIES: Nettle is ruled by Mars and the Fire Element, which is funny because its sting is somewhat fiery and weaponized! However brutal the sting, Nettle is the Sacred Mother and has our nourishment in mind. Nettle helps with transforming lower energies into high vibrations, and is a Threshold Guardian between the realms. Nettles cares about sacred boundaries and helps you be mindful. It makes a perfect tea to drink before meditation, centering and stimulating intuition.

MAGICAL USES: Nettle in the home keeps away sickness. This is a plant of transformation and reclamation. Nettle has been used for ages in magic for protection, banishing, and healing the entire body. Use it to return unopened any negative energy, reversing curses or anger spears sent your way. Sprinkle powdered herb or plant Nettles around the house to keep away ghosts and as a protection against lower entities (and window peepers!). Carrying Nettle increases virility in men, and wrapping a leaf in green or purple cloth in your wallet brings abundance. Nettle was burned with other incense plants for exorcism ceremonies to reclaim the peace. Tossing Nettle into a fire averts imminent danger and protects against lightning. Use in a bath if you feel you have been "slimed" with another's dark energy. Nettle is one of the sacred plants in the **Nine Herbs Charm** for healing the sick, used by the Anglo-Saxons in the 11th century. Here is a quote describing it: *"A vexation to poison, a help to others. It stands against pain, it dashes against poison, it has power against three and against thirty, against the hand of a fiend and against mighty devices, against the spell of mean creatures...."*

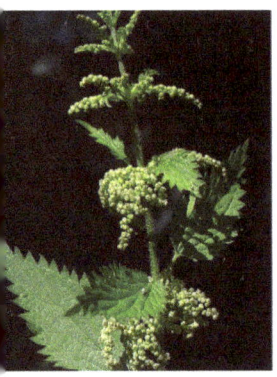

FLOWER ESSENCE: Perfect for brain fog, deteriorating memory and poor cognition, Nettle Flower Essence stimulates the brain for better focus, recall, and concentration. It helps when you are distracted and spacey. It makes a great study or testing remedy for kids and adults alike, as it soothes the nerves but keeps the brain sharp. Helps you transform prickly or heated situations for the better. Helps you stand up and fight back when you have been stung. Recommended to nourish underweight or convalescing people, and may help with pain from rheumatism and arthritis. Provides resilience, adaptability, and inspires respect.

PREPARATIONS: Collect young shoots when about 6 inches high and cook like Spinach. Later in the Summer, pick the top 4-6 pairs of leaves from the top of the plant. You can steam them, saute them, bake them into quiches and other dishes, just remember to gather a lot because they cook down to half their volume. Juice the whole plant for superior nutrition. Puree it and add to salad dressings, sauces, soups, pesto, hummus, and zucchini bread recipes. Dry the leaves and flowers for a sweet flavorful tea. When camping you can wilt the stalks and leaves next to the campfire until they dry out — herbal potato chips! Make a Nettle tea and use it as a hair wash for hair loss, dandruff, and to enhance shine and dark lowlights. Tea is supportive and nourishing for pregnant Mothers. It is recommended that you drink Nettle tea in the afternoon for its most powerful effect.

OTHER EDIBLE "NETTLES" (THAT ARE ACTUALLY MINTS):
Dead Nettle (Henbit), *Lamium amplexicaule*, **LAMIACEAE** ~ In this case, Henbit Dead Nettle is a sting-free, odorless Mint with purple-tinged leaves and glorious little flowers that can be freely eaten all the way through to late Summer. Early shoots, stems and leaves are great in salads, fresh and raw, or it can be used like spinach in cooked dishes and casseroles. When blooming, the upper parts and pretty pink-purple tubular flowers have a more mature peppery taste and look awesome as edible garnishes.

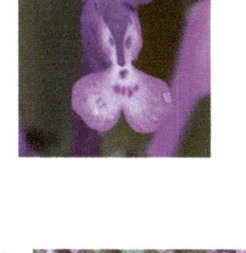

Purple Dead Nettle (Purple Archangel), *Lamium purpureum*, **LAMIACEAE**
This is the very first wild edible to cover the hillsides and lawns in early Spring here in Tennessee. Its abundance as a Weed is always a good indicator of its benefits. It has a beautiful Ombre style with purple leaves that fade to grey-green leaves at the bottom of the plant. Flowers are purple and in whorls at the top of the stem like all mints. Like Henbit, this is also an odorless Mint and a Nettle with no sting. Harvest leaves and use as you would any other Mint for tea and enjoy fresh leaves in salads and smoothies. Use DeadNettle to make the less abundant herbs in homemade Pesto or Chimichurri go further.

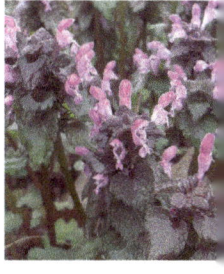

LAURA: Be brave and work with real Nettles! You can avoid the sting with gloves and reap the bounty, I promise. Let this plant nurture and nourish you with all she offers. Your body's energy, stamina and vitality will be vastly improved.

Brigitte always made things from the huge patch of Nettles she cultivated in her yard from a single plant a kind old German lady gave her. She believes the plants now number upwards of a thousand! You could always count on fresh Nettle Juice and Pesto and Nettle Tea warming on the stove. I hope to live near my own patch of Nettles someday so I can utilize them DAILY like she does. She is even so brave as to pick Nettles with her bare hands, and she attributes her complete recovery from arthritis to this practice. This may be the secret of, and reason for, ancient Urtication. The needles of Nettle do have Formic Acid in them, the same irritant employed by the sting of Fire Ants and Bees. Formic Acid has been proven to be a counterirritant that does resolve inflammation of the joints. Nettle stings, like them or hate them, energize the nerves, provide pain relief, move lymph, cause the body to release antihistamines, and greatly improve circulation. The sting is also a remedy for erectile dysfunction - but the application - ouch!!!!

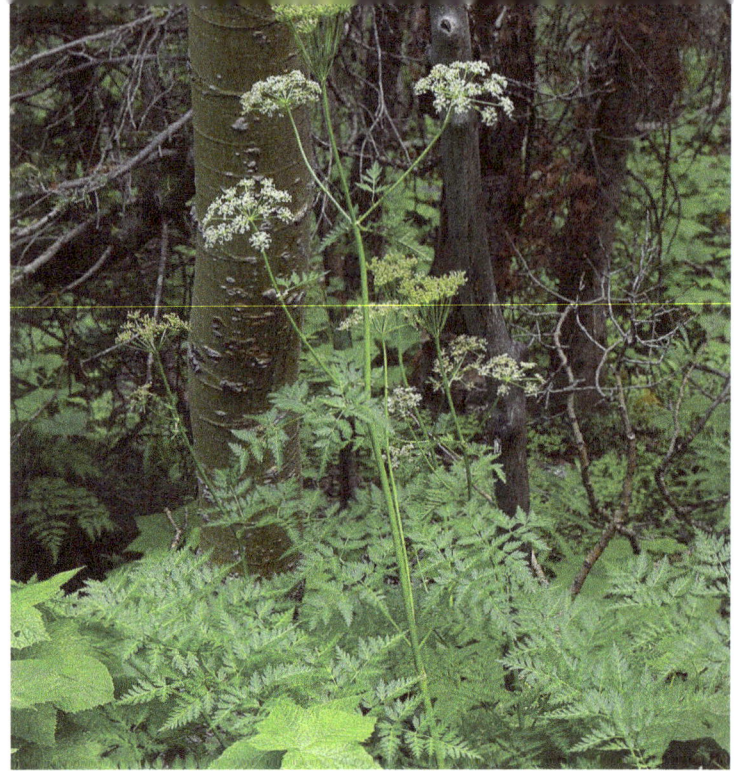

OSHA

Ligusticum porteri   Carrot Family / **APIACEAE**

FOUND: Osha can be found abundantly in the Rocky Mountain west from British Columbia to New Mexico, growing in Aspen & Lodgepole Pine groves above 7500 feet. It is native to Eurasia and North America, and prefers slopes and mountains, shade and high altitude moist soil.

IDENTIFYING FEATURES: Osha leaves are very lacy and fern-like and smell distinctly aromatic like a spicy celery, on a regular thin, hairless, green stem. They are mostly at the base of the plant but you find some clasping the stalk. Large but delicate, round compound umbrella-like white flowers are made of many smaller umbrellas of tiny white flowers, and have long pistils with knobs on the ends. Seeds have narrow wings. Brown hairy aromatic roots are found 1-3 feet deep into the soil. The leggy plant above grows to about 2-5 feet tall on very thin, not spotted stalks.

CAUTION OSHA RESEMBLES POISONOUS WATER HEMLOCK and other Hemlocks, always confirm with a few sources what you have collected before using it or sharing it. Smell helps confirm it. **Water Hemlock** smells musty & nasty with more of a flatter, serrated compound leaf. Most Hemlocks have a large, thick hollow stem that is **mottled with purplish red spots** and they stink. Hemlock is very poisonous, fatal at the smallest amount, do not even touch. Children have died making flutes out of the hollow stems.

FOOD: Leaves are edible as a spicy green, and the edible root must be cooked and has a taste similar to spicy celery when ground chopped, boiled or baked. Make tea with the dried or fresh root and reuse it many times, then use it as a vegetable or spice (see below in Preparations). Seeds are edible and make a flavorful spice similar to Caraway seeds. Osha is a potent medicine plant, with a very strong flavor and action, but you can make a delicious edible treat from the glorious root.

CONTAINS: Silicon, Essential Oils (Ligustilide, Terpenes), Lactone Glycoside, Saponins, Flavonoids, Coumarin, Ferulic Acid, Phytosterols, Oxytocin.

BODY BENEFITS: Osha is stimulating to the circulation and chi (vital energy) of the body and strengthens the immunity, having been used in Traditional Chinese Medicine for over 2000 years. It is soothing to the sinuses, warming to the digestion, phlegm-clearing, lung-nourishing and strengthening. Osha relieves nicotine cravings and sucking on a small piece of the root can help you quit smoking. It can be utilized to treat altitude sickness (interesting because it grows at high altitudes), help allergies, fever, coughs, headaches, herpes, indigestion, sore throat, laryngitis, lung infections, sinus infections, rheumatism, and toothache. Avoid in pregnancy, much too strong.

QUALITIES: Osha Root is pungent and bitter, warming, drying, yang, masculine and pushy in Nature. Osha Gets What It Wants. It is alterative, analgesic, anesthetic, antibacterial, antihistamine, antirheumatic, antispasmodic, antiviral, aromatic, bronchodilator, carminative, circulatory stimulant, diaphoretic, diuretic, expectorant, hypotensive, immune stimulant, mucolytic, stomachic, and a vasodilator.

FIRST AID USES: Keep a small root in your first aid kit like Dave Allen does - when I discovered this, I knew he was the man of my dreams! Bite a bit off and chew if you have a toothache, lung complaints, allergies, or feel phlegmy, or chew and wet with saliva to place into wounds. Powdered root can also be used as a drawing poultice or an antibiotic on a wound. Use tincture or powder on a herpes sore for faster healing. Gargle with tea or suck on the root for laryngitis and sore throat.

SPIRITUAL PROPERTIES: Osha is ruled by several strong planets Sun, Mars and Jupiter and the Fire Element. The action of Osha in the spiritual realm is purifying, protective and expansive, bringing with it the Love of the Creator. This is one of the powerful Spirit allies. When you meditate on it, don't be surprised to see bears lurking around, or you may witness the Plant Spirit as a bear. This Spirit also seems to work with all the Chakras as it traverses the gamut of energetic effects.

MAGICAL USES: Considered sacred and carried by many Native Americans in their medicine pouches to potentize all the other medicine herbs and ward off sickness. Osha is worn around the ankle to repel rattlesnakes. Burned as a purifying incense or smudge before rituals, Osha may increase psychic impressions and stimulate more lucid dreams. It can be smoked, added to Damiana, Mullein or other herbs for a sacred smoke in rituals and ceremony, and can be especially helpful for quitting nicotine. Osha helps bring the rain when it is washed in a nearby stream. If you are going to meet any Indian Elders, bring them Osha as a gift.

FOLKLORE: Folk names Porter's Lovage, Bear Root, Love Root, Colorado Cough Root, Deer Eye, Wild Parsnip, Wild Celery, Empress of the Dark Forest, Chuchupate, Indian Parsley, Mountain Ginseng, Porter's Licorice Root, Raíz del Cochino, Scottish Licorice Root, Guariaca, Mountain Carrot, Oshala, Nipo, Wild Lovage, Chuchupa, Liveche Ecossise, Wasia, and Bear Medicine. The genus Ligusticum was chosen as a tribute to the italian city of Liguria. Most indigenous tribes in North America use Osha medicinally and ritually. Apache scouts and runners would chew the root to enhance their energy and stamina. The Zuni use the root tea for body aches. Bears seek the plant out first thing in Spring to stimulate their appetite and produce needed energy for foraging. They eat it, spit some out and rub it all over themselves.

FLOWER ESSENCE: Opens the heart center and eases breathing and lung complaints, as well as pushes open the Crown Chakra to higher energies. Osha Flower Essence is especially helpful for anything that is "stuck" like lingering grief, guilt or heartbreak. Helps you deal with the emotional blocks to Love, and returns your Heart and ability to Love to full power.

PREPARATIONS: Leaves are a great spicy additive to salads, and can be dried for seasonings. Roots can be boiled with meat like the Apaches do. The roots of Osha are so potent and filled with essential oils that it is said you can boil them **FIFTY times for medicinal teas**. After all that, you can still dry and grind the remaining root into a spice for baked goods, salads, and fish, or add to bitters or honey for an easy throat spray or syrup.

LAURA: Osha is on my list of Most Favorite Plants, and I used to dig one root every year in Colorado. For some reason, Osha is one weed that just won't be cultivated or moved, and it is hard to grow out of the wild. It is likely that it enjoys special mycorrhizal relationships from fungi in the soil, with which Osha works her magic. I imagine this Wild Weed just likes what it likes - it thrives in the high alpine forest and that is that. Because it cannot be grown commercially, there is concern the plant will one day be overharvested. Ironically, some plant specialists have noted that careful harvesting of Osha seems to *renew* the community in which it grows, which seems to become *more prolific* after sensing it is needed to be of service. What a beautiful Plant Spirit! When harvesting Osha (and any root), remember you only need a little bit, and that you are removing an entire plant that can never grow again. Give thanks for its medicine, scatter its seeds before you go, offer your respect and honor this very special plant each time you see it.

Volume Two should have been sponsored by **Joe "Geronimo" Zapf-Kent's** handmade **Living Love Root Osha Candy**! I have eaten several pounds of it (literally) in the writing of this book. His is the best preparation of Osha I have ever tried, sliced and cured in wild Arizona honey, and I am completely in love with it! Genuinely Obsessed, more like. I find it very interesting that Native Americans used Osha to ward off rattlesnakes, and Geronimo had a very challenging time with a rattlesnake bite! He became stronger and now makes this amazing medicine with the Osha Spirit. Find this and his whole wild and extensive mineral collection at **www.thegoodmedicineshop.com.**

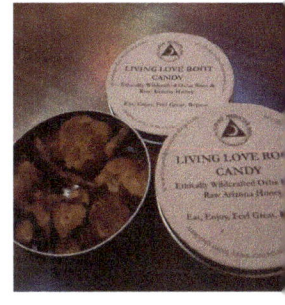

I never understood why Osha's common folk name was "Love Root." But upon doing a months-long dieta with Osha, I can say I definitely felt it! I'd always felt a discernible *loving* energy while eating Osha, and I fell directly in love with the plant after digging it. But with daily tuned-in use, I noticed a very available sensual/sexual energy building deep underground in my Root Chakra. It provided that "extra energy" that is necessary for good sex. Osha also opens the Heart Chakra, bringing with it LOVE, stronger, deeper breathing and a heartfelt energy boost. Just rack up the benefits!

The lung-clearing effects of Osha are noticeable and the strong antiviral action was exactly what I was looking for to keep me strong. But I did not expect the energy and the focus-stimulating effect. It really helped me stay in the zone while writing. I think the pushy and pungent essential oils in this herb are determined to get you to perform well! And I did feel they opened my Crown Chakra up to higher knowledge and helped me trust my intuition and my own voice while writing.

Here is a renowned Osha Champion and Hero, our friend Ethnobotanist **Shawn Sigstedt**, teaching how to harvest Osha easiluy and sustainably. This helpful image shows what Osha looks like at harvest-time in Colorado.

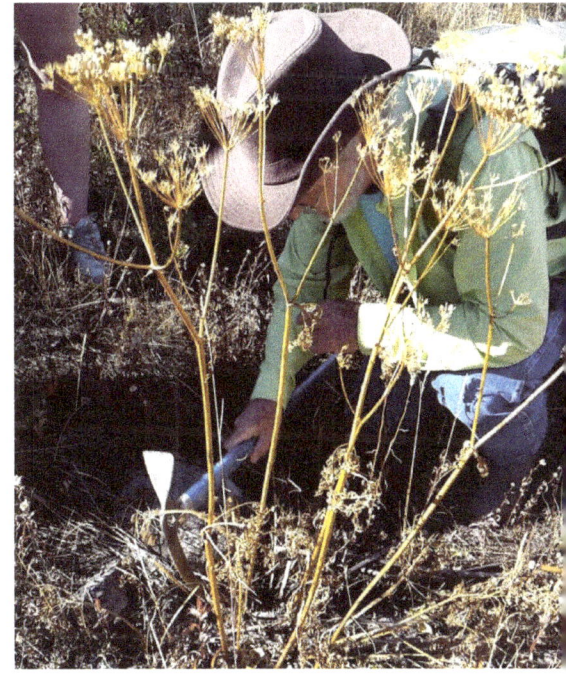

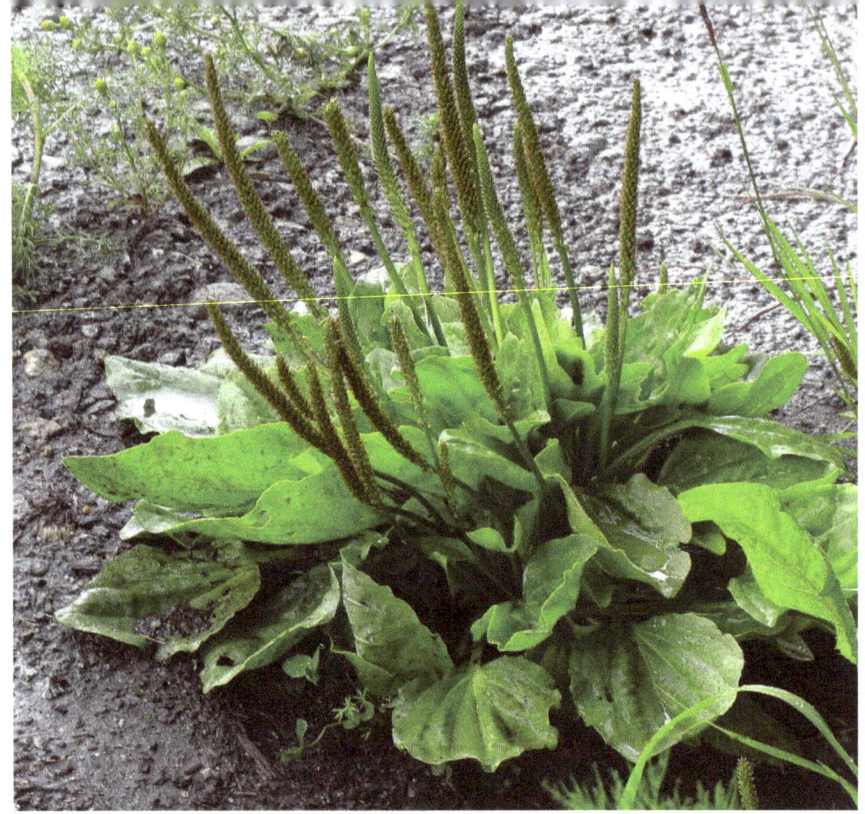

PLANTAIN

Plantago major   Plantain or Fleawort Family / **PLANTAGINACEAE**

FOUND: Native to Europe and Northern and Central Asia, Plantain has naturalized itself, growing in all 50 states, Canada, and all over the World. Plantain is an opportunist, it will grow equally well in lawns, gardens, roadside ditches and cracks in the sidewalk, and it can be happy in shade and in the Sun. The tropical Banana Plantain is not related but delicious as well!

IDENTIFYING FEATURES: Big basal rosette of shiny, large, deeply-veined, almost ripple-y leaves with many flower spikes on tall central stems. Veins extend from tip to tip. Brownish-green flower spikes can grow as tall as 15 inches. The spike explodes into white microflowers, leaving behind tons of seeds. Plantain is a good neighbor and does not crowd, squeeze out or inhibit the growth of other plants, so it is not considered an "invasive weed."

FOOD: This easily identifiable, *incredible* survival plant can be found growing **all year long** in many places, so it can be harvested and utilized at any time of the year. Plantain leaves are an awesomely-flavored vegetable similar to Spinach. Young flower heads taste like Mushrooms and add a deep umami flavor to every dish to which they are added. The seeds are high in Protein, nutritious and delicious, and are highly adaptable and a radical source of dietary fiber. Beyond its extensive food uses, Plantain is like a first aid kit growing everywhere, with many amazing topical and internal uses.

CONTAINS: *Leaf:* Vitamin A, C, K, Iron, Calcium, Magnesium, Allantoin, Aucubin Glycoside, Silicic Acid, Oxalic Acid, Flavonoids, Tannins, and Mucilage. *Seed:* Protein, B Vitamins, Starch, Oils, and Mucilage.

BODY BENEFITS: This humble ground weed is a Superior Healer. Its main function is to reduce inflammation and clear heat, treat infection, move digested material, and soothe and repair tissues. Internally, it is useful for AIDS, allergies, asthma, bedwetting, blood poisoning, bronchitis, earaches, fever, IBS, laryngitis, staph and salmonella, sore throat, neuralgia, psoriasis, thirst, ulcers, UTI's, and weak vision. It can be supportive for leaky gut syndrome and most intestinal issues. Topically it acts as a drawing agent and can pull out splinters or toxins. Its soothing and antiseptic action is helpful for burns, beestings, boils, poison ivy, swellings, toothache, ulcers, hemorrhoids, bruises, eczema, ringworm, mastitis, and spider and bug bites.

QUALITIES: Plantain is sweet, salty, and bitter, cooling, drawing, moisturizing and yin. It is also alterative, anti-allergy, antibacterial, anti-inflammatory, antiseptic, antispasmodic, anti-venomous, astringent, anti-toxic, antimicrobial, anti-inflammatory, antihistamine, decongestant, demulcent, diuretic, expectorant, kidney yin tonic, ophthalmic, mucilaginous, refrigerant, restorative, styptic, and vulnerary. Seed is demulcent, soothing and a fiber laxative.

FOLKLORE: Folk names Cuckoo's Bread, Ripple Grass, Englishman's Foot, Ribwort, Snakebite, The Leaf of Patrick, Snakeweed, Rat's Tail, Patrick's Dock, Slan-lus, Che Qian Zi, Lahuriya, Waybread, Wegbrade, Waybroad, White Man's Foot - many of the names reflect that the broad leaf looks like a foot. Native Americans called it "White Man's Foot" because the foreign settlers seemed to have brought the plant with them and it followed their footsteps and wagon trails across the country. The Latin root planta means the "sole of the foot." The Chinese have traditionally used Plantain for resolving dry hot conditions, liver fire, phlegmy coughs, and skin conditions.

FIRST AID USES: Chew leaves when you are thirsty out in the wild, they will provide electrolytes and thirst-quenching relief. Plantain is called Nature's Band-Aid. **For Poison Ivy:** Stack a few leaves together and tear open, rub edges of leaves all over the exposed area and allow to dry. To stop bleeding and soothe wounds, chew leaves (or grind between 2 smooth rocks) into a paste and apply directly to bee stings and insect bites, Nettle stings, Poison Ivy rash, boils and blisters. Top with a whole leaf and wrap in place with a bandana or tape it to the skin. Combine leaf mash with salt for a drawing poultice. Consider adding Plantain to the *Heals It All Comfrey Salve* (on pg. 164) and use it for everything! For constipation, steep a small handful of Plantain seeds in a cup of boiling water for 10-15 minutes - drink tea and eat some of the seeds as well with lots of extra water. For a Plantain Remedy you can always have in hand year-round, try the following awesome, all-purpose, frozen miracle medicine!

QUICK RECIPE: Instant Owie-Fixing Plantain Cubes

- Blend a few handfuls of **Plantain Leaves** in a food processor or blender with 1-2 cups **Aloe Vera Gel** (depending on the size of batch you want to make). Add 10-20 drops of **Lavender Essential Oil**. Freeze into ice cube trays. Grab a cube when you need fast and effective relief for **bug bites, bee stings, Poison Ivy, Nettle stings, skinned knees, itchy skin, blisters,** and especially for **burns & sunburn**.

SPIRITUAL PROPERTIES: Ruled by Venus and the Earth Element, Plantain plant is all about being grounded and connected to the Earth while you cosmically journey far and wide. This plant reminds us we are able to sense deep spiritual truths *because* we are in our bodies, close to the Earth, and can employ our body's sensing mechanisms for feeling. Our spiritual antennae, like the many Plantain stalks, reach right to the heavens to connect us.

MAGICAL USES: Used extensively (probably because it was so available) for healing, strength, protection and snake-repelling. Binding the leaves to the head with red wool will cure a headache. Place leaves in the shoes for weariness. Hang a bouquet of Plantain in the car to keep out evil spirits. A piece of the root is carried in the pocket to ward off snakebites. Plantain (Waybread) is also one of the sacred plants in the Nine Herbs Charm for healing the sick, used by the Anglo-Saxons in the 11th century. This completely authentic verse reveals just some of what was said about Plantain:

> "And you, Waybread, Mother of Herbs, open from the east, mighty inside. Over you chariots creaked, over you queens rode, over you brides cried out, over you bulls snorted. You withstood all of them, you dashed against them. May you likewise withstand poison and infection and loathsome foe roving through the land."

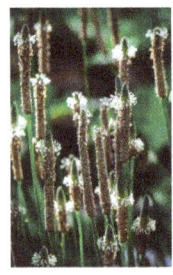

FLOWER ESSENCE: Plantain is the perfect *dissolving* remedy for releasing bitterness, obstacles, the desire for vengeance, old trauma, rigid beliefs, resentment, and pain. It roots out what's no longer needed, healing old wounds, and placing a protective covering over you and your heart. Use this remedy to restore peace, impart a sense of justice, and to cool down heated emotions. Plantain offers you a surrender flag, and seeds in you many wonderful possibilities for enjoying the future beyond every emotional injury.

PREPARATIONS: For Herbal Potato Chips which taste better (and grow in the yard FREE compared to expensive Kale Chips), pan-fry individual leaves in butter or olive oil until crisp - or paint with olive oil and bake in a low oven. Gather smaller leaves raw for salads (remove longer stems like Spinach). Leaves are also delicious sauteed, creamed, or steamed. Use in place of grape leaves for delicious Dolmas. Juice the leaves and stir into Honey for coughs and tickly throat. Gather the multitudes of seeds and dry them thoroughly - then use as a spice, add to oatmeal, cookies and cakes, or powder to make a flour for baking and to thicken sauces. Seed powder can be added to water as a Psyllium-relative fiber remedy, or included in baked goods for nutrition and extra dietary fiber. Leaf and flowers can be made into extracts and salves for harnessing Plantain's super healing power.

LAURA: Plantain is simply **always there**, every day in Tennessee in every month of the year, growing abundantly bright green and wild and all over my front yard and driveway. It's a genuine relief to know there's wild nutritious food and reliable medicine at the ready for me if I need it, in all seasons. I use it a lot when I run out of salad greens in the winter between shopping trips. Or if I want to make the Basil go further in Pesto, or in my Chimichurri recipe (found in the Purslane section).

Plantain holds itself close to the ground and is always underfoot and at the ready. Keep your eyes open for it wherever you go. It is your own healing army, and you will find it waiting to serve you anywhere and everywhere.

Psyllium, *Plantago ovata,* is the world-famous fiber herb that has recently seen great press in the Ketogenic Diet as an alternative, carb-free flour for bread-making and gluten-free thickening. Our humble and abundant Plantain is a relative of Psyllium and works exactly the same way, swelling and sweeping through the bowels like a broom to promote cleansing and regularity. You can use Plantain the way you would Psyllium in recipes and remedies. Remember to always drink an additional amount of water when using fiber or clay remedies internally, as you don't want to wind up with a fiber block in your gut!

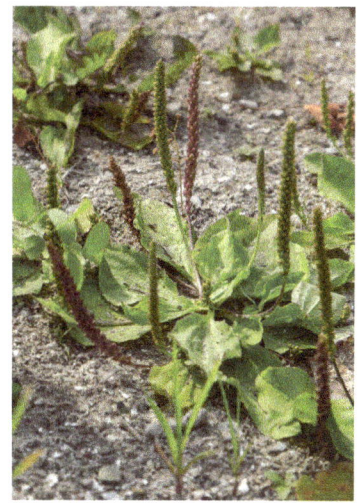

Horses love Plantain leaves, once they discover them it can spoil them for Alfalfa. Plantain is a major service-to-others plant. Even though the flowers are so small, they provide wonderful nectar for Pollinators and make tons of seeds to spread their goodness around mightily. Plantain helps the soil decompress and aerate, providing necessary functions in the ecosystem, making even the *land* healthier.

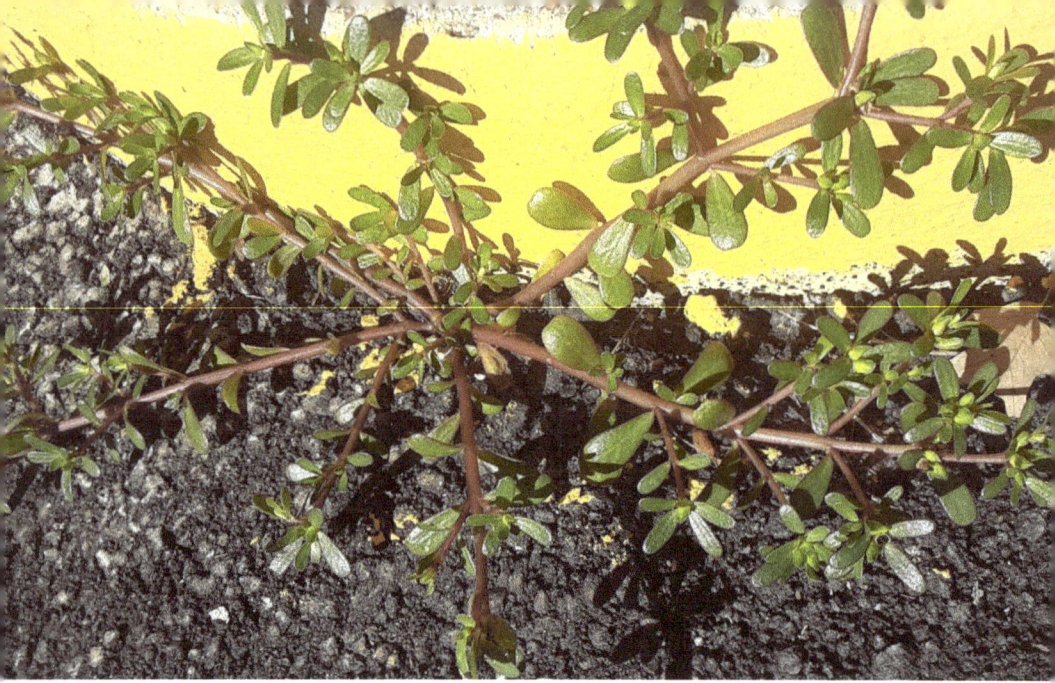

PURSLANE

Portulaca oleracea   Purslane Family / **PORTULACACEAE**

<u>FOUND</u>: All over the World (except Antarctica), growing abundantly in fields and gardens, roadsides, trails, sidewalks, driveways and disturbed places. Grows well in a drought and can switch to different kinds of photosynthesis to adapt to climate conditions.

<u>IDENTIFYING FEATURES</u>: Reddish, smooth, forked stems look like copper pipes, oval, tongue-like leaves look like jade plant leaves (it is considered a succulent). Leaves cluster at the end of branching stems and are fleshy, thick and smooth, full of an aloe-like gel. Small, yellow flowers have 5 regular parts but look like they don't open fully. Has a deep taproot for accessing soil, often found growing through cracks in pavement. **Clear sap is the positively identifying feature**, Purslane stem sap is totally clear, it does NOT have white sap when broken. Purslane forms a rosette-shaped, mat-like covering that can be as large as 3 feet in diameter.

There is a very similar looking plant called "Spurge" that is not edible, poisonous and could be mistaken for Purslane. It sometimes even grows right alongside, but the main differences are easy to spot. Spurge is always **smaller, the stems are **thin & woody**, the **leaves are flat & thin**, opposite and toothy and have **spots** in the middle sometimes, and there are lots more of them appearing all along the stem; **there's no yellow flower, no fleshy thickness to the leaves like succulents**, and the stem exudes a **bad, milky white sap. POISONOUS, do not eat.** Purge the Spurge.

<u>FOOD</u>: Purslane tastes like Lemon Pepper, slightly spicy and sour. Evidence of

European and Native American cultivation of Purslane is present in fossil records that confirm it has been grown and eaten for over 4000 years. Purslane rivals Spinach in nutritional value, and is widely known and loved in Mediterranean countries. And in this country, by smart foragers!

CONTAINS: More Omega-3 Fatty Acids than Fish Oil or Vitamin E, the most Vitamin A of all leafy greens, Vitamin C, E, Folate, Magnesium, Iron, Manganese, Calcium & Potassium, Copper and Phosphorus, Bioflavonoids, Antioxidants, Lithium and Melatonin. Purslane is 93% water for superior hydration, and is low in calories and high in fiber. *The plant does contain a high amount of oxalates and should be consumed in moderation by those who form kidney stones.

BODY BENEFITS: Superior nutrition boosts the immune system. Soothing and useful in urinary tract infections, diarrhea, IBS and digestive issues. Also a great heart tonic as it lowers cholesterol and blood pressure and decreases risk of heart attack and stroke. Useful in treating depression, lupus, and arthritis. Great for the brain and memory, supports neural connections and may help prevent migraines. Purslane stabilizes blood sugar and insulin levels. High levels of Omega-3 Fatty Acids prevent leukotriene production (which cause inflammatory skin conditions like psoriasis) so this is a perfect food for people with skin issues. Omegas also nourish brain health in children and may be of benefit in ADHD and hyperactivity. Lithium promotes mood-balancing and Magnesium reduces anxiety so this is a great mental health herb.

QUALITIES: Feminine, cool, hydrating, sour and salty taste, mucilaginous, fatty and soothing. Abundant and self-renewing, Purslane has a plan to provide. It is antibacterial, antioxidant, anti-inflammatory, antiulcerogenic, antiscorbutic, diuretic, a febrifuge (reduces fever), and wound-healing.

FOLKLORE: Folk names Golden Purslane, Garden Primrose, Duckweed, Little Hogweed, Pigweed, Fatweed, Luni-Bhaji, Pursley, Pourpier, Regelah, Verdolaga, Wild Portulaca, Khorfeh, Portulak, Andrachne, and Krokot.

FIRST AID USES: Crush leaves and apply to sunburns, burns, and bug bites. Mucilage in leaves has similar soothing properties to Aloe Vera. Eat as a cooling food in the hot Summer. Eat raw leaves for dehydration to replace electrolytes. Purslane Tea before bed will provide Magnesium and Melatonin for deep sleep. Purslane's nutrients act like an antidote to Coffee, if you have consumed too much caffeine and have the jitters, it will soothe you right down.

SPIRITUAL PROPERTIES: Ruled by the Moon and the Water Element, works specifically with the emotions for easy peaceful flow and the washing away of what is not needed. Fluidity, connection and satiation are offered. Mahatma Gandhi ate it and he called it Luni, most likely in devotion to the Moon. Henry David Thoreau consumed it at Walden Pond. Purslane is comforting to the Spirit, reveals magic about Abundance in small and simple places, and is Peace-inspiring.

MAGICAL USES: Lay Purslane on the bed to stop nightmares and assure a good night's sleep. Pliny the Elder suggested Purslane should be worn as an amulet to ward off all evil spirits. It was carried by soldiers to protect them in battle, and worn to draw love and luck to one. Sprinkling it through the home spreads happiness and joy.

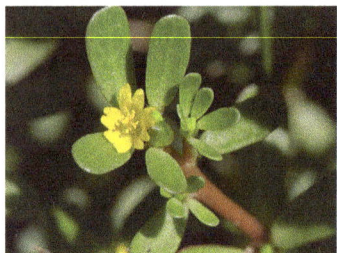

FLOWER ESSENCE: Purslane helps connect you to the Plant Spirits and Devas, and the other Realms. It taps into your nurturing essence and magnifies it. This is a wonderful children's remedy for any need, as it is soothing, nourishing, and protective. Purslane helps you resolve insomnia and nightmares, and process extreme emotions. It inspires tenacity, constancy, support, and abundance.

PREPARATIONS: Eat right out of the Garden or off the trail. *AVOID cement-harvested Purslane if possible. sidewalks and driveways may be treated with pesticides and contain oil or heavy metal residue, so look for it growing in dirt instead. This awesome vegetable needs to be soaked and washed thoroughly, as it is often gritty with ground dirt. Leaves, stems and flowers are delicious raw, cooked, sauteed or stir-fried, or baked into casseroles. They make great pickles or faux capers, and their flavor pairs well with garlic, dill and other herbs. Blanch quickly and freeze extra plants for exceptional nutrition all year long. Seeds can be ground into a flour for pancakes and muffins. Unlike spinach, Purslane does not shrink when cooked, so a small amount can provide many servings. Use like Okra as a thickener for soups and stews. Makes a great fermented kraut vegetable full of Vitamin C. Traditional Greek salads contain Purslane with Feta, Tomatoes and Herbs. Boil stems and leaves for 3-5 minutes and drink for a soothing and sleep-enhancing bedtime Tea.

LAURA: You can transplant Purslane anywhere in your yard. See one coming up in the driveway? Pull it up gently, with the whole deep taproot, and place it in the Garden! Purslane is known to be a great Companion Plant because it holds moisture in the soil creating its own microclimate, and its taproots tunnel down deeply. It is especially helpful when grown with Corn, as its deep roots bring up moisture and nutrients, and break through soil that Corn roots would not have been able to penetrate alone. Much like all succulents, even a few rogue stems will probably root themselves and multiply, and the tiny seeds will burst out when mature to grow more. To keep it from spreading where it is not needed, harvest before flowering - because each plant produces about 240,000 seeds! Make something great with it, preserve the rest for Winter and enjoy!

Purslane was Gandhi's favorite food. Throughout his life he recommended it to many people because he knew it could feed everyone. He instinctively knew that it would give people a sense of empowerment to harvest their own free, fresh food. All they needed was to know what to look for and how to prepare it - just like you.

Euell Gibbons called Purslane *"India's Gift to the World,"* as this is where the plant most likely originated. Euell says that with careful harvest, JUST A FEW plants can provide abundant nourishment for a ***whole family, through every season***. One source even calls Purslane the *"greatest terrestrial source of Omega 3 Fatty Acids"* and the *"greatest superfood to never be marketed"* because it grows right in your driveway! This humble little plant, hidden right underfoot, has been used for thousands of years to prevent hunger and scurvy, and most people don't even realize it exists. Purslane deserves to be recognized and eaten now! You might have even thought Purslane was just a driveway or garden nuisance. But once you learn more about it, you can realize what is right there in front of you: **REAL FOOD that saves lives**.

Here is my most favorite way to use Wild Weeds - in whatever combination is handy.

Wild Weed Chimichurri

A flavor firecracker! This wild plant take on the delicious Argentinian sauce brings a perfect flavor punch for BBQ, steaks, poultry, sandwiches, tacos, popcorn, pasta, baked potatoes, tofu and more. I actually put it on everything.

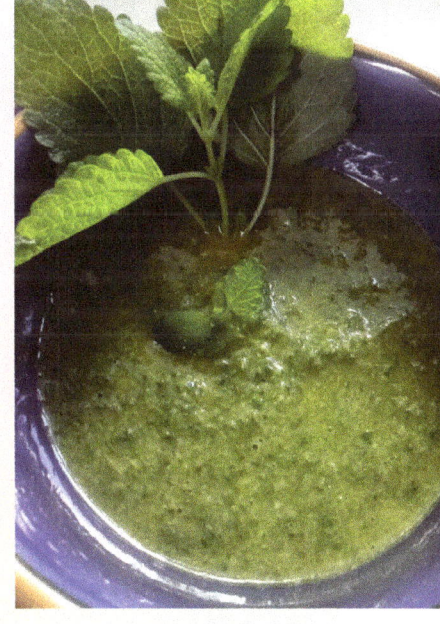

In a food processor or blender, pulse together 1 cup each **Purslane** and any other Wild Weed greens like **Lemon Balm, Plantain, DeadNettle, Violet Leaves** or **Lamb's Quarters**. Add small bunches of fresh aromatic herbs like **Italian Parsley, Cilantro, Oregano** and **Basil,** and 4 cloves of chopped **Garlic**, 1 deseeded **Jalapeno Pepper** or **Red Chile** (or ½ tsp. **Red Pepper Flakes**), 1 teaspoon **Capers**, ½ cup **Olive Oil** and 2-4 Tablespoons **Red Wine Vinegar**.

Process just until loose and still a little chunky, sauce should be runny and juicy. Taste often and adjust ingredient amounts for intense flavor and the texture you desire, add **Hot Sauce, Salt & Pepper** as needed. Allow to sit at least 10 minutes to 2 hours before serving to blend flavors. Serve in little bowls with spoons. Store in a glass jar in the refrigerator for up to 1 week, or make extra to freeze into ice cube trays for a quick flavor booster for soups and sauces.

Needless to say, I freeze a bunch in small cubes, but once I have made this it doesn't last long! It is delicious on everything. Varying the recipe with the Weeds I find in my yard seasonally, adding a little grocery produce, and I can make this fresh year-round.

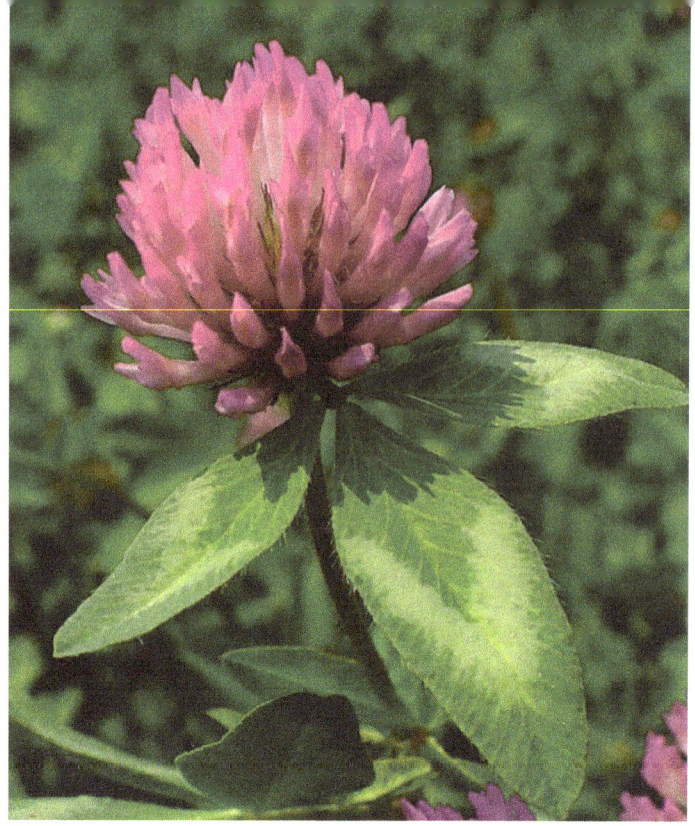

RED CLOVER

Trifolium pratense   *Bean & Legume Family* / **FABACEAE**

FOUND: Originally from Europe, Africa and Western Asia, this hardy plant spread itself around Worldwide. Prefers to grow in meadows, fields and lawns, but frequents disturbed areas, dry roadsides, and abandoned sites. Prefers full sun and likes to spread.

IDENTIFYING FEATURES: Three leaves (tri-folium), are dark green, with lighter arrow heads on them, and a deep pink globe compounded of many tiny flowers. Usually fairly close to the ground, Red Clover grows in large patches, but groups of it have been seen to top 18 inches. It has hollow stems with little hairs, and micro hairs on the leaves.

FOOD: Flowers are beautiful and edible, they taste a little nutty and sweet. Because they are compound, I like to break them up when I use them in salads. Whole tops of the plant can be eaten raw or cooked like spinach, the leaves are the best before it flowers. Seeds can be gathered and sprouted for delicious young greens. The root can be cooked like a root vegetable. Ground seeds and flowers can be used to make flour.

CONTAINS: Protein, Beta-Carotene, B-complex Vitamins, Vitamin C, Calcium, Chromium, Copper, Iron, Magnesium, Manganese, Selenium, Silicon, Isoflavones

(Genistein, Daidzein, & Biochanin-A among others), Flavonoids, Phenolic Glycosides (Salicylic Acid), Essential Oils, Polysaccharides, Salicylates, Coumarins, Cyanogenic Glycosides.

BODY BENEFITS: Useful for menopause symptoms especially hot flashes and night sweats. Helpful for fighting and preventing cancer, lowering high cholesterol, treating asthma & whooping cough, and soothing skin complaints (eczema and psoriasis). Red Clover enhances the flexibility of arteries, increases HDL (good) cholesterol, and thins the blood to prevent heart diseases. It strengthens the hair, skin and nails with naturally occurring Silica, and reduces inflammation in arthritis. Red Clover helps maintain bone density, its mineral matrix has been shown to slow bone loss and is consequently helpful for osteoporosis. As it is a member of the Bean Family (Fabaceae), Red Clover is very nourishing but it can also cause gas. ****Not recommended in pregnancy.** Avoid it if you take methotrexate injections or blood thinners, or have estrogen-sensitive cancers. Stop taking a week before any surgical procedure so your blood will not be affected.

QUALITIES: Sweet and salty, cooling and moisturizing, nourishing to the yin, Red Clover is alterative, antibacterial, anti-inflammatory, antispasmodic, antiseptic, antitumor, antitussive, cardiotonic, diuretic, expectorant, galactagogue, nutritive, phytoestrogenic, and sedative.

FOLKLORE: Folk names Cow Clover, Wild Clover, Bee Bread, Purple Clover, Cow Grass, Honeystalks, Marl Grass, Meadow Trefoil, Three-Leaves Grass, Triolet, Trebol Rojo, Trepatra. Red Clover is the Vermont State Flower, and the National Flower of Denmark.

FIRST AID USES: Flowers make a delicious sweet tea that can help hot flashes. Add flowers to a tea made with Nettle, Horsetail and Yellow Dock. Drink liberally, also cool and apply to itchy or inflamed skin, and add to a bath with some Ginger Powder.

SPIRITUAL PROPERTIES: ruled by Venus or Mercury and Earth, Wind, Fire and Water Elements! With such varied correspondences and properties this plant is a spiritual powerhouse that supports fidelity, beauty, prosperity, protection, and success in love. Red Clover is also good for releasing other people's energy, and negativity in general.

MAGICAL USES: Red Clover is worn for protection in an amulet. Add it to bathwater for financial success. The tea sprinkled around the house removes evil spirits. Red Clover keeps snakes off the property where it is grown and allowed to prosper. Four Leaf Clovers are one of the most magical fresh plant talismans, and can be worn to prevent drafting into military service and to ward off madness. They are the Lucky Shamrock and grant wishes and fortune to the holder. Sharing one in a ritual between lovers seals their mutual devotion (split it and both eat half).

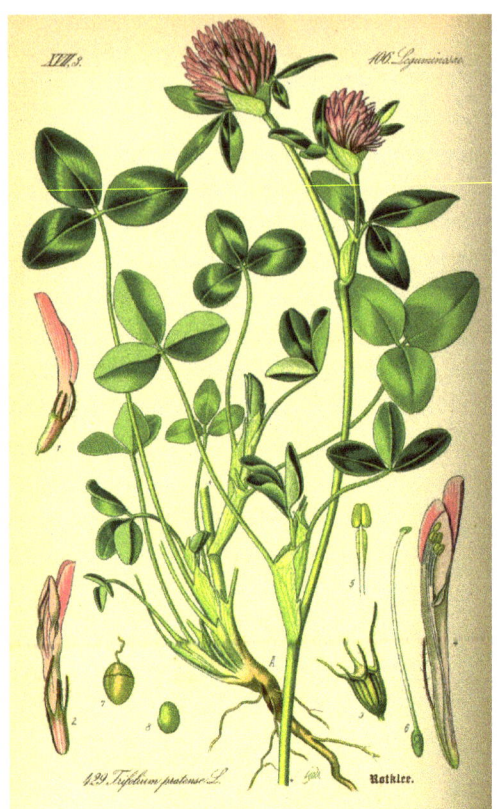

FLOWER ESSENCE: Red Clover is a first responder, emergency essence that helps you stay calm in the face of fear, misfortune, or dangerous incident. It helps with panic attacks, offers you the opportunity to let things go, and brings you back into a whole protected unit. It helps you maintain individual discernment within a field of "mass consciousness" that feels infectious or damaging. The Flower Essence is good for soothing animals for vet trips, or after scary altercations with other animals.

OTHER USES: In agriculture, Red Clover makes a great green manure. With its deep taproot, as it pulls up and deposits Phosphorus into the soil. It also fixes Nitrogen into the soil and can be used successfully as a rotation crop to remediate tired and mineral-poor fields or plots. Animals love to eat it. It is a great erosion-control plant for stabilizing soils and saving ground. Clover Honey is delicious and is usually made from White Clover. Bees LOVE Clover! This is one of the most important reasons to keep it growing where you find it - leave patches of it in your lawn for all the Pollinators. The butterflies and moths flock to it as well, and all your plants will benefit.

LAURA: I will never forget the day when Dave Allen found me a Four Leaf Clover in 10 seconds flat. We were wandering through the grass in the front yard of our Nashville home, while I told him how I had never, ever found one myself. I had never in all my years even *seen* a real one. Dave Allen proceeded to reach down into a Clover patch and literally just pick one out of nowhere for me! With no thought or searching his hand went directly to it, and I now have a pressed and preserved, magical Four Leaf Clover of my very own. With this ability (and oh, so many more) my husband is truly a walking good luck charm!

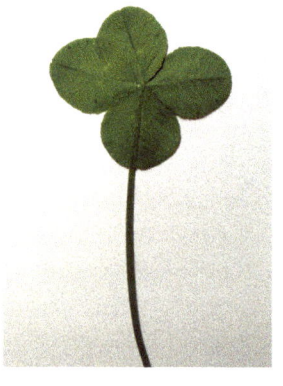

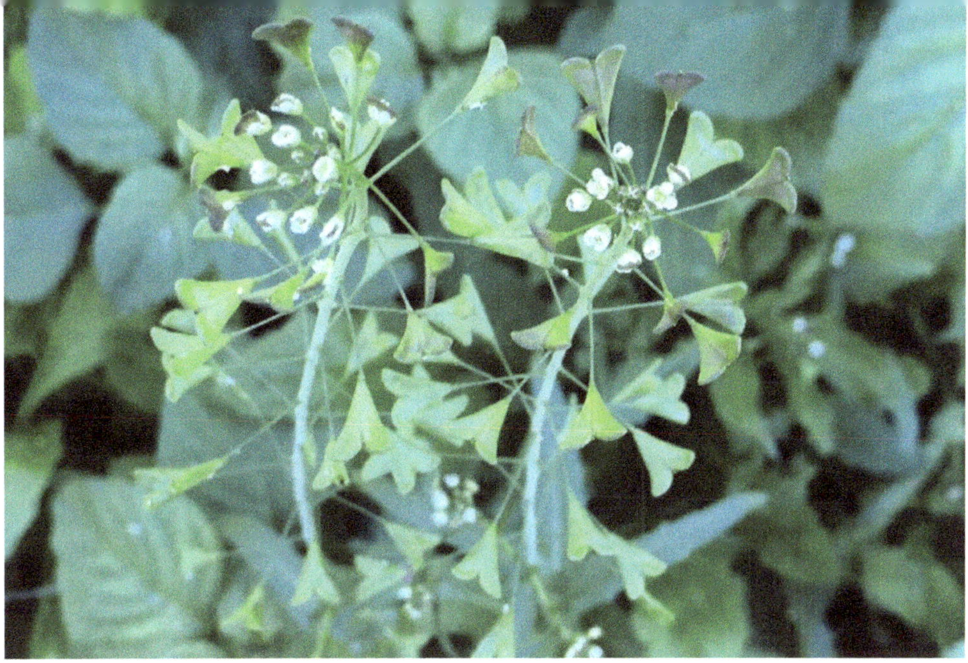

SHEPHERD'S PURSE
& THE WILD MUSTARDS

Capsella bursa-pastoris   Mustard Family / **BRASSICACEAE**

FOUND: On riverbanks, in fields, and on vacant land in rural and urban areas in all 50 states and Canada. Grows wild in the Mediterranean, and all over Europe. In Asia it is grown as a food crop.

IDENTIFYING FEATURES: Heart-shaped seed capsules! Thin stalks are dotted with tiny stems that terminate in these beautiful seed capsules that form from each individual flower. Lance-like leaves grasp the stalk. Larger very lobed leaves are found in a basal rosette on the ground from which the plant grows - looks almost like a Dandelion. The compound flower grows right up from the center of the plant on a thin stalk, and is white, 4-petaled in a cross. Flowerhead blooms at the top like a thin, miniature broccoli head.

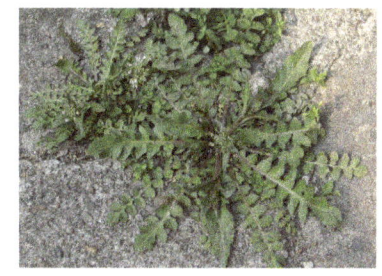

FOOD: Before flowering the leaves are great as salad greens, after flowering it is best to cook leaves like spinach. In Korea they use the root, which is small but flavorful, and is nutritious for soups and stir fries. Once they turn brownish, seed capsules can be burst and the seeds are small but very tasty as a spice or ground up for flour. The seed capsules are a great trail snack that gives you energy and nutrition to keep going, and they are fun to use as mustard spice when cooking outdoors. a great addition to salads. Plant is highly nutritious and can be eaten in moderation for survival.

Shepherd's Purse Flowers are a spicy and a great addition to salads. Plant is highly nutritious and can be eaten in moderation for survival.

CONTAINS: Beta-Carotene (Vitamin A), Vitamin B-complex, Vitamin C, Vitamin K, Calcium, Iron, Potassium, Flavonoids (Quercetin, Rutin, Luteolin, Diosmin), Amino Acids (Proline, Tyramine, Ornithine), Acetylcholine, Histamine, Malic Acid, Fumaric Acid, Saponins, Mustard Oil, Essential Oils (Camphor), Phenolic Acids (Vanillic Acid, Fumaric Acid).

BODY BENEFITS: Better to use the plant fresh as it is much less effective after drying. Shepherd's Purse constricts blood vessels to reduce high blood pressure. It also moves blood, so it is helpful for blood circulation, internal and uterine bleeding (especially postpartum hemorrhage), and can be helpful for regulating periods and relieving menstrual cramps. All wild Mustards help the digestion, and emmenagogue, febrifuge, hemostatic, hypotensive, oxytoxic, styptic, urinary antiseptic, vasoconstrictor, and vulnerary. Shepherd's Purse has been used as a remedy for acid reflux, indigestion, diarrhea, UTI's, bedwetting, organ prolapse and intestinal cramping. This pungent spice is a warming, anti-inflammatory pusher like Ginger, and the root can be used similarly in its absence. It is helpful for strengthening the blood and resolving anemia with its high Iron content. It regulates blood pressure and may lower thyroid hormones. It helps the body excrete uric acid so it's helpful for gout and arthritis. It is diuretic, so Shepherd's Purse can help resolve water retention and swellings.

QUALITIES: Sweet, spicy and pungent like all Wild Mustards - Shepherd's Purse is warming, stimulating, drying and yang. It is alterative, anti-inflammatory, antioxidant, antiseptic, anti-tumor, astringent, detergent, diuretic, emmenagogue, febrifuge, hemostatic, hypotensive, oxytoxic, styptic, urinary antiseptic, vasoconstrictor, and vulnerary.

FOLKLORE: Folk names Blind Weed, Purselet, Saint James' Wort and Weed, Pickpocket, Sanguinary, Shepherd's Sprout, Rattle Pouches, Lady's Purse, Life-Preserving Plant, Old Man's Pharmacetly, Case Wort, Purse of the Father, Mother's Hearts, Pepper & Salt, Bolsa de Pastor, Bourse a Pasteur, Blutkraut, Clappedepouch, Picklooker, Toywort, and Witch's Pouches. As it staunches wounds and stops bleeding, Shepherd's Purse was used successfully as a liquid extract on the battlefields in World War I. It makes a great chicken feed that may increase Activator X in the eggs, making the yolks a deeper orange color, full of antioxidants, and much more nourishing.

FIRST AID USES: Make a juice or tea from the Shepherd's Purse and soak a cotton ball with it, put in the nose for nosebleeds. Or rub on Poison Ivy rash to remove the itch. Apply to wrists to lower a fever. Make a thick paste from the dried seeds, use as a plaster on the chest for bad colds & coughs, or on burns or injuries, cramps or bruises. Prepared Yellow Mustard with water (or Pickle Juice) can be used internally and externally for relieving muscle cramps and burns. Mustard Tea makes a great mouthwash for gingivitis. Brigitte recommends gathering Mustard seeds and placing them in small bowls with water all around where you need to repel bugs - their mucilaginous gel traps mosquitoes and harms their larvae.

SPIRITUAL PROPERTIES: Ruled by Saturn and the Fire Element, this is a plant that has foundational mineral nutrition for the Body and Spirit. Its medicine for the Spiritual Heart spreads like a wildfire and brings comfort to those who are afraid. The many hearts on the stem are like badges of hard-won, heartfelt wisdom that come through growth. Shepherd's Purse can help you stop the emotional bleeding, assisting you to constrict and contract the proper amount for energetic shielding. This plant creates a matrix of spiritual support.

MAGICAL USES: The taller the plant the more heart-centered wisdom it contains. Bring a tall cutting onto your altar when working with Love issues. Shepherd's Purse concentrates the heavenly energies and brings them down to you for support - and opens the Heart Chakra. All Mustard Seeds hold the energy of Abundance and were used as currency in ancient civilizations. They hold such potential in their tiny form, Jesus used them as a metaphor for great things coming in tiny packages. Use the stalks with many seed pods, especially Penny Grass, to decorate prosperity shrines.

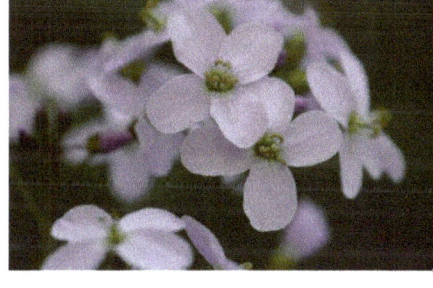

FLOWER ESSENCE: Shepherd's Purse has a particular affinity for the Feminine Energy and Reproductive System. It can be helpful for soothing the adolescent Spirit, and releasing fear and negative feelings around menstruation or pregnancy. This is a perfect blessing essence for preparing for Motherhood, as it supports fertility and the contracting inward to hold a child. As it helps you to draw in and nurture, Shepherd's Purse also helps you to let go of everything that is of no use, that is not worth seeding, growing or creating.

PREPARATIONS: Fresh leaves, flowers and seeds are delicious in moderation. Use the fresh plant when making a tea, or an extract or tincture as most of the potency is in the essential oils and volatile constituents. Clean dried seeds can be sprinkled on foods, or ground into a Mustard paste and used as a condiment. The root is very spicy and can be used as you would fresh Ginger. *Avoid during pregnancy.*

LAURA: With over 4500 seeds in one plant, and HEART-shaped seed packets, this plant has a PLAN - **to spread Love far and wide!** Shepherd's Purse may seem like a humble and unassuming ground cover - but it absolutely reflects what it means to be "tiny but mighty!" All Wild Mustards are great for the environment as they help reclaim the soil, absorb heavy metals and turn sandy soil into fresh growing material. They provide seeds for many wild birds and small animals, and abundant flowers for Pollinators. Truly another AMAZING Weed.

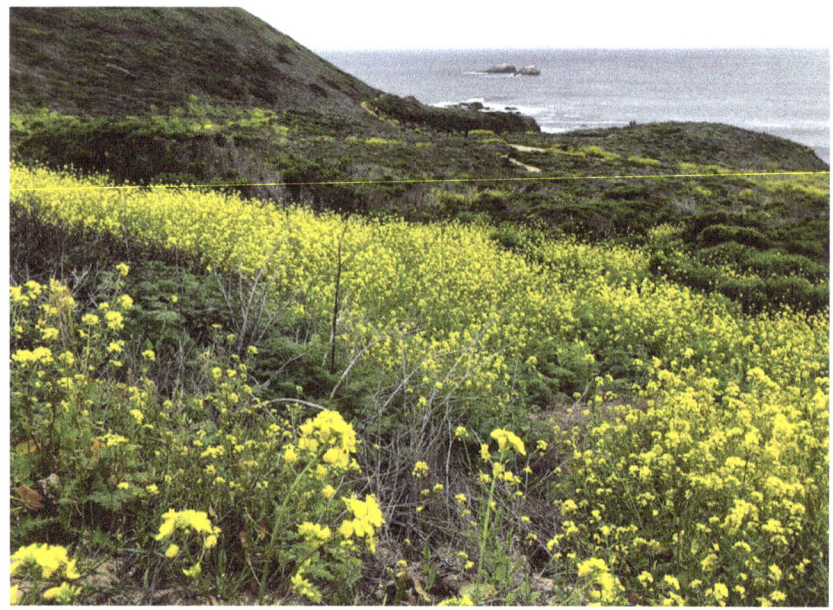

Just like Jesus said, although each Wild Mustard may seem small, they contain a world of nutrients, incredible numbers of seeds, and everything needed to spread the great gospel of faith far and wide. Mustards take over entire hillsides with their vibrant, expansive nature as they willingly provide exactly what we need in a grand and glorious supply. Some call this "invasive" especially when non-native Mustards go wild, but I just call it ABUNDANT FOOD.

Euell Gibbons calls Wild Mustards ***"Nature's Finest Health Food,"*** and teaches that there are few foods that surpass them for nutritional value. As he points out, this Family of Brassicaceae contains some of our most beloved and nutritious vegetable food staples: **Broccoli, Cauliflower, Brussels Sprouts, Kale, Radishes, Turnips, Cabbage, Maca, and Collard Greens**.

EXPLORE THE MANY SPICY FORMS
~ There are tons of Wild Mustards (more than 4000, to be a bit more exact) and **they are ALL EDIBLE**. They grow profusely and can cover enormous fields in a carpet of yellow. Look for the characteristic peppery taste from visible seed packets, the 4-petaled cross flower, and the ever present Mustardy scent of the whole plant. Seek out **Dame's Rocket (with a bright fushia-colored Mustard flower), Yellow Rocket, Yellowcress, Watercress, Field Mustard, Black Mustard, Garlic Mustard, Rock Cress, Pepperweed, Penny Grass, Tumble Mustard, Wintercress, Sea Rocket, Wild Radish, & Sweet Rocket.**

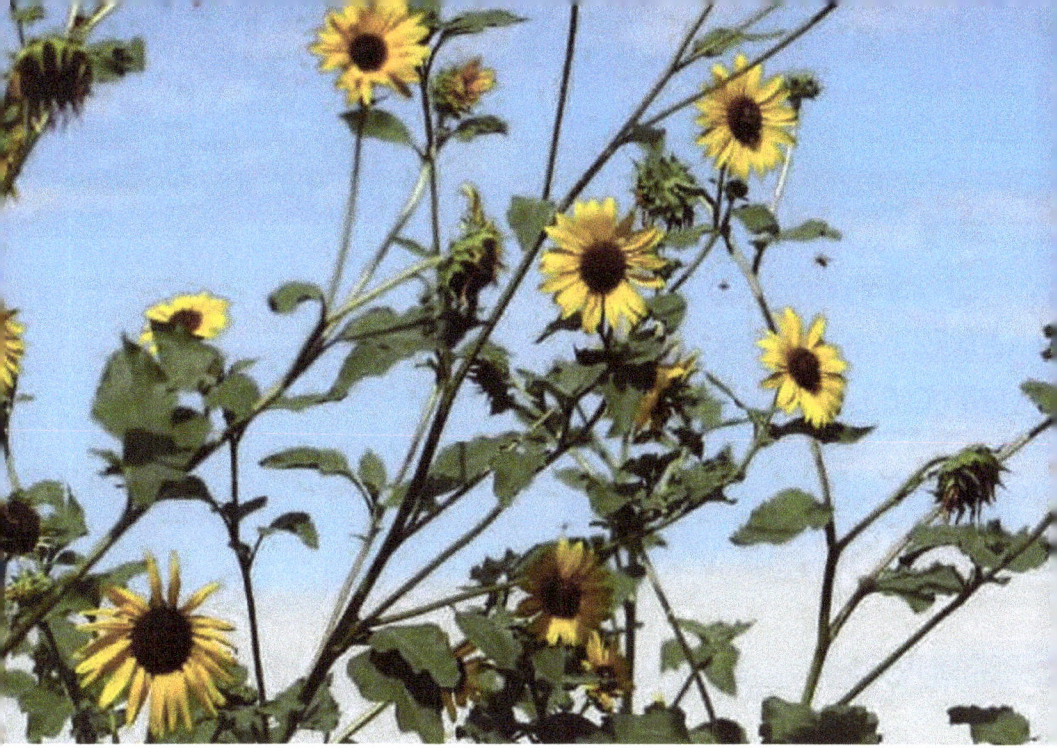

SUNFLOWER

Helianthus annuus   Daisy Family / **ASTERACEAE**

FOUND: Wild Sunflowers are found in the Sun on prairies, in plains, mountains, roadsides, and in disturbed ground. It grows abundantly wild from Mexico to Canada in North America, and all over Europe and Asia in well-drained, fertile soils.

IDENTIFYING FEATURES: Wild Sunflowers are branched with many yellow flowers, the cultivated variety has but one giant flower. The flowerhead of Sunflower is actually an enormous compound flower with thousands of blooms that turn to seed. With its large, deep taproot as a balance, it can grow from 3-9 feet tall, but the tallest Sunflower on record was 30.1 feet tall.

FOOD: Seeds are the Fruit of the Sunflower, and are a remarkable food for Humans, and feed many creatures as well! A coffee substitute can be made of the discarded shells. The nut butter made from Sunflower is delicious (especially for peanut sensitives) and is easily made in a blender or with a mortar & pestle. The top commercial growers of Sunflower for seeds and the valuable oil are Ukraine and Russia, Argentina, China, and Romania, but most of the seeds sold all over the world are roasted and salted.

CONTAINS: Protein, Vitamin B-complex, Vitamin E, Folate, Calcium, Iron, Magnesium, Manganese, Phosphorus, Selenium, Sodium, Zinc, Cadmium, Fiber, Chlorogenic Acid, Linoleic Fatty Acids, Phenolic Acids, Antioxidants, Phytosterol Beta-sitosterol.

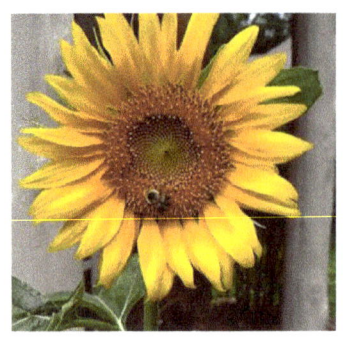

BODY BENEFITS: High in Zinc and Selenium, raw Sunflower seeds (and oil) are superior immune-boosting foods. Fiber, and the good fats in the Seeds, help lower cholesterol. They are gluten-free, and they improve brain power, digestion and elimination. Sunflower is the best food source of Vitamin E, the antioxidant nutrient that protects cell membranes and brain cells. Seeds are considered cardioprotective as regular eating can benefit and reduce arrhythmias and high blood pressure. Beta-sitosterol from the seeds can prevent breast cancer. Sunflower seeds are one of the best foods for managing diabetes, providing high fiber and protein to keep blood sugar stable. The energy pick-me-up from the Seeds is reliable, and you often see athletes chewing them. They contain so many nutrients, especially minerals, and are easy to eat regularly to dramatically enhance the potency of your diet. The seeds act preventively, reducing the risk of major diseases including most cancers (especially breast, prostate and colon cancer), asthma, arthritis, constipation, and nervous issues. The Magnesium content in Sunflower seeds is helpful for leg cramps, migraines and anxiety. The oil has sunscreen properties and is nourishing for the skin. Because they are addictive and high in calories, it is best to keep each serving size below ¼ cup for optimal health. Eating the seeds with shells you must crack slows down consumption.

QUALITIES: This plant is warming, nourishing, masculine, supportive and filled with Sunlight. It is anti-inflammatory, antioxidant, antimalarial, hypotensive, immune-building, nervine, oxygenating, and soothing.

FOLKLORE: Folk names Corona Solis, Marigold of Peru, Solo Indianus, Flower del Sol. Flowers yield a beautiful golden and orange dye with applications from textiles to warpaint. The domesticated Sunflower was bred to have only one enormous seed head, and it is thought to have been cultivated this way in Mexico around 3000 BC. Fossil remnants of the plants have also been found in Tennessee and Kentucky from 2300 BC. The Inca, Aztecs and otomi peoples worshiped the Sun and therefore revered the Sunflower as a major symbol in their culture. Native Americans planted Sunflower along the north edges of their gardens, as the "fourth sister" (in their gardens of the other "three sisters" - corn, beans and squash). The Pueblo Indians used the seeds and flowers as decorations for ceremonial dances and feast ceremonies. They made flutes from the hollowed-out stalks, and used the smaller stalks for arrow shafts and bird snares. In the 1500's, explorers brought Sunflower seeds to Europe where they were widely cultivated. It is the national flower of Ukraine, the state flower of Kansas, and one of the city flowers of Kitakyushu, Japan, as well as the symbol for the Vegan Society. The Chinese use a fiber from the stalks as a paper and textile material. In its native Americas, Sunflower fiber was reputedly used as a building material and an additive to mud bricks. Sunflowers were a major theme in the work of famed artist Vincent Van Gogh and he loved them. Peter the Great also loved Sunflowers, and

Russia is credited with much of the popularity of this plant.

FIRST AID USES: Chew raw seeds for energy. Sap from the Sunflower stalk can clean and disinfect wounds. A tea made from the petals is good for lung complaints and can be used topically for bee stings and bug bites (chew a few petals and apply if you are out in the wild).

SPIRITUAL PROPERTIES: Rather obviously ruled by the SUN, and the Fire Element, Sunflowers represent vitality, Midsummer and the Golden Ray. They are symbols of loyalty and honesty. Sunflower relates to the Solar Plexus (3rd) Chakra and helps restore this energetic source of personal power. Meditate with a flower on this Chakra, on your diaphragm below your breastbone, and feel its solar warmth returning your lightforce vitality.

MAGICAL USES: Blessings from the Sun are bestowed on all who grow Sunflowers, and they are considered to bring good luck, abundance, self-confidence, joy, and positivity. Eating the seeds during the Waxing Moon can reportedly help women to conceive (likely the nutritive support is a factor). Necklaces made of the seeds were said to ward off smallpox. Sunflower is also traditionally used for protection, loyalty and fertility. Picking a flower at sunset and wearing it will offer you good luck for the following day. Sleep with a flower under your pillow and you will have the truth revealed before the next sunset. In HooDoo, the Sunflower is associated with great joy. Use Sunflower petals and flowers in a ritual bath to restore a sunny attitude.

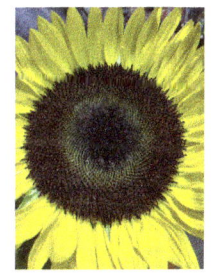

FLOWER ESSENCE: Sunflower is warming and brings the great Golden Light of the Sun with it. It is specifically supportive for low self-esteem and people who lack the ability to let their real Sun shine forth. It can also be used for people who have an inflated sense of self, are overly vain or believe the Sun rises and sets by their decree. It helps harmonize issues of masculinity and heals concerns relating to the Father. The themes this essence can treat are universal and foundational, and it can support everyone on their emotional journey to self-actualization.

PREPARATIONS: THE BEST SPROUT EVER. They are so easy to grow on cookie sheets in a window or on a deck - see *Sprouting* page 95. When eaten as a sprout, there is considerable added nutritional value from the chlorophyll in the early leaves. Raw Sunflower seeds can be added to every salad, smoothie, oatmeal and vegetable you make to increase their nutritional content many times over. For outrageous snacking, toss raw seeds with spices like Dill or Garam Masala or Lemon Pepper and serve in tiny bowls with spoons. Hulled seeds can be ground into paste for a really delicious nut butter, or parched and powdered for flour with multiple uses in breads, desserts, vegetable dishes, soups and to thicken sauces. Sunflower Seeds may turn blue when baked in desserts and breads, due to a chemical reaction of baking soda and the Sunflower's Chlorogenic Acid.

LAURA: One large Sunflower head can contain more than 2000 seeds, and some *giant* cultivated Helianthus have thousands more. This abundant harvest is *designed* to feed a village. But this beauty has many more properties that make it valuable.

Sunflower plants have been used in **PhytoRemediation** for cleaning up toxic ingredients from the soil (lead, arsenic and uranium) and can reduce radionuclides and harmful bacteria from water, and even dry up marshy areas that are flooded. Sunflowers were grown to remove caesium-137 and strontium-90 from a nearby pond after the Chernobyl disaster, and a similar campaign was mounted in response to the Fukushima Daiichi nuclear disaster.[17] So their value for the environment is still being discovered, and is likely inestimable! Not such a lowly weed after all.

I love going to Brigitte's house to eat our way through her wild foods. She always had trays of Sunflower seeds sprouting on her deck and we'd graze through heart-shaped Sunflower sprouts in their miniature dark green forest. She even named her first daughter Sunflower Sparkle Mars! Sunny remains a dear friend of mine to this day, and has a beautiful, wild, spirited Family of her own. Just like her namesake, Sunny continues to spread seeds, smiles and joy.

Here are some Wild Sunflowers growing plentifully at well over 9000 feet altitude, in the Flat Top Mountains near Yampa, Colorado. Hardy! These withstand feet of snow in the Winter, only to come up tall and proud each Spring.

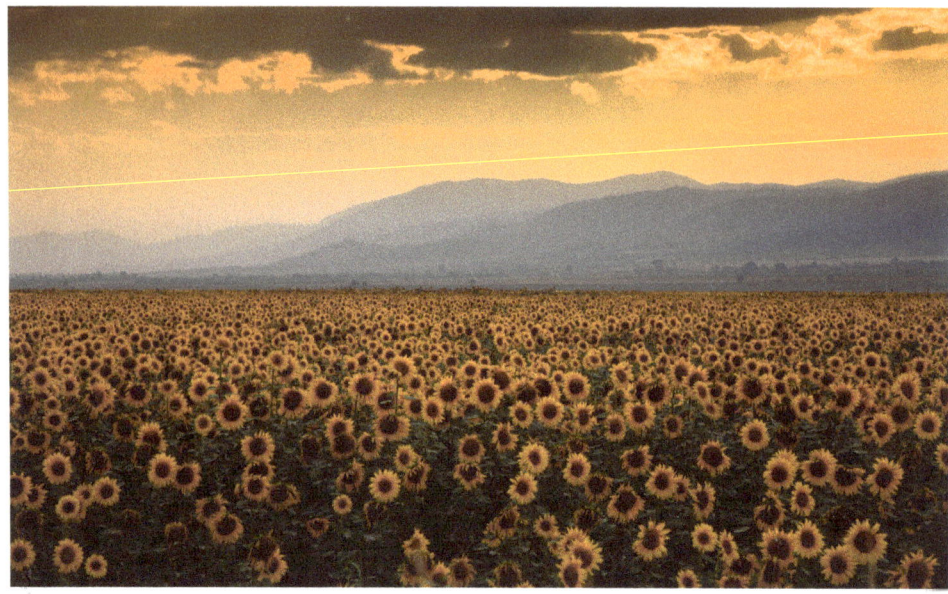

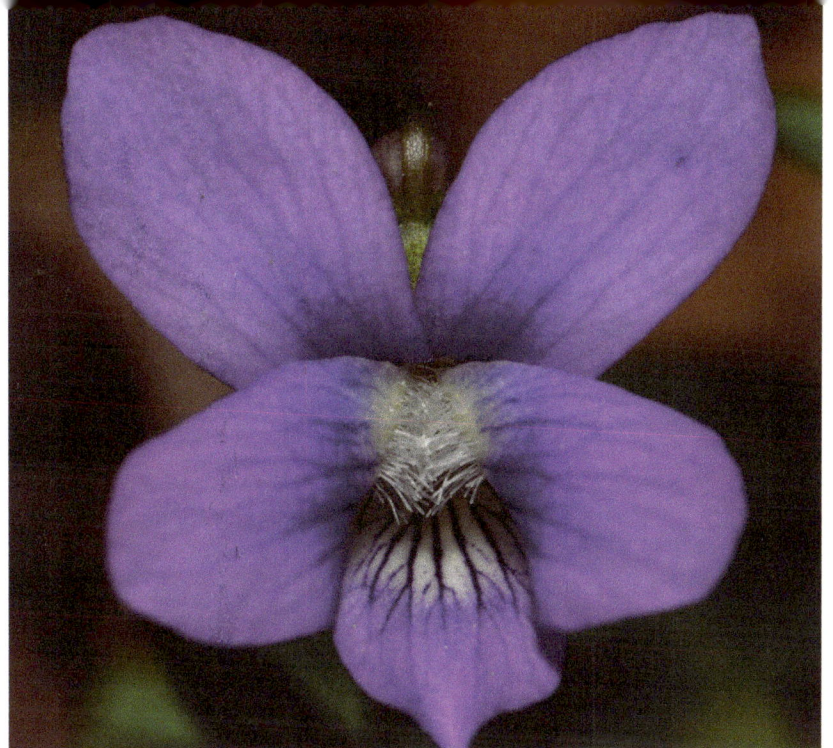

VIOLET

*Viola odorata   Violet Family / **VIOLACEAE***

FOUND: Originally found in Europe and Western Asia, now Violet is a wild weed (as well as a cultivated shade garden plant) and loved the World over. Violet prefers full shade and lots of water, spreading readily over forest floors and shady groves.

IDENTIFYING FEATURES: Violet has evergreen, heart-shaped leaves that uncurl from the center, and provide food all year long. On a single leafless stem perches a beautiful purple, five-lobed single flower, blooming early and abundantly in Spring. It may reach six inches tall, and grows in large communities. Violet has a secret - that its self-pollinating, seed-bearing flower also grows hidden in the foliage in late Fall, to set it up abundantly for the Spring. So look for it secreted under the leaves in all seasons.

FOOD: Leaves and flowers are **completely edible** and quite delicious. Tea can be made with the entire aerial part of the plant. Violets grow abundantly and provide some of the earliest Spring nectar for butterflies and bees. Pansies are edible flowers as well, (that look like large violets) and are in this same Violaceae Family.

CONTAINS: Beta-Carotene, Vitamin C, Salicylates, Saponins, Alkaloids (Violene), Flavonoids (Rutin), Essential Oil, Mucilage, natural Blue Dye.

BODY BENEFITS: Half a cup of Violet leaves has more Vitamin C than four oranges, and more Vitamin A than the recommended daily allowance. Violet cools everything down and saves the day to relieve the body of excess heat. The lobed flower resembles and supports the lungs, and helps relieve congestion, expectorate phlegm, and soothe the bronchial passages for bronchitis, pneumonia, asthma and sinus conditions. The leaves are full of natural anti-inflammatories, useful for relieving dry and sore throats, laryngitis, acne, ulcers, UTI's, headaches, swellings and heartbreak, as well as heated and angry emotional conditions. Violets induce a restful sleep cycle, and are soothing and helpful for nervous conditions as well. They are blood-cleansing and helpful for stimulating and clearing the lymphatic system. Soluble fiber from the mucilage in the leaves is helpful for lowering cholesterol.

QUALITIES: Violet is feminine, sweet, pungent and bitter, moist, watery and yin, with cooling and soothing qualities. The plant is alterative, antifungal, anti-inflammatory, antioxidant, antiseptic, anti-tumor, astringent, demulcent, diaphoretic, diuretic, emetic (root), emollient, expectorant, mild laxative, nutritive, restorative, vulnerary.

FOLKLORE: Folk names Heartsease, Sweet Violet, Blue Violet, Violetta, Violette, Viola, Fialka Polevaya, Johnny-Jump-Up (*Viola tricolor*). You can make ink with the crushed up flowers, and a dye from the flowers is used in making litmus paper to determine acid or alkaline pH. You can find Violet-scented candies, perfumes and syrups everywhere in France. Gourmet stores in the US usually carry Violet Pastilles or gum, and I have seen them in the Vermont Country Store catalog and other fine establishments. Violet is a very old-fashioned perfume-style ingredient similar to Rosewater, and it was very much in vogue in the Victorian Age, where they really celebrated Flowers in art, food and fashion. In fact, Violet was one of the very first flowers grown for cosmetic, culinary, perfume, and medicinal use. Hippocrates prescribed Violets for bad eyesight, melancholia, headaches and inflammation of the chest. Ancient Britons used Violets steeped in goat's milk as a beauty remedy for the complexion. In Greece they wrote of using Violets to control anger, bring restful sleep, and benefit the heart.

FIRST AID USES: Use Violet leaves as tea or salad for vertigo and dizziness. Washcloths soaked in Violet tea may be helpful for headaches, breathing difficulties, fever and inflamed conditions. Leaf tea is safe and gentle enough for children, and can be sipped instead of baby aspirin when feverish. Violet is cooling and NOT recommended in cold conditions such as the chills or colds. Chew Violet flowers to relieve thirst, freshen the breath or to calm a ticklish throat while hiking. Topical compress or poultice of Violet may help with breast cysts, relieve hemorrhoids, shrink lumps, swelling, and calm skin eruptions.

SPIRITUAL PROPERTIES: Ruled by Venus and the Water Element, Violets confer peace, beauty, protection, and Love from the Goddess to the wearer. Violets are Elemental - they say Violet cannot be smelled until the Fire of the Sun warms it and the Air brings its glorious scent up with the wind. They are thought to bring great favor and magic wherever they are honored. Violets are nourishing for the Pineal Gland

and Third Eye as well as Crown Chakras. This high vibrational Plant Spirit gives your energy a spiritual upleveling. Violet represents the Violet Flame in physicality.

MAGICAL USES: Carry Violets to change your fortune, or to call on Lady Luck, The first Violet of the Spring can be gathered and wished upon, and your dearest wish will be granted. Violets inspire and symbolize faithfulness. Violets symbolize life, Love and beauty, and were dedicated to the goddesses Persephone and Aphrodite, and the god Pan. Carry the flowers to ward off "wicked spirits." Violets represent innocence, and a tradition was started in Roman times of planting them on a child's grave. The blossoms can be worn to calm angry energy. Use Violet in Love and lust spells, and for twilight or sunset ceremonies. Violet can be successfully used in heartbreak to change the tide for new love. If you dream of Violets your life is about to change.

FLOWER ESSENCE: Violet is a *Transcender.* It helps you rise above the noise by raising your vibration. It offers you an elevated spiritual perspective. Violet Flower Essence is a great break-up remedy, and for grief (nicknamed Heart's Ease for a reason!).

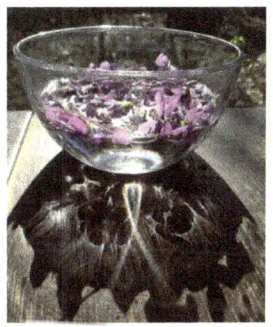

The Flower Essence promotes easy communication that stays firmly rooted in personal truth. It is specific for people who feel lonely even in a crowd of friends. This is a perfect remedy for stage fright, fear of public speaking, or social awkwardness - perfect for "the shrinking violet." People in need of this essence may display outer "cool" and could even be cold to the touch, lonely, shut down and isolated. Violet helps them to open, bloom, and warmly express through sharing of themselves. It is a great addict's remedy for the social involvement of meetings and counseling. Violet helps you to trust others, to stand your ground while expressing yourself, and to emerge victorious with abundant rewards.

PREPARATIONS: EAT THE LEAVES AND FLOWERS FRESH! They taste faintly of Wintergreen (due to the Salicylates). Juice the whole plant for super nutrition! Violets are perfectly paired with fruits in sweet dessert dishes, and they are standout gorgeous in salads and savory applications as well. Flowers can be candied, jammed, jellied, syruped, made into ice cream, cordials, concentrates, spirits, bitters and wine - and used as edible decorations. Top breads and meats, cookies and cakes with the flowers before baking. Violet Honey (see recipe below) is a magical way to concentrate the many healing properties of this plant. Leaves make a wonderful and abundant salad green for which you can forage during the whole year in warmer climates. Leaves are similar to Spinach and can be cooked, steamed, sauteed, and added to soups, veggies, and casseroles. Violet flowers will make a deep turquoise cold water infusion, perfectly cooling and quite stunning for a Summertime drink. A wonderful and medicinal hot tea can be made with the flowers and fresh leaves. Make a strong infusion of Violet leaves in Castor Oil as a massage oil for resolving breast cysts and for encouraging breast health. Make Tea with two teaspoons of dried leaf per cup of boiling water and use for gargling to soothe sore throat or a tickle. Sometimes called Wild Okra, Violet is similarly mucilaginous and can be used to thicken and extend soups and sauces. Violet Vinegar is incredible, made with the flowers packed into jars with champagne or white balsamic vinegar. Stuffed Mushroom caps can be made with the chopped flowers and greens, with some spices and breadcrumbs. Flowers can be added to pesto, omelets, pancakes, muffins, crepes and curries. Place a couple of flowers in each ice cube before freezing, and serve with drinks or float in punch bowls. Use Violet leaves and flowers in lip balms for moisturizing action, and make into salves for eczema, bug bites, hemorrhoids, varicose veins and swellings.

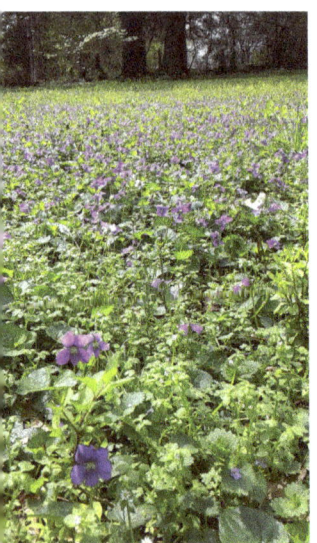

LAURA: You know how I maintain that Nature will show up, show out, and grow for you what you most need? In the Springtime my ENTIRE backyard is VIOLETS! Solid purple - what a show for me. Every year more Violets grow and I sing their praises even louder. I try to make new wonderful products every year from the embarrassment of riches right outside my door. Violet Honey is one of my favorites. The sweet aromatic perfume of Violets is heavy in the taste and aroma when I open the Jar in midwinter. Since Violets are so good for the Heart and Lungs, you can modify the Honey recipe below for a great Lung Healing Syrup with Violet Leaves (and the Violet Vodka is yummy, too). I also made Violet Brandy and used the Violets in Bitters. I've candied the flowers with egg white and raw sugar for cake decorating and to put over ice cream. I've made syrups and teas and used them in my breakfast fruit salad. I am ever grateful for my vital, Violet wonderland.

When you need to gather a lot of flowers, you can drag your fingers gently (like a rake) through a Violet patch to pull off just the flowerheads. Because the real seeding flower does not come out until the Fall, you can feel justified in picking more Violet flowers than you normally would with other plants. However, *sparingly gather the leaves*, and take only one or two per plant, cutting above the stem and roots. The leaves provide needed nourishment for the plant and are necessary for its abundant growth.

★ **Witness the "Litmus Effect"** (pH measuring) of the Violet's dye! Make a water infusion (tea) of the Flowers. Strain when deeply colored, and place in a clear glass. Add lemon juice (acidic) and watch the color change. Add baking soda (alkaline) and watch it change again! This can be used as a teaching device for homeschooling.

★ **Violet Lung-Healing Syrup** can be made in the early Spring using Violet Leaves & Flowers, Spruce Tips, and **Local Honey**. Add some **Osha Root** if you have it, and consider adding **Garlic Cloves** as well, for anti-viral support and extra immune action. You can strain and rebottle, but I usually leave all the herbs in the syrup.

Violet Honey

1. Gather fresh **Violet Flowers** just before or on the New Moon, and gently wash. Leave for a few hours on a clean towel, to dry and wilt a bit.
2. Warm 2 cups of **Local Honey** gently in a small saucepan, stay nearby and do not overheat. It should be runny, but not steaming or bubbling from heat.
3. Pack the flowers into your wide-mouthed, clean, sterilized glass jars. Leave a ½ inch space at the top.
4. Fill with Honey, drizzling it warm over the Violets. The smell is heavenly as they release essential oil in the process. Cover the flowers completely with warm honey, and cap the jars quickly to preserve the precious scent.
5. Store in a pantry or cool, dry, dark spot. Swirl around often for best flower infusion. Taste after the first 2 weeks to see if the flavor is to your liking, or if it could use another month to strengthen.
6. Sometimes I add another harvest or two of Violets, in successive days, on top of the old, as demonstrated in the image below. Make sure to get all flower matter down below the liquid line, and swirl around often.
7. Strain and bottle after the Full Moon. I usually leave mine for 6 weeks, then strain and bottle after the 2nd Full Moon. Or (most of the time), I leave the flowers right in there and use in one season.
8. Decorate with a nice homemade label, ingredients and date. Give the extras away, or stash a jar for the perfect present you just happen to have on hand when you need it!

★ Add the **Violet Honey** to cocktails or mocktails, or use it to make your own sweet Liqueur Syrup by adding it directly to a Spirit or Wine.

VIOLET VODKA, Brandy, or Gin:

Procure a **High-Quality Spirit** of your choice, set up your supplies, and pick your **Violet Flowers** on or before the New Moon. When dry-ish, pack flowers into your jars. **DO NOT HEAT alcohol,** just pour directly over flowers, to completely cover, then cap and shake 100 times. Store in a cool dry place, and shake daily. Allow to infuse for 2 weeks to several months. Strain (if desired), and place into fancy bottles, make your own cool labels, and try to save for gifts! Delicious and floral, super great in seltzer, and for fancy cocktails and mocktails.

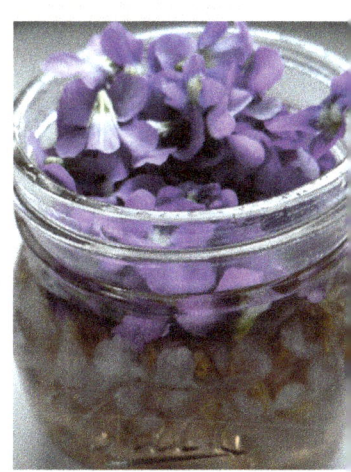

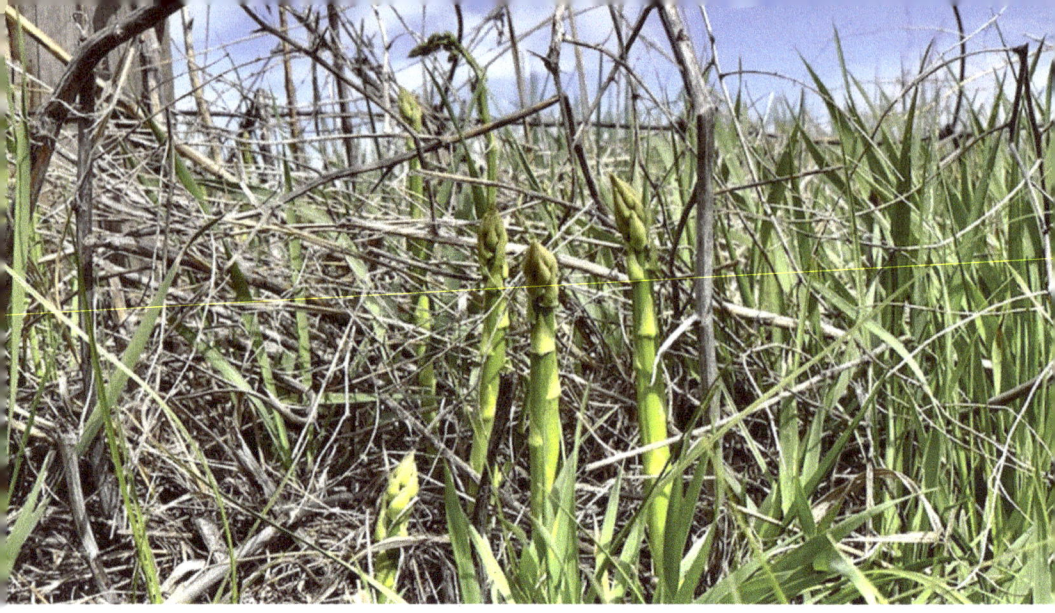

WILD ASPARAGUS

Asparagus officinalis   Asparagus Family / **ASPARAGACEAE**

FOUND: *"In fence corners and hedgerows"* as Euell Gibbons says. Asparagus grows in old fields, along country roads near irrigation ditches, and in and among fence lines in all 50 US states and Canada. It was a native of Europe and temperate Asia, but now, as with most of our weed friends, it grows all over the World.

IDENTIFYING FEATURES: Early Asparagus spears with their thick stalks are instantly recognizable, rising fully formed right up out of the ground and can grow up to 10 inches in 24 hours. Small ivory-colored flowers dot the edges of the plant in the middle of the Summer, and its red seeds in Autumn are popular with sparrows. Its roots penetrate deeply into the ground, an old perennial Asparagus may have an 18 foot taproot. When it matures it looks like a super scraggly Christmas tree. It is most easily found looking for last year's straw-like branches, through which Asparagus usually grows.

FOOD: Spears showing first are the highly nutritious vegetable and can be eaten raw or prepared many different ways. Seeds make a great coffee substitute when roasted in an iron skillet for a few minutes, although raw seeds should not be eaten. The tubers can be eaten as well, but are mainly used in Chinese Medicine and Ayurveda as a medicinal herb.

CONTAINS: Vitamins A (Beta-Carotene), B-complex, C and K, Folate, Potassium, Copper, Iron, Zinc, Fiber, Chlorophyll, Lutein, Silica, Molybdenum, Chromium, Phosphorus, Magnesium, Selenium, Steroidal Glycoside (Asparagoside), Essential Oil, Asparagine, Arginine, Tyrosine, Flavonoids (Quercetin, Rutin, Kaempferol), Mucilage, Resin, and Tannins.

BODY BENEFITS: Asparagus is anti-aging, inhibits toxins, and is highly alkalizing for the body, preventing and encouraging recovery from nerve disorders and every kind of cancer. It is organ and blood-cleansing, and is one of the most supportive foods for adrenal exhaustion. It helps the body fight stress and fight off disease. Asparagus is a testosterone and libido-boosting Aphrodisiac food that nourishes the body's vital force and sexual energy on a very deep level. It also has various phytochemicals that help dissolve uric acid for the prevention of gout and kidney stones. Asparagus treats and prevents neurological disorders. It is diuretic and helpful for the urinary tract, and is heralded as a kidney yin tonic for people who burn themselves out. It is also considered a galactagogue (stimulates lactation), and is on my List of Lactation Foods. Asparagus is a full body tonic, but especially moisturizing and rejuvenative for the heart, lungs and reproductive systems. It flushes out toxins, heavy metals and unwanted acids, and then inhibits damage from any new toxin, which makes it a perfect for treating and preventing cancer. Asparagus is so good for the body that it is recommended for anyone who is ill or convalescing, and it even relieves the side effects of chemotherapy, helping the body to return to optimal health quickly. Use it for poor memory and to stimulate focus while working. Asparagus works exceptionally well to treat viruses like EBV and chronic fatigue, shingles, herpes and mononucleosis, and mysterious diseases like fibromyalgia, Hashimoto's, Grave's and Meniere's. It can be of great use in fibroids, hernia, muscle spasms, sleep apnea, pelvic inflammatory disease, migraines, TIA, celiac disease, neuropathy, kidney stones, PMS, twitches, tinnitus, ovarian cysts, canker sores and infertility.

QUALITIES: Sweet with a slight bitter taste, the action is cooling, sedative, moisturizing, and yin. Asparagus is alterative, aphrodisiac, brain tonic, cardiotonic, demulcent, diaphoretic, diuretic, expectorant, female tonic, galactagogue, mild laxative, lung tonic, nutritive, refrigerant, rejuvenative, reproductive tonic, & sedative.

FOLKLORE: Folk names Shatavari, Points d'Amour, Sparrowgrass, Sparrergrass, Satavar, Hundred-Rooted Vine, Many-Haired Vine, Longevity Vine, Challagadda, Esparrago, Asperge, Tenmendo, Tian Men Tong (sounds like "Ten Men's Dong" to me, advertising its most famous erectile action). Asparagus increases the milk output of cows and can be used as a graze feed. You can find Asparagus carved into Egyptian architectural friezes dated from around 3000 BC. Emperor Augustus, the first Roman Emperor loved it so much he had a whole "Asparagus Fleet" just for hauling it around, and he coined the phrase "velocius quam asparagi conquatur" translated to "faster than cooking asparagus" to mean something that was speedy. The Perfumed Garden of Sensual Delight, a 15th century Arabic sex manual, mentions Asparagus contains "special phosphorus elements" that are aphrodisiac and counteract fatigue.

European settlers apparently brought Asparagus to North America, and in 1685, William Penn advertised Asparagus as one of the crops that would grow well in his new land of Pennsylvania.

FIRST AID USES: Tea made with the young shoots can be relieving for digestive distress and soothing symptoms of colds and flu. A poultice of the leaves, shoots and root will relieve muscle cramps or spasms, and painful stiff joints. Try a bite of fresh Asparagus (or tea) for acid reflux.

SPIRITUAL PROPERTIES: Ruled by Venus and the Water Element, Asparagus revives the Spirit and raises the will. It works through the application of sacred healing waters and the action of levitation. Eating it when you feel down will give you a lift. It helps you stand up for yourself and feel confident in public.

MAGICAL USES: Asparagus has always been known as a magical life extender. Toaist texts from 300 AD tell of Tu Tze-Wei who drank Asparagus tea everyday and was able to satisfy his 80 wives, walk 50 miles a day, and live to be 145 years old. It is often used in fertility charms and as a food for male potency and virility.

FLOWER ESSENCE: This remedy helps you stand up for yourself, perfect for people who are shy and self-conscious. Asparagus Flower Essence wills you to claim your place and break out of your shell. It helps agoraphobics and people with extreme social awkwardness feel comfortable in public. Asparagus is useful for relieving stage fright, and enhances teaching and public speaking. Helps you have a spine.

PREPARATIONS: There are so many ways to prepare Asparagus - it can be eaten raw, roasted, steamed, sliced in salads, made into chips and flash fried, and cooked by a campfire on a hot rock, to name a few. You can juice it with other veggies (a perfect thing to do if you have some that is old). Quick-broiling with a splash of Olive Oil is my favorite method. Asparagus is a no-fat food with zero cholesterol, it is filling and does lower the appetite, so it is a great weight loss food. Refrigerate unused spears in a glass of water like a flower bouquet to keep them fresh and supple.

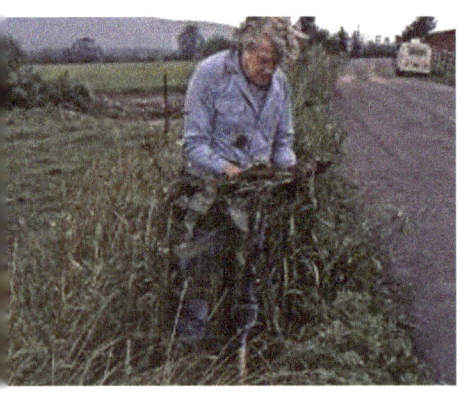

LAURA: Euell Gibbons named one of his greatest books *Stalking the Wild Asparagus* after this plant. He said every time he was out foraging for it, he felt like he was a child again, with wide-eyed wonder, curiosity and an unlimited zest. He tells a story about being somewhere around age twelve and finding a small patch of Wild Asparagus on the way to fish a nearby stream. He cut some of the tender young shoots, and as he walked further on he found more. Full of awe - he decided to sit down and spend some time really looking at last year's dead growth under which the new shoots were sprouting. He spent five full minutes training himself in **every feature of the old and new plant growing side by side**. He compared colors to the surrounding foliage and really noted the qualities of the plant. When he stood up and looked back he discovered *dozens* of plants he had walked by without seeing before! Euell describes how the old growth gets tall and spindly on its stalk, almost like a straw Christmas tree with no needles, and looks like old hay but lighter and much more thread-like. This is where you will find the new spears if you root around a little bit. That day when he really discovered Asparagus, he gathered a whole pailful of spears and tips, and then filled his shirt with them as well. The family ate Asparagus prepared every different way possible for a week, and he was a hero! His successful trips back every Saturday kept the family well-fed for a whole season. **Nature is the Great Provider, and his family was nourished because one curious little boy cared enough to discover it!** The "eye training" he gave himself that day when he was twelve years old set in motion a radical love for the wild things, and an entire life of foraging and living off the land for which he will be forever known.

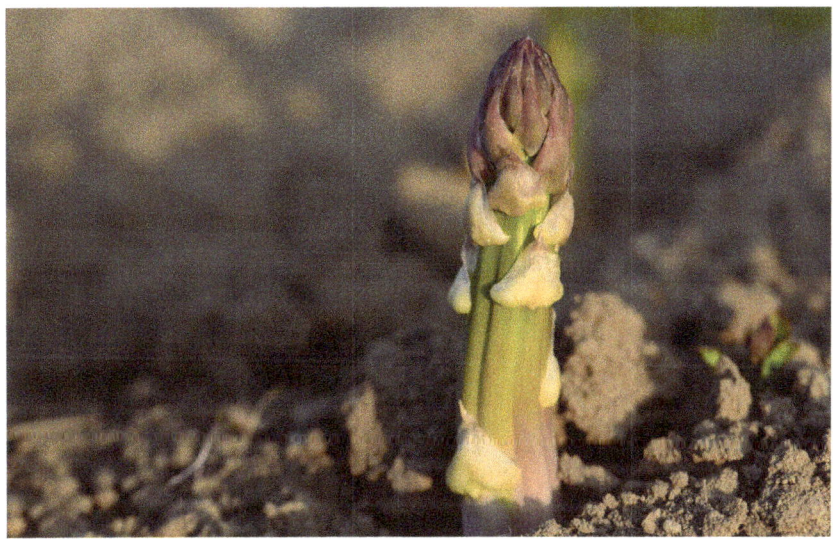

Anthony William (the Medical Medium) says that Asparagus is the ***"Fountain of Youth!"*** He explains that in the first few weeks of Asparagus growth, as each spear *intends* to grow into a small tree, it contains a **remarkable amount of vital force**. He compares it to being in the youthful prime of life, full of potential, and this food brings you that same feeling. He says the plant has "propulsive energy that is transferred to us" which nourishes our ability to stand tall and flourish. This is the kind of energy that keeps us young - exactly like the Fountain of Youth! And very obviously, this energy and this food would make men more **virile!**

He also teaches that the Lutein and Chlorophyll in Asparagus scour through the organs, cleansing them of toxins, and gently removing heavy metals. Anthony recommends eating a bunch of Asparagus every single day all through April and May, for a powerful Spring tonic and organ detox. Find yourself a wild patch (or plant one!) and start cleansing!

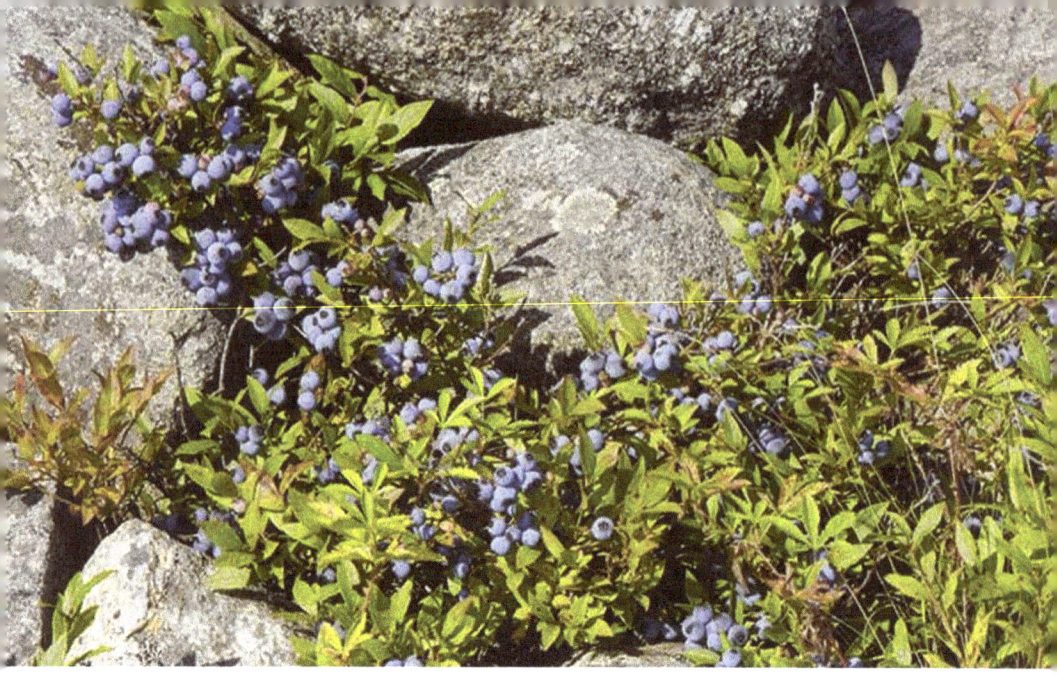

WILD BLUEBERRY

Vaccinium angustifolium   Heath Family / **ERICACEAE**

FOUND: Wildly prolific in New England, Maine and Canada, and from the Great Smoky Mountains to the Great Lakes and Minnesota. Wild Blueberries are one of North America's oldest native berries (of which there are only three). They prefer thin glacial soils and rocky outcroppings on coastal hills, ridgelines and fields, especially burned out areas. Inquire at your State Forestry office for sites of fairly recent forest fires - you could check there for new growth.

IDENTIFYING FEATURES: This is the lowbush variety that stays close to the ground. Leaves are ovate, glossy green and abundant, and turn red in the Fall. Flowers are off-white and shaped like a bell with triangular petals that curl backwards, growing in little clumps just like the future fruit. Berry is dark blue-black with a waxy, powdery white coating and a star-shaped top. A Blueberry barren can dominate the terrain, spreading over many acres and exploding into roughly 150 million blossoms per acre.

FOOD: Pick when perfectly ripe because the Wild Blueberry does not ripen any more off the branch. It only takes a small handful to rival the nutrition of any other food on Earth. If you can't find them growing in the wild, find Wild Blueberries in the freezer section at grocery and health food stores. Ironically, and quite magically, freezing makes their potent medicines even stronger. Look for frozen Wild Blueberries from Maine (like Wyman's), Canada and Nova Scotia.

CONTAINS: Vitamin C, Fiber, D-Mannose, Polyphenols, Tannins, Anthocyanins, Anthocyanidins, Antioxidants, Dimethyl Resveratrol, Flavonoids. Highly concentrated nutrition with no fat, sodium or cholesterol. In a USDA study, Wild Blueberries were found to have the highest level of Antioxidants of all 40 fruits and vegetables tested. It has been reported that they may have the highest level of antioxidants (proportionately) of *any food* on the Planet!

BODY BENEFITS: Anthony William says, *"There is not a cancer that Wild Blueberry cannot prevent, nor a disease known to Humankind that Wild Blueberry cannot protect you from."* That pretty much says it all - but to expound a little bit: vision is improved by Wild Blueberries (they look like little eyes) and the brain is greatly nourished, enhancing memory, cognition, and focus. Eat Wild Blueberries first thing in the morning (after your Lemon Water) to nourish the brain and even support mental health. They remove radiation and detoxify heavy metals, xenoestrogens, pesticides and other chemical toxins and pollutants from the blood, supporting and helping to feed and restore the liver. The nerves are healed and renewed with Wild Blueberry - use them for neuropathy, Parkinson's and sciatica. Freezing the fruit only INCREASES its potency and antioxidant count. These plants grow in punishing climatic conditions, and have been adapting to climate change for 10,000 years at the very least. This is the ultimate survivor plant, truly an adaptogenic plant, and it will help you survive just about anything. As with other high-tannin berries in the same Family (think Cranberry) this Berry will fight recurrent urinary tract infections with its high D-Mannose content (for nonadherence of bacteria). Blueberries are a great food for relieving teenage angst and promoting better mental health at any age. Wild Blueberry is especially supportive for extreme athletes and people with extra physical jobs, as it enhances visual perception, offers heroic nutrients for performance and stamina, protects the cells and speeds recovery from overexertion.

QUALITIES: Cooling, feminine, nurturing and soothing, cleansing and yin. Wild Blueberries are adaptogenic, antibacterial, radically antioxidant, antipathogenic, moisturizing, nervine, nutritive, and universally healing.

FOLKLORE: Folk names Star Berries, Wild Lowbush Berry, Dwarf Blueberry, Brulis. Blueberries were probably the most important fruit for the Native Americans. They relate that Wild Blueberry was the first plant to grow back after wildfires, and it grew back much healthier and more resilient than before. Rabbits, birds and many small animals find Wild Blueberries a welcome food source, but so does our biggest animal, the Grizzly Bear! Some tribes called the fruits Star Berries, and believed they had magical properties. They tell fables of how the Star Berries were delivered to them from the sky by the Great Spirit, in a time of starvation, to relieve the hunger of his children. This is one of many stories associating Wild Blueberries with Great Spirit, Great Mother and Divine Nourishment. Wild Blueberries were first harvested commercially in the modern age for the Civil War, during which they were canned and distributed to feed the Union Army. It is the state fruit of Maine and the Nova Scotia Provincial Berry (Nova Scotia is known as the Wild Blueberry Capital of Canada).

Caterpillars love the leaves and this is a Butterfly food plant. Blueberries are one of the crops that growers hire traveling Honey Bees to pollinate for two weeks a season. Sometimes they also use Bumble Bees, who pollinate the flowers in a different way. This is called Sonification, or "buzz pollination," that vibrates the pollen grains into place to produce fruit. Wow.

FIRST AID USES: Take a baggie full of dried Wild Blueberries everywhere you go, and keep in the glovebox for survival food. Squish a cold or frozen Wild Blueberry on a burn. When you feel a urinary tract issue coming on, eat them daily, in good therapeutic doses for a few days to a week. Eat Wild Blueberries regularly when fighting any disease or cancer, or recovering from literally *anything*.

SPIRITUAL PROPERTIES: Ruled by Venus and the Water Element, this is a plant that simply loves all creatures like a Great Mother! This Plant Spirit wants to feed the World, and to spread even further than it has already. Wild Blueberry contains Divine encodements for Humankind's evolution and survival. It has a protective energy and spiritual intelligence that everyone needs. Especially in trying times, the right foods can elevate you, and Wild Blueberry is one of them. The deep blue color corresponds to the Third Eye Chakra and the Pineal Gland (for which it is a cleansing food) - so Wild Blueberry enhances your Spiritual Sight as well.

MAGICAL USES: Place a few fruits under the doormat to protect the home and keep intruders and undesirables from entering. Blueberry repels psychic attacks, eat it when feeling vulnerable and to reverse the energy. String the dried fruits into necklaces and headwear, add to medicine bags, amulets, and anointing oils for protection. Use a few Berries as an offering to the Wild Ones when hiking outside. Baking with Blueberries is said to reinforce your psychic shield, and to help return curses and angry messages unopened. You can blend the dried berries into a powder and use in face masks, incense, ritual protection baths, and to sprinkle on thresholds in protection ceremonies. Eat fresh Wild Blueberries on the Full Moon to strengthen the aura and energetic body. Utilize Wild Blueberries in abundance rituals for manifesting and nurturing your wildest dreams. They bring positive results.

FLOWER ESSENCE: Provides healing on an emotional level, as all Flower essences do, but this one takes it personally. Wild Blueberry is the hero who rescues you from feeling rejected, over criticized, overlooked, mistreated, underpaid, discredited or neglected. Use when you have been leveled by something or burned to your core. Its strong Spirit entices you to rise from the ashes and become who you were meant to be. It offers inspiration, healing, recovery, and a creative force from the Divine that grows wildly.

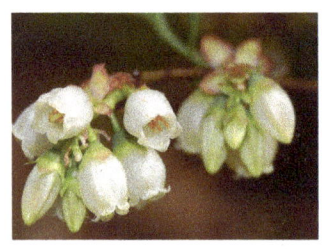

PREPARATIONS: Wild Blueberries are smaller and contain less water than their cultivated cousins, but have much more flavor and are actually better suited to baking. Eat fresh, juice with other fruits, or turn into concentrates or syrup. Use fresh berries for fruit salads, muffins, scones, pies, jellies and jams, berry cobblers, or fold into whipped coconut cream for a real treat. Berries can be blended with coconut water for a nice pick-me-up drink. Fresh-picked berries can be stored in Mason jars in the fridge and will last for more than a month. When they get close to looking old throw them in a ziploc in the freezer for instantly adding to smoothies. Berries can also be canned with much success. Dry Blueberries in the Sun or a hot attic for about a week to ten days, and store them for winter fruit. Stew them with meat and greens like the Indians did, and add a small handful to soups for a surprisingly rich flavor.

QUICK RECIPE: WILD PURPLE SYRUP & Vinaigrette

Muddle, grind or blend a few handfuls of **Wild Blueberries** into 2-4 cups of **Pure Maple Syrup** or **Local Honey**. Pour into small jars. This makes an incredibly simple and highly nutritious topping for ice cream, pancakes, cheesecakes, biscuits, scones, fruit salads, goat cheese, and to glaze barbecue meats, vegetables & veggie burgers.

Divinely Wild Blueberry Vinaigrette - Add a nice amount of
Wild Purple Syrup to 3 parts **Olive Oil** and 1 part **Vinegar**. Add fresh herbs, spices, pepper and salt to taste. Shake well and use liberally.

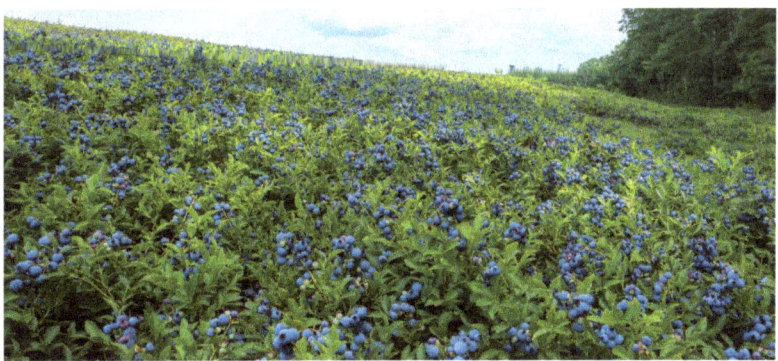

LAURA: I think the "purple berries" in the Crosby, Stills, Nash & Young song, *Wooden Ships*, are Wild Blueberries! The story tells of two soldiers on opposite sides of a war, who meet by chance and find common ground:

> "Say, can I have some of your purple berries?"
> "Yes, I've been eating them - for six, seven weeks now -
> Haven't got sick once."
> "Probably keep us both alive."

And he's right. You could live on these amazing purple berries for many, many weeks, only getting healthier! Remember to dry some for the future each time you harvest.

Anthony William calls Wild Blueberry a **"Resurrection Food"** and he says *"There is more information in one Wild Blueberry plant than there is on the entire internet."* He maintains that Wild Blueberry has a sensing mechanism (an "innate intelligence" much like our own) that scans the body, and searches for the areas and conditions that need the most support. It monitors your toxicity and stress levels to *tailor* its actions to your most prioritized needs. Wow, just wow.

Apparently, there is no other food on Earth that works with our bodies in this fashion, doing so much good work for our health. Much like **Nettle**, Wild Blueberry can be used medicinally for **all conditions and all symptoms**. It is Universally Healing. It conquers Fire and Ice and rises up stronger and more able to nourish your body than nearly any other food. This indestructible energy is yours for the eating.

Wild Blueberries really ARE Star Berries!!!

Apparently the Wild Blueberry only grows where it wants to - I would too if I was this big of a Star - so it has not been able to be cultivated for home growing. However, these berries are widely spread by birds, animals and brush fires.

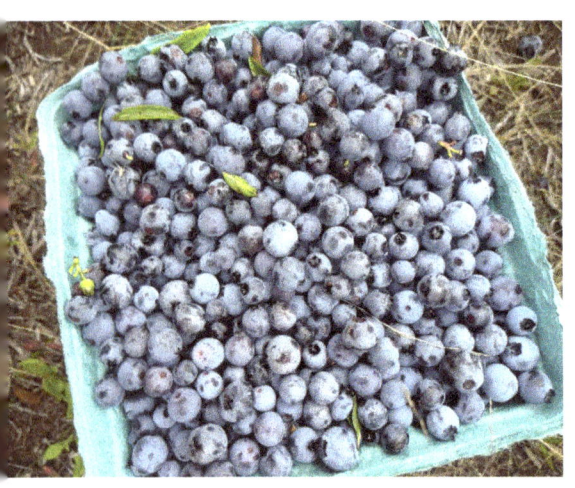

There is so much recent interest in the health benefits of this plant, a **Wild Blueberry Association of North America (WBANA)** was created to fund research and support native growers. Each year, they present a Wild Blueberry Health Research Summit in Bar Harbor, Maine for "a worldwide gathering of renowned scientists and researchers from leading institutions representing broad disciplines - from cardiovascular health to cancer to heart disease, osteoporosis, neurological diseases of aging, and more. Their work is leading the way to learn more about the health benefits of Wild Blueberries, and their findings, which use rigorous methodology, are documented in a growing number of published studies on the potential health and disease-fighting benefits of Wild Blueberries." Their website has informative scientific papers and some really great research:

https://www.wildblueberries.com/health-benefits/research/

https://www.wildblueberryassociation.ca/contact-us/

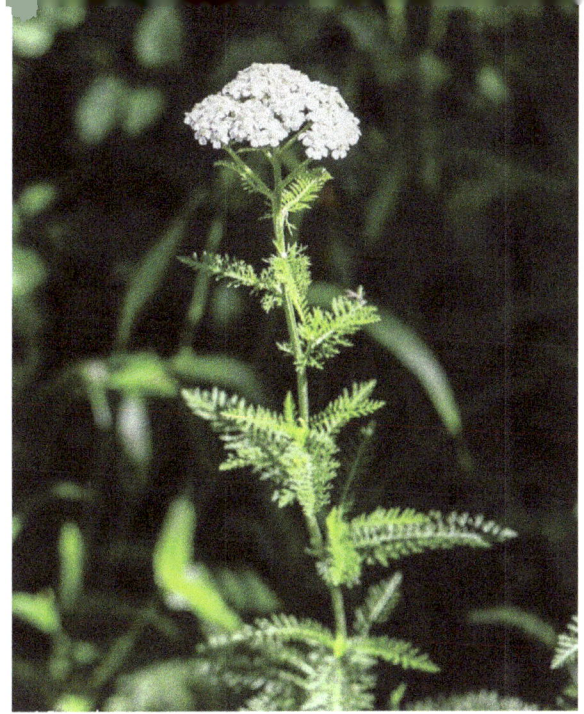

YARROW

Achillea millefolium   Daisy Family / **ASTERACEAE (COMPOSITAE)**

FOUND: In fields and forests, in all 50 states & Canada, as well as native Asia and Europe. This "Weed" is now cultivated and hybridized as a perennial garden flower.

IDENTIFYING FEATURES: Feathery, fern-like, grey green leaves are very fragrant, and flowers are usually white and many 5-petaled blooms in a flat umbrella-like flower. The individual petals are squarish and have a double cleft. Some domesticated varieties are pink, golden or red. It usually grows about knee-high, from 1-3 feet tall. ****Be careful not to mistake a poison look-alike for Yarrow. Poison Hemlock, Conium maculatum is a taller plant, but with large, broad leaves and large similar flowers (but they usually grow 5 or 6 feet off the ground). It has large, hollow stems that are spotted with what look like purple ink, and it smells super funky** - giving you some major clues that it is deadly poisonous. CONFIRM **Yarrow is a shorter plant with FEATHERY leaves,** flowers no more than 2-3 feet tall, with solid, small thin stems, and smells deliciously like Sage.

FOOD: The fresh leaves are a Sage-y addition to salads & stir-fries, great with turkey, but they are bitter so use sparingly. Flowers are a beautiful edible for desserts and special salads. Yarrow is a great livestock feed and a food source for insects and small animals, but it is considered toxic to horses, dogs and cats because of the strong essential oils.

CONTAINS: Beta-Carotene, B-Complex, Vitamin C & E, Choline, Inositol, Calcium,

Copper, Magnesium, Phosphorus, Potassium , Silicon, Essentials Oils (Azulene, Pro- Azulene, Borneol, Pinene, Linalool, Eugenol, Camphor, Cineole, Thujone, Achillein), Formic Acid, Salicylic Acid, Sterols, Flavonoids (Quercetin), Coumarins, Tannins

BODY BENEFITS: A cup a day keeps the doctor away, literally! One cup of Yarrow tea every day is an incredible way to heal the body, feed the organs, stabilize the blood sugar and balance the hormones. It brings alertness and action to your mind and also to the body's many systems, so it is a great wake-up substitute for coffee. Use it to alleviate allergy symptoms, keep you from catching everything that comes around, and to completely banish early cold and flu discomforts. Many people think this is too simple a remedy to be effective - just try it. Yarrow stops bleeding, reduces fever, is good for cold sores, and healing and repairing tissues all over the body. It is nourishing for the brain and nervous system and can be a preventative as well as treatment for Alzheimer's and Parkinson's. Yarrow kills microorganisms on contact and is considered a strong immune mobilizer to help the body fight off viruses and bacteria. It promotes circulation and helps ease muscle cramps, spasms and menstrual cramps. Its bitter digestive action is strong medicine for digestive issues like excess gas, ulcers, IBS, Crohn's and sluggish metabolism. Yarrow stimulates bile production, nourishes the liver, and helps move lymph through the lymphatic system. It balances the blood sugar and can keep it balanced through the night if taken as a tea before bed. It is a female tonic, balancing the cycles and nourishing the reproductive organs, and can help with many issues including PMS and extreme hormonal and mood swings. Yarrow can stop urinary tract infections in their tracks, and nourish the kidneys and soothe the bladder at the same time. It is one of Lalitha Thomas' 10 Essential Herbs because it offers so many positive attributes for the body. She likens its cleansing abilities to cleaning up oil spills, as the constituents trap. package and remove toxins from the blood in a way that is unique and remarkable. Drink several cups a day when fasting and detoxing for just this kind of support. *Avoid in pregnancy.

QUALITIES: Feminine, soothing but pushy, drying, purifying, and healing in so many ways. Yarrow is analgesic, antifungal, anti-inflammatory, antiseptic, antispasmodic, aromatic, astringent, bitter, carminative, cholagogue, circulatory stimulant, diaphoretic, digestive stimulant, diuretic, emmenagogue, expectorant, hemostatic, hypotensive, nervine, styptic, urinary tonic & antiseptic, uterine stimulant, vasodilator, and vulnerary.

FOLKLORE: Folk names Sanguinary, Soldier's Woundwort, Carpenter's Weed, Nosebleed, Old Man's Pepper, Staunch Weed, Life Medicine, Seven Year's Love, Knight's Milfoil, Millefolium, Millefoille, Gordaldo, Hundred-Leaved Grass, Military Herb, Thousand Seal, Military Herb, Plumajillo. There is evidence that the Neanderthals used Yarrow over 50,000 yeast ago. Yarrow was given its botanical name in 1753 by Linnaeus, after the great warrior Achilles. The legends say that Achilles was instructed by Chiron (the Centaur and Wounded Healer) to apply Yarrow to heal his

"Achilles Heel" wound during the Trojan War in 1200 BC, and to use the plant in battle to stop bleeding. The Druids used the sticks to foretell the weather. Navajo Indians say it is a *"Life Medicine"* and the Ojibwe smoke the flowers in shamanic rituals. The essential oil of Yarrow has been used to flavor soft drinks. The powder has been used as a tobacco additive and also in fancy snuff mixtures. A yellow and green dye can be made from the flowers. Birds line their nests with Yarrow to act as an antiparasitic to keep their homes pest free.

FIRST AID USES: Make a poultice of fresh leaves (chew some up in your mouth), place on bug bites and stings and pack into wounds. Make a tea and use it as an eyewash or cold compress for styes, irritated and allergy-swollen eyes. Styptic - keep the dried powder in your first aid kit to stop bleeding. Use poultice of the leaves and flowers for toothache, blood blisters, hemorrhoids, migraine and varicose veins. Yarrow will staunch the blood flow of wounds and act as antiseptic and antibacterial. Boil Yarrow on the stove with Ginger, Cinnamon, and Peppermint for a fever-reducing, flu-busting tea. Inhale the steam of Yarrow for asthma and hay fever. Drink Yarrow tea hot to increase body temperature to promote sweating, and cold to act more as a diuretic.

SPIRITUAL PROPERTIES: Ruled by Venus, the Water Element, and White Light. Yarrow is helpful for shifting times and ages, in other words, right now! It provides Divine reassurance and the protection of all the positive forces of Light so Humans and Gaia can ascend to higher states. It brings healing, courage, fortitude, strength, and protection. The Tea of Yarrow can be taken ritually to increase divination powers and psychic abilities.

MAGICAL USES: "A shining shield of light," used to banish evil, enhance love spells, bring Love, friends, and initiate contact from distant relations. Place a few stalks under your pillow and you will dream of your true love. Use it for courage, psychic powers, and in Love rituals. Forty dried, bare stalks are used to throw the I Ching, an ancient-Daoist divination system. Useful in love sachets, hung over the bed, in wedding decorations and wedding ceremonies for keeping the happy couple together for at least seven years. Yarrow is also a strong banishing herb for exorcizing evil or negative energies from places, things and people. Place Yarrow over the doorways to keep negative entities from entering the home. Holding the herb to your eyes is reputed to confer Second Sight.

FLOWER ESSENCE: Yarrow is a white flower that **strengthens your radiance** and aura, bringing benevolent healing forces. It can be helpful for sensitives and autistic spectrum people. Yarrow helps birth the light of the Spirit into physicality. It knits the energetic field together, and stops energy leaking. It protects you from environmental toxins and negative influences like a Divine shield. Use this Flower Essence if you work on computers, near electromagnetic fields, or under fluorescent lights.

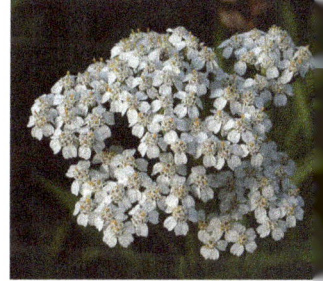

PREPARATIONS: Eat fresh Yarrow leaves on hikes for a pick-me-up, and add to salads for a very aromatic green. Flowers are beautiful and tasty in salads and for edible decorations, especially on wedding cakes. When making tea, use a covered pot or place a lid on your cup to contain the volatile and potent essential oils. You can cook the younger leaves and flowers or saute in stir fries. Swedish Beer uses Yarrow as an ingredient, and it is a perfect and traditional herb for Bitters and Liqueurs. Dry the leaves and powder for instant tea, and to use directly on wounds to stop bleeding. Make an extract of Yarrow with brandy or glycerine to rub on baby's gums for a remarkable teething remedy. The essential oil of Yarrow is blue, and used as an antiinflammatory in natural body care much like other Azulene-containing oils like Blue Chamomile and Blue Cypress. Use the stems and leaves in a wonderful ritual bath for resolving any inflammation, detoxing and enhancing Yarrow's magical properties.

LAURA: Yarrow was another of my first Wild Weed allies. Once you start to see it, it is everywhere! Yarrow is very refreshing to snack on while hiking, and always steers the conversation to plant identification and survival. I have used Yarrow successfully for bug bites, especially after scratching too much, and found real itch-relief and the bleeding stopped. I am always so grateful each time I see it, because I know how many wonderful things this plant can do - and it is always RIGHT THERE.

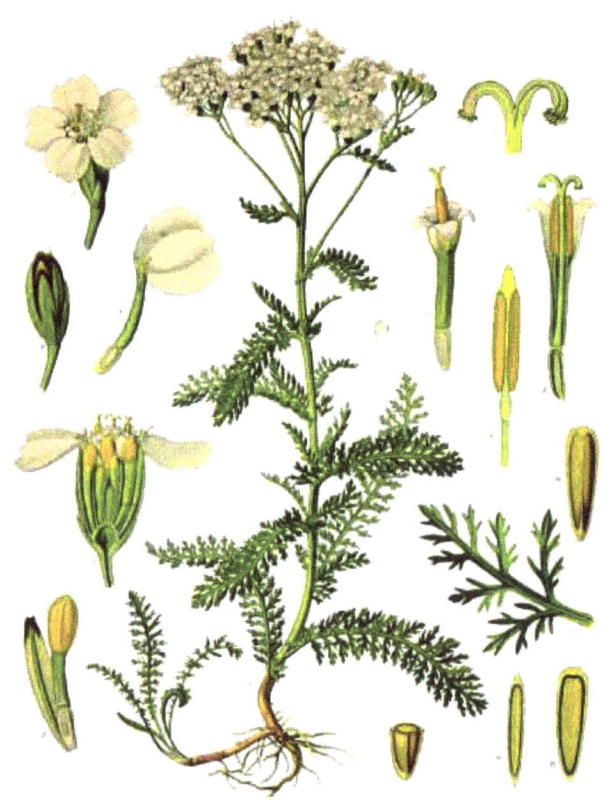

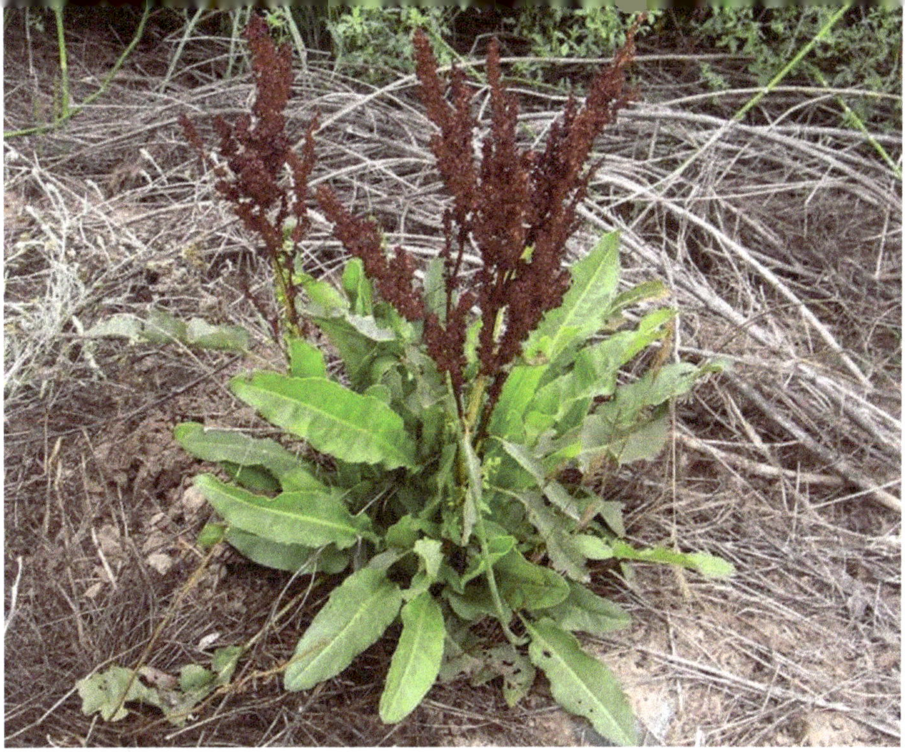

YELLOW DOCK

Rumex crispus   Dock Family / **POLYGONACEAE**

FOUND: Like so many of the Wild Weeds, Yellow Dock is native to Europe and Western Asia, but has spread itself into Ireland, into North America in all 50 states and Canada. It grows in full Sun and part shade on roadsides, trails and in open fields.

IDENTIFYING FEATURES: A basal rosette of narrow, hairless, long leaves, curly and ruffled on the edges, alternating and decreasing up the stem until it is bare to the flower. Flower grows in whorls is a long, green and reddish compound seed panicle that turns a deep rust red in the Fall, when it is time to harvest the root. Whole plant can reach 1-5 feet tall. Yellow Dock Root looks like a little yellow man. It runs deep into the ground, and retains its golden, yellow hue when dried.

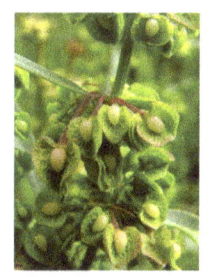

FOOD: Leaves can be foraged year-round and are easy to spot in cold seasons by the giant rusty seed cluster above that stands out in the field. Seeds can be dried and used the way you would whole grains. Yellow Dock is a relative of Buckwheat and has similar food characteristics. The root is used medicinally and must be dug by making a deep hole next to the plant to access the deep taproot.

CONTAINS: Vitamin A & C, Calcium, Iron, Magnesium, Potassium, Sulfur, Anthraquinones, Glycosides, Flavonoids (Quercetin), Mucilage, Tannins, Resins, Oxalates.

BODY BENEFITS: Yellow Dock is a cleansing, rebuilding tonic for the blood and body, full of Iron and other helpful minerals to remedy anemia. It inhibits the growth of E. coli and staph infections. The bitter root of Yellow Dock supports Liver functions and helps clear the blood of toxins. With cleaner blood comes clearer skin and this plant is also helpful for acne and eczema. It improves appetite, remedies constipation, encourages healthy peristalsis, invigorates the colon and supports better digestion of fats. It also soothes and cools inflamed intestines due to food allergies and an acidic diet. It is eminently useful for urinary tract infections, stones and bloating. The syrup or Honey (see below) can be used for energy, anemia, bronchitis, asthma and to soothe a scratchy throat. It boosts lymphatic clearing and is wonderful for resolving swollen glands and issues of the lymph nodes. Yellow Dock moves bile, and can help with gallbladder congestion. It soothes rheumatism and arthritis and other inflammatory conditions. The golden color principle Antioxidants make this root a cell-protector and anti-tumor cancer fighter. *Not for use in pregnancy.*

Because this plant is high in oxalate, it impairs calcium absorption and is best avoided by those prone to kidney stones, arthritis and gout.

QUALITIES: Masculine, bitter, cooling, drying, and yang, with a downward motion. Yellow Dock is alterative, anti-inflammatory, anti ascorbic, antioxidant, antiseptic, astringent, blood tonic, cholagogue, diuretic, laxative, and tonic.

FOLKLORE: Folk names Dock, Curly Dock, Field Sorrel, Garden Patience, Narrow Dock, Sour Dock, Sheep Sorrel, Acedera, Churelle, Amlavetasa, Erba Britannica. The roots when boiled will produce a dark brown or grey dye. The Navajos used the whole plant as an emetic to prepare for visions and ceremonies. The Zunis used a poultice of the fresh root for healing sores, rashes, and foot fungus and to disinfect wounds.

FIRST AID USES: Make a poultice of the bruised leaves for soothing Nettle rash, varicose veins and any infected wounds. This poultice is also helpful for horses, mules and donkeys for treating saddle sores. The tea taken internally and poured into the bath will help with inflammatory skin conditions such as eczema, psoriasis, sunburn, and bug bites and stings.

SPIRITUAL PROPERTIES: Ruled by expansive Jupiter, but some associate Yellow Dock with Saturn and Mars as well - and the abundant Air Element. Many call Yellow Dock the "Herb of Understanding" and it was used by Native Americans before entering the sweat lodge to bring wisdom and visions. Yellow Dock cleanses the aura and makes way for higher vibrations to be attained so helpful energies can reach you.

MAGICAL USES: The seeds are useful for money charms, as incense, and in medicine pouches. Sprinkle Yellow Dock seeds around the property and place of business, to attract customers. Use a strong tea to rinse the door knobs, wash the floor and wipe down the cash register regularly to increase sales. Tie the seeds in a cloth to the left arm to encourage conception. Make the seeds into an eye pillow for revelatory dreams. To find the perfect mate, drink the tea while daydreaming about attracting harmonious, mutually beneficial Love.

FLOWER ESSENCE: Yellow Dock flower essence helps you to **stand tall** and assert your true self, strengthening your will and confidence. It helps you cut ties and binds that no longer serve you, cleansing the mind and the Spirit as well as the body. It assists with the release and purging of old emotional waste, and helps you resolve issues. It clears space and opens the floodgates for what comes next and erases the boundaries between inner and outer space. Yellow Dock Flower Essence offers support for working in groups toward a common goal, and for doing anything new.

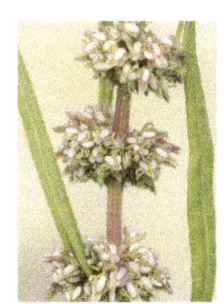

PREPARATIONS: Harvest young leaves before the stack shoots up. They are lemony and sour-tasting and can be eaten fresh, used to flavor food or made into tea. Leaves and peeled stems are delicious and nutritious, eaten like a vegetable in Spring (and Late Fall after a hard frost) and chopped and pickled. You can use the tangy leaves like Rhubarb in pies. Root can be roasted and used as a coffee substitute with Dandelion or Chicory. Grind the seeds (after you crush a bit and winnow away most of the chaff) for a gluten-free flour, to add to sauces to thicken them, to add fiber and for use for baking into breads, veggie burgers and pancakes. Large amounts of the leaves should be boiled to remove excess oxalic acid. Yellow Dock Root is the perfect strong herb for making into nourishing Extracts and Bitters. To make a tea, because it is a tough root, you must make a boiled decoction of the plant instead of a simple infusion. Use ½ cup fresh root (or 3 tablespoons dried root) in 3 cups water, bring to a boil on the stove and simmer for about 30 minutes. Strain out what you need and leave the herbs in the water until well cooled. Store unused portion in the fridge. Add Yellow Dock extract to Molasses to make an iron-rich syrup, or ferment fresh root in Honey for a sweet, blood-building tonic. This is a perfect herb to use with Nettles for every ailment.

LAURA: I am nurturing a solitary Yellow Dock plant that comes up every year right next to my garden. It was a weedly volunteer who showed up one year out of the blue, so now I water it and care for it like the other plants. I understand Yellow Dock can help fix nutrients into the soil for its friends the other plants, so I know it is enhancing all the plants my garden. One day, before we move, I do plan to harvest the root and make a lovely tincture from it, and take a cutting or seeds with us to our next place. For now, I honor this regal Weed every year I see it return to its honored garden spot.

*****

The next chapter offers helpful suggestions for how to use our new Weed friends, how to derive the most nutrition from our Natural Foods, and how to optimize our health with all of the wonderful bounty this Garden provides.

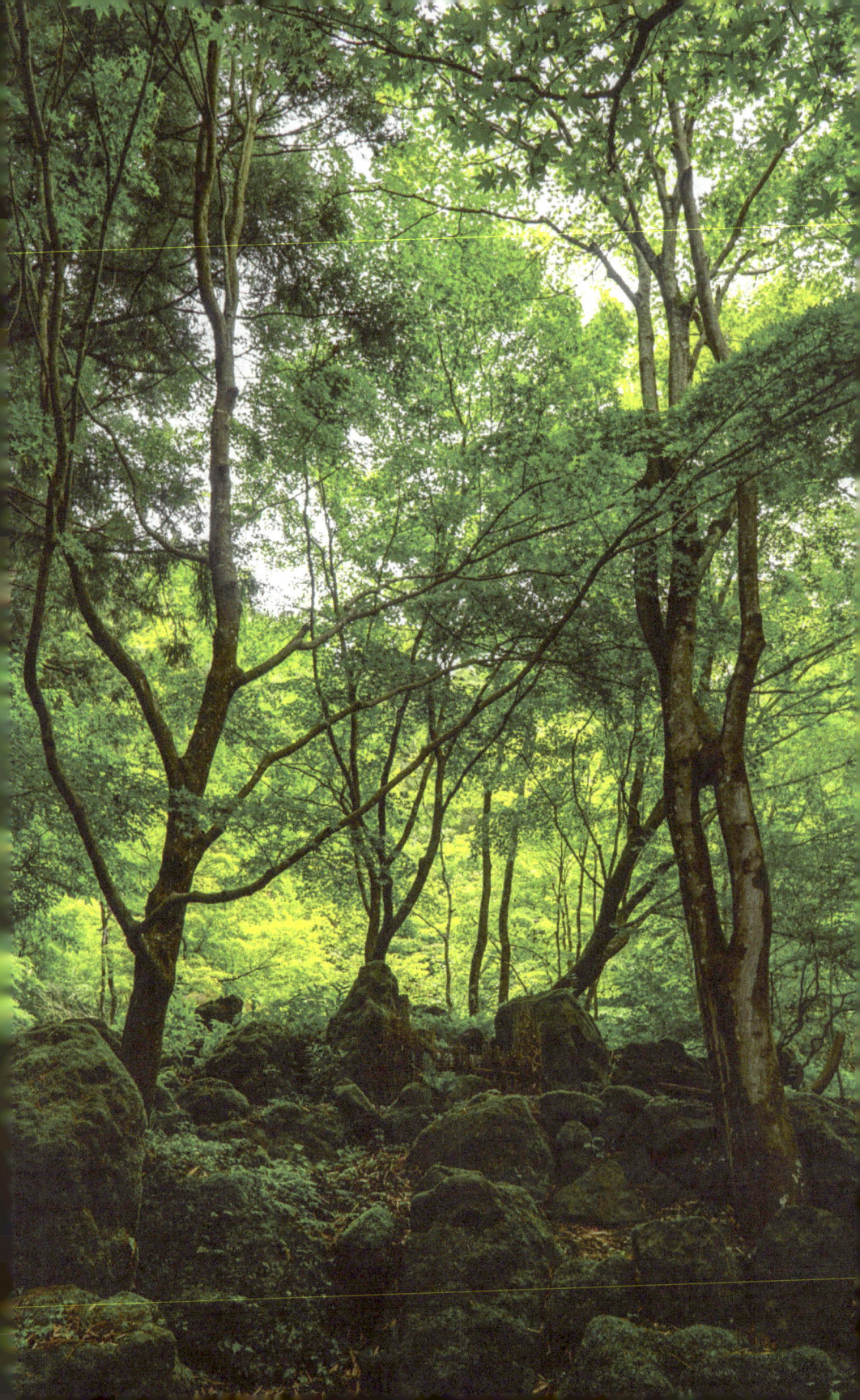

~ the garden of earth ~

~ Chapter 3 ~

GIFTS OF THE GARDEN

"Keeping your body Healthy is an expression of Gratitude to the whole Cosmos - the Trees, the Clouds, Everything."

~Thich Nhat Hanh

MAKE YOUR CONTRIBUTION

What a concept - that you might be "giving back" to Everything by taking care of Yourself!? What if your gift to the World *is* your Radiant Health? Like so many Buddhist teachings, this kind of a mind-blowing concept is worth meditation and contemplation. It seems too easy (and maybe even self-indulgent?) to concentrate on your own needs to such a degree. Do you have time? Will it help anything? Are you "worth it?" The whole Cosmos is chiming in, "Yes, Yes, Yes!" Deep inside, you know this is true: Self-Care is necessary to insure your Health, and nobody benefits if you lose your Health. It's the old warning, "Put your oxygen mask on first, and then assist others." Your body needs all the healthiest foods and best-ever body care, plus healing time, nourishing time, quiet time, play time, living and dancing and just being you time - specifically so you can be at your best for everyone else.

My dear friend and director Paula Kalustian is the one who taught me to **"Pre-Tend."** She had an intuitive feeling one day that she needed to remind me to take care of myself (*pre-tend*) before I sought to go out and heal the World! Right on track with directing yet again, Paula was prescient in reminding me to concentrate FIRST on my own tending and healing within. It's much the same with Acting, too - you must first deeply feel your character and inhabit it completely. Acting is resonating and broadcasting the character's different vibration in order for others to feel it with you. Becoming the character first - you pretend. When YOU are in need of life support - Pre-Tend. Once the Pre-Tend Concept was named for me by Paula, I couldn't forget it. I am now able to remind myself to take care of me first, with that one simple word signal. Remind yourself regularly.

Now, we all know this is an ongoing practice. Our whole lives-long our Mothers harped on us "Take care of yourself!" We know we should. But to stop at all for a few minutes for ourselves can be hard, while life makes ridiculous demands on us, our children need our guidance, our relationships need tending and our worldly responsibilities increase. I completely agree, it takes WORK to heroically do all you do out in the World, and to ALSO take care of yourself.

BUT, if caring for yourself comes in LAST place, that is the first sign of burnout. Take action before you (and others) start to see the dangerous consequences of letting your Self-Care slide. When you are working as a vital cog in a system, you naturally need to be in top form to make your grandest contribution. Let's all just make a pact that our top form needs a sturdy foundation. That starts with You taking care of You!!

Widening your concept of Self-Care, and why you do it, could be the key to your own inspired improvements. You may be the kind of person who is more motivated if you realize that **your personal acts can help others**. It may be easier to accomplish regularly, if you recognize that all of your choices for personal health will positively affect those around you - and indeed, the whole World!

You are here by Design, your Energy matters, and your own Personal Vitality has a direct effect on EVERYTHING.

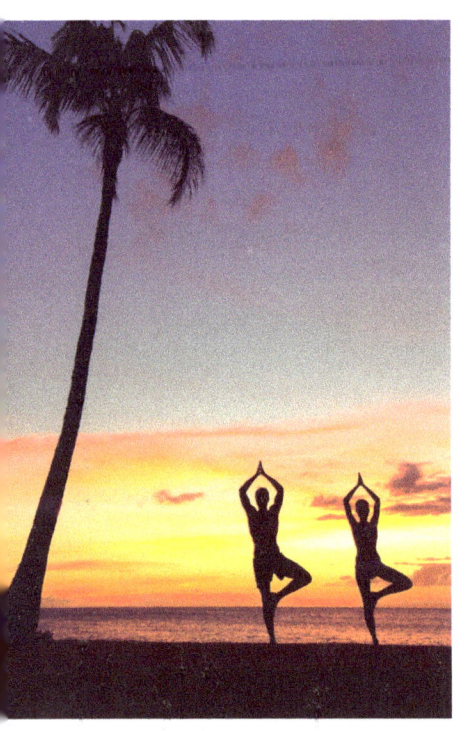

Shifting your mindset to include the fact that **Your Health is benefitting the whole Planet**, makes it so much easier to accomplish. And it begins to feel a bit more noble and joyfully inclusive to take personal time when you need it. Your body is an amazing, wonderful temple that responds quickly when you give it the attention it needs. It doesn't take a long time to make personal improvements that have exponential repercussions in the World.

This harmonizes perfectly with the holistic concept with which this book is inspired: **we are, each of us, truly a vital part of the natural scheme of things, chips off the same crystal, flowers of the Garden of Earth.** Living in such an interdependent natural system means we all have to do our part for the whole. Personal Health is a Sacred, Universal Responsibility. We need to be shining our brightest at all times! We all want to be an energy resource for our families and friends and co-workers and students and our Planet. To assure this, let's focus on utilizing the Gifts we have been given to heal ourselves - so we can be a gift to the Garden and everyone else! Each one of us, receiving, healing and contributing. As Joey says, "Having and giving, and sharing and receiving...." (so many *Friends* jokes).

"Giving back" implies we have already been given a Gift. Indeed - **SO MANY GIFTS**. The entire, beautiful Planet Earth is full of them and we are here now, free to explore and utilize them. What follows in this chapter are some of the radical remedies, natural food sources and mind-blowing resources with which Gaia has gifted us! Hopefully you'll find some ideas here for working on your personal health and vitality. And for preserving and enhancing your Family's health in both lean times and abundant times.

SHINY HAPPY PEOPLE

I think of some of my most radiant teachers - **Brigitte Mars, David Avocado Wolfe, Steve Adler, Juilano, Elaina Love, Happy Oasis** - these Sparkling Beings all had their own lifetimes of challenges. They learned from intense hardships, and each had to create health with Nature and within their own bodies first, before they could share it with the rest of the World. And if you know any of them, their vibrant, light-filled presence alone speaks volumes about what they learned to create from within! Vitality, wildness and magic shines out through their laughing eyes - belying the deeper stories of their **overcoming**. I always wanted to be a better, healthier, kinder person because of these walking angel examples. I could sense they had found a treasure trove of secrets with which to treat their bodies better. And it turns out that many of those secrets are about **CARING FOR YOURSELF NATURALLY** with **EXCEPTIONAL LIVING FOODS**. Their gift was showing this to me, living it in plain sight, so I knew it was possible.

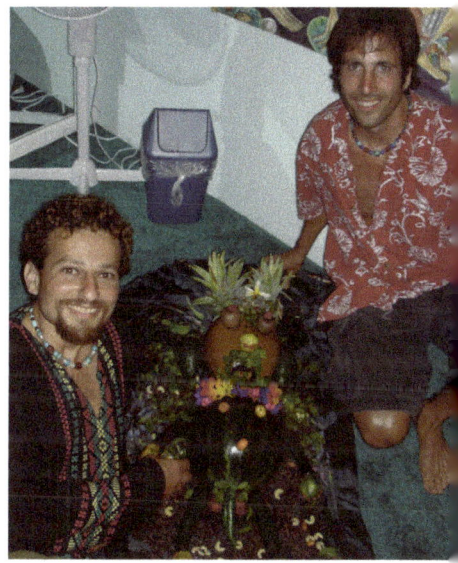

FOOD IS MEDICINE

The Plants we eat are also doing their very best in this natural system to be of help and of service. Plants know what we think and can respond, and will dynamically grow to please us and nourish us! They participate in the making of nutrients, medicines and chemical reactions which lead to the changing of our Biology. Our Food is our Best Health Partner, and we should enjoy the joy of growing it and derive comfort from the eating of it, as well. When you interact with the Plants you will later eat, they come to know you and grow specifically to heal you and will be truly helpful for your energy on all levels. The energy you give the Plants will return to you a thousandfold.

Since many modern medicines are based on such plentiful, helpful chemicals in Nature, how did we ever evolve away from using the actual Plants for medicine? That is just a long (and not admirable) story of economics and greed. Money-hungry people found a way to engineer artificial substitutes that cost less and could be produced anywhere, at any time of the year. A plant can't be patented, but a product can. They began to turn their backs on Nature because they believed in their power to improve upon it. They genetically altered our plants and filled even natural medicines with preservatives, and then put our plant remedies into toxic plastic bottles. Well, many of us make a growing, remembering force who simply won't stand for that kind of abuse anymore! We want our Nature back! We are crusading for the preservation and naturalization of our Natural Remedies! We will grow our own.

We may not always be able to get the most basic essential oils - what a privilege we enjoy now to be able to have vials of these oils made for us from all over the World. This is why I wrote so much about Living Remedies in Volume 1. It is important for us to find and cultivate **Living Sources** for our Aromatherapy and Herbal needs. The same goes for our Food, Vitamins, and Medicines.

We may not always be able to buy big plastic bottles of vitamins or herbs (and maybe that's a good thing). At one point in Spring of 2020, I could not get ANY Vitamin C or Zinc or D to sell in the store in which I worked, not a single bottle. If you didn't have a stash of medicinals, you couldn't get them anymore. My friends living in foreign countries couldn't get any more supplements when they ran out, and there was no more to be sent to them. So they HAD to resort to using Foods to attain their nutrition, and treat their ailments, just like the old days.

We may not always have such luxurious access to electricity for ordering online, and sometimes the trucks might not be able to deliver! Farmers may not be able to grow crops profitably or they may not be able to grow certain foods in their fields at all anymore in locations with climate changes. In the same way, we may not always have access to the food we like, or more importantly, the food we NEED! As I said in Chapter 2, we cannot be solely dependent on the farming, delivery, import, trucking, or transportation systems. **We may not ALWAYS be able to rely on someone else to feed us, isolate vitamins for us, or make our medicines!**

Experiencing such a real shortage of supplements convinced me it is high time we RE-EDUCATE ourselves to **derive better nutrition from the Food we eat.** We ought to know what our food DOES and what is IN IT. We need to know *where* we can get Vitamin C to prevent colds or what foods are high in Zinc to boost our immunity. We need to know which spices are helpful and used in all major cultures, and why it is important to combine foods correctly when you eat.

THE BODY TEACHES YOU

Did you realize that many times you are drawn to foods because of their healing purpose, something your body needs right now, a nutrient you are lacking? Do you honor your internal feelings about food? Do you follow your body's Innate wisdom whispering to you? Your body does make suggestions based on the nourishment to be obtained from a certain food. Like craving **Chocolate** at "that time of the month" - without realizing it is providing the muscle-cramp-relaxing **Magnesium** you need. The body will send you messages about what it requires. Once I hear something internally twice, I realize my attention is being sought and I better notice!

If you are craving Blueberries, eat them as often as your body craves them. Trust the signals your body gives you about food! Kids do. They do say that when children have food obsessions for one food (mono-dieting) it is often a direct message from their body to nourish themselves more fully based on the foods they know. The food they craved was later found to be improving their health in a specific way, providing additional nutrients they needed in abundance for proper growth. Kids are too smart to resist their Innate Knowing, LISTEN to them! They have a direct, open connection and can surprise you and teach you when they say what they need.

One of the many things that were revealed by the latest health scare is the amount of "comorbidity" illness and obesity that afflict our population. Our society as a whole doesn't work at true independent health. Our advertising media constantly convinces us to take a pill to mask the symptoms we feel. We have discovered how surprisingly few people know how to **EAT for HEALTH**, or how to enhance their own super-strong Immune Systems. The same media has been mysteriously absent when it comes to natural remedies and nutritional support. We have to change this!!! Why aren't there enormous gatherings at the Fairgrounds with smiling healthy people dispensing Vitamin C, D and Zinc and proper Immunity Nutrition and Education, instead of vaccines?! **Why don't we have clinics DISPENSING HEALTHY LIVING FOOD WITH ZERO SIDE EFFECTS?!**

There are so many amazing ways to support the body's ability to adapt and heal itself, and our most foundational opportunity to do that is with the Foods we choose to include in our diet and eat everyday. I like to stand in front of my refrigerator and see which way and to which foods I am drawn first. It is usually toward an Apple. When researching Apples, I was absolutely blown away at the many issues I have suffered with that they help heal. Watching how our bodies teach US what we need through food is astounding, we all need to pay attention in class! Find and listen to the Foods that call to you to nourish your body deeply. The Best Foods Ever will help you make NATURAL health choices a top priority.

> **"If you keep adding in the Good Stuff (fresh fruits & vegetables) soon there won't be any more room for the Bad Stuff."**
> *~ David Avocado Wolfe*

He also says, **"Nothing tastes as good as Good Health feels."**

~ the garden of earth ~

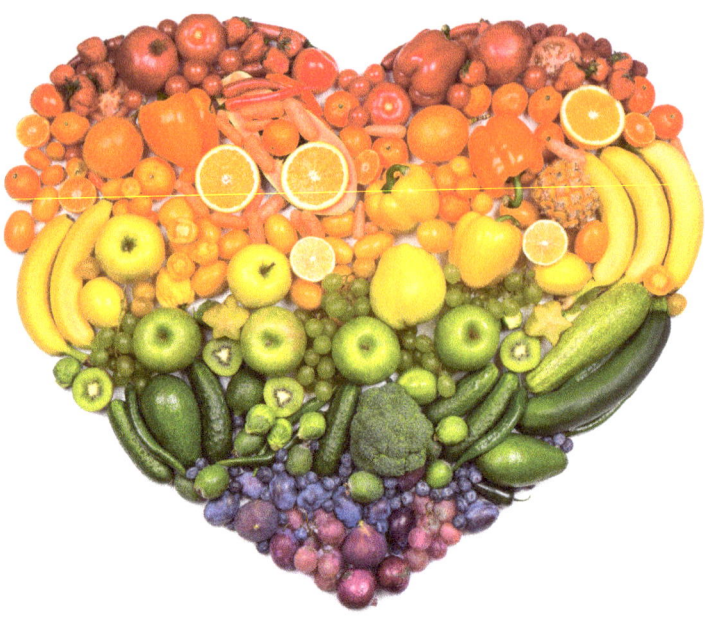

FOOD SOURCES FOR MAJOR NUTRIENTS
living vitamins and minerals

"I believe we would be better off, both financially and nutritionally, if we still procured as many of our Vitamins and Minerals as possible from wild green plants, rather than depending on synthetic products dispensed by a druggist."

~ *Euell Gibbons*

This is a guide to help you discover **real absorbable nutrition** from *Foods,* for optimal health & true longevity. Use your own innate wisdom about how and when to eat them, or use these lists to help you follow the suggestions of your nutritionist or medical professional. I have purposely not listed any "recommended dietary intake" amounts for these nutrients for supplementation. This information is widely available on the internet and on supplement bottles. Here instead, I offer many ways you can receive your nutrients directly from natural living sources.

This list is by no means exhaustive, nor represents all foods with these nutrients - just the ones we have the most access to in the modern day. Consult this list when you are under the weather so you can add certain nutrients you know you may need for what they provide. Notice the foods that are repeated over and over again in many different nutrient profiles, these are our true **Multitasking Superfoods!** These are the heroic foods you want to add to the diet regularly. For example, start eating a small handful of **Sunflower Seeds or Sprouts** every day (you can add to salads, smoothies, oatmeal or stir-fries) and you'll receive nearly the same nutritional value as if you took a multivitamin! Use your **FOOD** as your **Nutrient Source** and your **Medicine.**

Vitamin A:
A group of **fat-soluble** vitamins, which means they are not excreted in the urine like vitamin C but stored in the liver for when they are needed. This also means they need other fats, zinc and enzymes to be properly absorbed. Vitamin A is antioxidant (cell protective) so it lowers the risk of many types of cancer, particularly helpful for lung cancer and reversing precancerous growth. It is an eye nutrient that ensures proper vision, counteracts night blindness and eye weakness, regulates growth, reproduction, stem cell differentiation and immunity. As a baby develops in the womb, Vitamin A is like a Director, telling the cells how to specialize and form the strongest organs, and may increase chances of becoming pregnant. Vitamin A lessens the effect and mortality of the measles in children. It helps the bones, hair, skin and nails to grow strong. People with Crohn's or Celiac disease who have poor lipid absorption may be less able to store and utilize Vitamin A, and need to consume more of it. This amazing Vitamin can also stop the spread of skin diseases, relieve itchy skin, and shows great promise in skin-care for preserving youthful wrinkle-free skin and treating acne. It is essential in the body's hormone production. Vitamin A is responsible for the health of epithelial tissue all over the body, including the glands, lining of the stomach and other hollow organs, and all along the respiratory, gastrointestinal and urinary tracts. Vitamin A strengthens the body against infections, sore throats, frequent cold & flu and most importantly, all respiratory illnesses including allergies and sensitivity to environmental pollution. While there are many forms of active Vitamin A present in animal liver tissue and dairy, there are plenty of vital vegan sources for its precursor Beta-Carotene as well.

Vitamin A Food Sources: ORANGE & YELLOW FOODS
Carrots, Oranges, Cantaloupe, Papaya, Sweet Potatoes, Pumpkin, Mango, Peaches Apricots, Avocado, Goji Berries, Passion Fruit, Guava, Acorn & Butternut Squash, Pink Grapefruit, Paprika, Pistachios, Olives, Spinach, Purslane, Watermelon, Broccoli, Kale, Celery, Nettles, Peas, Collard Greens, Black-eyed Peas, Red Bell Pepper, Tomatoes, Lettuce, Turnip Greens, Peanut Butter, Seaweed Greens, Yams, Tofu, Ghee, Beef Liver, Eggs, Dairy, Halibut, Salmon, Tuna, Cod Liver Oil, Organ Meats, Roe, Shrimp, Clams

<u>**To increase absorption:**</u> Combine with healthy fats (hemp, coconut, flax, avocado). Don't consume or combine with fiber (so consuming fresh juices are better). Fermenting increases bioavailability of carotenoids.

Plants contain the *Beta-Carotene* form of Vitamin A, and Animal sources contain the *Retinol* form. You may have seen people who juice a lot of carrots for their health (or to fight cancer) begin to have orange hands, or an orange tint to their skin. This is called carotenemia, and is a harmless condition caused by carotenoid pigments. If you see this, it is an indicator that the body has enough Vitamin A from the beta-carotene in plants, and does not need to convert it anymore so it is storing it in the skin. This indicates it a good time to cut back for a while.

Vitamins B:

The B vitamins are an enormous group of **water-soluble** nutrients, which means they are not stored, but need to be replenished daily with foods. They are also fairly delicate and are mostly destroyed by cooking. All the B's work on the metabolism, converting food to energy. They also combat stress, relieve anxiety, provide mental and physical energy, work on muscle health, support brain function and focus, and stimulate nerve health. Some of them are used individually for their special effects, like the ability of Biotin to thicken and support hair and nail growth, or Folate to support brain health, fetal development in pregnancy (preventing birth defects), and red blood cell production.

Many "fortified" breads, cereals and milk contain B vitamins because most people simply don't get enough in a regular diet. **Brewer's Yeast or Nutritional Yeast** contain nearly all the B vitamins except for B12, and can be very supportive and effective for Vegans and Vegetarians and others who don't eat red meat. You can see other repeating foods that contain multiple B's and the diet should be rich in them. Herbs with high yellow pigment content are usually full of B vitamins.

Vitamins B Food Sources: YELLOW FOODS and many more

B1 (Thiamine) - *"The Morale Vitamin"* - **Pine Nuts, Coriander, Acorn Squash, Artichokes, Broccoli, Brussel Sprouts, Sunflower Seeds, Sesame Seeds, Lentils, Macadamia Nuts, Soybeans, Beans Watermelon, Whole Grains, Rice Bran, Goji Berries, Wheat Germ, Tahini, Spirulina, Plums, Prunes, Brown Rice, Pecans, Peas, Beans & Nuts, Asparagus, Brewer's Yeast, Hibiscus, Organ Meats, Fish, Pork, Eggs**

B2 (Riboflavin) - **Almonds, Brewer's Yeast, Sesame Seeds, Avocados, Asparagus, Broccoli, Buckwheat, Whole Grains, Mushrooms, Goji Berries, Quinoa, Soybeans, Spinach, Purslane, Beet Greens, Leafy Greens, Lucuma, Buckwheat, Prunes, Organ Meats, Dairy, Yogurt, Meat, Poultry & Fish, Caviar, Eggs**

B3 (Niacin) - **Peanut Butter, Almonds, Avocados, Bananas, Brewer's Yeast, Tahini, Spirulina, Rice Bran, Mushrooms, Durian, Millet, Chia, Potatoes, Goji Berries, Purslane, Legumes, Buckwheat, Tomatoes, Carrots, Peas, Buckwheat, Lucuma, Whole Grains, Chiles and Chili Powder, Sesame Seeds, Sunflower Seeds, Barley, Cheese, Poultry, Fish, Beef, Eggs**

B5 (Pantothenic Acid) - Brewer's Yeast, Sunflower Seeds, Broccoli, Brown Rice, Avocados, Paprika, Whole Grains, Beans, Lentils, Mushrooms, Buckwheat, Rice Bran, Royal Jelly, Shiitake Mushroom, Sweet Potatoes, Tomatoes, Yams, Soy, Egg Yolks, Organ Meats

B6 (Pyridoxine) - Bananas, Brewer's Yeast, Buckwheat, Pineapple, Soy, Oats, Almonds, Chickpeas, Brussel Sprouts, Hemp seeds, Chia Seeds, Sunflower Seeds, Rice Bran, Avocados, Legumes, Nuts, Brown Rice, Wheat Bran, Sweet Potatoes, Spirulina, Watermelon, Peanut Butter, Purslane, Figs, Pistachios, Potatoes, Yeast, Garlic, Sage, Prunes, Wheat Germ, Tofu & Soy, Spinach, Walnuts, Plantains, Heart of Palm, Garlic, Peppers, Kale & Collard Greens, Water Chestnuts, Broccoli, Squashes and Pumpkin, Green Beans, Turkey, Chicken, Fish, Beef, Liver, Organ Meats, Eggs

B7 (Biotin) - Almonds, Peanuts, Oats, Onions, Chocolate, Beans, Chia Seeds, Tomatoes, Carrots, Brewer's Yeast,,Walnuts, Egg Yolks

B9 (Folate) - Spinach, Kale, Asparagus, Broccoli, Brewer's Yeast, Mung Bean Sprouts, Lettuce, Artichokes, Soy, Yeast, Walnuts, Lentils & Lentil Sprouts, Wheat Germ, Chickpeas, Tomatoes, Broccoli, Beans, Mangoes, Oranges, Purslane, Beets & Beet Greens, Basil, Flax, Sesame, Cauliflower, Leeks, Turnip Greens, Chestnuts, Okra, Peas, Celery, Hazelnuts, Avocados, Whole Grains, Peanuts, Cantaloupe, Tahini, Sunflower Seeds, Mint, Celery, Dark-Green Vegetables, Liver

B12 (Cobalamin) - *"The Energy Vitamin"* - Seaweed Greens, Soy, Spirulina, Honey, Nutritional Yeast, Probiotics & Elevated Biotics, Beef, Poultry, Salmon, Liver, Lamb, Shellfish especially Clams, Shrimp, Crab, Oysters, Trout, Sardines, Mackerel, Herring, Organ Meats, Egg Yolk, Cheese, Fermented Foods like Tofu, Kombucha & Yogurt

B17 (Amygdalin)* - *"The Cancer Remedy Vitamin"* - Bitter Almonds, Apricot Seed Kernels, Millet, Buckwheat, Barley, Flax Seeds, Cashews, Macadamia Nuts, Raspberry, Strawberry, Currants, Elderberries, Bamboo Shoots, Alfalfa Sprouts, Cassava, Spinach Watercress, Black Beans, Sweet Potatoes, Lima Beans, Lentils

*Note that B17 is not a "nationally recognized" B Vitamin. But it is a part of this family of nutrients and is vital as a pain-reliever, antioxidant, for regulating hypertension. B17 (laetrile) is a popular alternative cancer treatment, sought out by smart health enthusiasts and worth noting for overall immune enhancement. Eating these foods are highly recommended for anyone working with this ailment. Watch the movie *"A World Without Cancer,"* written and directed by G. Edward Griffin.

To increase absorption: *B12 absorption can be interfered with by pharmaceutical drugs (like Metformin for diabetes, and antibiotics, ulcer medications and acid reflux medicines). If you HAVE to take these, make sure you do so with lots of spinach and*

other dark leafy greens and the high Folate (B9) foods which increase B12 absorption rates. Biotin (B7) can also be lost due to low-fat diets and over-reliance on egg whites alone, so increase egg yolks or other Biotin-rich foods if you are looking for healthier skin, hair and nails. Alcohol reduces Thiamine (B1) absorption, so eat more of these foods if you drink.

When wheat is processed into white flour, 68% of the Folate is removed. Likewise when rice is polished into white hulless grains, nearly 90% of the B vitamins are tossed out as trash. You will see "rice bran" often in these lists, because it is where most of the nutrients in rice exist. When they first began polishing rice to make it nice and white, they fed the bran they removed to the animals who grew thick beautiful coats and all were very healthy, while the people eating the polished rice were all pale, sickly, and lacking energy and strength.

Niacin (B3) and the mineral Chromium were found by Wayne State University to reduce cholesterol by 30%. B12 keeps homocysteine levels down which cause inflammation. The body can make its own B12 with the help of "Elevated Biotics" (see pg. 264 *Probiotics*) that are found in the biofilm of organic produce. This type of self-made B12 is particularly important to brain health as it nourishes our neurotransmitters which boost the mood and keep depression away. It also contributes to healing digestive issues and "autoimmune" disorders.

Vitamin C: *"The Protector Vitamin"* - A **water soluble**, strong antioxidant cell protector that increases longevity, and is our finest immune-stimulating vitamin. Vitamin C is best known for preventing colds and flus, scurvy (and death) and destroying viruses! This versatile, truly essential vitamin also protects cellular integrity, defends the heart from disease, helps the body repair damaged tissues, prevents hair loss, creates gum health, feeds and maintains connective tissue by supporting collagen production, helps bones heal and prevents osteoporosis, modulates the inflammatory response and damage, increases iron absorption in the body, reduces the 'bad" (LDL) cholesterol and triglycerides, protects the body from free radicals and cancer and can mitigate the side effects of chemotherapy, prevents oxidative stress, and also helps neutralize the damaging effect of nitrites and other preservatives. It can reduce the risk of developing diabetes and insulin resistance. It lowers the cortisol stress response and inflammation, can reduce wrinkles in the skin and other signs of aging, and may help correct arrhythmia and prevent strokes. Vitamin C controls alcohol cravings, and reduces withdrawal symptoms from alcohol and drug use. It supports Iron deficiencies and is helpful (with Bromelain) for easy bruising. Vitamin C may prevent or treat Alzheimer's disease and improve cognitive functioning. It can support the healing of and slow cataracts, treat and prevent gout, reduce the severity and duration of colds, viruses and sepsis, and contributes to the health of EVERY body system. It protects the body from radiation poisoning, heavy metal toxicity, and environmental pollution.

Vitamin C Food Sources: ALL COLORS, PRIMARILY SOUR & SPICY FOODS

Citrus Fruits - Oranges, Lemons, Limes, Grapefruit, Green Chiles, Green Tea, Kiwi, Red, Orange & Green Bell Peppers, Jalapenos, Yellow Banana Peppers, Amla (Indian Gooseberry), Acerola Cherry, Acai, Apricots, Avocados, Broccoli, Kale, Violet Leaves & Flowers, Rosehips, Tart Montmorency Cherries, Sea Buckthorn, Pineapple, Tomatoes, Potatoes, Brussel Sprouts, Zucchini, Cantaloupe, Chard, Kohlrabi, Cabbage, Lucuma, Baobab, Cauliflower, Papaya, Mango, Hibiscus, Peaches, Black Currants, Strawberries, Goji Berries, Greens, Spinach, Mung Bean Sprouts, Jujube Dates, Dried Coriander, Lychee, Persimmons, Guava, Black Currants, Yellow & Dill, Apples, Berries, Melons, Asparagus, Orange Peel, Red Raspberry Leaves, Dark Greens, Peas, Saffron, Bay Leaf, Chives, Basil, Thyme, Parsley, Bergamot, Cilantro, Rosehips, CamuCamu, Persimmon, Cranberries, Tamarind

To increase absorption: Consume in raw food form, or cook minimally with very low heat, in low amounts of water for best absorption. Vitamin C is destroyed by heat and light. Drinking the cooking water or adding it to the meal or juices is also suggested. Lower doses of C taken more often are said to enhance absorption, so food sources provide that perfectly. I always recommend 4 oranges a day (from Anthony Williams) to someone fighting something off and needing more C.

Liposomal Vitamin C is a form in which a higher dosage of the nutrient is enrobed in a lipid or fat sphere so its high dose is better tolerated by the digestion. High doses of Vitamin C can be cancer-preventative and are usually administered intravenously so the body does not reach saturation in the digestion and can handle higher levels in the blood. This Liposomal C is the next best thing to an IV and can provide high concentration. However, for people with too much iron (hemochromatosis) or with kidney stone risk this form is not recommended. Stick to food sources.

The way the body tells you if you are at it's limit of Vitamin C (oral intake) is through "bowel tolerance" which means you get diarrhea if you have taken more than you need. However, the excess is excreted quickly and some believe taking right up to this tolerance is helpful for a cleansing, healing reaction in certain circumstances. This is unlikely to happen with food sources alone.

Vitamin D:

Vitamin D is much misunderstood! It is actually a **fat-soluble hormone** and chemical messenger that your body produces in the skin, with exposure to UVB rays in Sunlight. You absolutely need vitamin D to absorb and utilize Calcium, Magnesium and Phosphorus for healthy bones and teeth, and to prevent osteoporosis, but it also nourishes and protects all the cells, muscles, and the very delicate hormone balance. While it is so valuable and essential, *there are not a lot of food sources for this nutrient.* It is perfect that your body would have a process for making it! Vitamin D also prevents cardiovascular disease, reduces cholesterol, benefits those with breast cancer, rickets, diabetes, lupus, crohn's, parkinson's, dermatitis, kidney disease, multiple sclerosis, rheumatoid arthritis, and gum disease. Vitamin D controls hundreds of genes for skeletal and endocrine health that relate to cancer, autoimmune disease, nervous system optimization and immune response in infection prevention. Another reason to seek Sunlight and Food Sources for this nutrient is that many supplements contain Vitamin D from Lanolin which is the sebaceous gland oil washed from sheep's wool (not vegan and....yuk).

Vitamin D Food Sources: SUNSHINE & OILY SEAFOODS
Fortified Nut Milks, Leafy Greens, Lichen, Mushrooms (especially Portobello, Maitake, Morel, Button & Shiitake), Oats, Orange Juice, Tofu, Salmon, Tuna, Swordfish, Mackerel, Halibut, Herring, Sardines, Cod & Fish Liver Oil, Yeast, Beef Liver, Egg Yolks, Yogurt, Cheese, Butter

*To increase absorption: Get several minutes of exposure to the Sun everyday on at least the arms and face, as Sunlight can provide ALL the Vitamin D your body needs. Obviously where you live and the seasons will hamper this, but many studies show Vitamin D is stored from the Summer months, exactly so it can be used for the Winter months. Discontinue using sunscreens unless absolutely necessary for your skin type (one SPF 10 application blocks UVB light and reduces Vitamin D production by 90%) or get some short exposure **without** them first. UVB light from the Sun is also helpful for lowering the blood pressure and creating testosterone.*

Dr. Ryan Cole, a Mayo Clinic-trained, Board Certified Pathologist who is an expert on immunology and virology, says, **"There is not a cold and flu season, there is a deficiency of Vitamin D season."**[18] Combine lower Sunshine exposure and cold weather with all the "candy and cookie holidays" that start in October, and you have a fabulous recipe for illness. If we are more conscious of our Sunshine exposure, diet choices and food sources, we might eliminate the need for such a bad "yearly" experience as a cold or the flu. Let's eradicate them!

I have noticed that over-supplementation with Vitamin D (in viral-scare concerns) gave me hot flashes, reinforcing its role as a hormone that can cause ripple endocrine effects. Especially with Vitamin D, *more is not always better.* And let me remind you yet again, **Food and Sunshine Sources don't have these side effects.**

Vitamin E:
"The Anti-Aging Vitamin" - Vitamin E is the designation for a group of eight **fat-soluble** nutrients. One of our most powerful antioxidants, Vitamin E is tasked with protecting the nerves and cellular integrity, healing wounds and supporting cell regeneration, preventing cardiovascular disease, cancer, macular degeneration and cataracts. It is valuable for supporting brain function and reducing cognitive loss, helpful in Alzheimer's and Parkinson's disease. Vitamin E acts as an

anticoagulant and vasodilator to fight blood clots and heart disease. Vitamin E has been known to improve balance and reduce muscle weakness and may support and heal neuropathy. There is evidence that chronic "incurable"diseases like arthritis, lupus, parkinson's and MS are benefitted by Vitamin E. It is an effective hair-loss nutrient as it stimulates and protects hair follicles for better growth. Taking 400 i.u of Vitamin E daily makes tender breasts, as a characteristic of PMS, go away. Some experts say that without Vitamin E, our bodies would turn rancid and oxidized. It literally preserves US! Vitamin E helps to block the activity of many inflammation-producing enzymes, decay-causing organisms and free radicals. Oxidation by free radical damage causes cancer and many of our most degenerative diseases, which this nutrient helps resolve. Vitamin E stimulates the immune system and supports better cell signaling. This is THE *Anti-Aging remedy* as it slows down degeneration in the skin, cells and organs. Vitamin E Oil is found in nearly every skin care product as a cell treatment and as a great natural preservative to keep the products from spoiling.

Vitamin E Food Sources: BROWN and GREEN FOODS

Sunflower Seeds, Many Seeds & Nuts, Coconut Oil, Wheat Germ Oil, Almonds, Apricots, Hazelnuts, Pecans, Peanuts & Peanut Butter, Olives and Olive Oil, Avocados, Wheat Germ, Beet Greens, Chocolate, Collard Greens, Kale, Tomatoes, Soy, Spinach, Avocados, Safflower-Grapeseed-Corn-Soybean-Sunflower Oils, Kiwi, Asparagus, Swiss Chard, Walnuts, Whole Grains, Broccoli, Cranberries, Mango, Red Bell Pepper, Fish

To increase absorption: Healthy fats increase the uptake of Vitamin E, and conversely a fat-free diet virtually starves the body of it. Vitamin C may increase Vitamin E absorption and foods rich in both should be consumed regularly if one smokes.

Take with Selenium for enhanced activity. **Selenium**-rich foods include: **Bran, Brewer's Yeast, Broccoli, Cabbage, Celery, Corn, Cucumbers, Garlic, Mushrooms, Nuts, Onions, Oysters, Seaweed Greens, Sesame Seeds, Tuna, Wheat Germ and Whole Grains, Organ Meats, Fish**

*****TOPICAL** usage of a good, pure Vitamin E oil can reduce scar tissue and stretch marks, and can also be used preventively on the skin during pregnancy and for premature aging. It helps the body regenerate and produce skin cells to repair damage. Vitamin E Oil is a natural preservative. You can prick a capsule or softgel with a pin and squeeze the oil out to use in preserving homemade body care products and extracts.

Vitamin K:

Another **fat-soluble** set of nutrients especially helpful for making the proteins responsible for blood-clotting, proper scab formation, and maintaining bone strength (the K came from the German word Koagulation). The body recycles this nutrient in order to use it many times, and also produces its own source of it in the intestines. Vitamin K can heal broken blood vessels in the eyes, reduce excess menstruation, and stop bone loss. The Liver is especially affected by Vitamin K, and uses it as a source for healing jaundice and cirrhosis.

K1 is found in **Vegetables, and from plant sources**. K2 is of **microbial origin**, meaning it is a cultured nutrient (made with bacterial and fungal help) and normally found in **Fermented Foods and Animal products**. But it is also produced by our healthy gut flora, in our own body. It can be useful in preventing osteoporosis, but is most usually supplemented in people with a high bleeding risk. It also seems to play a part in a healthy heart and cardiovascular system. Natto (a fermented soybean product) is highly suggested for heart disease and high blood pressure healing regimes.

Vitamin K Food Sources: DARK GREEN FOODS & BUBBLY FERMENTS, YOGURTS and VINEGARS

K1: Cabbage, Spinach, Sprouts, Broccoli, Cauliflower, Nettles, Oats, Parsley, Kale, Collard Greens, Avocados, Tomatoes, Strawberries, Molasses, Watercress, Brussel Sprouts, Mung Bean Sprouts, Dark Green Lettuces, Sea Vegetables, Turnip Greens, Soy(Edamame) & Soybean Oil, Olive and Olive Oil, Whole Wheat

K2: Fermented Foods, Kombucha, Vinegar, Tofu, Natto (Fermented Soybeans) Liver, Lean Meat, Egg Yolk, Seafood, Yogurt, Kefir

To increase absorption: Eat with healthy fats to enhance uptake - like eating good olive-oil based salad dressings and avocado with your greens. The darker, outer leaves of greens contain more Vitamin K1.

Antibiotics and other prescriptions destroy the bacteria that assure the body's ability to make this nutrient in the gut. This blocks Vitamin K uptake, so eating dark greens is a must if on these pharmaceuticals. Birth control pills taken with too much Vitamin K supplementation (from pills not foods) may increase the incidence of blood clots.

David Avocado Wolfe calls **K2** the "Anti-Ahrimanic" Vitamin, the "**anti-mind control vitamin**," that can protect us from negative and demonic influence. He widely discloses that K2 helps clear pineal gland calcification, remove oil-based poisonous toxins from the body, and cancels the negative programming of demonic thought.

Vitamin CBD:
The Endocannabinoid System is one of your body's *major* functional systems like the Circulatory System, but it was only discovered in the 1990's! I believe if it had been discovered earlier, we would all be taking our recommended daily allowance of **Vitamin CBD!** This fat-based nutrient is THAT vital in BALANCING the body, reducing whatever is excessive, increasing what the body needs more of, and supplementing all body systems so that they can work better. There are so many life-promoting effects of CBD, I stand firm that it should be **reclassified as an essential Vitamin**. Incredible, life-altering results have

been experienced with using CBD for PAIN relief and the remediation of crippling anxiety. It also assists recovery from excess exercise and reduces inflammation. The tremors and convulsions from Epilepsy and Parkinson's can be instantly improved or eliminated altogether. This nutrient can lower blood sugar, lower blood pressure, maintain healthy stress responses, soothe nerves, boost brain power and focus, reset the sleep cycle and circadian rhythms, lower inflammation, treat cancer and toxic side effects from chemotherapy, and promote the healing of other deadly diseases. Plus it makes you FEEL GOOD, with virtually no side effects. People always facetiously ask me if it is a miracle remedy and I always say, "Yes."

CBD Food Sources: GREEN & BLACK FOODS

Marijuana & Hemp, Magnolia, Echinacea, Electric Daisy, Helichrysum, Black Pepper, Chocolate, Black Truffles, Chinese Rhododendron, Kava Kava, Liverwort, Orange Peel, Hops, Yeast, Sunflowers, Tea, Acetaminophen (Tylenol fills your body's endocannabinoid receptor sites like CBD, and stimulates a similar effect which may account for its effectiveness in stressful and painful situations. I have been more likely to recommend it in urgent situations since I learned this).

To increase absorption: Some believe mycellized water extracts are better absorbed. For fastest effect, take oil, extract or bite a gel cap, swish in the mouth and **hold under the tongue** for at least a full minute for sublingual absorption into the bloodstream, bypassing digestion. If using candies or gummies, allow them to linger in the mouth for as long as possible.

*TOPICAL use of CBD Oil products is exceedingly effective in an oil or salve base. Adding Menthol, Castor Oil or Cayenne to any topical remedy will drive it deeper into the tissues, Magnesium Oil will help relax the muscles. Consider formulating your own topical relief remedy with CBD.

Cannabinoids are particularly well-absorbed by the lungs through smoking, so this is an instance where a pipe or joint smoke, or an all natural live resin vape-pen is very effective, and especially fast-acting for anxiety. Because there are so many CBD products in the market today, it can be daunting to choose. Research brands and look for companies from reputable sources like health food stores and friend's companies on the internet (not so much from the gas station).

DOSAGE - stick with 1-10 milligrams for anxiety, generally lower doses with a fast-acting liquid are much better. Higher capsule doses of 20-50 mgs per dose for pain relief can be taken every few hours as often as needed, although less is best with CBD. Take the lowest effective dose, but make sure you take enough to feel a grand difference in stress level or reduction in pain. If you don't feel a difference you may need a higher dose; the relief should be not subtle, but profound.

Calcium:

Calcium is the most abundant mineral in the body, **every single cell needs it to survive**, and our bodies contain nearly 3 pounds of it! About 99% of it is stored in the bones and teeth. The other 1% circulates through the blood and tissues supporting electrical signals that are essential for life. This mineral is so important that the body will rob it from the bones if necessary to maintain an ideal level. It activates enzymes for fat and protein metabolism, in order to produce energy. Calcium also figures as a vital nutrient to prevent colorectal cancers, treat pre-eclampsia and lower high blood pressure (especially in pregnancy), and even to moderate PMS symptoms. Calcium works with the constriction and relaxation of blood vessels, causes muscle contraction, the transport of nerve impulses, and supports blood coagulation. Calcium makes stronger bones and forms a crystal matrix upon which they grow. This mineral also treats depression and anxiety, nourishes the nerves, ensures good sleep.

Calcium Food Sources: GREEN & ORANGE FOODS

Apples, Leafy Greens (but not Spinach), Grapefruit, Kale, Lamb's Quarters, Nettles, Bok Choy, Broccoli, Cabbage, Flax, Nuts & Seeds, Sesame Seeds & Tahini, Watercress, Chamomile, Valerian, Pau D'Arco, Winter Squashes, Chia Seeds, Molasses, Nori, Carrots, Edamame, Alfalfa Sprouts, Chickpeas, Chocolate, Legumes, Oranges, Tofu, Figs, Lucuma, Lentils, Pinto White and Kidney Beans, Collard Greens, Mustard Greens, Clams & Shellfish, Canned Fish, Sardines, Shrimp, Dairy, Fortified Milks

To increase absorption: Vitamin D from Sunlight enhances Calcium uptake into the bones. A low-Sodium and high Potassium diet enhances Calcium absorption. Juicing, fermenting, and blending all liberate more bioavailable Calcium from plant source foods. Soaking sprouts, nuts and seeds reduces the phytates and lectins which inhibit Calcium absorption.

Spinach and other oxalate-rich foods (Chard, Rhubarb, Cashew, Quinoa) **inhibit** Calcium digestion and uptake, and may contribute to the body forming stones in the kidneys and gallbladder. Phosphoric acid (found in most sodas) lowers uptake of Calcium and leads to a bone-leaching of the nutrient, as do corticosteroid use, chemotherapy, and alcohol. If you feel you need to supplement Calcium beyond these foods, or are recommended to do so, take it with Magnesium in a 2:1 ration (like a combination with 400 mg Calcium to 200 mg Magnesium).

Iron:

Iron is the trace mineral that makes blood Red, and it carries oxygen to every tissue in the body. It supports the body's ability to synthesize DNA, make collagen, promote wound-healing, strengthen immunity, produce amino acids, neurotransmitters and hormones. It is found in 2 different forms in our food, "Heme Iron" found in meat and blood of animals, and "Non-Heme Iron" found in Plants. A diet that is too low in Iron causes anemia, or iron-poor blood, characterized by low energy, paleness, lightheadedness and hair loss, and this is the most common nutritional deficiency worldwide. Children, menstruating and pregnant women need to be especially careful of anemia, and also athletes and vegetarians need to consume a great deal of iron-rich food. Iron keeps your hair color vibrant and the body strong. Iron is the 4th most abundant mineral in the Earth's crust, and is essential for all living organisms.

Iron Food Sources: RED FOODS & DARK GREENS
Alfalfa, Beets, Bilberry, Burdock, Catnip, Strawberries, Raspberries, Cherries, Red Cabbage, Grapes, Red Wine, Red Bell Peppers, Cranberries, Chocolate, Goji Berries,Tomatoes, Sun-Dried Tomatoes, Dried Apricots, Sunflower & Sesame Seeds, Molasses, Peas, Prunes, Leafy Greens, Black Beans, Spirulina, Figs, Raisins, Hazelnuts, Quinoa, Yellow Dock, Prune Juice, Oatmeal, Lentils and Legumes, Steamed Spinach, Lucuma, Dried Parsley, Soy, Dried Thyme, Wheatgrass, Dark Leafy Greens, Whole Grains, Nettles, Kale, Yellow Dock, Watercress, Sarsaparilla, Red Meat, Bison, Red Fish, Eggs, Tuna, Poultry, Chicken Liver, Sardines, Oysters, Clams, Mussels, Poultry

To increase absorption: *Vitamin C increases absorption of Non-Heme Iron (found in plants) and may prove very important in CV-19 treatment for its ability to help the body receive more iron and fix oxygen in the cells. However, bran fiber, supplemental calcium and some phytates and tannins in plants can reduce absorption. Soak nuts and grains before using to reduce phytates.* **Foods to increase absorption** *include Blueberries, Onion, Bell Peppers, Cauliflower, Lemons, Garlic, and Kiwi.*

Sometimes, in a true Iron Deficiency Anemia, or with endurance athletes or children who are overly fatigued, supplementation is necessary and can be instantly helpful. I recommend *PlantForce Iron Liquid* by Gaia Herbs. I have also met a few people who suffer from Hemochromatosis - which is an *overabundance* of Iron in the blood. These people are usually bright red! Having blood drawn on a regular basis and **avoiding** meat, Iron and Vitamin C-rich foods help them dramatically.

Magnesium: - *"The Muscle Mineral"* - Magnesium is present in every
cell in your body and it regulates over 325 enzymes for hundreds of bodily functions! Magnesium relieves leg cramps, restless leg syndrome, tremors, muscle spasms, and acid reflux. Good levels of Magnesium actually promote athletic endurance. It is the mineral which relaxes the muscles that Calcium contracts. Anxiety attacks are a signal the body is low in Magnesium, and the same goes for Chocolate cravings - your body knows what it needs! But this mineral is also vital for nerve function, and can make a marked difference in neuropathy, anxiety, and sleeplessness. Low Magnesium on a drastic scale contributes to schizophrenia and other serious psychiatric problems. Stress leads to lower Magnesium levels in the blood, and poses a higher cardiovascular

disease tendency in 'Type A" people. Magnesium counteracts stress, balances irregular heartbeat, relieves depression and supports emotional stability. This may also be one of the reasons women get such serious PMS tension and irritability, and why Chocolate always helps during the cycle! In 2017, a study found more than two out of three Americans are Magnesium deficient - so most people suffer from problems that are remedied with this mineral. Magnesium will settle down hyperactive children, support alcoholism recovery, relieve fibromyalgia and asthma.

Magnesium Food Sources: DARK BROWN FOODS
Dark Chocolate, Blackstrap Molasses, Wheat Germ, Chia Seeds, Buckwheat, Raisins, Soybeans, Almonds, Avocados, Bananas, Cashews, Dates, Potatoes, Pumpkin Seeds, Sunflower Seeds, Brown Sugar, Lucuma, Seaweeds, Spinach, Swiss Chard, Hot Spices, Black Beans, Peanuts, Seeds, Oatmeal, Millet, Cornmeal, Brown Rice, Whole Grains, Tofu, Dairy, Meat, Poultry, Seafood, Fatty Fish

To increase absorption: DE-STRESS! Avoid Calcium-rich foods for 2 hours on either side of eating Magnesium-rich foods. Don't smoke - this leaches Magnesium from the body. Avoid dark-colored sodas at all times as their phosphates bind with and leach Magnesium from the blood. Refined sugar in pastries, candy and cakes reduce Magnesium uptake and leave your body deficient. Alcohol also leads to Magnesium deficiencies.

*TOPICAL: Magnesium Oil is an amazing muscle-soothing remedy for pain and inflammation, absorbing through the skin and relaxing the muscles. You can also use Magnesium Oil to remove ticks by dabbing it right onto their bodies. **Epsom Salts** are **Magnesium Sulfate**, another form of Magnesium that soothes sore or cramped muscles. The mineral is absorbed through the skin in footbaths and whole-body baths. Helpful for migraine headaches and tension, and superior for supporting the nerves.

There are many different chelated forms of supplemental Magnesium today, which basically means the Magnesium has been bonded to an amino acid molecule for better absorption. Research each kind if you decide to supplement, some are easier on the digestion and better absorbed like Magnesium Glycinate. Magnesium relaxes the muscles of the colon as well, causing bowel evacuation (remember the famous Milk of Magnesia?) - needless to say, too much causes diarrhea. Oral contraceptives, diuretics, and cyclosporine drugs are known to cause magnesium deficiencies (and can also be the reason blood clots are more apt to form on these drugs). Alcoholics, bulimics and diabetics are also at risk for lower magnesium levels. I recommend a Magnesium powder, like ***CALM*** by Natural Vitality for nightly use before bed or when particularly stressed. It is great for leg cramps, insomnia and acid reflux, too.

Potassium:
One of the three vital Electrolytes of the blood (along with Sodium and Chloride, and also Calcium and Magnesium but to a lesser degree), this

water-soluble vital mineral actually carries a small electrical charge and conducts electricity. Our cells contain more Potassium than any other mineral. It regulates the functions of the heart, the cells, our enzymatic reactions, hormone secretion, contraction of the muscles, and the electrical functions of the nerves. It keeps the balance of minerals and fluids in the body, maintaining normal blood pressure and hydration, and preventing strokes. Low potassium levels can cause organ damage, abnormal heart rhythms and ultimately death. Potassium helps oxygenate the brain for clear thinking when people go on low-carb or keto diets, they often get the "keto-flu" or a crappy, lightheaded, weak and even faint feeling, as a result of lower potassium levels. The food sources below are a great antidote, along with increasing your water intake significantly.

Potassium Food Sources: ORANGE, YELLOW & GREEN FOODS
Bananas, Basil, Blackstrap Molasses, Celery, Chocolate, Coconut Water, Coriander, Cumin, Ginger, Hot Peppers, Dill, Kiwi, Paprika, Parsnips, Broccoli, Brussel Sprouts, Sweet Potatoes, Spinach, Parsley, Lettuce, Pistachios, Almonds, Most Nuts & Seeds, Acorn Squash, Artichokes, Oranges & Citrus, Beet Greens, Sunflower Seeds, Peas, Legumes, Lima Beans, Potatoes (especially the skin), Peaches, Prune Juice, Pumpkin, Tarragon, Tomatoes, Turmeric, Seaweed Greens, Cucumber, Zucchini, Eggplant, Butternut Squash, Lucuma, Cantaloupe, Cashews, Root Veggies, Apples, Avocados, Raisins, Dried Apricots, Seeds, Wheat Germ, Whole Grains, Dairy, Meats, Poultry, Fish, Salmon, Eggs

To increase absorption: One of the best-absorbed minerals at about a 90% success rate, potassium comes packaged with what it needs to get the job done. Magnesium helps keep this mineral balanced, transporting it in and out of cells, so it probably influences its absorption rate as well. Alcohol, coffee, caffeine, sugar, steroids, laxatives and diuretic drugs all cause potassium losses. It is also easily destroyed by cooking and boiling, so make sure to eat plenty of raw sources.

Prebiotics:
These are the **food-source for Probiotics** and healthy gut flora, that which keeps them vital & living. **Prebiotics are usually starch, fiber or sugar-based.** I teach that you can remember this because the prefix "pre-" always means before, like before there is a Probiotic there must be the pre-nourishing food of the Prebiotic. **Chicory** (see Weeds) is the premiere source of **Inulin**, which is one of the most popular Prebiotics. You may also see **FOS** - the Prebiotic *fructooligosaccharides* - combined with Probiotics in supplements. When they are formulated together the products are called Synbiotics. Prebiotics do not take the place of Probiotics at all! I find some people think they are interchangeable, or their doctors have told them they only need a Prebiotic (I hear this all the time) - who knows. Prebiotics are just the *precursors* to the helpful bacteria you really need. Supportive Prebiotic foods are best consumed raw, and are very helpful when eaten with Probiotic foods.

Sour drinks like Lemon Water and Apple Cider Vinegar Water create a more hospitable pH for Probiotics to thrive within, so they have a nourishing Prebiotic effect.

Prebiotic Food Sources: BROWN & BEIGE FOODS
Chicory (Inulin), Under-ripe Bananas, Apples, Raw Honey, Raw and Cooked Onions, Psyllium, Oat Fiber, Slippery Elm Powder, Cassava Garlic, Leeks, Raw Dandelion Greens (or lightly steamed), Acacia Fiber, Asparagus, Artichokes, Jerusalem Artichoke (shredded in salads), Cacao, Almonds, Jicama, Radishes, Potatoes, Burdock, Flax Seeds, Beans, Whole-Grains (Barley, Oats, Wheat Bran),Sprouted Grains & Seeds, Berries, Shirataki Noodles or Rice, Konjac Root, Shiitake Mushrooms, Seaweeds

To increase absorption: Eat raw, take with a Probiotic source.

Probiotics:
The word probiotic actually means *"for Life"* - and the Probiotics in your digestive system embody that and assure it. You have enormous colonies of these helpful, healthy bacteria in your gut. Probiotics populate this vital intestinal ecosystem which is called your microbiome. This community contains over 100 trillion "friendly bacteria," yeasts, and other helpful microorganisms. Your microbiome is assisted and enhanced by eating foods high in supplemental "healthy flora" called Probiotics. These are the living cultures, the essential helper bacteria that create fermentation and help with digestion, and many other bodily functions. Probiotics are essential for the body's "in-house" production of Vitamin K and B vitamins including B12, so they affect the mood and stress-response, but also play a pivotal part in proper organ function, immunity, pH, weight maintenance, bowel health, and nutrient assimilation. Benefits from eating Probiotics include an easing of lactose intolerance, bowel regulation, digestive peace, better response to stress, candida overgrowth-resolution, increased immunity, lowering of overblown autoimmune responses, and a very helpful lowered incidence of colds and flus. Use them to treat yeast infections, improve digestion and regulate hormonal balance. **"Elevated Microorganisms"** or **"Elevated Biotics"** as Anthony William calls them - are present as a film of Probiotics on raw, gently washed ORGANIC produce (like from your Garden). They survive the digestive process to make it to the small intestine ileum, which uses them to create vitamin B12. Probiotics can make an enormous difference in your mental health, well-being and ability to adapt to stress.

Probiotic Food Sources: BIOFILM ON FRESHLY HARVESTED LIVE FOODS, ACTIVE CULTURED FOODS
Kombucha, Sauerkraut, Pickles, KimChi, Pickled Veggies, Yogurt (low or no sugar best, plant-based are great, must be labeled "active cultures"), Vinegar, Miso, Umeboshi Plum, Apples, Green Peas, Celery Juice, Algae, Spirulina, Coconut Kefir, Tempeh, Brined Olives, Sourdough, Natto, Dairy Kefir, Raw Cheeses, Goat Milk & Cheese, Sour Cream, Buttermilk, Belgian Beer

To increase absorption: Freshly-picked **ORGANIC** fruits and veggies have millions of naturally-occurring Soil-Based Probiotics (SBO's) growing on them, don't wash them too much, if at all - *"Eat the Dirt, the Dirt Don't Hurt."* These are some of the most easily tolerated Probiotic sources, so if you are extra sensitive, fresh organic food is a great Probiotic source for you. Eat with one or more of the Prebiotic foods for best microbiome support.

Antibiotics, excess alcohol, hormones and stress destroy the microbiome. Supplementation at high doses (90- 400 Billion CFU's per day) for 5 days is advised after any round of antibiotics to restore your essential community after it has been wiped out. After this, regular supplementation with a 30 Billion probiotic with strains that suit you is a must for restoring the foundation of good health in your gut.

Bizarrely, I found out through my own body's reaction that not all Probiotics are the same. I was on a low or NO histamine diet, and was still having inflammatory symptoms. I got some great tips from an amazing natural doctor that **certain strains of Probiotics were actually histamine-PRODUCERS**. I had cleared every triggering source EXCEPT a complex Probiotic blend that included six of the offending bacteria, which I had been taking everyday. When I changed to an **all Bifido-bacterium Probiotic** supplement, I saw marked results in my symptoms within a day or two. Choosing the right Probiotics if you have histamine intolerance could be a real key to feeling better.

★ <u>Histamine-Producing Probiotics to AVOID if sensitive</u> include: *Lactobacillus casei* (produces histamine and tyramine), *Lactobacillus bulgaricus* (in some yogurt), *Lactobacillus helveticus*, *Lactobacillus reuteri*, *Lactobacillus lactis*, and even the most familiar, all-purpose *Lactobacillus acidophilus* can cause symptoms in sensitive people.

<u>Quercetin:</u>
Vital nutrient for lowering the body's allergic response, and reducing excess histamine and leukotriene production that lead to chronic inflammation, Quercetin is actually a **pigment-based phytochemical** in the family of Flavonoids. I always speak about the Color Principles in food that are our cell-protecting antioxidants. And Quercetin is their Queen! Sunlight stimulates Quercetin production, so the fruits and veggies that get the most light are highest in this pigment, and can be most repairing to the DNA. Used by the body for brain, respiratory, and heart health, and for reducing free-radical damage, this is one of the body's strong Protectors. Thus, it is a natural for reducing tumors, protecting healthy cells and eliminating cancer. Quercetin also neutralizes spike proteins.

Quercetin Food Sources: DARK RED & YELLOW FOODS
Red, Purple & Yellow Onions, Red Apple Peels, Honey, Red Grapes, Cherries, Green Leafy Vegetables, Horsetail, Kale, Spinach, Berries, Asparagus, Brussel

Sprouts, Citrus especially Blood Oranges, Pumpkin Seeds, Capers, Watercress, Red Leaf Lettuce, Red Wine, Black and Green Tea, Chili Peppers, Cherry Tomatoes, Broccoli, Blueberries, St. John's Wort

To increase absorption of Quercetin: Eat the **raw peels** *of fruits & veggies, where the highest concentration of these colorful pigments are found. Eat with Bromelain rich foods like:* **Asparagus, Bananas, Ginger, Kimchi, Kiwi, Pineapple, Sauerkraut, & Yogurt.**

Zinc:
Zinc is a trace mineral (which means your body needs less of it), but it is vitally important for over 100 functions in the body including strong immunity, building enzymes, cells and proteins, healing damaged tissues, creating hormonal balance, reproductive health, and the production of DNA in your body. It causes the cells to grow and multiply, so it is especially important for growing children in adolescence, and in pregnancy to prevent birth defects. Zinc is intimately connected with the senses of taste and smell. Taken at the early stages of colds or flus it is highly possible to shorten the duration and severity of symptoms. Viral cases in the early 2020's, in which people lost their sense of taste and smell, were directly related to the body **robbing itself of vital Zinc** to increase immune fighting power. Regular Zinc supplementation can be key to restoring these functions, and in this case I definitely recommend taking about 15-23 mg of Zinc supplement after every meal in the form of a lozenge or drops until senses return. Zinc causes nausea in even small doses, **always take AFTER a meal**, or specifically eat the food sources for better absorption and less symptoms. Zinc also protects the body from harmful effects of lead, cadmium and other heavy metals from treated drinking water and pollution. There has been proven a significant connection between zinc deficiency and the onset of anorexia nervosa, which also depletes the body of this and every other mineral. Zinc supplementation improves this disease and would likely play a role in preventing it. This mineral also seems to enhance the activation of Vitamin A for the eyes, and the highest content of Zinc is found in the retina and iris of the eye. Zinc plays a role in night and color blindness as well, and both of these improve when proper levels are maintained. Impotence and sexual function seem to also be a concern that improves with Zinc, and men are particularly suggested to eat Pumpkin Seeds (and all these other great foods) for more Zinc. It is also considered to be a brain food, it stimulates alertness and focus and helps control mental disorders.

Zinc Food Sources: BROWN & BEIGE FOODS
Brewer's Yeast, Caraway Seeds, Chickpeas, Pumpkin Seeds & Oil, Hemp Seeds, Soybeans, Tempeh, Tofu, Oats, Spinach, Broccoli, Cashews, Chocolate, Almonds, Goji Berries, Sunflower Seeds, Shilajit, Poppy Seeds, Pumpkin Seeds, Chia Seeds, Buckwheat, Sesame Seeds, Peanuts, Whole Grains, Mushrooms, Pistachios, Beans, Pecans, Brazil Nuts, Pine Nuts, Lentils, Nuts, Blackberries, Watermelon, Wheat Germ, Kidney Beans, Lucuma, Herring, Oysters, Eggs, Poultry, Beef, King

Crab, Liver, Lobster, Oysters & Shellfish, Pork, Dairy

To increase absorption: Do not eat with corn, cereals and rice which are high in phytates which inhibit absorption of Zinc. Alcohol, cigarette smoking, steroids, diuretics, and oral contraceptives all interfere with the body's proper absorption of Zinc. DO eat with Quercetin-rich foods as these pigments help fix Zinc into the cells. Stress, both physical and mental, reduces zinc levels, so practice relaxation every day.

*TOPICAL application of Zinc Oxide is helpful for burns, eczema, diaper rash and aids in the renewal of healthy tissue for wound-healing. But many over the counter Zinc Oxide ointment products contain petroleum products and poisonous preservatives. Find a source for cosmetic Zinc Oxide powder and add it to your salves and oils to make your own Zinc remedies & sunscreens. Zinc is a popular natural sunscreen ingredient because, as a metal, it reflects and scatters UV light to prevent sunburn, without being a toxic chemical, impacting your body, or destroying coral reefs.

*****

Let's go through the garden gate, and see what else we can do with the *many* Gifts we receive from Nature. There are so many Remedies, and so little time! But as you'll see with the **Mudras** - sometimes the medicine is literally within your **own two hands**.

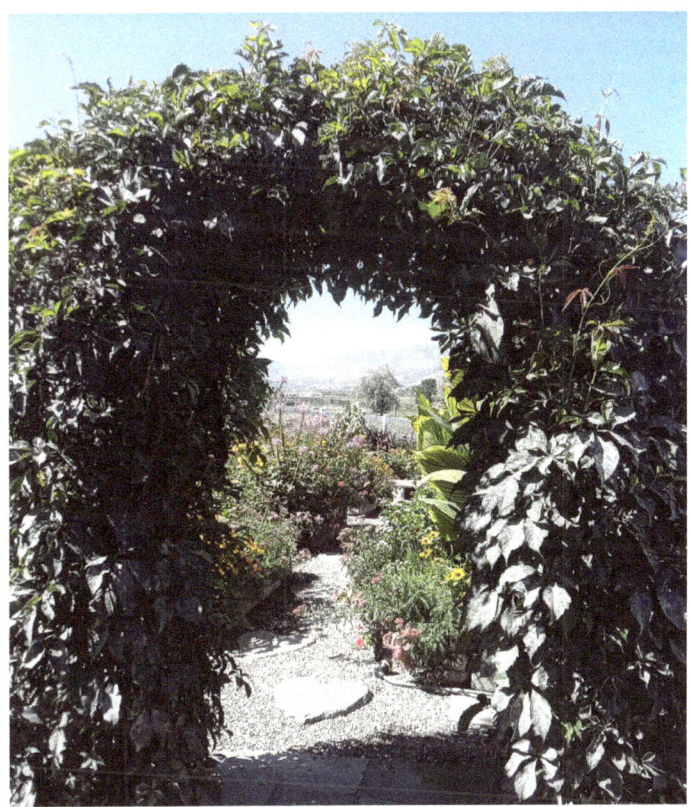

~ the garden of earth ~

LIFE-SAVING PRACTICES
from first aid for heart attacks to boosting testosterone

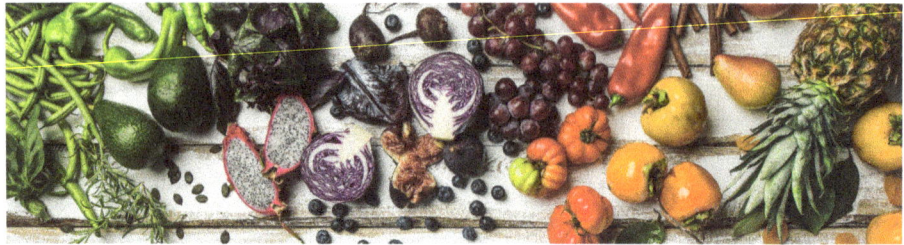

LIVING FOODS LIVE ON

Health ALWAYS begins with what you eat. I wrote a lot about my journey going Raw and being a Raw Foodist in my first book. I was honored to be a part of the adventure - speaking at retreats, selling Little Moon goods, the boundless physical energy, watching countless Avocado lectures you wish would never end! All these years later, the facts remain: **Raw Living Food can absolutely cure ailments, increase physical, mental, *and* spiritual energy, promote joyfulness, and enhance longevity.** I can personally attest to it. There is so much living proof, as well as outstanding research, documenting the absence and reversal of diabetes, cancers, high blood pressure, and many of our other "killer diseases" with a Living Food Diet. Scientific proof for over two hundred years certainly legitimizes the idea the eating Raw is not just a "trend." Take, for example, the work of Dr. Francis Pottenger studying four generations of cats:

> "One such early pioneer was a medical doctor by the name of Dr. Pottenger. He performed a TEN YEAR EXPERIMENT whereby 900 cats were fed controlled diets. The cats eating raw food produced healthy kittens from generation to generation. Those on cooked food developed modern Man's ailments: heart troubles, kidney and thyroid disease, pneumonia, paralysis, loss of teeth, difficulty in labor, diminished or perverted sexual interest, diarrhea, irritability. By the third generation, a great percentage of cats were infertile. This was written up in the American Journal of Orthodontics and Oral Surgery in August of 1946."[19]

The Living Food Lifestyle is based on the concept that optimal health comes when you make an effort to consume more foods in their **natural alive state**. Fresh-picked produce grown in organic soil is IDEAL for your health, and the reason this book spends so much space talking about gardening and harvesting wild foods.

While some enthusiasts may get caught up in needing to be 100% Raw or grow everything they consume - not everyone can do that yet. What matters is that you just ramp up the amount of Fresh, Vibrant, Raw Food you DO eat. Everyone should try eating more living food, or at least have Raw Days in your month during which your body gets a break and gets more Light from raw food. Sometimes I eat the first 2 meals of the day as raw as possible and enjoy some cooked food at night.

Raw Food needs no repackaging or mechanical processing into plastic or cardboard, due to its ingenious, God-given "wrapper," which is brilliantly designed to prevent exposure to heat, light and air, retaining nutritional value and shelf-life. Every bit of the natural packaging is compostable and will return to the Earth as nourishment instead of garbage and poison. Choosing natural food with no packaging is an Earth-Honoring Practice in and of itself. Like **Juliano** says about Raw Food, *"Don't trust the Man - trust the Mom. Mother Nature!"*

Raw foods are naturally digestible as they bring along their own digestive enzymes. When you eat something in its natural raw state you are receiving the **Exact Intent of the Plant Kingdom** to nourish with a 7-Fold Purpose, designed by Gaia to provide instant life force energy, and all you need to unpack it. Living plants contain the energy of the Seed, the energy of fractal expansion, encouraging expansion and the fruition of Life. Cooked food contains the energy of ash, fire, breaking down, and decay, and the food is stripped of many nutrients that are destroyed by heat. Some foods *do* need to be activated with heat (like certain Mushrooms, see Volume 4), or heated to kill parasites. But for the most part, Fire is a destructive force and damages vitality in food.

Living Foods gather Sunshine, Moonshine and Starshine - **stellar cosmic light** - which may account for how quickly they spark the body up with a new, noticeable energy (at the speed of Light!). Many times I am asked where I get all my energy - and the truth is Raw Food is a big part of it. I receive an abundance of Photons from my food! People will literally tell you you are "glowing" when you eat this way.

The Living Food Lifestyle also promotes Juicing, Sprouting, Cleansing and increasing Water intake daily. Read the works of: **David Avocado Wolfe, Gabriel Cousens, Juliano, Brigitte Mars, Jay "The Juiceman" Kordich, Patricia & Paul Bragg, Victoria Boutenko & Family, Jameth Sheridan, Edward Howell, Elaina Love, Anne Wigmore, Anthony William, Cherie Soria, Sarah Glover, Paul Nison, Norman W. Walker, Maximilian Bircher-Benner, Eugene Christian,** and **Joel Gazdar.**

JUICING

Juicing is a really enjoyable way to bring more Raw Food into your life. *Drinking* your vitamins and minerals is so easy, and fresh juices can be such a premier source for delivering living nutrients to your body. Every time we drink raw juices we can feel our CELLS begin to SING and shout for joy!! You can truly feel the increase in light, enzymes, and living activity (Vital Life Force) right away. All that, plus superior nutrition becomes yours when you drink these beautiful plant elixirs. They are quite literally Liquid Cosmic Light.

In particular, drinking a Green Juice is said to be akin to taking a blood transfusion, as the chlorophyll molecule is nearly identical to our hemoglobin molecule except with a Copper (blue-green base) versus our Iron (red) base. Beet juice along with green juices can provide the Iron molecule to build up the blood and be as near a match to our own blood as anything! Next time you feel low, remember to try a **fresh live juice** - and watch your energy return. As you will feel, we are deeply and instantly nourished at a blood and cellular level by the minerals and nutrients in fresh juices. JUICES are the Lifeblood of Plants delivering to us their perfect Plant Medicines -which become our Lifeblood. Mind-boggling.

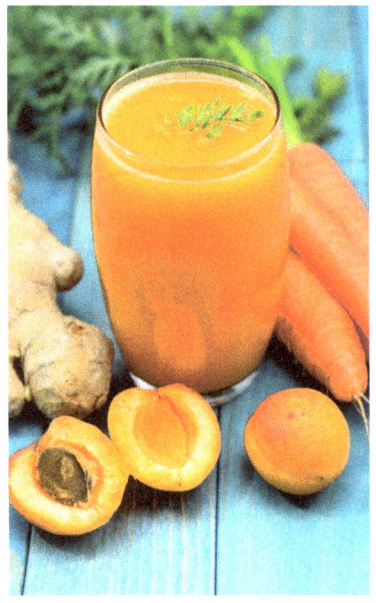

One of my dear Raw Family friends, **Steve Prussack**, and his wife **Julie** have written a wonderful guidebook about Juicing called *Juice Guru*. Their belief is that you can completely transform your life and health by adding just **one living Juice a day**. He proved his concepts with his own body, restoring his energy levels, purifying his body, raising his testosterone and literally "cleaning his engine" with a regular juicing habit. He found he no longer craved sweets and fast food, unwanted weight was shed without difficulty or denial, and his age-old addictions disappeared. Reuniting with his high school sweetheart after 20 years, she remembers it was so easy to fall for him all over again because he looked just like he did in high school - youthful, vital, full of energy and glowing! The two of them married and dedicated themselves to Juice Guru, the first ever juicing-related show syndicated worldwide on iHeartRadio. They share great resources for education, started a consulting and coaching business, and continue travel to trade shows and health events spreading the good word of JUICING! We reunited at Expo West recently and it was a joy to see him so vibrant and passionate after so many years - Juicing WORKS!!! Fresh juices provide an enormous supply of powerful plant chemicals, enzymes, antioxidants (and Sunshine!) that instantly satisfy hunger as they energize and revitalize the body.

> "With Daily Juice you will absorb more nutrients every day than most people do in a week!"
>
> ~ *Steve Prussack*

These phytonutrients are broken down, and somewhat pre-digested by the juicer, making them much more bioavailable for instant use by the body. Steve writes that juices spend less than 15 minutes being digested because they are in a perfectly prepared form to deliver nutrition to your hungry cells. **For children with focus problems, beginning the day with a fresh juice improves their concentration and energy in the classroom**. For elderly people, Juices offer much more premium nutrition than pharmaceuticals, and solve many problems for which they thought they needed medicines. Chronic problems can disappear, and the immune system is given the supplementation it needs to be strong and resilient. The body receives better hydration as well, and an enormous amount of minerals are available through juicing that the body can put to good, immediate use.

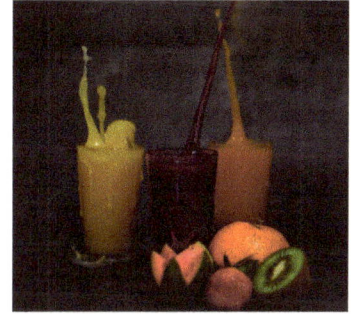

The **Color Principles** in foods are the **Antioxidants**. What they do in the body is essential, protecting the cells and enhancing their function and stability. Juicing is an amazing way to provide the body with loads of antioxidants in a mostly effortless fashion. Antioxidants protect the body from premature aging and from cancer and other cell damage as they miraculously revive cell growth and renewal.

Juices are **detoxifying, anti-inflammatory, lower cholesterol, provide essential fatty acids, boost productivity, boost body alkalinity, balance hormones, regulate blood sugar, prevent kidney stones, provide soluble fiber and promote youthful vitality** you can really feel. To read more amazing stories and great research about the power of Juicing, get their book! It is a wonderful resource with tons of delicious recipes and brilliant suggestions for true, lasting health.

SAVE THEIR TEETH

Did you know there are vital resources in your child's baby teeth? There are special STEM CELLS in each baby tooth that could be grown and utilized as donor stem cells to repair defects or injuries later in life. Stem cells are naturally programmed to cure many illnesses and promote tissue repair. The smallest baby teeth have the strongest, most abundantly proliferating stem cells, so keep every tooth you can (after the Tooth Fairy pays her due).

Older teeth that have lived longer in the mouth lose these particular stem cells as they age, so it is the younger first teeth that must be saved. Stem cells from this type of personal source donation are most likely to be accepted by the body, so the fear of rejection is eliminated. This could mean the difference between the Life and Death of a child. From now on, tell everyone you know to save their kid's teeth! Make sure to label them with the child's name and store them somewhere away from heat and air.

USING HERBS WISELY

One of our greatest gifts on this Planet is the diversity of species - especially in the Plant Kingdom! It is incredible how many Herbs and Spices we all have access to now, even at the local grocery store. We are so blessed to have so many herbs to turn to in times of need, they are our truest Plant Allies! Learning to use (and make) Plant Remedies has been the most important and life-changing education of my life. In Volume 1, I wrote about how passionate I was about moving back to Colorado in the late 80's to "learn ALL the plants" and study with some of the world's most esteemed Herbalists. Well, it worked - I have been hooked on Herbs ever since!

It is actually very easy to self-educate when it comes to plant lore and herbal medicine, I did it for years: **READ**. I'd consume herb books like chocolate! Some of my favorite Herbalist-Authors are: **Brigitte Mars**, **Roy Upton**, **David Wolfe**, **Rosemary Gladstar**, **Feather Jones**, **Jeanne Rose**, **Susun Weed**, **Michael & Leslie Tierra**, **Mindy Green**, **Sayer Ji**, **"Herbal Ed" Smith**, **Ric Scalzo**, **Christopher Hobbs**, **Richo Cech**, **Eliot Cowan**, **Stephen Harrod Buhner**, **Dr. John Christopher**, **Jethro Kloss**, **Dr. David Frawley**, **Dr. Vasant Lad**, **Hanna Kroeger**, **James Green**, **Michelle E. Lee**, **Euell Gibbons**, **Scott Cunningham**, **Paul Bergner**, **Matthew Wood**, and **Linda Page**.

These books and many more have helped me maintain a whole lifestyle of health with my many Herbal Allies. It should be clear by now that I like to Stay Well. If I ever do get sick, I seek out Food Cures first. I search out foods and Herbs that will have the desired healing effect for my body ailments, and which will enhance any supplement I may take. I will look for Essential Oils that will complement my therapy and diffuse them into the air, or make an essential oil blend I can rub on my body, spray into the air, add to a mineral bath, or apply to my feet if it is too hard to eat. If I am ever under the weather, I go after it on many levels and consequently I always heal quickly and completely.

Another AMAZING book I highly recommend is called *10 Essentials Herbs* by **Lalitha Thomas**. I found this book early in my herbal education quest, and it still blows me away every time I pick it up. There is something to be said for befriending and learning everything about a small set of herbs, that you can stock and always rely on for their benefits. She details literally HUNDREDS of ways to use just these ten herbs, demonstrating their versatility and ability to treat and heal almost everything!

★ **Lalitha's 10 Essential Herbs:** Cayenne, Chaparral, Cloves, Comfrey, Garlic, Ginger, Onion, Peppermint, Slippery Elm and Yarrow

I have gifted this book to many people, most recently to my friend Addie Ruth when she was traveling to live in Ecuador, because I knew she would be able to find these herbs there, too. These are remedies you can find most anywhere on Earth that might make a big difference to your health. Because of Lalitha Thomas, I keep a vial of **Cayenne**

Powder in my car, backpack, and first aid kit. I can use it to stimulate alertness when I am tired (adding a couple of grains or up to ⅛ tsp **Cayenne Powder** to water or juice can provide more energy than a Red Bull, and is an old trucker's remedy). It's a wonderful herb to start utilizing daily in juice or water - *cold preparations only* - from a few grains, up to ¼ teaspoon at a time as a body and circulatory tonic. I love how it makes me feel so sparked-up

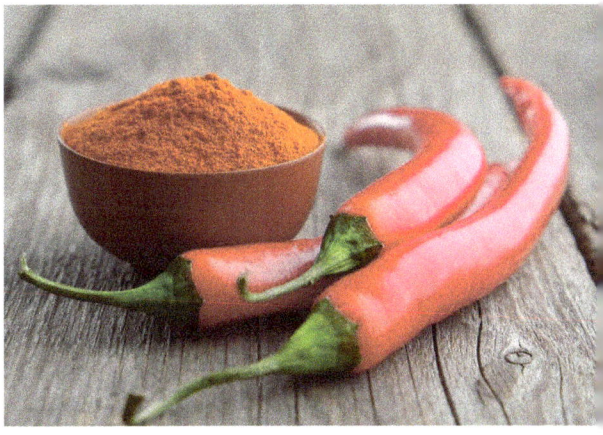

and aware. There's a jar of it right here on my desk for writing days! I only use the tiniest pinch, but it packs a powerful punch.

Cayenne is also a wonderful first-aid remedy to soothe shock, restore equilibrium, stop anxiety attacks, heal digestion, and cure bleeding ulcers. Cayenne Powder will stop profuse bleeding, even stop internal bleeding in animals hit by cars, and can possibly prevent a heart attack. Uncooked, dried **Cayenne Powder** has an amazing heart-balancing and blood-regulating action that helps to normalize circulation.

The following amazing life-saving remedy comes from one of Lalitha's stories. I have used it when I had heart palpitations, and also when I was in an anxiety moment, with great results. ***This in no way replaces medical attention, and the fact is that any person suffering in this manner is in an emergency, and they should be seen and medically evaluated.**

FIRST AID FOR HEART ATTACKS

If someone believes they are having a heart attack, or if you think YOU are, **act fast with Cayenne Powder:** Immediately apply a tiny pinch of Cayenne directly on the tongue. As you await medical attention, or are being driven to the hospital, sip on juice or water that has ¼ teaspoon Cayenne Powder added to it, or you can continue with a pinch on the tongue as needed every minute to every ten minutes. In Lalitha's book she details how she has seen this remedy literally save people's lives *"by stimulating and balancing the heart and circulation and preventing shock from setting in prior to medical treatment."* Sometimes an anxiety attack could be the culprit, and Cayenne quickly snaps the body out of that fear pattern, and could save a needless hospital visit.

Did you know you could prevent a heart attack using your fingers?

The **Life-Saver Mudra**, or *"First Aid For Heart Attack Mudra,"* is a hand position that can be gently performed to soothe heart symptoms, regulate heartbeat and improve circulation complications. It can **ward off a heart attack**, yogis say maybe even faster than traditional nitroglycerine. If you are far from help, or awaiting medical assistance, or on the way to the hospital, place hands in this position and take Cayenne as above.

LIFESAVER MUDRA
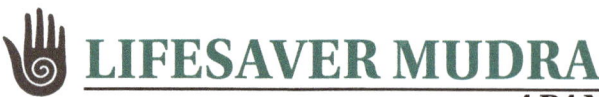
APAN VAYU MUDRA

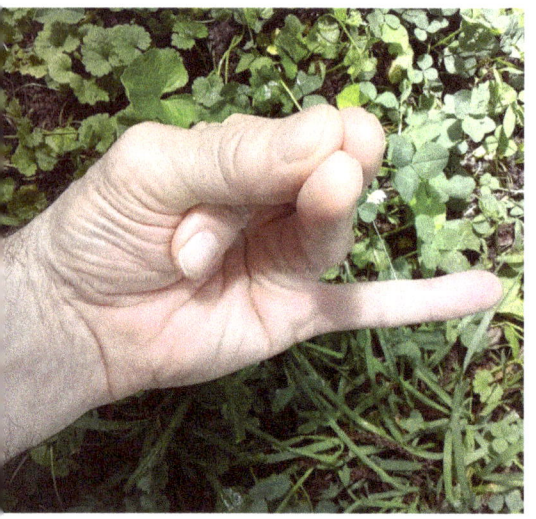

Bend the Index (2nd/pointer) finger gently inside the hand to touch the base of the Thumb. Bring together the tips of the Ring-finger and Third-finger right on the tip of the Thumb, (the Index finger reaches down to the palm through the circle they make), stretch the little Pinky-finger outward. Hold as needed, with both hands if possible, breathing deeply, until peace and a calm heartbeat are restored.

This is also a very powerful **ANXIETY-REDUCING MUDRA**. I use it when I feel anxious, have little heart flutters or heart palpitations, or feel the paranoia of health hysteria. It always makes me feel better right away. This Mudra can always be used for emergencies, but when practiced regularly, it will heal and strengthen the heart. Work up to holding it three times a day for 15 minutes each time. It can also be used as a **painkiller**, and can be practiced for **headaches, stomachaches,** and **toothache.** This Mudra increases the **Earth Element for grounding,** and **decreases Air and Fire.** It can remove blockages, anchor you to reality, and help detoxify the body.

✌ MUDRAS: THE MEDICINE IN YOUR HANDS ✌

Mudras are Yoga postures for the hands, specific positions or gestures of the fingers that have remarkable, health-altering effects on the whole body and mind. Your hands provide a remedy you can make for your body, anytime or place! Mudras have an instant physiological effect that you can usually feel right away, similar to the postures or asanas in Yoga. Brain chemicals and other hormonal secretions are released that alter your chemistry, energy and mood, so they affect your feelings quickly, as well. You can perform Mudras while walking, waiting in line, reading, meditating, watching television, falling asleep, doing breathing exercises, or any time your hands are free! There are Mudras for so many things, including **mental focus, circulation, energy, peace, better breathing, for remembering things**, and even to **enhance sexual performance** - read on! Mudras keep your hands strong and flexible, and can combat arthritis and strengthen hands after injuries. Doing the postures occupies your hands so they make a great substitute for smoking, eating, or scratching! Mudras work.

LAURA's LISTS

During the many years I worked in health food stores, I compiled Shopping Lists for customers for their health needs. I'd research their conditions and recommend specific **Healing Foods** for them to add to their daily regimen. I got to see first-hand the power of Food! I found that most people would make a new **food choice** to affect their health, before they would take a chance on a new herb or supplement. Sometimes **food changes** are exactly what the body is asking for, and it will re-balance quickly without the need for any medicating. Small and simple changes, like adding supportive foods, multivitamins or herbs can make *great* changes in the body's physiology. Here I have added a whole new layer to the Lists. For each condition, we will also learn to make healing changes to the body with **Mudras** and your own two hands! Some people are mysteriously drawn to **Essential Oils** like I am, so I have also included my favorite Oils to utilize for each need. The best idea is to do it all! These suggestions should help you treat minor issues for yourself and your Family, in simple, natural ways, and will decidedly kickstart your efforts toward lasting health improvements.

✍ MENTAL ENERGY & FOCUS ✍

One of the most prized feelings in life is having an abundance of alert mental energy and strong brain power on which to rely. Everyone I know would like to have sharper cognitive functions, always have a bright outlook, and have a much better memory. These foods bring it! They offer your brain the *nutrition* it requires to be able to handle many mental tasks and to keep focus all day long, so you can keep on working and playing.

While writing this book, I utilized many of the following remedies and maximized my workspace for personal brain support. I filled it with little bottles of Essential Oils, snacks, candles, signs, cards, Osha candy, stimulating mists, colors and Sunlight! Use what helps you to feel

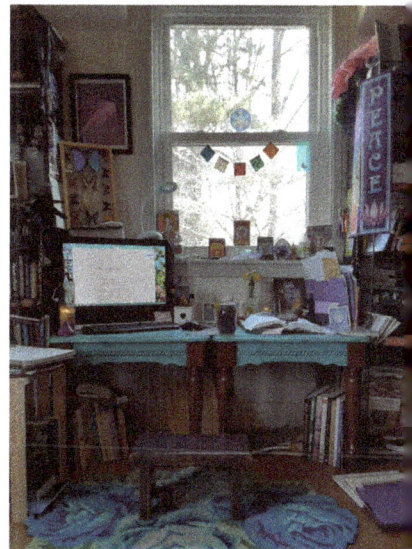

expansive and energized and on top of your game.

The brain is mostly composed of Fat - **Omega 3-6-9 Fatty Acids** and other healthy fats are essential for its proper functioning. Low-fat diets affect your brain. **Hydration** has a huge effect on the brain's ability to process. Drink more water during the day then you usually do, and you will see your brain power improve dramatically. **Chia Seeds** (a great source of brain-boosting Omegas) are the Superfood that powered the whole culture of the Aztecs. They offer a sustaining physical energy that lasts all day long - and a discernible improvement in attention and focus as well. **Honey** is a wonderful energy food, and eating just a Tablespoon a day by itself is a small adjustment that will provide huge energy and focus rewards for your brain, as well as your body.

FOODS & HERBS FOR MENTAL ENERGY & FOCUS

Acetyl l-Carnitine	**Cayenne**	**Gotu Kola**	**Peppermint**
Almonds	**Chia Seeds**	**Grapefruit**	**Pumpkin Seeds**
Ashwagandha	**Chickpeas**	**Greek Yogurt**	**Quinoa**
Avocado	**Coconut Oil**	**Green Tea**	**Reishi Mushroom**
Bacopa	**Coffee**	**Herring**	**Sage**
Bananas	**Dark Chocolate**	**Holy Basil**	**Salmon**
Blueberries	**DHA & EPA**	**Honey**	**Sardines**
Broccoli	**DMAE**	**Kale**	**Soy**
Brown Rice	**Edamame**	**Lemon Balm**	**Spinach**
Brussel Sprouts	**Eggs**	**Maca**	**Sprouts**
B Vitamins and Vitamin A, C & E	**Fresh Juices**	**Matcha**	**Sweet Potatoes**
	Ginkgo	**Nuts**	**Turmeric**
Cabbage	**Ginseng**	**Omega EFA's**	**Walnuts**
Cacao Nibs	**Goji Berries**	**Osha**	**Whole Grains**

Diffusing **Essential Oils** into the workplace is a pleasant and sneaky way to raise the level of brain functioning in the whole office. Casinos use aromatherapy all the time to secretly enhance energy, mood and spending! Diffuse your favorites into the air, smell right out of the bottle, make a roll-on for yourself, or simply place a drop into the palms, rub together, and take deep inhalations for 30 seconds. Your productivity will instantly increase. When I need some instant "brain juice" or inspiration or fatigue relief, I just smell the ones that call to me! I can attest, by the writing of this book, that Black Pepper gives you the "pep" you need to keep thinking and expressing with clear, boundless mental energy. Whenever I lost focus, a good few whiffs of Black Pepper or Eucalyptus would get me right back on track.

~ the garden of earth ~

ESSENTIAL OILS FOR MENTAL ENERGY & FOCUS

Balsam Fir	**Clove**	**Grapefruit**	**Peppermint**
Bergamot	**Coffee**	**Holy Basil**	**Rosemary**
Black Pepper	**Cypress**	**Lemon Balm**	**Sage**
Cardamom	**Eucalyptus**	**Lime**	**Spearmint**
Cedarwood	**Frankincense**	**Menthol Crystals**	**Sweet Orange**
Cinnamon	**Ginger**	**Nutmeg**	**Tangerine**

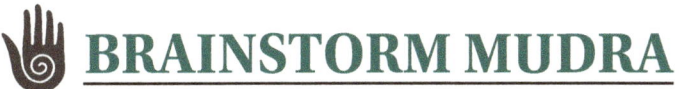

BRAINSTORM MUDRA
HAKINI MUDRA

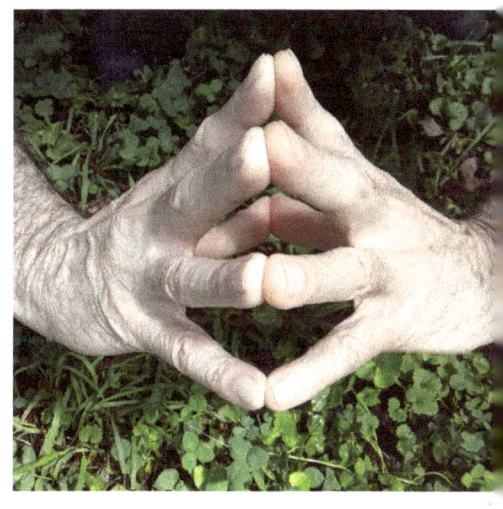

Press the tips of all fingers of both hands together and hold in a relaxed manner. Breathe deeply. Focus the eyes upward for a few moments. Hold this Mudra while public speaking, when searching for words, or to open the mind and stimulate ideas when working on a mentally taxing project. Uncross your legs when brainstorming or doing **intense mental work for optimal energy flow**. Witness the lighting-up of your mental abilities, as your Third Eye opens, begins to receive impulses, and shines more brightly. Oxygen concentration goes up to dramatically increase brain function and thinking is fast and effortless.

This is the **I'VE GOT IT! MUDRA**. You'll find this is an instinctive hand position you go to naturally when speaking. You will see many public speakers using it unconsciously when they speak to an audience. Turns out it is a superior tonic for Brain Function, as it energetically unites the two hemispheres and speeds up their interactive impulses. This position opens greater access to the right hemisphere where memory is located. It is a blood-flow renewing remedy, and can be significantly helpful for brain injuries and memory loss. The Hakini Mudra aids concentration, retention and memory and can help you become inspired, or think of a word you have forgotten! To find something you have lost, take a moment to slow down, close your eyes and do this Hakini Mudra. It also deepens the respiration to build lung energy, and brings more oxygen to the brain for healing and increased brain power. Hakini (the namesake) is the Hindu god of the Forehead, Pineal Gland, & 6th Chakra.

~ the garden of earth ~

✳ HANGOVER REMEDIES ✳

HYDRATION, ELECTROLYTES and **B VITAMINS** are the most important principal remedies for treating a hangover. As soon as you can stand to drink something, especially if you wake up in the middle of the night, start taking in water. Even better, drink water with **B and C vitamins, Baking Soda** or a pinch of **Salt**. I love the *Trace Mineral Research PowerPak*, it is kind of like an Emergen-C version 2.0 with less sugar, more minerals, electrolytes, Vitamin C and B vitamins. Take it with water, water, water. Hydration is exactly what you need the most. **FRESHLY-MADE JUICES** are perfect remedies in this case, add a little **Coconut Water** or **Salt** to your juice, and consider using **Green Apples**, **Celery**, and **Spinach** (or **Carrot**) for best effect.

A half a teaspoon **Baking Soda** in water before bed will soothe acidity and begin rebalancing your body pH while you sleep. Drink some, and also swish it around your mouth as a great mouthwash and hangover treatment the morning after. **Activated Charcoal** 2 caps before sleeping and 1 capsule upon waking can help you feel tons better (or sober you up quickly in an emergency). When you do get up, drink **Lemon Water** first thing using a small wedge to ½ Lemon in a large glass of Water. Then some **Dandelion Root Tea** will flush away toxins with **Peppermint** or **Ginger** to help your belly feel better. Forage and make some tea with wild **Wood Sorrel**. Then a **Banana** or an **Apple** would be the best *first food* to eat, supplying your hard-working liver with the glucose it needs after a long night of processing alcohol. See Volume Three for a

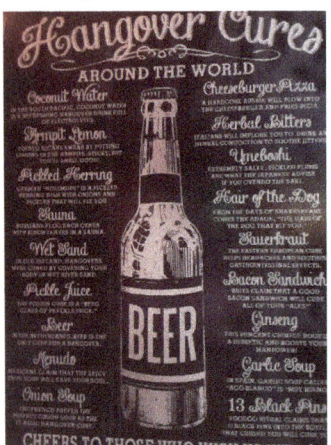

deep dive into Activated Charcoal's amazingness for soothing alcohol poisoning and so much more. Like a nagging Mother I tell you again, drink LOTS of extra water, add a few pinches of salt for fast rehydration.

Here are some other crazy ideas, seen in a bar in rural Tennessee. Some of the suggestions are actually spot on - especially **Coconut Water** to increase hydration, and **Bitters, Umeboshi Paste**, **Plums** or **Plum Candy**, **Sour Pickle** or **Lemon Juice** to nourish and soothe the Liver. Sometimes the old folk remedies become traditional medicines because they are so successful!

Essential Oils offer fast relief and are super easy-to-use medicines when hungover. No need to *ever* take them internally, **just smelling them alone** is restorative and alters your brain chemistry instantly. Or you could rub your chosen oils (always diluted in a little vegetable oil) on the feet, or pulse points like wrists and neck, or right on the head. Get your partner to rub your back and neck with a blend of these for instant relief, and the wonderful endorphins released by Human touch. Here are some of my super-helpful favorites to use when you feel less than stellar.

HANGOVER-RELIEVING ESSENTIAL OILS

Black Pepper	**Grapefruit**	**Marjoram** (relieves headache)	**Sandalwood**
Cardamom	**Juniper**	**Peppermint** (nausea & brain fog)	**Spearmint**
Fennel	**Lavender**	**Rosemary**	**Tangerine** (mood-elevating)
Ginger	**Lemon** (for nausea)		

 ## LIVER-LOVE DETOX MUDRA
VISHUDDHA MUDRA

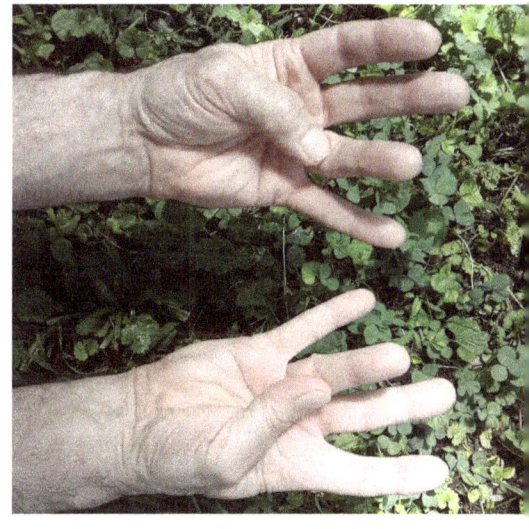

With both hands, touch the Thumb pad to the inside of the lowest Ring-finger joint, closest to the palm and hold. Also - perform the Ring Finger *Jin Shin Jyutsu* exercise of alternately enclosing each of your Ring-fingers in the fist of the other hand, holding it like it's a battery cable, recharging yourself and your Liver. Visualize a strong supportive energy coursing through your whole body. When I have a pressing need for peace or serenity, I like to perform this with every finger to calm down quickly.

This is the **LETTING GO MUDRA**. This position of the hands enhances circulation to neck and brain to increase mental clarity, purify thoughts. Causes the release of toxins, purification that supports the Liver, the organ most affected by drinking binges and chemicals in the blood. The Ring Finger holds the Liver energy, which can be powerfully healed with Mudras, whenever it has been impacted (pretty much daily!).

Did you know there is a remedy you can take WHILE you are drinking (if you have to overindulge, or drink some night when you normally wouldn't) called **PartySmart** by **Himalaya Herbal Healthcare**. It is a natural Ayurvedic herb supplement that destroys the acetaldehyde from drinking which causes much of the discomfort and acidity. I have found it is great for histamine-sensitive people who find themselves drinking wine in a social situation and wish later they hadn't! PartySmart can help your body recover and make you feel much better than you would without. Especially when traveling, or on a business trip, this could make or break how you feel in the morning! Use every nutritional resource available, to set the "future you" up for success.

✹ VIRAL IMMUNITY ✹

Viruses thrive on nutrients from Eggs, Dairy, Gluten (Wheat), Sugar, Pork and Corn. **Remove these from the diet when challenged with a virus.** Exosomes, toxins, spike proteins, and traces from childhood ailments like chicken pox and mononucleosis leave residues that build up in the body causing a "viral load." This load can compromise your immunity, increase susceptibility to additional virus colonization, elevate your allergy sensitivity, stir up mysterious diseases and cause flaring inflammation symptoms. Reduce and detox your everyday viral load by eating these vital fighter foods, all of which strongly build Natural Immunity and disrupt viruses.

ANTI-VIRAL FOODS & HERBS

- Active-Culture Yogurt
- Almonds
- Andrographis
- Apricots
- Arugula
- Asparagus
- Astragalus
- Beets
- Blackberries
- Black Cumin Seed & Black Seed Oil
- Black Pepper
- Broccoli
- Brussel Sprouts
- Burdock
- Calendula
- Carrots
- Cat's Claw
- Celery Juice
- Chaga, Reishi, & Shiitake
- Cherries
- Chicken Soup
- Cilantro
- Cinnamon
- Coconut Oil
- Colloidal Silver
- Cordyceps
- Cucumbers
- Echinacea
- Elderberry
- Fennel
- Garlic
- Ginger
- Goldenseal
- Grapefruit
- Grapefruit Seed Oil
- Green Tea
- Honey
- Kale
- L-Lysine
- Lemon Balm
- Lemons
- Licorice Root
- Maitake & Other Mushrooms
- Melatonin
- Mesclun Lettuce
- Milk Thistle
- Moringa
- NAC
- Neem
- Olive Leaf
- Oranges
- Oregano
- Osha
- Papaya
- Parsley
- Pau D'Arco
- Pomegranates
- Potatoes
- Pumpkin
- Pumpkin Seeds
- Quercetin
- Raspberries
- Red Marine Algae
- Schisandra
- Seaweeds - Dulse, Kelp, Nori
- Sesame Seeds
- Spinach
- Spirulina
- Sprouts & Microgreens
- Squash
- St. John's Wort
- Star Anise
- Strawberries
- Sweet Potatoes
- Tomatoes
- Turmeric
- Vitamins A, B6, B9, B12, C & D, Zinc
- White Pine Needle Tea
- Wild Blueberries

If you have a stomach virus, it may be difficult to eat. Make yourself an **Antiviral Massage Oil** with a base of 4-8 ounces of Black Seed Oil, Hemp Oil, Sesame Oil (or any other good oil you have on hand, Olive Oil would work great). Use 10-40 drops of any oil on this list (except Cinnamon or Clove Oil, which I would only recommend you only smell, as they are very strong). Choose as your inner guidance prompts you, use 3-8 of your favorites and blend as you feel (see recipe below for suggestions). Shake or stir your remedy oil well, and apply to the bottoms of your feet. Massage your neck and shoulders with it, and draw down the sides of the throat to milk the glands. You could also make a great full-body massage blend for any viral-related disease: Lupus, Parkinson's, Epstein-Barr, Chronic Fatigue Syndrome, Chicken Pox, Shingles, Mono, etc. Just research a bit about which Essential Oils suit your purpose the best, and always use the scents in those categories that you like the most.

ANTI-VIRAL ESSENTIAL OILS

Basil	**Clove**	**Lemongrass**	**Peppermint**
Bay Laurel	**Cypress**	**Manuka**	**Pine**
Bergamot	**Eucalyptus** Radiata	**Melissa** /Lemon Balm	**Ravensara**
Black Seed	**Frankincense**	**Mountain Savory**	**Red Thyme**
Cedarwood	**Grapefruit**	**Myrrh**	**Rosemary**
Chamomile	**Ho Wood**	**Niaouli**	**Sandalwood**
Cinnamon	**Juniper**	**Oregano**	**Spearmint**
Citronella	**Lavender**	**Palmarosa**	**Spruce**
Clary Sage	**Lemon**	**Patchouli**	**Tea Tree**

IMMUNE-BOOSTER MUDRA
PRANA MUDRA

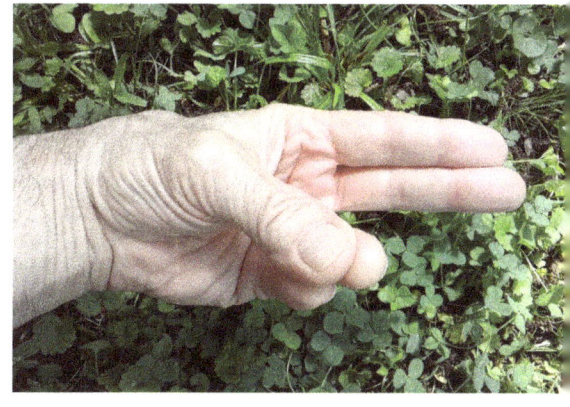

Place the Ring Finger and Pinky fingertips on the Thumb pad, with other fingers extended and held together. You may also place the Thumb on the fingernails of those two fingers, closing them toward the palm. Hold Mudra for 5-30 minutes, or as long as you can. It can be used several times a day. This Mudra also joins the hemispheres of the brain to harmoniously work together. And it can help you Sleep, too!

This is the **CURING MUDRA**, also called the *"Mudra to Cure 100 Diseases"* or *"Elixir* of Life" or *"The Healing Mudra of Life."* Prana is another name for Life Force, Chi or Qi. This Mudra lives up to its name by strengthening the immune system and raising that vital, healing life force energy, while it lowers body inflammation. It is a very energizing Mudra, great to use anytime to relieve fatigue, and can be used when fasting or hungry to nourish yourself with energy instead of food. Regular daily use is especially beneficial, and brings resistance to disease. It greatly increases mental and physical strength. It can even improve eyesight or eye problems, if practiced regularly. Prana Mudra can also reduce nervousness and increase self-confidence. As it reduces the Fire Element, it may also cool the body when overheated. It activates the Root Chakra, our very root to the Earth, keeping us fully grounded and powerful.

Special Secrets For Working With Viruses

- Viruses are drawn to feelings of **Unworthiness** - work on Self-Esteem, Personal Value, Approval of Self, Release of Vampiric or Parasitic Energies, Strong Boundaries, Restoral of Sovereignty, and Self-Sufficiency. Be self-sufficient, don't parasite others!

- **FEAR** creates a negative stress response in the body, which will eventually create weakness in every body system, especially your Immune System. **JOY** raises your immunity! You can definitely convince yourself you are ill and **will have made it so by fearing it so much**. Viruses are drawn to **Negativity**, and in that stress state the body is a weak defender and vulnerable on all levels. **Shame** lowers immunity.

- **Viruses crave sweets** and can cause your body to feel it needs to eat them. Similar to fungal ailments like Candida, they can chemically compel you to stop taking your supplements or medicine, and to geek out on sugar or breads to assure their own survival. Been there, felt that! If you are no longer in control - take back your power.

- Many viruses have a **protective lipid envelope** that soap will break down, which is why *regular* soap (no need for harsh antibacterial soap) will work to kill them.

- **Viruses seek living cells** for replication and must invade and take command of our cells as the donor/host material for their existence. *"Viruses are microscopic parasites, generally much smaller than bacteria. They lack the capacity to thrive and reproduce outside of a host body."***[20]**

- **Viruses are NOT malevolent by Nature, should not be feared or hated**, they seek only to live. Viruses are accelerants, why going "VIRAL" happens quickly. Viruses and flus usually come on quickly like a freight train, which is how you recognize and differentiate them from colds. They rapidly take hold and cause havoc.

- **Viruses are Fragile - they can be destroyed by Heat, Sunshine & Ultra Violet Light, Plant Medicines** and **Chemicals.** They have protein spikes with which they attach to our cells. These spikes are vulnerable, they can be altered and broken with phytochemicals, especially those within **Elderberry, Burdock** and **Cat's Claw**.

Many believe it is better to preserve the skin's **natural microbiome** by NOT using sanitizers. But if you are in a situation where you need to be more careful, I suggest you make your own gentler version and use sparingly.

Hand Saver Sanitizer

- 16 oz. **Isopropyl Alcohol** 70% or higher (or **Vodka**, or **Everclear** above 100 proof)
- 2 oz. **Aloe Vera Gel or Juice**
- 1 teaspoon **Vegetable Glycerine**
- 1.5 oz. **Rosewater** (or 2 oz **Rosewater & Glycerine** by Heritage Store)
- **Glass Mister-Top Bottles**, amber or cobalt
- 1 - 1 ½ teaspoon (100-150 drops) total **Essential Oils**

Prepare all your bottles and make sure all your mister tops are cut to the appropriate length to just touch the bottom of the bottle but not bend.

Combine all ingredients in a big glass jar. Add Essential Oils of your choice, you could include: **Oregano, Lemon, Tea Tree, Lavender, Rosemary, Peppermint** or **Lemongrass,** or all of them! Most Essential Oils are anti-bacterial and anti-microbial, but the ones above are the best Anti-Viral Essential Oils to use. In my personal blend, I used 13 different Essential Oils. I ascertain which quantity of oils to add by deciding what action, as well as scent, I most wish to employ at what level. Plan a **hierarchy** of the most important oils that you want at the highest concentration, and other lesser amount/helper oils in lower amounts, gauging your recipe by how much help you need from each. For this particular blend we want the KILLERS here, powerful antibacterial and antiviral essential oils. Their maximum effectiveness enhances, and will make up for, any lower alcohol content.

Shake Liquids and Essential Oils together briskly for more than 100 shakes, vortex the liquid in both directions and let it sit (we call it "cook") for at least an hour. Strain through a wire mesh strainer to remove any Aloe chunks that could clog your misters. Pour 8-12 oz. into a measuring cup at a time, and be diligent about shaking and stirring with a spoon as you pour into the bottles. Shake again and stir again each time while filling until your bottles are all nicely topped off. This product has a distinct moisturizing effect and doesn't destroy the skin as much as store-bought!

Makes 5+ bottles at 4 oz. each, 10+ bottles at 2 oz. each. Use the extra to top off any old sanitizers you may have hanging around. Wipe the counters & surfaces with the rest! If you leave out the Rosewater, Glycerin, and Aloe, and add 4-6 oz. of **White Vinegar** this would make a wonderful **Disinfecting Household Surface & Glass Cleaner,** as well.

LACTATION SUPPORT

Breastfeeding is the most natural and beautiful act of Love, and every woman can do it. Breast-feeding provides a type of nutrition that is clearly **supernatural** - beyond what regular feeding could provide, even with the best of ingredients. Breast Milk is even referred to as "Liquid Gold."

The composition of Breast Milk changes with EVERY SINGLE feeding as the Mother's body adjusts to the changes in her baby. Yes, the Milk is altered in response to the baby's saliva to create a perfect-for-the-moment formula, exactly what the baby needs. There are many benefits beyond bonding (which is significant) and nutrition. Studies show breastfed children have better learning abilities when they become of school-age, demonstrate advanced brain development, perform skills sooner, and have much greater disease resistance.

The goal is to INCREASE MILK PRODUCTION & SUPPORT BREAST-FEEDING. All of these foods would be great to add to your diet to increase and fortify your milk, while supporting and deeply nourishing the Mommy as well as the Baby all through the Pregnancy. If milk production is an issue, increasing water intake and adding more juices alone may solve the problem. The super helpful foods make a real difference.

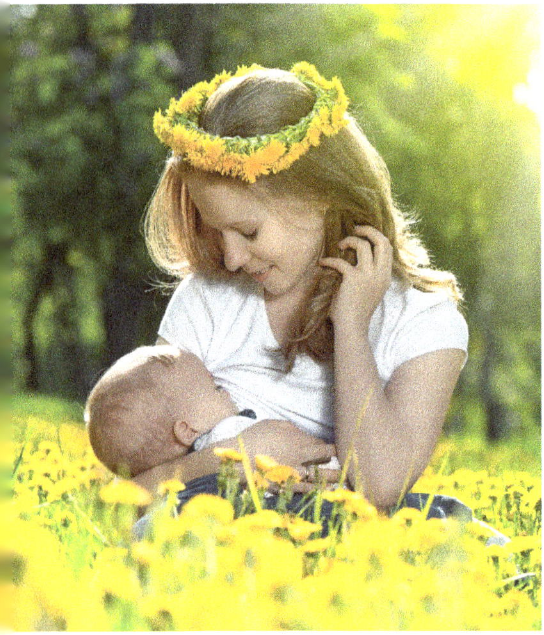

Breast Milk is made of mostly sugar and water (LOTS OF WATER), with vital minerals and nutrients, including only about 1-2% protein content. It is very high in carbohydrates and glucose, which assure healthy brain development. Excessive protein and fats consumed by the Mother will *not* stimulate better Milk, and may actually decrease production. If you are craving sweets, then you need more Fruit and Potatoes along with the supportive foods below. Breast Milk alone can feed and sustain a baby for over a year. It is absolutely your most natural source for **foundational, PERSONAL nutrition** that is vital for creating a healthy new person. Feel the power of being a Provider for your baby. Use your imagination to picture your breasts (gently and comfortably) **full of UNLIMITED, ambrosial, nutrition-filled Liquid Life**. When you speak of it, always affirm out loud that **"I always have more than enough Milk for my babies."** Deeply nourish your own remarkable body, your baby and your Milk.

FOODS & HERBS FOR LACTATION NUTRITION

- Alfalfa
- Almonds
- Apricots
- Asparagus
- Avocados
- Bananas
- Barley
- Barley Grass Juice & Powder
- Basil
- Beef
- Beet Greens
- Beets
- Bell Peppers
- Blessed Thistle
- Blueberries
- Brewer's Yeast
- Broccoli
- Broccoli Sprouts
- Brown Rice
- Butternut Squash
- Carrots
- Chia Seeds
- Chicken
- Chickpeas
- Cumin
- Dark Chocolate
- Dark Leafy Greens
- Dates
- Dill
- Fennel
- Fenugreek Seed & Tea (only after baby arrives)
- Freshly Sprouted Sunflower Shoots (keep milk ducts from clogging)
- *Gaia* Lactation Support Tea & Caps
- Garlic
- Hemp Seeds & Oil
- Holy Basil
- Kale
- Lentils (& Lentil Sprouts)
- Millet
- Moringa
- Mother's Milk Teas
- Oats (in muffins & cookies) & Oatmeal
- Oils & Good Fats (Avocado, Coconut, Olive)
- Okra
- Oranges
- Organ Meats
- Poppy Seeds
- Pumpkin Seeds
- Quinoa
- Raw Honey
- Root Veggies
- Russet & Yukon Gold Potatoes
- Salmon
- Sardines
- Sauerkraut & Kimchi
- Seaweeds
- Shellfish
- Spinach
- Sprouts & Microgreens (nourish New Growth)
- Sesame Seeds (Black & White)
- Strawberries
- Sunflower Seeds
- Sweet Potatoes / Yams
- Tofu
- Unripe Green Papaya
- Winter Squash

Bathe in, use a hot compress, or try Breast Massage with **Anise, Dill** or **Fennel Essential Oil** highly diluted **(to 1.5% concentration to be safe)** to relieve pain and help milk expression. This works out to be about **1-1½ drops of total essential oils** (no more) **per teaspoon** of carrier oil or Aloe Vera gel.

My awesome Jackson friend, **LOLO (Lauren Pritchard)** world-famous Superstar, Broadway baby and Grammy-winning singer/songwriter, had her baby boy, **Xander**, in 2020. She had a brief challenge with breast-feeding and sought my help. When she added foods and herbs from this List, she told me the breast milk was always there, and that *she* felt so much better. *"It all really worked! I feel like **I am finally getting the nutrition I need as a Mom**, as well. I eat so much better because of that List!"* Pregnancy is exceedingly "draining." Moms need nourishment, and deep nurturing for themselves

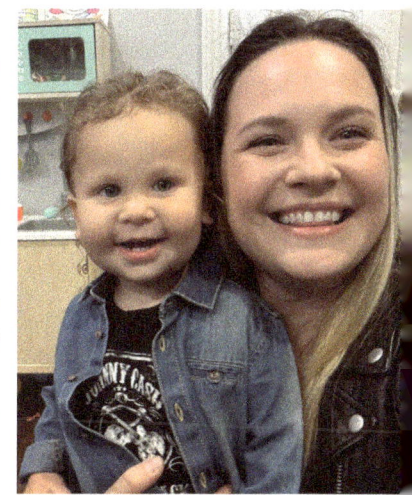

at this time more than ever! Even postpartum depression can be reduced with the use of fresh foods and good nutrition. Give yourself and your baby the very best.

WATER-GIVING MUDRA
VARUNA MUDRA

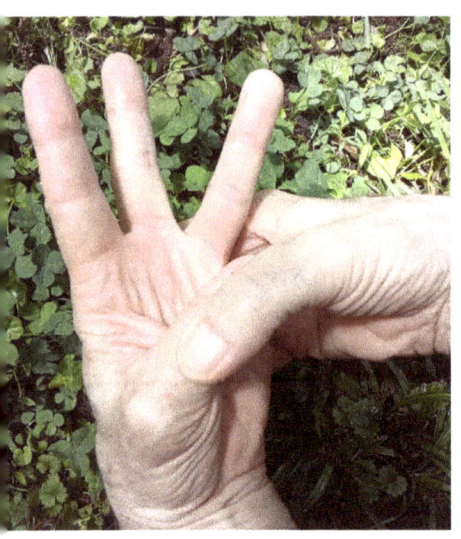

Open the hand, place the tip of the Thumb on the fingernail of the Pinky finger pressing it closed, and hold other fingers out straight, gently relaxed. Apply a gentle pressure. Hold around it with the other hand, Thumb on top over the Thumb & Pinky, and the other fingers gently cradling the hand. Try to work up to holding for 10-15 minutes. Think about FLOW and liquid support raining down on you bringing superhydration. Varuna means "rain" in Sanskrit and is also the Rain God of the Water Element.

This is a **CLEANSING NECTAR MUDRA**. It increases the Water Element in the body, to nourish and supply a Mother's Breast Milk. But it is also great for anyone with dehydration, dry skin, dry mouth, joint pain, psoriasis, tendon inflammation, constipation, loss of taste, and skin, lymph or tongue disorders. This Mudra inspires confidence and helps release inner turmoil. It washes away negative emotions as it removes toxins and pernicious water. Water is the essential fluid in our 70% Water bodies. Visualize the steady flow of water that waves in and out of every cell of your body, reviving and plumping them up with moisture. Imagine perfect skin, perfect moisture balance, perfect health with abundance to spare. If you are nursing, imagine and affirm your Breast-Milk is plentiful, nourishing, and can be endlessly given and replenished. Give gratitude for your body and this resource.

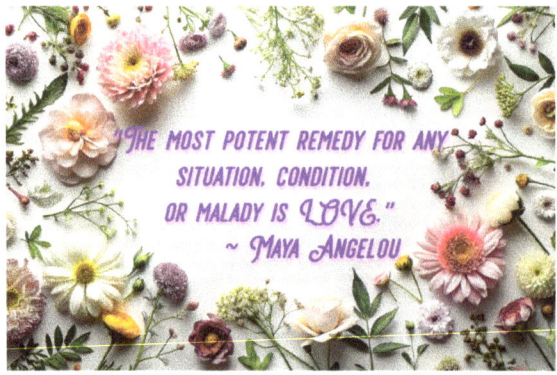

"The most potent remedy for any situation, condition, or malady is LOVE."
~ Maya Angelou

PREGNANCY SAFETY

PREGNANCY PAUSE: USE ESSENTIAL OILS A LOT LESS

I do not normally recommend Essential Oils for use in Pregnancy or Nursing (*and never for internal use*) because they are such concentrated medicines that will travel through the bloodstream or Milk directly, and can overwhelm a growing baby. This is a good time to **step back from strong-smelling medicines** and use only the gentlest of remedies in teas and infusions. **"Babying"** both of you is the idea. And remember what you put IN your body, as well as what you put **ON** your body will get into the **bloodstreams of BOTH of you**. Search your house and eliminate unnecessary household chemicals and poisonous cleaners, as well as personal care products with devious preservatives and harsh chemicals. Use only the most organic, non-GMO, all-natural and gentle body care for the whole family.

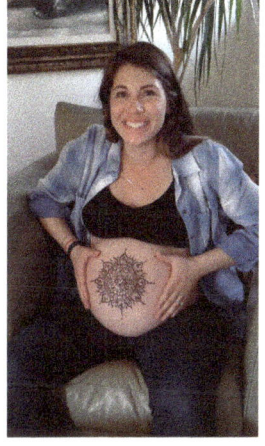

The exceptions within Essential Oils would be the use gentle Floral Essential Oils like **Lavender, Chamomile, Tangerine,** or **Ylang-Ylang** in no more than a **1.5% dilution,** for topical use only. A gentle topical salve or massage oil can serve many purposes: prevent stretch marks, condition perineum for birthing, treat cracked nipples, and soothe cradle cap and diaper rash on the baby. If you choose to vaporize them in the air, single drops only of the gentlest Floral essential oils like **Lavender, Ylang-Ylang,** and **Chamomile** would be the safest for atomization use. **Definitely unplug, remove (or never buy) artificial fragrance atomizers (air fresheners) if you have a new baby at home. They are very overwhelming, poisonous and damaging to the baby's lungs and developing organs (dangerous as well for adults).**

It is always wise to have on hand a List of Herbs & Oils that should be avoided because they could be harmful to pregnancies. Just to be extra safe, **stay away from these Plants as foods, supplements, essential oils or in tea while you are carrying a child**. Many of these herbs have a *downward motion energy*, or are simply much too stimulating. This is exactly the opposite of the supportive, secure, calm, containing energy a Mother needs.

Remember, as a Mother, your responsibility is to nurture, and to provide a safe, secure Sanctuary for your little one. Guard your thoughts as well as your physical environment. **Don't dwell in fear, anger, doubt or worry. Those frequency waves of negative emotions will travel to your baby.** Work every moment to be Mindful, filled with JOY and Gratitude, for their sake!

HERBS TO AVOID DURING PREGNANCY

Angelica	Devil's Claw	Motherwort	Rue
Barberry	Dong Quai	Mugwort	Sage
Black & Blue Cohosh (except for last month)	Epazote	Nutmeg	Saw Palmetto
	Ephedra	Oregano	Senna
	Fenugreek	Oregon Grape Root	Shepherd's Purse
Black Walnut	Feverfew		Tansy
Borage Oil	Ginseng	Osha	Thuja
Cascara Sagrada	Goldenseal	Passionflower	Tobacco
Cat's Claw	Hops	Pau D'Arco	Uva Ursi
Cayenne	Horseradish	Pennyroyal	Vitex
Clover	KavaKava	Rhubarb	Wild Yam
Comfrey	Lady's Mantle	Roman Chamomile	Wormwood
Concentrated Aloe Vera Juice	Licorice		Yarrow
Damiana	Maidenhair Fern	Rosemary	Yohimbe

ESSENTIAL OILS TO AVOID DURING PREGNANCY

Angelica	Clary Sage	Marjoram	Sage
Aniseed	Dill	Mugwort	Star Anise
Basil	Eucalyptus	Myrrh	Tansy
Bay Laurel	Fennel	Myrtle	Tea Tree
Birch	Feverfew	Nigella	Thuja
Bitter Almond	Frankincense	Oregano Parsley	Thyme
Camphor	Ho Wood	Pennyroyal	Wintergreen
Carrot Seed	Hyssop	Peppermint	Wormwood
Cayenne	Juniper	Pine	
Cedarwood	Lemon Balm	Rosemary	
Cinnamon	Lemongrass	Rue	

In all these ways you will influence the very primordial waters running through both you and your baby. Reading, singing, telling stories and playing lullabies for the baby in the womb bring amazing results. Encourage all members of the Family to introduce themselves and converse with the baby. This produces instant recognition when the baby hears their voices outside the womb! Treat the entire Family to the beauty of gestation - a growing phase of connecting through music, words, and positive vibrations, with time for the fondest and most devoted, loving care.

~ the garden of earth ~

✺ EFFORTLESS SLEEP ✺

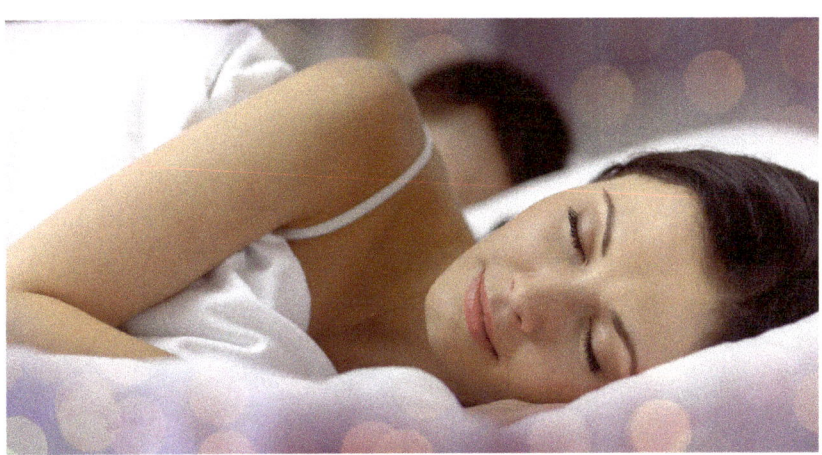

Peaceful, thorough and restful Sleep is so important. It is generally foiled in three different ways: by **overfiring nerves**, a **restless mind**, or a **hyperactive body**. It can be helpful to treat sleep disruption and insomnia on *all levels*, and also identify which type of insomnia or night-waking you have, and its pattern. If you awake at the same time every evening, check a Traditional Chinese Medicine clock for what hours you are most disturbed. This is a good indicator of areas or organ systems you might want to treat first. For example - **"Liver Time" is 1-3 o'clock in the morning** - a very popular night-waking time, which indicates the Liver needs some love. Sleep-supporting foods and soothing, dark, before-bed relaxation practices can greatly influence a good night's sleep. Some Eastern cultures suggest a *"Golden Hour"* during which you drink hot Golden Milk (Turmeric, Cinnamon, Cloves and other spices in Coconut milk) and wind down with calming, non-electrical influences only, for the last hour before bed. Put your electrical clocks and devices far from the bed and have no electrical stimulus nearby. Dim the lights and prepare for Perfect Sleep.

I have read recently that you can't be in a sleep or deep meditation state while your brain and visual states are still engaged and hard at work. That doesn't mean you go blank or fight what comes through, but the idea is to disengage your mind and let everything flow and go. I drain my brain, and make lists of all the things I need to think about while I am still preparing to go to the bedroom. I leave all my worries behind before I get to bed. The time for thinking is over once I cross the threshold into the bedroom.

Visualizing Green Landscapes can soothe you and help you fall asleep. Slowly repeating the Mantra "Sleep, sleep, sleep," can help. A nice soothing Aromatherapy Bath with any of the Essential Oils above works wonders, especially with Epsom salts (which are muscle-relaxing magnesium sulfate). I created a wonderful formula for Little Moon Essentials called *"Sleep Comes Easy"* and it is available in Bath Salt, Salve, Spray and Lotion at **www.littlemoonessentials.com/**.

Eat some of these foods later in the day. Make teas of the herbs or get tea blends, and dedicate your last few hours before bed to soothing yourself, slowing everything down.

SLEEP-PROMOTING FOODS & HERBS

Almonds	**Hops**	**Oats**	**Turkey**
Bananas	**Kiwi**	**Passionflower**	**Turmeric/Golden Milk**
Black (Forbidden or Purple) **Rice**	**Lavender**	**Peppers**	
CBD Oil or Caps	**Lemon Balm**	**Reishi Mushroom**	**Valerian**
Chamomile Tea	**Motherwort**	**Sleepytime Tea** (double-bag)	**Vitex**
Cherries	**Magnesium Caps, Powder, or Foods (pg. 262)**	**Tarragon Tea**	**Walnuts**
Cloves		**Tart Cherry Concentrate**	**Warm Milk with Clove Powder** (plant-based better for acid-prone people)
Fish	**Milk & Eggs**		
Homeopathic *Ignatia Amara* (for grief & constant mind-churning)	**Mushrooms**	**Tension Tamer** (Tea, double bag)	
	Nutmeg	**Tomatoes**	
	Nuts & Seeds		

Personal rituals have a lot to do with sleep quality. Essential Oils offer many wonderful ways to prepare for bed. A fast-working remedy is to massage the feet with one or more of the following sleep-inducing Essential Oils, diluted in a Tablespoon or so of carrrier oil. The skin of the feet is so thin that the potent medicines can easily penetrate and sweep through the bloodstream quickly, relaxing muscles, calming the mind, and causing chemical changes that support the body to fall asleep naturally.

SLEEP-PROMOTING ESSENTIAL OILS

Bergamot	**Coriander**	**Neroli**	**Chamomile**
Cedarwood (for restless legs)	**Frankincense**	**Peppermint** (tiny sniffs may prevent sleep apnea and snoring)	**Sandalwood**
	Jasmine		**Sweet Marjoram**
Clary Sage	**Lavender**		**Ylang-Ylang** (calms mind)
Clove	**Lemon**	**Roman**	

Binaural beats, relaxing music, ocean or bird sounds or white noise helps some people fall asleep. Writing out a list of things you want to do the next day, or writing in your journal can help the mind to let go. Any practice that lowers anxiety like deep breathing, meditation, yoga, tai chi, or gentle stretching can support sleep relaxation.

~ the garden of earth ~

SLEEP ANTENNA MUDRA
SHAKTI MUDRA

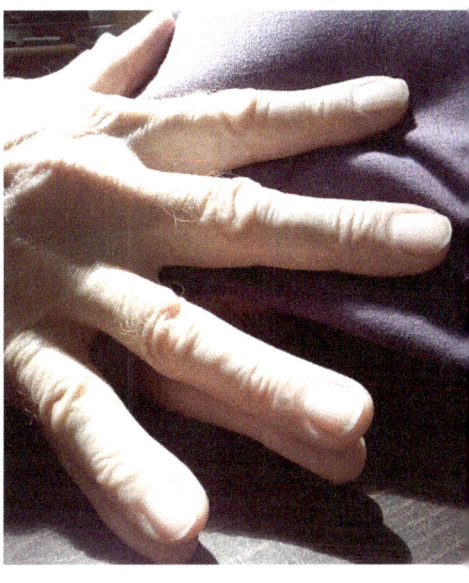

Place the hands together with the tips of Ring and Pinky fingers touching while you hold the pillow or blanket between the other fingers. Or drop your other fingers loosely toward the palm with the thumb inside. Let go of all thoughts, cares and worries. Look up toward your third eye with your closed eyes and feel the day slip away as your consciousness shifts. Slow down and rest here, as you let yourself drift peacefully away.

This is the **CREATING THE SLEEP VIBES** Mudra. I think of this one as an *"Antenna to Dreamtown."* It is practiced to slow the mind and the breathing, which relaxes the body, to foil insomnia and induce sleep. But it is also good during the day for relieving menstrual cramps, intestinal spasms, and pelvic tension, and to promote deep breathing. This Mudra soothes mental stress, and can also be used when you need to chill out and to relieve impatience. Naturally, holding the Mudra for too long can cause sleepiness and lethargy.

A bizarre sleep remedy is to **moisten the outer and inner sides of both legs with a damp cloth and go to bed without drying them**. Don't ask me why this works!

Second Sleep - sometimes it is worthwhile to sleep in segments. The idea of two separate sleep sessions has been studied, and shown to provide some people with better rest. If you wake up enough to get out of bed, do so - and use the time to read, write in your journal, drink a cup of tea, eat an apple, meditate, express, play music, or relax until you feel another natural call to drowsiness begin to come on. Then follow your night-time routine again and sleep for a second segment. I appreciate knowing this can be good for the body, because I often sleep this way and really enjoy it. I find that secret time perfect to play with the animals, and set up for my day. Segmented sleep requires acceptance (not getting bent out of shape that you are awake) and can really work. The magic comes with what other cool things you do with the time.

We like to have some **"24-Hour Time"** during each week when we can detach from the clock and follow our body's own urgings and rhythms all day and all night. Natural sleep patterns emerge and you can feel your body relax into its own pace. Sometimes the body wants a nap and it should be able to get it whenever, at whatever time! With so little we can control these days, it is nice to have some TIME OFF THE CLOCK.

▲ TESTOSTERONE-BOOSTING ▲

Men need special nutrition for optimal hormone-production. It might be hard to hear, but it all starts with **the diet and your habits**. It is imperative for men to **lower or eliminate sugar intake** as they get older. Sugar lowers Testosterone by 25%. Smoking and alcohol intake will lower it even further. **Cut out Seed Oils** (*Canola, Soybean, Safflower, Flax, Cottonseed*) and processed food. Examine and optimize the diet and exercise regimen for healthy lower weight if it seems necessary. **Sunshine** stimulates Vitamin D (actually a hormone) which in turn supports other hormones for testosterone production. So get Sunshine every day if possible, and supplement with **Vitamin D Foods (page 256)** and **D3. Sun directly on the genitals** is very nurturing and can be very helpful. Testosterone is made from cholesterol, so ensuring fat intake is vital from nuts, fish and the good oils in avocado and coconut. It is important to refrain from junk-food, trans fats (bad fats), and to try not to eat plastic-packaged items. Also, **stop using conventional Mouthwash** - it kills the oral microbiome and lowers nitric oxide which affects testosterone and erectile function.

Organic produce only is recommended, as there are xenoestrogens in pesticides, and all the fruits and veggies you eat must be free of them. These estrogen-mimicking chemicals (found in most plastic) disrupt the natural hormone balance in the body and can even cause male breasts to swell. **Sleep** is an important factor in hormone production, too, and more sleep will boost the T-levels immediately. **Stress lowers Testosterone**, but participating in enjoyable, non-work projects for several hours each day will raise it. Sometimes emotional issues of submission and feeling "depants-ed" or emasculated by another will cause hormonal changes that affect virility. **Stand up for yourself** and assert your glorious masculinity in a non-threatening, mature and loving way. Adding extra **physical activity** raises your Testosterone levels as well, so does **physical touch**. The hormones and bodily responses can all be positively affected by the many benefits found in quiet time, meditation and visualization.

Medicinal Use of Your Imagination

*Raise your own Testosterone levels with Concentrated Visualization. Picture a dial in your brain labeled **TESTOSTERONE**, and simply turn it up to a higher amount. Command that the release of Testosterone be at YOUR most perfect level for optimal health. Witness this chemical release happen in your bloodstream, know that it will be so in your body. Imagine flawlessly performing at your highest level. Visualize yourself doing everything you want to do, with power and vigor, including effortless, virile performances.*

This is so effective because it is scientifically proven that the brain doesn't really discriminate between real life and imaginary thoughts. They **both** stimulate cells, actions and hormonal secretions in the brain and organs. Picture what you want, see it clearly, and declare it to be - and your body will make the necessary chemicals to make it so. Affirm your Testosterone levels are **Optimum for Health, Sex and Energy**. Give gratitude for your body and nourish yourself with your own positive thinking.

Another interesting factor for sexual health is that sexual energy is EXTRA energy. If you feel worn out from work, run-down, overtired, or even didn't eat well or hydrate that day, you might not have the physical energy for sex. This of course applies to both sexes, but I think men are less likely to realize when they are exhausted. Which is why awareness of what is going on in your body, and with your health and nourishment is so important. It affects the VITAL abilities of your most precious resources! Hormonal health is a reflection of how you take care of the whole system.

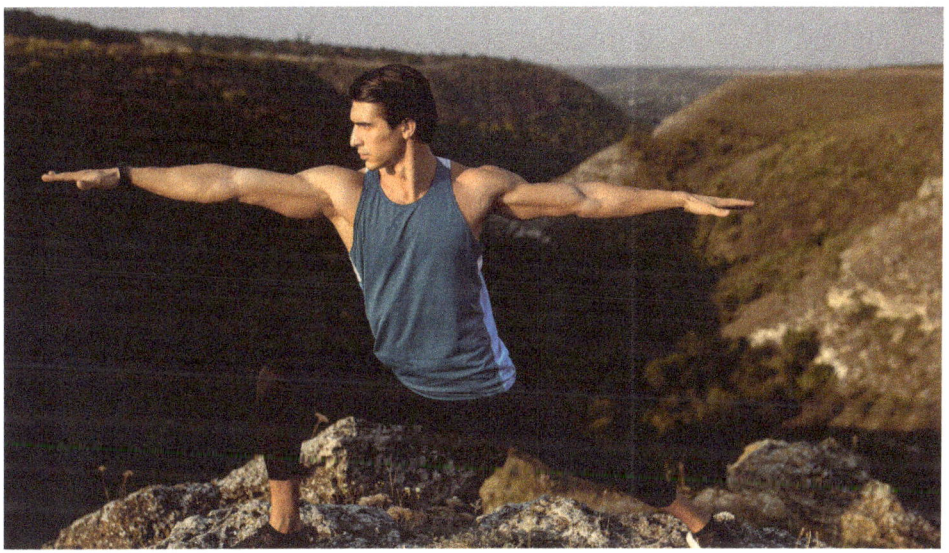

Sexual energy is considered the source of regeneration and creation. Healthy sex is a mutually beneficial action, releasing pleasure chemicals and cleansing actions that are essential for the health of both men and women. A Yogi told me the act itself is like an acupuncture treatment for both partners, with profound physical benefits.

The Spiritual Creation energy released with sex is transformative for our World, whether procreation takes place or not. If you are not making babies with it, dedicate this life force energy from your orgasms to the Earth, or for the Healing of Mankind, or for special dispensation where it is needed. This is a powerful practice.

The next step is to really focus on the diet. Make a daily effort to hydrate, quit sugar, get outdoors for daily Sunshine, get quality sleep, and support with Vitamin D foods. Eat as many of the Foods, Herbs And Superfoods on this list as you can. You'll notice that many of the items on are round (ball)-shaped, or elongated and phallic. This is no accident and is again the proof of the Doctrine of Signatures, the ancient but accurate theory that foods look like parts of the body for which they are beneficial!

Eat several foods from this list every day, add them in to your routine.

TESTOSTERONE-BUILDING NUTRITION

Almonds	**DMG**	**Lentils**	**Raw Milk** & Cheese
Ashwagandha	**Eggs** (dark yolk best)	**Licorice Root**	**Sardines**
Astragalus	**Epimedium** (Horny Goat Weed)	**Lobster**	**Sarsaparilla**
Avocado		**Maca**	**Saw Palmetto**
Bananas	**EV Olive Oil**	**Mucuna**	**Schisandra Berries**
Barley	**Fenugreek**	**Muira Palma**	
Beans	**Fermented Dairy** (Yogurt, Cheeses)	**Mushrooms**	**Shellfish**
Bison		**Mustards**	**Soy Protein**
Bone Broth	**Fish Oil/Algae Oil**	**Nettles**	**Sprouts/ Microgreens**
Brazil Nuts	**Fo-Ti**	**Nitric Oxide**	
Broccoli	**Garlic**	**Oats & Oatstraw**	**Sweet Potatoes**
Brussels Sprouts	**Ginger**	**Olives**	**Tongkat Ali**
Cabbage	**Gingko**	**Omega-3 Fatty Acids**	**Tribulus Terrestris**
Cauliflower	**Ginseng**		**Trout**
Cayenne	**Goji Berries**	**Onions**	**Tuna**
Celery	**Grapes**	**Oysters**	**Turnips**
Chia Seeds	**Hawthorn Berries**	**Pine Bark Extract**	**Veggies**
Clove Tea	**Herring**	**Pine Pollen**	**Vitamin C, D, & E**
Coconut	**Honey**	**Plant Milks**	**Walnuts**
Coconut Water	**Kefir**	**Pomegranates**	**Whole Grains**
Crab	**L-Arginine** (amino acid)	**Poultry**	**Wild Salmon**
D-Aspartic Acid	**Leafy Green Vegetables**	**Pumpkin Seeds**	**Yogurt**
Dark Chocolate		**Quinoa**	**Zinc**
DHEA	**Lean Red Meat**	**Radishes**	

I notice more bike racers in the Tour de France, Giro and Vuelta, and other extreme sports, using cotton **Essential Oil** plugs in their noses before competition, because they work so well for stamina and athletic performance! It is the same for low Testosterone. Chemical messengers in the Essential Oils will begin right away to support Testosterone production and all the other helpful hormones. All that is really necessary is that you *smell* one or more of these great scent remedies for a lift. A Massage Oil containing one or more of these oils would be wonderfully stimulating, though do AVOID CINNAMON altogether for topical use (too spicy) - smell or diffuse it only! Use 1-10 drops total in 2 ounces of carrier oil. Many of the oils with this particular stimulating action are the high florals and spicy, sensual Aphrodisiacs which are very effective for enhancing the sensual mood for both sexes!

For fastest results: place a drop or two of any one of the oils below in your palms and rub together. Inhale the scented vapors deeply and practice the Mudra below.

TESTOSTERONE-BOOSTING ESSENTIAL OILS

Balsam Fir	**Frankincense**	**Nutmeg**	**Rosemary**
Black Pepper	**Ginger**	**Patchouli**	**Sandalwood**
Blue Spruce	**Jasmine**	**Roman Chamomile**	**Vanilla**
Cinnamon	**Myrrh**	**Rose**	**Vetiver**
Clary Sage	**Neroli**	**Rose Geranium**	**Ylang-Ylang**

RISING ENERGY MUDRA
KUNDALINI MUDRA

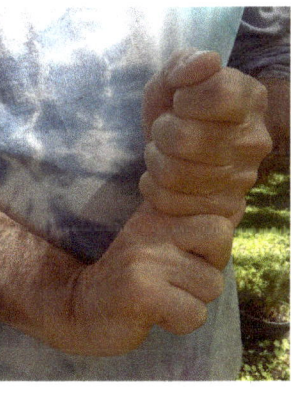

Make loose fists with both hands. Extend the left index finger and place it into the right fist from below. Place the right thumb tip on the tip of this left index fingertip. Hold the Mudra down low in front of the abdomen, visualizing red root energy rising up from the base of your spine. Allow the Kundalini to rise upwards and fill you with physical and spiritual energy.

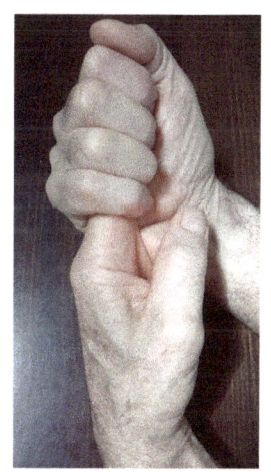

This is the **ASCENDING ENERGY MUDRA**. It is a strong activating Mudra, useful for awakening sexual desire, increasing vital Testosterone, and gently drawing Kundalini energy up the spine. It acts as a unifying force, bringing together polar energies into partnership: uniting masculine and feminine energy, individual soul with cosmic soul, physical body with the Divine. The nervous system and the endocrine system get more balanced with this posture, so hormones raise to more optimal levels. Physical energy, mental clarity, self-confidence and intuition are also strengthened, and the chakras are all activated and balanced.

*****

More Lists in the books to come. Next we meet and celebrate some very special, rebellious Plant Heroes who forever changed the way we look at the Natural World.

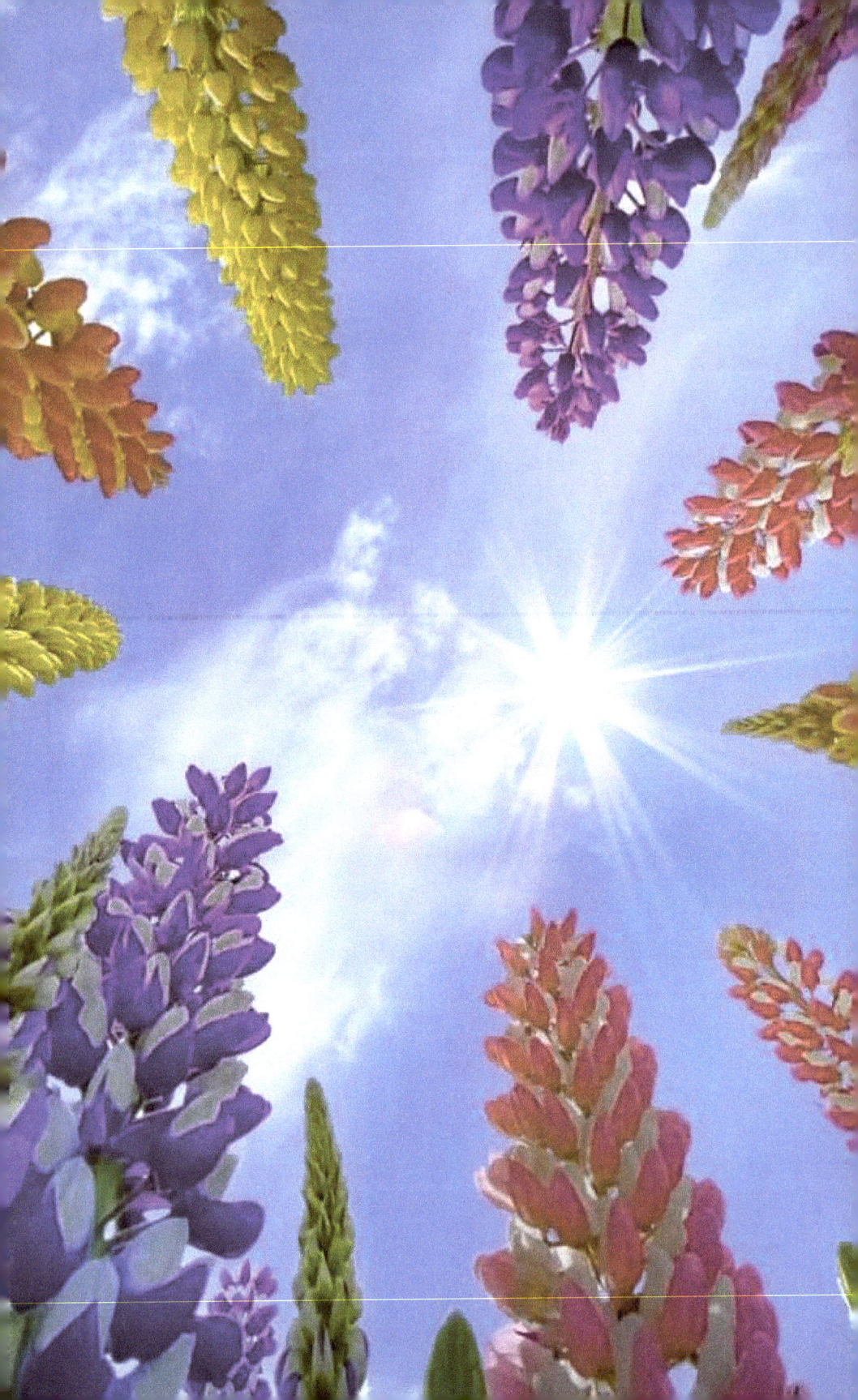

~ the garden of earth ~

~ Chapter 4 ~

REBELS OF THE GARDEN

> "These people have learned not from books, but in the fields,
> in the wood, on the river bank. Their teachers have been the
> Birds themselves, when they sang to them, the Sun when it left
> a glow of crimson behind it at setting,
> the very Trees, and Wild Herbs."
>
> ~ Anton Chekhov

REVOLUTION OF THOUGHT IS AFOOT

It sure is exciting to be alive, to witness so many discoveries in Nature, Science and Spirituality, happening all at once! Truths about the Planet we live on are being revealed every day. I am intrigued by the young (and veteran) Scientists, brave thought pioneers, stretching the boundaries of what we can discover and become as Humans. I love reading the work of these Rebels, who not only think outside of the box, but refuse to believe there needs to be a box! We all benefit from such brilliant thinking.

But my favorite stories are the ones where a great explorer found their *heart touched deeply* by the creatures they studied. They were MOVED by the Plants they befriended, or the Spirit of Mother Earth revealed. The following Rebellious Experts discovered the **MAGIC of NATURE** in their own unique ways. You will never see the World the same way after reading about these beautiful people, and their work. They are true ***Earth Heroes***, worth recognition, celebration and discussion. Their research has changed *me* to the point I felt compelled to write about them and share their mind-blowing findings with you. I rejoice in their LOVE for Earth's creatures, and continue to be ever thankful for the drive that causes people like these to REBEL!

Many of their trailblazing theories point to the conclusion that the Earth is a ***Living Being***. Journalists are even writing about it in the *Sunday New York Times!*

> **"If Earth breathes, sweats and quakes - if it births zillions of organisms that ceaselessly devour, transfigure and replenish its Air, Water and Rock - and if those creatures and their physical environments evolve in tandem, then why shouldn't we think of our Planet as ALIVE?"**
>
> *~Ferris Jabr, NYT*

This truth springs from the foundational wisdom revealed by the progressive (and persistent) **James Lovelock,** our first featured Rebel/Hero.

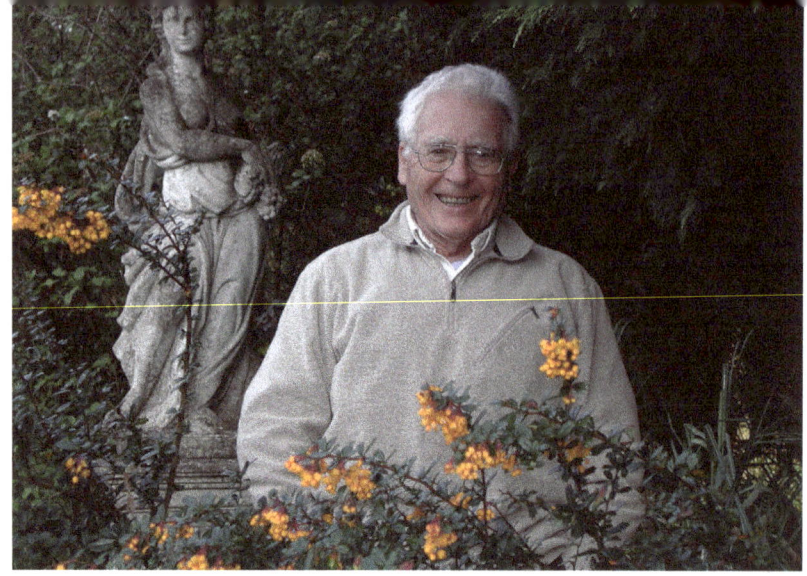

JAMES LOVELOCK

FATHER OF THE GAIA THEORY, INVENTOR, & THE ORIGINAL ENVIRONMENTALIST

Thanks to James, **we *know*** **that the Earth is alive**. He published his most famous work, *The Gaia Hypothesis*, in 1979, originally called the "Earth Feedback Hypothesis." It states that our Planet is an **interactive, dynamic, self-regulating SuperOrganism,** that is very much a functioning *living creature*. It explains that the Earth responds to what we do, with feedback we can measure. Improving the conditions here is the only way to assure our continued Life. In his words:

> **"Perhaps the greatest value of the Gaia concept lies in its metaphor of a Living Earth, which reminds us that we are part of it, and that our contract with Gaia is not about human rights alone, but includes human obligations."**

Being a part of the Gaia System has its responsibilities. At the time, his research was the very first scientific proof that the Earth was actually ***alive***. While I completely agree, many scientists of his time, and for decades, refused to accept his insight. Still today, many scientists refuse to use the word Gaia because they think it is "new agey" and unscientific. Little did they know that Lovelock named his theory after the Greek deity **Gaia** (from *Ge = Earth*, and *Aia = Grandmother*, essentially Earth GrandMother). He chose this deliberately to recognize not only her Divinity and her Feminine Goddess energy, but her vast Intelligence, Authority and **Motherly Love**. He *wanted* us to associate the Planet Earth with Family, and to feel responsible and connected to her in that very personal and beloved way.

He was publicly ridiculed for *most* of his career (until he was proven correct). The way his theories were received, it is no wonder he preferred to work alone in his lab and with Nature! He wrote more than 200 scientific papers, authored five books, received three advanced degrees as well as eight Honorary Doctorates in Science, including one from the University of Colorado, in Boulder. He held over 40 patents for his inventions, all with the intent of supporting and revealing a self-balancing Gaia. James could not be deterred by negative press and he would not relent. Eventually his outspoken rebellion on Earth's behalf paid off. It took more than 40 years, but his Hypothesis was finally accepted and is now **quite revered**. Science now recognizes Lovelock's **truth** as *The Gaia Theory* or *The Gaia Principle*.

James has since proven nearly every one of his other theories, and won many awards, citations, and worldwide recognition. He continues to express his disdain for the ever-increasing pollution of our atmosphere. He now speaks up for returning the Soul, the Divine, the Creator God to our concept of Science as well as to Gaia. He has become a surprising advocate for the unknown and the *magical* in our Universe. Love him.

But he knows, and tells everyone he can, that our actions will ultimately determine our future on Earth. For years he has been warning whomever will listen that we are breaking the fine balance of the self-regulating Earth System. Humanity's ability to grow food and sustain Life on this Planet will suffer irrevocably if we don't make radical adjustments.

> **"We need to understand the consequences of adding greenhouse gasses to the air and equally the consequences of removing natural forests for farmland; each of these acts disable the Earth System's capacity to regulate itself."**
>
> ~ *James Lovelock*

Some see him as a doomsayer, as his vision for our future without radical change is somewhat bleak. I see him as a visionary and a voice for Gaia. James Lovelock made a lifelong commitment to serve Gaia, to be the one to speak up for her, to be the Scientist Who Would. Without brave champions like James Lovelock, with his inventions as well as his desperate, persistent and passionate feelings for Gaia, we might never have understood the extremity of the damage we were doing to the Earth System. We certainly could never have measured it.

His discovery of the Electron Capture Detector *"made possible the detection of CFCs and other atmospheric nano-pollutants (DDT pesticide residues) in the air."*[21] Measuring particulates in both water and the atmosphere with gas chromatography, he was able to *illustrate* environmental impacts on this Planet for all to see. This led to the first-ever study of "air quality" and commercial emissions. His work lead to uncovering dangerous airborne poison pesticides and chemicals, which resulted in a ban of chlorofluorocarbons for the recovery of the ozone layer. He has always been a crusader for water purity, forest preservation, ocean pollution remediation and atmospheric integrity, working his whole life for our Earth.

James Lovelock's original thought, and loving connection with a Living Earth was unique in his field. But he has paved the way for other Living Earth Rebels like you and me in our own fields. It is our duty to continue his good work to find sustainable and balanced ways to work WITH and FOR our Gaia as though we were related, because we very much are. Our microcosmic needs are much the same as those of the macrocosmic Earth - when we take care of her, we meet our own needs as well. Again, as above, so below. As James so eloquently proves, we are - all of us, the Planet included - Living Relations who deserve protection, support and honor.

> **"We are the intelligent elite among animal life on Earth and whatever our mistakes, Earth needs us. This may seem an odd statement after all that I have said about the way 20th century humans became almost a planetary disease organism. But it has taken Earth 2.5 billion years to evolve an animal that can think and communicate its thoughts. If we become extinct she has little chance of evolving another."**
>
> *~ James Lovelock*

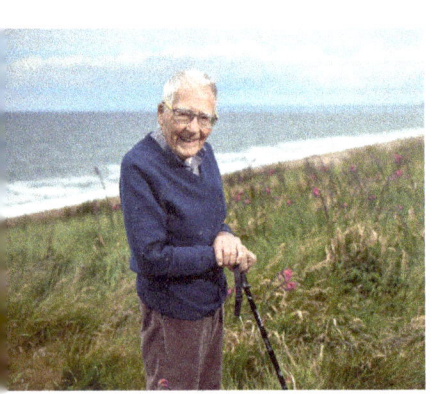

Here is James at the beach at 100 years old! We just recently lost this angel/rebel at a ripe, old 103 years of age, but he will forever be remembered as the true **Father of Environmentalism**. He is also credited with showing NASA the similarities between Earth, Mars and Venus (he invented the machines to analyze them) for which they gave him three NASA Certificates of Recognition. He said he loves to look up at Mars, knowing that his palladium-based data gathering devices (from the Viking lander) have a permanent home there. **James Lovelock**, you live on, here on Gaia, on Mars, and far, far beyond! Thank-you for everything. We hear you, and I promise we will improve as Earth Stewards.

> **"Nature favors those organisms which leave the environment in *better shape* for their progeny to survive."**
>
> *~ James Lovelock*

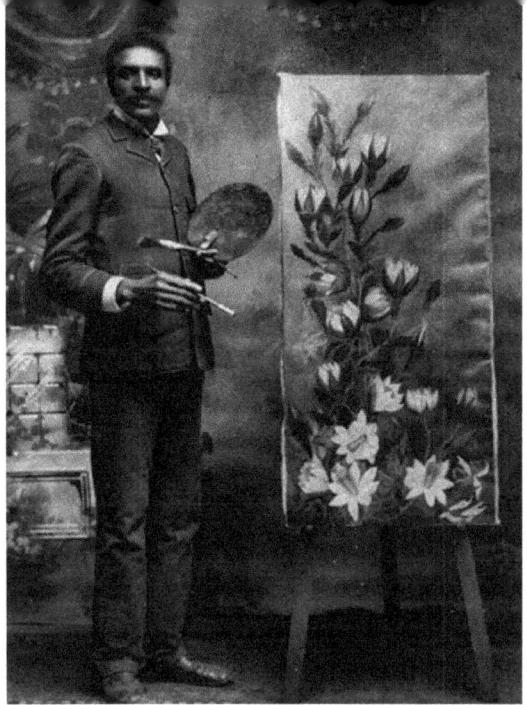

GEORGE WASHINGTON CARVER

PLANT DOCTOR & COMMUNICATOR, FOOD INVENTOR, CHEMIST, FARM PIONEER, TEACHER & ARTIST

"I wanted to know the name of every Stone and Flower and Insect and Bird and Beast. I wanted to know where it got its color, where it got its life - but there was no one to tell me."

He was born a slave on the Carver Farm, in Civil War-torn Missouri in 1860 - or maybe it was 1864, nobody knows for sure. George's Father had recently died, when he and his Mother were abducted by bandits in the night. A few days later, a rescue party found the infant child, and bartered a $300 race horse for his return. They brought George back to the plantation unharmed (though they never found his Mother). Directly after the ordeal, he was taken very ill with whooping cough (and some other undiagnosed ailments) that impaired his vocal cord growth, leaving him with a distinctive high-pitched voice. George was nursed back to health and fostered by the man who owned the farm, Moses Carver, and his wife, Susan. Moses was a friend of **Abraham Lincoln**, which may have had an effect on his kindness and willingness to raise George as his own son, instead of as a slave. They named him **George Washington** because he seemed to have an uncanny knack for speaking the truth in all situations! Moses offered him his last name Carver, and his home.

George was a special miracle even then, but he was fragile in health and needed much rest and care. He was too weak to work in the fields, so he helped in the kitchen gardens, where his mother Susan taught him to make herbal remedies. He used his leisure time to learn to sew, cook, knit, crochet, draw, play the piano and paint. At age six, he gathered wild plants and flowers from the forest to plant in his own personal botanic garden. He was known to have a special sense of color, and could draw accurate botanical portraits of the plants he loved at a very young age. He spent many hours in Nature in the forest and fields, and spoke often about his communications with Nature and with God. People say he spoke more to the flowers and animals than he did to anyone, probably because he was full of questions no one could answer!

As a child, and all throughout his life, George would have visions. The earliest vision he could remember was regarding a pocket knife he desperately wanted but could not afford. He dreamed about it one night and saw it in one of the fields on the Moses farm. The next day he walked right to the spot he saw in the dream, and found an abandoned pocketknife in an old watermelon. He soon trusted that when he had a dream or a vision, he must pay direct attention.

He was not allowed to go to school, so he taught himself to read after finding an "old blue speller." Susan Moses taught him how to write and helped him improve his reading. He began to devour books on his own, until at ten years old he found a school in the next town that he could attend. He walked eight miles to get there and home, several times a week, until he finally was taken in by some kind people and boarded for the term. He learned everything the school could teach him in one year, so he decided to hitch-hike to Kansas to go to school. There he worked as a cook, dishwasher, laundryman and housekeeper for seven years until he received his high school diploma.

George continued to watch Nature for hours after school. He talked to every flower and leaf and suggested that everyone do the same. Based on what he could see, and by doing what the plants told him, he began to devise ways to cure the sickly ones, and protect them from pests. When he was just a teenager, the neighbors would bring him their troubled plants to save, calling him the Little Plant Doctor.

"If you Love it enough, anything will talk with you."

~ George Washington Carver

He overcame many personal hardships, not the least of which was the challenge of being an educated Black Man in the South looking for colleges to attend in the 1880's. All the Southern schools would not permit him to attend, so he applied to a Northern school. He was accepted right away for his grades and was granted a full scholarship, only to be turned away the day he arrived, for his color. Hard to believe, but it was a much more cruel and segregated world back then, and George spent several years recovering from the disappointment and the rejection. But a force within him would not allow him to stop seeking.

He took many odd jobs to survive, working as a chef and even as a singer for a while, as he traveled around the Midwest. He had a chance meeting with a couple in Indianola who urged him to apply to Simpson. He was accepted and welcomed as their first "Black Student" (as they called him). George spent three years there, learning everything he could, studying piano and art. It was his art teacher who saw his botanical paintings and suggested he study agriculture at a bigger school, figuring he could make a better living teaching than painting. He transferred to Iowa State, where he was awarded his Bachelor's of Science. Then in an unprecedented move, George was invited to join the agriculture faculty (as their first "Black Teacher"), while he worked on his Master's Degree.

Always trying to be of service, George worked as a masseur for the football and track team, and developed new recovery oils to relieve their sports injuries. While teaching at Iowa, he was discovered by **Booker T. Washington**, who recruited him to run the entire agriculture department at his Tuskegee Institute, in Alabama. George meditated on his decision, and he had a vision where God told him he would be teaching great numbers of African-Americans, doing something for his people, and that Tuskegee would make that a reality. He took the position, and it was said that when a group from the school came to welcome George at the train station, they found him on the other side of the tracks talking to the flowers, stopping at every plant to introduce himself.

His true life's work began in his laboratories and farms at Tuskegee. Except that when he arrived there, they had no laboratory and no equipment and no farm from which he could teach. George built his own lab from discarded things he found: he made his own beakers from old glass bottles, fashioned crucibles out of hubcaps, and made alcohol burners from old lamps. He bought his own farm, 19 acres of the worst land in Alabama in order to study exactly how he could make it profitable (which he did in two years). He would bring his farm discoveries back to the laboratory and his students, and then consult with God and the Plants to establish details. In this unconventional way he was able to invent many natural fertilizers, fungicides and pest repellants, and make green grass grow in the arid clay of Alabama. But his greatest contribution was the concept of **crop rotation**, which single-handedly saved the Farmers, the harvests, and the fields of the South.

George's observations proved that the heavy reliance on mono-cropping, growing ONLY Cotton in the fields, was robbing the ground of vital Nitrogen and causing dead soil. He counseled that one year of rotating Peanuts into the fields as a recovery crop would remediate the soil with new Nitrogen and enhance its ability to yield a much more abundant, future Cotton crop. He encouraged the farmers to plant Sweet Potatoes, Soybeans, Pecans, and Peanuts, which provided nourishing food to the farms and their workers while revitalizing the fields.

He started a free mobile school in a schoolbus, he called the *Jesup Agricultural Wagon*. He traveled in it all over the South delivering tools and techniques, and teaching

Farmers to compost and rotate their crops. In an effort to educate every Farmer about how to approach Nature in the most successful way, he wrote more than 44 famous Bulletins and distributed them for free.

> "God is going to reveal to us things He never revealed before, if we put our hands in His. No books ever go into my laboratory. The thing I am to do and the way of doing it are revealed to me. I never have to grope for methods. The method is revealed to me the moment I am inspired to create something new. Without God to draw aside the curtain, I would be helpless."
>
> ~ *George Washington Carver*

In 1921, George successfully testified before the House Ways & Means Committee **on behalf of the Peanut**, for which he won the case and earned himself a national reputation. **Thomas Edison** became interested in his brilliant mind and offered George a six-figure salary to work with him at Menlo Park (a fortune in those days) which he turned down so he could stay in service at Tuskegee. In World War I, he was asked by **Henry Ford** to make a rubber substitute from the Peanut! He developed over 30 different dyes from clays he found locally in Alabama, which supported the textile industry during the war. He discovered a brilliant blue mineral pigment that he created via chemical reaction that appears to be exactly like the deep blue paint found in King Tut's tomb! He developed a massage oil using Peanut oil that helped heal infantile paralysis, and he replied by hand to over 3000 inquiries from worried parents to describe its simple and effective use.

Carver was a **Weed Crusader**, too; his museum features many, many products he developed using Weeds and agricultural castoffs. He showed farmers how to make positive use of their Weeds and how to eat many of them! During the Depression, his conservation ideas and wild food advice helped many families survive, and his expert guidance saved many farms. He even went to India to consult with Mahatma Gandhi about wild food sources for his people (I am sure they spoke about Purslane). Gandhi asked him what he might need to supplement his vegetarian diet and George developed a new soybean food (quite probably a tofu-like protein) he offered to Gandhi to build his strength.

George rebelled against the way *people* had always done things. He let Nature teach him new and better ways. He rebelled against the idea that race mattered at all. He just tried to be of service to everyone. He rebelled against poverty and slavery and lack of education, and he personally transcended all that and more. He believed that EVERY Human need could be met by creating products from the raw materials Nature provides. And then he'd prove it to you, by making you something naturally perfect!

Some of the items George created from PEANUTS:

Vinegar, instant coffee, candy, cheese, milk, butter, cereal, pickles, chili sauce, flour, starch, shampoo, lotion, shaving cream, soap, antiseptic and laxative medicines, remedies for goiter, cosmetics, glue, shoeblack, creosote, insulation, ink, library paste, paper, wallboard, wood stain...the list goes on and on. George Washington Carver invented over 300 products from this one plant.

They said he always wore a flower in his lapel, the love of God in his heart, and a contented smile on his face. He died in 1943, after which he left his entire life savings ($60,000) to establish the **George Washington Carver Institute for Agriculture at Tuskegee,** and a museum for his findings.

Carver's headstone says, *"He could have added fortune to fame, but caring for neither, he found happiness and honor in being helpful to the world."* It is no wonder his story lives on! Teach your children about this amazing Human Being. And please teach them to talk to Nature, as was his everlasting wish.

> **"To those who have not yet learned the secret of True Happiness, begin now to study the little things in your own door yard."**
>
> ~ *George Washington Carver*

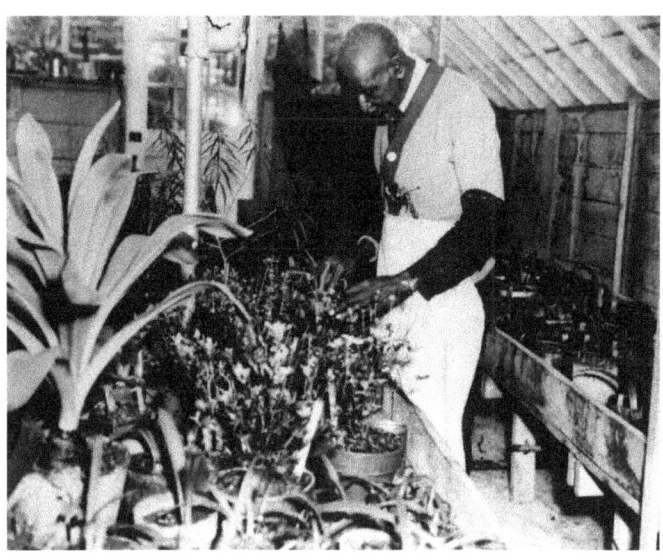

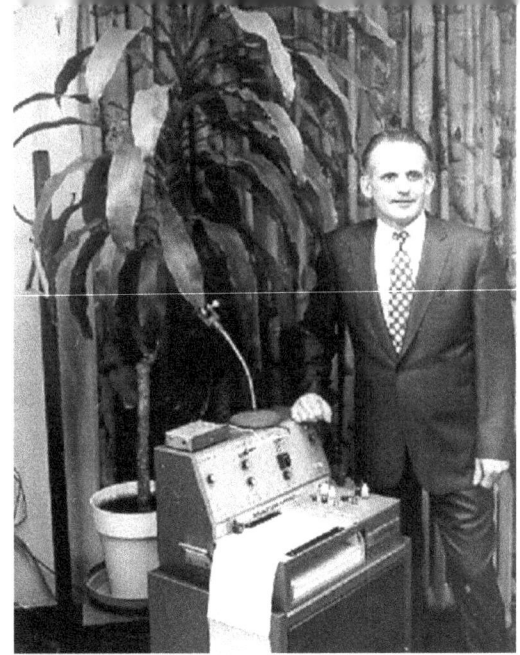

CLEVE BACKSTER

BIO-COMMUNICATIONS EXPERT
& PLANT ENERGY BIONEER

> "The Western scientific community, and actually all of us, are in a difficult spot, because in order to maintain our current mode of being, we must ignore a tremendous amount of information."

Cleve was an Interrogation Specialist for the CIA, already well-known for inventing the Backster Zone Comparison Test. This is what we laymen refer to as the **Lie Detector Test**, which is used to this day, all over the World, as the "truth" standard. Examination with his device records the body's galvanic (electrical) skin response to stress and the threat of danger, comparing it to the way the body responds to non-stressful questions. It displays the results on a long read-out tape for evaluation.

The defining moment of Cleve Backster's life came on February 2, 1966. On this momentous day, Backster was messing around in his lab in Manhattan and noticed some plants his secretary had purchased that needed watering. After deeply soaking them, he wondered how long it would take for the moisture to reach the top of the plant. He decided to use his own invention to measure a *Dracaena Cane* plant's galvanic response! He hooked the tree up to the machine, just as you see pictured to the left. To this day, Cleve Backster himself wonders why he did it, and if maybe it might have been a nudge from his subconscious. We are all very glad he listened.

One thing he knows for sure, while measuring from the plant what looked like a normal Human reading on the polygraph, he got an *enormous* response at the same moment he thought about **burning** the plant. He didn't touch it or actually burn it, he simply *thought* about it in his head. He witnessed an undeniable violent reaction (like a scream) from the plant, registering on the graph. It persisted while he got some matches, and acted as though he would burn it. The plant only calmed down when he put the matches back in the desk. He says, ***"From that moment on, my consciousness has never been the same."*** He said it was so emotional, he never tried to burn or hurt or not water another plant again. The *Dracaena* revealed that it could feel him and even hear his *unverbalized* intent. Then Cleve Backster proved we could measure it.

Plants are telepathic. He realized that Plants have a means of perception - even if we don't think they have a "brain" - that is far more sensitive than our own! They can even read our thoughts! He called this capability "**Primary Perception**," and from that day forward he devoted his life to understanding and researching this mind-blowing phenomena. He believes it is an **elemental and basic ability of all Plants**, and probably all living things, one that informs them and connects them to the Living Nature System of Earth.

Probably his most impressive case was proving the Plants could identify a killer. He had a lineup of research assistants spontaneously and randomly parade in front of a few plants as a control. Then he sent one of them out to be "the bad guy" and destroy a plant *outside* of the facility. When the researchers were paraded back in one by one, in front of the Plants hooked to the polygraph, all the Plants screamed when the perpetrator entered the room. This proved that Plants have *extrasensory* cognizance and memory, as well as a way of organizing data and processing lightwave frequencies like vision. In other words - they can recognize faces **even when they don't see them do the damage**! They can even identify the color of your hair.

Cleve discovered that the "screams" or shock event effects are only repeatable if the plant (or other subject) does not go into protective shock - and if its stimuli has been SPONTANEOUS. He proved that the observer can affect the result as well, obviously with his thoughts (when he simply thought about burning the plant he got the result). If the researcher had big plans in advance and tried to trick them, or harm them unduly, the Plants somehow knew it and would flatline. This made it difficult for others to repeat his findings, but Backster wasn't fazed because he knew what he'd discovered. He kept experimenting and validating and understanding.

Backster tested many items on the polygraph and noted their effects: egg embryos, ivy plants, yogurt, brine shrimp, flatworms, and living Human cells. In every case, he discovered that the Plants and the living Cells ***do not like anger, ugliness, violence and harm,*** and they respond profoundly. He found the Plants were overly sensitive, and became disturbed when some yogurt was dosed with alcohol (a after-hours vodka & tonic experiment) and its bacteria died, or when hot water was poured down a sink killing the microbes in the drain. With two yogurt dishes side by side, he proved that one would respond when the other was fed, in an effort to ask to be fed as well.

He tested Human cell samples that were as far as 300 miles away from their donor, and found that they would have the exact duplicate emotional reactions, regardless of distance. He proved Nature is **connected and alive and reactive** and knows what you do! He says, *"I have file drawers full of high-quality anecdotal data showing time and again how Bacteria, Plants, and so on are all fantastically in tune with each other."* The signal from the plant or cell can not be blocked by walls or lead cages, and as Backster wrote, *"it is dependent on neither time nor distance."* So it is impossible to explain - except perhaps in the realm of magic (or perhaps quantum physics).

As with most Rebels, he was highly ridiculed. His work was trivialized, and because of its sensitivity it was misrepresented as "unrepeatable" - the death knell in Science. The problem was that most testers would not reproduce his careful sequestering and skill in eliciting spontaneous reactions. The researcher has to remove his consciousness from the equation, and when you start talking like that, Scientists flee! But Backster listened to his detractors and took great pains to prove them wrong, installing switches he could hit when he performed tasks in other areas of the building, and automating tests and timing from afar. His findings *have* since been duplicated, even recorded and verified on camera for posterity. Rebel vindicated.

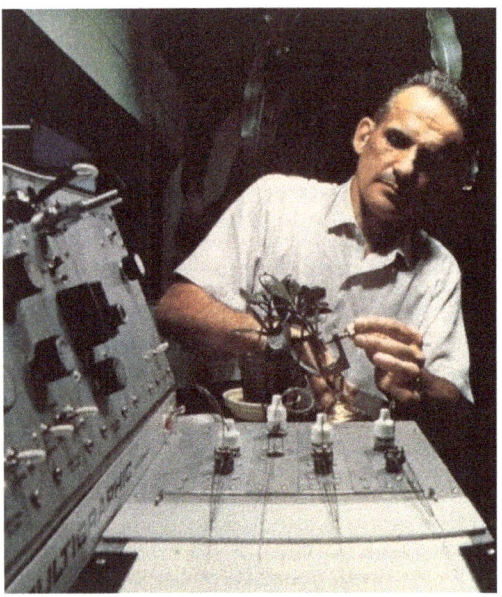

Years later, many researchers admit that Cleve Backster changed their thinking for good. They never looked at Plants the same way again. Cleve never claimed to know HOW it works, which is one of the reasons he can't be attacked. He simply performed the experiment. He devoted his whole life to proving that his results were true, he would even ultimately pass his own Lie Detector test! In doing so, he helped wake us up to the fact that **Primary Perception is indeed very real**. And he changed Scientists forever.

"I have given up trying to fight other Scientists on this. But I know that, if they perform my experiment, even if it fails they will still see things that will change their consciousness. They will never be quite the same."

~ *Cleve Backster*

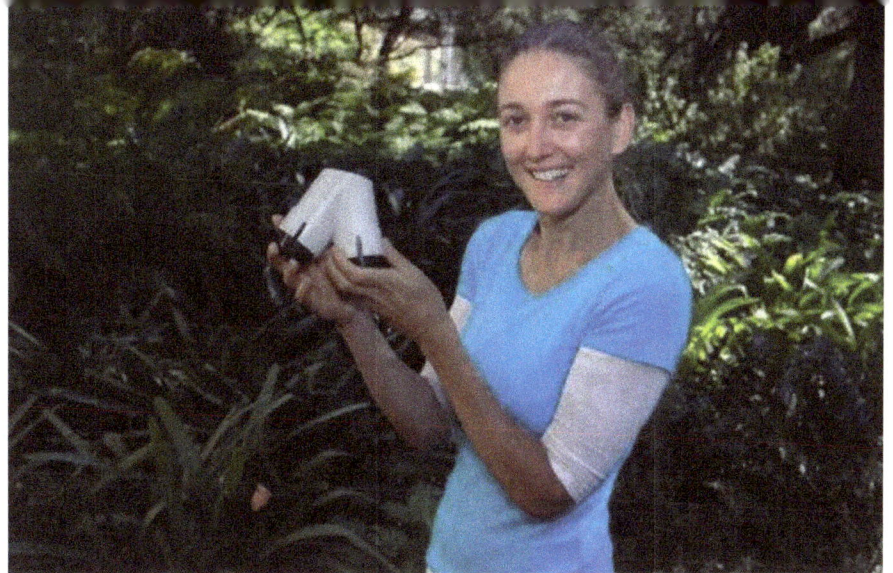

MONICA GAGLIANO

NATURE COMMUNICATOR, SENSITIVE, & COGNITIVE ECOLOGIST

"Allow for the Magical Absurdity of your subjective experience to walk alongside the objective reality of your logical mind."

Monica was originally trained as a Marine Animal Ecologist. She worked for years *underwater* at the Great Barrier Reef, off the coast of Australia. One particular Summer her life altered forever. She was tasked with documenting the mating and reproduction of pairs of Damselfish. One week into her study, she was already so non-threatening to the little fish, that they would greet her when she arrived, snuggle and gather in her hand. She was intimately close with them, studying their habits and habitat for months; she knew them and they knew her, and early-on developed a connection.

The morning before she was going to have to capture and destroy all the fish in the (murderous) name of Science, she visited them to say goodbye. Not a single fish came near her, there was not *one* Damselfish in sight. *"They knew."* It hit her like a ton of bricks; she was frozen there in the water. She realized that in her experience with the tiny fish there was a bridge between species, and a communication that actually was undeniable and real - as well as **telepathic!** They felt her, knew her mind, and realized what she had to do. That afternoon she was required to complete the study, but it was incredibly difficult. And it was her very last killing in the name of research, or for any reason. To this day, she thanks those fish for their sacrifice, revealing to her the need for **Living Research.**

She writes in her book, *Thus Spoke the Plant,* about some of the synchronistic turning points in her career. Almost overnight she was catapulted into studying the Plant World. She made a deal with the Plant Kingdom, she agreed to explore and listen in exchange for information, and many Plants called to her in the process. She realized through her many experiences (scientific, meditative, and tribal herbal rituals) that Plants will find whatever means necessary to work with you. **Whether it is through visions, dreams, imaginings, beauty, ingestion or inspiration they will find a way to *move you*.** Sometimes their messages are so magical, it is hard to believe they are real. She says Plants have never stopped teaching us, and we have never stopped learning from them.

One particular moment sparked her whole new realm of study. In 2011, in Bristol, England, scientists were studying living Corn plants, and they registered small "vegetal clicks" that the plants seemed to be making to each other. **The Corn was chirping**! They seemed to be relating information to each other with sound frequencies. Monica declared, *"And it was official. Plants emit sounds, they hear them, and on the basis of what they hear they modify their behavior."* Her inspiration to learn about this phenomena led her to a daring new field - the **Bio-Acoustics of Plants.**

She performed many interesting experiments over the last few years, delivering remarkable, groundbreaking revelations. **Plants have memory, they have feelings, they can imagine, they learn, they make choices, they communicate with sounds, they have photoreceptors to see colors, they have a value system, they make decisions, they play dead, and they can express intentions and preferences**. Because of her early horrific experience with the Damselfish, she had the experience to realize that this was not unique to Plants alone. More than likely, it was a principle of ALL OF NATURE. Once again, she thanked the Damselfish for letting her know.

It makes you realize we can hide from *nothing*, and we are being perceived by *everything*. Now that idea will blow your mind right open.

Her findings were much like Cleve Backster's, but Monica was able to regularly prove them in different ways in the laboratory. Like him, she got a tremendous push-back from the scientific community, who actually were afraid her work might be a prank or a joke. Her initial Plant Communication paper was rejected by *ten* leading scientific journals, and she wrote many papers that were laughed at by mainstream Science. She even says her colleagues would avoid eye contact with her in the halls, hoping to avoid her particular brand of infectious crazy! She lost funding and had to hope and pray for backing when she needed it most. **What could possibly keep you going** when no one believes you, and everyone ridicules you?

That you know you are right. As she so eloquently explains, there were *many* indicators she should continue her work, synchronicities that kept her going, and guidance that even came from the Plants themselves. At one point, she heard a **whisper** that she should study Peas and not Sunflowers for better results. She was shocked to find out that the Plants had been right. She tells of writing things in her diary when seeking the advice of her Plants, deep meditative insights that would later prove true - not only in the literature but in her lab. Since she made the deal with the Plant Kingdom, she realized it was her sacred duty to trust the Plants.

> "If you had this experience of connecting with Plants the way I have described - and there are plenty of people who have - the experience is so clear that you know that it's not you; it's someone else talking. If you haven't had that experience, then I can totally see it's like, "No way, it must be your mind that makes it up." But all I can say is that I have had exchanges with Plants who have shared things about topics and asked me to do things that I have really no idea about."[22]
>
> ~ *Monica Gagliano*

Most importantly, Monica was willing to listen! To rebel against what people think we know, to include the unknown and magical possibilities just like Cleve. She had to find a way to **reframe reality**, provided by her research and connection with Nature, Monica was able to open her own mind and utilize her imagination to bridge the gap between what we already know and the next amazing thing we *could* know. She had to actively engage in fantasizing *as though she was a Plant* in order to understand them better. **She had to believe they could speak, just like the fairy tales had told**. She had to be searching for their language to find it. And then, Communicating with Nature became one of the chief ways she discovered we could learn so much more, if we would only accept it is possible. In her words**:**

"You know, they just say plants do not learn and do not remember. Then you do this study and stumble on something that actually shows you otherwise. It's the job of Science to be humble enough to realize that we actually make mistakes in our thinking, but we can correct that. Science grows by correcting and modifying and adjusting what we once thought was the fact. I went and asked, can plants do Pavlovian learning? This is a higher kind of learning, which Pavlov did with his dogs salivating, expecting dinner. Well, it turns out plants actually can do it, but in a plant way. So plants do not salivate and dinner is a different kind of dinner. Can you as a scientist create the space for these other organisms to express their own, in this case, "plantness," instead of expecting them to become more like you?"

Rebelling against old thinking, releasing preconceptions, being truly open-minded is exactly what helps Scientists, and all of us, to make space for new discoveries.

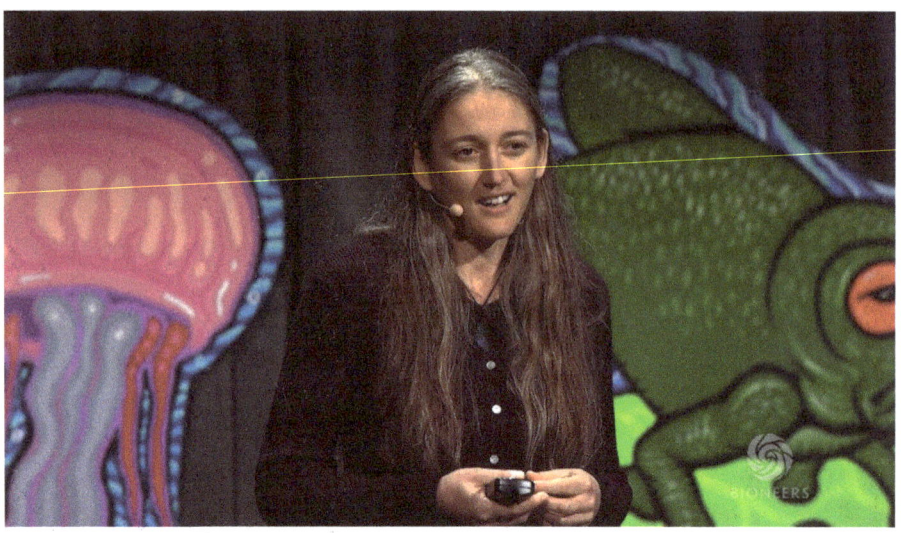

You must listen to her speak! I love everything about this **Earth Angel Rebel Rockstar** of the Natural World!

https://www.monicagagliano.com/

https://www.youtube.com/watch?v=90BUQoLu_Hg&t=727s

Her books are enchanting; her website is full of research and also full of MAGIC! This is one plant researcher who also understands, from first-hand experience in the deep jungles, the deep indigenous use of plant Entheogens. She has spent many years working with Plant Spirits, following their wild advice. Monica has so many wonderful tales to tell, and her writing is as poetic and beautiful as Nature itself. I appreciate her loving approach and her genuine surprise at the wonder of our Garden.

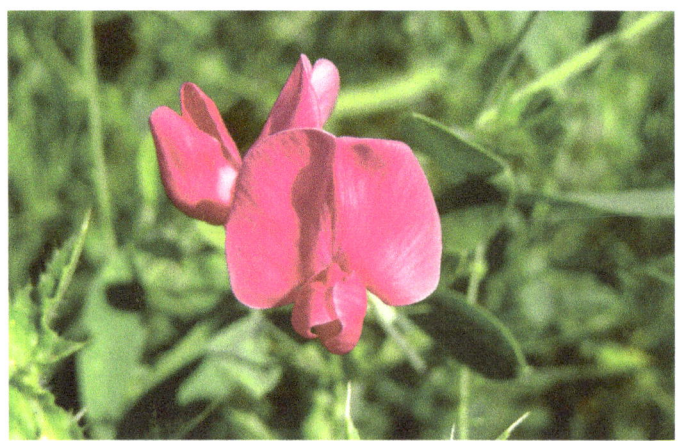

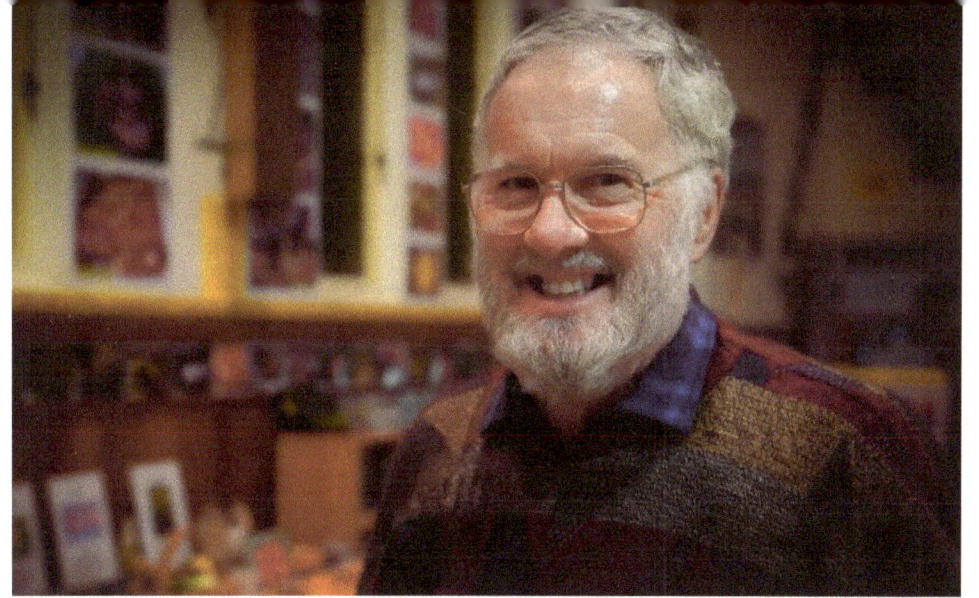

BRUCE FRENCH

OBSESSED TASMANIAN PLANT CATALOGUIST & REGIONAL FOOD REVEALER

"God has already provided the right Plants growing in their right places to sustain people in every place on his Earth."

With Collaborator and Wife **Deb French**, this wild Agricultural Scientist has identified and cataloged over **31,490** individual plants by nutritional qualities. He has compiled images and climactic details, noting the main vitamin, mineral and protein content of nearly **every plant, in every country on Earth**! His mission is to teach people to find the most nutritious plants naturally growing in *their* locations, and to give them the information they need to utilize them. He has dedicated his entire Life to *"Helping the Hungry Feed Themselves."*

Hunger is one of our most pressing Earth issues. I don't even want to cite the statistics of how many children die every day from hunger, so I won't. But these people have looked the problem straight in the eye and done something about it. Their work is an exceptional and desperate effort to avert hunger and malnutrition for **all children.** Through exhaustive and extensive research, education and information, the Frenches have saved many lives - as well as preserved *valuable* indigenous plant knowledge.

It is working! Their infinitely growing database is available online, and can save whole communities by revealing wild resources they didn't know they had, re-introducing many people to their nearby Native Food Plants.

It all began when Bruce was guest-teaching Agriculture in Papua, New Guinea in the 1970's. He discovered the Farmers (to their credit) wanted to know what **Local Plants** they could grow. Bruce was humbled to realize he had only been taught about growing Western crops, and had no real idea! At the same time, he was shocked at the level of hunger and malnutrition he saw in people living around perfectly good food sources. He set to educating himself, and in so doing, he found a true passion for identifying native plants and their nutrient profiles. As a former pastor and a man of God who was looking for what "good work" he could do here on Earth, he began to imagine a solution for *both* challenges.

> "Increasing the diversity of Food Plants available is the simplest solution to a balanced diet. What one plant lacks another will provide. Maintaining a diversity of Food Plants enhances food security. If some plants are affected by adverse weather and environmental conditions, others will still be there to provide food."
>
> *~ Bruce French*

French discovered a way to combine his interests into his mission. He looked for a wide selection of the best Food Plants in each country, the ones that could literally prevent hunger and save lives. He says it seemed like one country followed another, until he found he had researched them all! His obsessive devotion to the "undervalued and overlooked Food Plants" led him to educate people about how to eat them, as well as depend on them as a back-up resource in the case the current crops failed. He rediscovered what the Western world calls the **WEEDS!** He brought to light many THOUSANDS of little-known, HARDY native Weed species that have been, because of his work, rediscovered, studied and *eaten* as helpful foods all over the World.

> "I've been in Vanuatu and Cambodia and they have no idea their Local Plants are so good; they've got a mindset that everything that comes from anywhere else must be better. So when they suddenly realize how good their own Plants are they're delighted and they just about hug me because they like their own Plants better."
>
> *~ Bruce French*

Bruce is not so much a rebel as a **Revealer of what was always there**, a Native Plant Champion, a Food Saviour and a Weed Warrior. He showed all of us what was literally growing beneath our feet - the life-saving plants! **He rebelled against HUNGER!**

Bruce says he plans to work on his database until his dying day and he hopes to see an end to hunger. In his own humble words, *"I'm not trying to make fame or fortune. I'm interested in hungry kids not dying before they get to school."* This kind of faith-filled work for the Earth warms my heart, and deserves recognition. This man is a REAL HERO, and the *many* cultures all over the World he influenced that are eradicating hunger using their own Plants, are living proof.

Where do you keep 55 years of research? The physical sources for his online database, and thousands of his prized books and plant photos from all over the World are installed permanently at the old Gospel Hall in Burnie, Australia. You can visit and drink coffee or tea while you peruse this endless amount of vital information! This is now definitely on my bucket list.

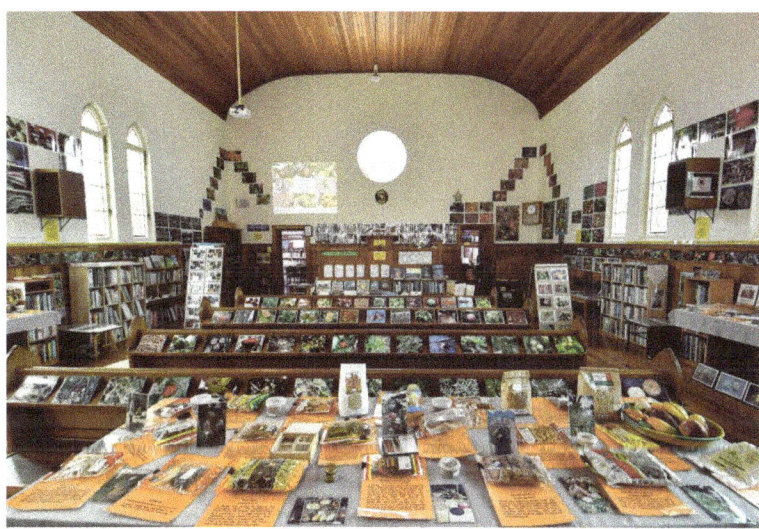

Find his extensive database here: **https://foodplantsinternational.com**

> "Commercial organizations try to make money and say, '*Keep going down the same road...using chemicals and monoculture crops.*' Non-commercial organizations say, '*No, we have to go in a different direction, holistic, integrated, sustainable food production.*' It's *these* individuals and groups who are fired up, and passionate, and love the Planet and Plants, who make me feel very optimistic about the future of the World."
>
> ~ *Bruce French*

Thank-you, **Deborah & Bruce French**, you make me feel very optimistic about the future of Humans.

*****

The next section offers many ways you can prepare, store, and keep the goodness of the Garden working for you all year long.

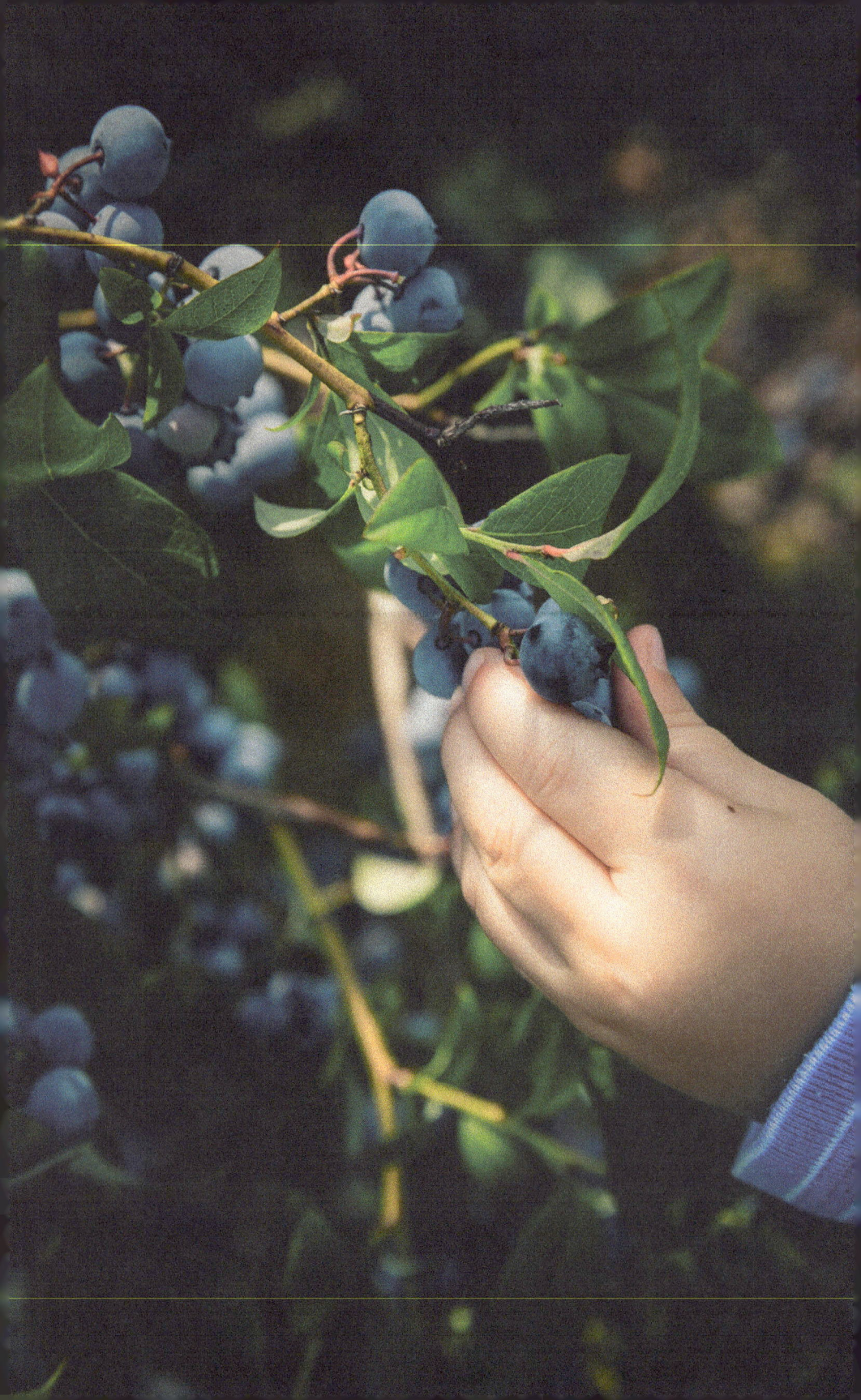

~ the garden of earth ~

~ Chapter 5 ~

PRESERVING THE GARDEN

> "We know there is a deep reservoir of Food Wisdom out there, or else humans would not have survived to the extent we have. Much of this Food Wisdom is worth preserving and reviving and heeding."
>
> *~ Michael Pollan*

STOCK YOUR SHELVES

I took a bigger interest in my *own shelves* when I found empty shelves at the stores. What did we have prepared for the Winter, let alone for some emergency? How much Food did we really have on hand? How long until we needed to shop, and would the store be open? It was humbling to realize that our modern, reliable way of life had not prepared us for any changes in access to our food. Even though just a few generations ago, our ancestors stocked and restocked their pantries constantly for just that reason. They knew it was smart to provide for themselves. **Practical skills** from their "days of old" need to be revived and preserved. In researching, I found there are many steps to Food Independence and Personal Sustenance. I wanted to take a few. What could we plant, then make from our harvest, then learn to preserve, to supplement our diet nutritionally? How could we be more independent and self-sustaining?

I found dozens of sources from the 1900's, from people living through both World Wars, where the prevailing thought was that each household needed to store and provide a **YEAR'S WORTH** of back-up food supply for themselves. Several Presidents of the United States recommended this kind of preparation for all people, and included it in their State Of The Union speeches. So this is not a new concept or a result of our own recent experiences. People of all cultures through history have learned they need to fortify their own Food Stores. Whole communities used to work together for the same. You can read ancient cultural references to the "city granaries" and still see water towers storing water all across the country. Farmers store hay for their animals for the times when the grass runs out, or is covered in a foot of snow. Being prepared is a wise and natural practice, that has simply fallen out of style for lack of any real need.

But I am encouraged that there are those who wish to revive the many great traditional skills required to preserve food, or nourish the soil, or keep "family stores." Recently, I have seen so many more books about self-sustainability and living off the land, in a wonderful resurgence of people writing about, and returning to, the Plants and their Remedies. Many highlight the ability to be able to feed your Family optimally when there's no fresh food growing in Winter, for which it is valuable to know some Food Preserving Techniques. This whole chapter is about reviving those practical preservation skills of our ancestors. I hope you will find some new inspiration in all the helpful "old" information here! These are natural skills that never go out of style.

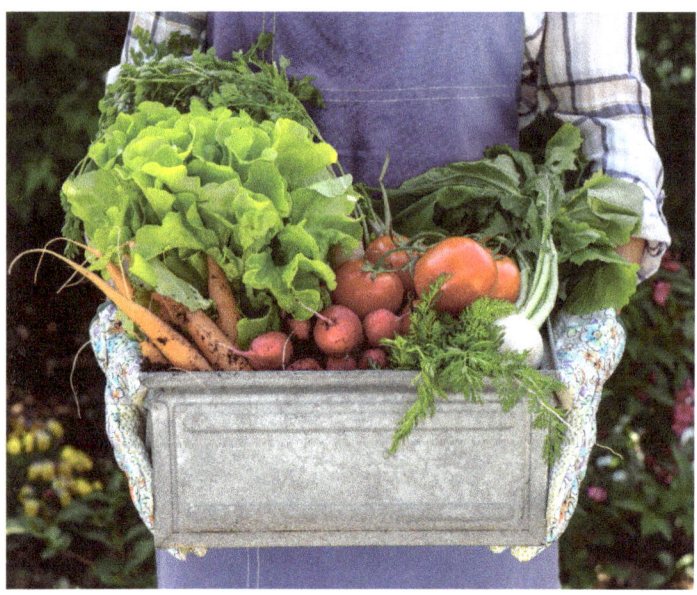

> "The kitchen is liberation. It's the conduit between the garden & the table; a ticket to self-sufficiency; a laboratory of nourishment; an upholder of food security. It makes a bold statement in a world drowning in consumerist ideals. And it's time to reclaim our ground here."
>
> ~ Jill Winger @homesteader

BEYOND SELF-SUFFICIENCY

You can easily learn how to harken back to some of your ancestor's skills for growing, preserving and storing food. I have suggestions for some cool ways of "putting up" your food. But **ask your Parents and Grandparents what they did**! Get some Generational Knowledge flowing in your Family! You want to record and preserve in some way their helpful folklore of wise old sayings and "life hacks" for your children. Get their recipes! Talk to your neighbors and friends and begin to study how other people handle their Garden's bounty. Ask the Master Gardeners at nurseries and seed companies. You know they will have wonderful ways of preserving all that they know and grow, and they would love to teach you! Be on the mission to preserve KNOWLEDGE as well as skills - and then utilize them, for the Garden's sake.

You never know what the next challenge might be. This is not meant to scare you or be a doomsday message at all, but realistic advice to help you be more self-sufficient. Everyday, things occur in our lives that we could never have imagined, bringing changes no one could have foreseen. Electricity can go out in a moment, shopping habits can be altered, storms pop up out of nowhere, fires take people unawares. You want to be prepared. When it comes to your Food Supply, keeping your families fed, it is important to try to be ready for anything.

I have fallen in love with the videos of the **Country Life Vlog (@country_life_vlog)**. In the mountains of Azerbaijan, these beautiful people gather everything they eat, and cook it over outdoor fires and in brick ovens. They gather herbs and flowers and make tea and dessert for each other. They preserve jars and jars of stores for the long Winter, all with their kitties and dogs and ducks and many wild creatures running around. These videos are truly a step back into the old ways, and watching them is one of my favorite ways to "escape to the country," relaxing with the sounds of the birds and the wild natural vistas. But I am most surprised by what I am learning from their traditional food preservation techniques!

You are the new Hunter-Gatherer. You are searching again for Food to feed your Tribe, striving to keep it healthy all year long. And by doing this yourself, you get to absolutely guarantee that all of your Food has been touched with Love and Kindness. Growing and preserving your own Food gives it the very Best Energy possible. When you co-create and interact with your Food, its very nourishment is increased, your absorption is enhanced, and much better health is the result. This is a provable fact, and is absolutely one of the reasons many cultures traditionally pray over their Food before eating. Adding your energy and your consciousness to any part of the process enriches the Food and its effects.

Assuring that you and your Family can eat abundantly and have good water is your first task. Collecting the *most nutritional value* from foods you can acquire and grow is the next step. Your pantry is your personal **health food "store"** - STOCK IT! No matter what, you will be glad to supplement your store-bought supplies with the Superfoods you are able to grow, and the many Medicinal items you can produce yourself.

I am suggesting it might be wise (and actually quite fun!) to view your food production, subsistence, health and well-being as lovingly in **your own hands**. Self-sufficiency is not just a "prepper's dream" or something for weirdos and survivalists only - it is the golden way we all lived before this age of easy-access. These are the old and wonderful ways of our ancestors, and they are skills we can learn now. Let's make a new effort to connect with Nature and let her supply our Food. And if ever we need to hunker down someday with what we have made and stored and kept at home to feed our Families - well, won't it be so awesome to have a pantry full of goodness?

At the very least it might mean the difference between serving freshly canned garden food instead of whatever artificial, shelf-life-infinite "boxed-up food" the store happens to have this week. It's always smart to be thinking about how to be more independent of unhealthy, vulnerable, unpredictable, and possibly unreliable systems.

PRESERVED NUTRIENT SOURCES

Your own homemade sauces and sauerkrauts and canned food will give you better quality, healthier Food choices than you can find in the stores, all year round. Their potent fresh nutrients will be so good for you! And, it's easier to accomplish than you think. You can make it a fun Family tradition, or a "weekend with the girls" project. I find it is very fulfilling to share with others the process of making Food exactly the way you want it! You can make it taste your way, or make it without any sugar, or tailor something specifically for your health. You can make sauces and stock that are more concentrated than store-bought, to add your own intense flavor when you need it. You can prep whole meals ahead of time and have easy-to-prepare food in your freezer. With a little extra effort you will find you have so many more options available to you.

Studying the skills and guidelines in this chapter will lead you to many discoveries: how you can feed yourself, invent new foods, provide nutritionally dense herbal remedies for your family's immune health, and increase your own pantry stores with ease. Besides what I have shared here, there are so many *other* ways to preserve your garden wares or prepare your pantry for winter: Brining (similar to pickling but requires refrigeration), Smoking, Salting, Freeze-Drying, Powdering, and many others you can research. While I haven't the space to go into *every* preservation method, all of these would be worthwhile to research and practice. I also share some of my favorite recipes so you can create Food Gifts for others with all of your Abundance!

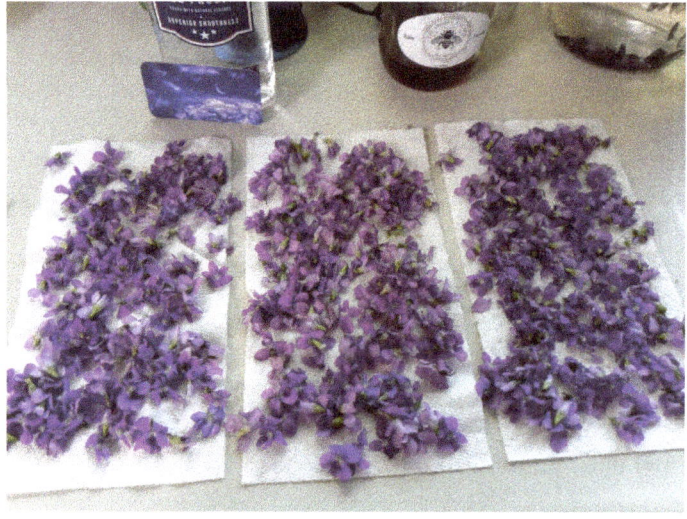

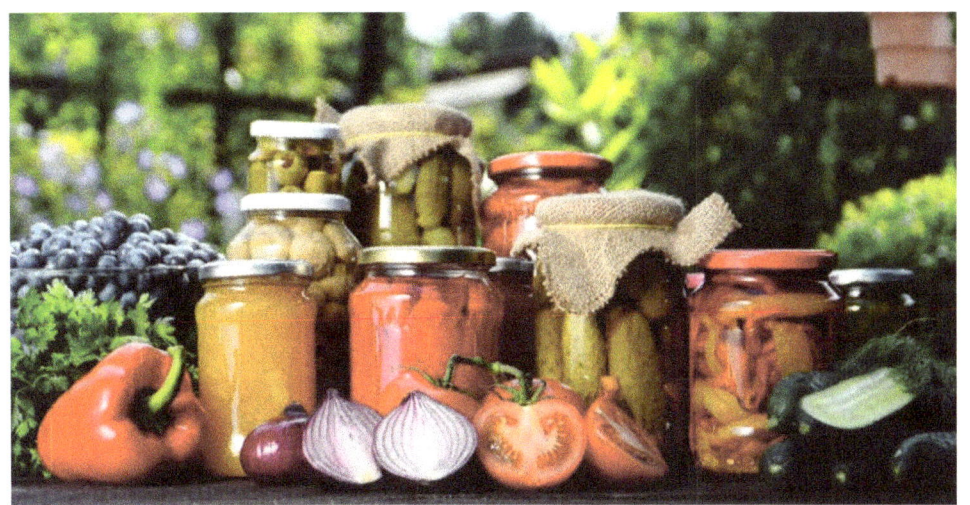

CANNING
produce your own abundant stores

When I was little, we had an enormous Golden Delicious Apple Tree in the backyard. When I think of it now, I can almost taste the amazing food it provided for us. But as a child of eight or nine, with my Little Sister LeeLee in tow - having to pick up the Apples was the *bane of our existence*. Oh I mean, we *hated* it. I personally complained to no end about the worms and the smell and the decaying apples being all schmushy - it sure didn't seem like a miracle to me. But then my Mother would take the bags full of apples we brought in, and turn them into Apple Pies and Applesauce and Clear Apple Jelly and deep Brown Apple Butter! My sister and I would watch in amazement as she made jars and jars of delicious stores from the fruits of our "hard" labor. The house would smell good for days. Because of her and that Tree, all through the Winter, everybody in our Family would be eating and shining in full Apple-cheeked glory. I remember thinking, even then, *"This is all free food we made ourselves! And from just one Tree!"* Somehow, the next year of apple-picking wasn't half as bad (I developed a quick eye for the good apples) and I knew what was coming when we brought in our bags. Now I wish for my own Apple Trees, I want an orchard! And a lot of canning jars.

Canning may seem a little old-fashioned, but it is having a popularity surge. During the pandemic you couldn't find canning supplies in the stores because so many people were doing it! I believe some people, having more time for themselves and also a greater need, started to revive the old ways. In fact, so many people decided to learn how to bake their own bread that there was no yeast in the grocery stores for months! Some great ideas never go out of style, and making and preserving your own Special Foods is one of them. Canning is a great way to take advantage of sale items at the Farmer's Market, your incredible overabundant harvest, or the bushel you "had to buy" of Peaches! And you usually make enough to share, which is quite nice, too.

For many gardeners and wild fooders, Canning is a welcome yearly practice to preserve all the beautiful fresh food they grow and forage. For others it may be something they do for neighborhood gifts or holiday presents. Some people are Canners because it is economical. We remember the older generations in our families Canning up a storm. This is surely because they learned, in lean war times and recovery boon times, too - that it *saves so much money* to make your own food.

Canning is a special skill you may never use, but if you do, watch out - you may become obsessed with it! Especially if you have abundant garden produce, it is a perfect way to save the nutritional value of your freshly-grown foods for later in the winter when there are none. One day you may feel inspired to "put up" some goods for your Family this way. When you crack open that jar of Homemade Heirloom Tomato Sauce, everyone will be glad you acquired this stunning ability.

IMPORTANT BASICS of CANNING

For many years the gold standard for canning instruction was the *Ball Blue Book: The Guide to Home Canning*, from the Ball Jar people. You can find the original as well as fully revised copies of it on the internet and in used bookstores. As more and more young writers are discovering the many benefits of Canning, beautiful new books are being written, too, with modern features like low-sugar and diet-specific recipes. Check out the National Center for Food Preservation site for some great suggestions, helpful pictures tables and tips at **https://nchfp.uga.edu/how/can**

Many blogs and websites will offer more detailed instructions and recipes, but below are the most important steps for putting up great food. It can be helpful to acquire special tongs and racks for this when you start doing it more often, as they make it much easier. Gather all your equipment and jars first. Sterilizing the jars and the boiling process after canning are SUPER important steps to insure your food is free of harmful bacteria that can not only spoil your goods, but cause serious botulism food poisoning (which kills people). There are responsibilities when you produce your own food stores, most importantly start with sterilized jars and keep things very clean.

Be Safe, Clean, Organized and Aware while Canning.

1. **STERILIZE THE JARS** - Some people run their jars through a high heat dishwasher cycle, some models have special settings for sterilizing. I have sterilized jars and lids in a bath of rubbing alcohol or vodka as well. Ideally, put all jars and lids in your biggest pan and let them boil in water (212 degrees F) keeping in mind you need 1-2 inches of headroom for the water to expand and boil. Or pour boiling water into and over the jars in the sink. If you save the water used for this step it can be used for

the processing step as well. Leave the jars in the hot water or dishwasher until you are ready to fill them. Handle the outside of the jars only - no fingers in the necks!

2. **CHOOSE THE END PRODUCTS** - Depending on your equipment and time commitment, make a plan for how to best use your items. You may want to make a sauce as well as a juice, a soup and a salsa all out of Tomatoes at one time. Or you may rather dedicate one day to a sauce alone. Study the old vintage time table below and get an idea about what time is involved, so you can plan for the processing after you have made all the wonderful stuff, too.

3. **WASH & PREPARE** - Choose the very best of your produce, a tad underripe is usually best. Wash gently, peel if necessary, cut away any bruises and remove pits. Cut into desired shapes and add to sterilized jars, or add to a saucepan if making sauces or preserves. This step is where you combine produce into a soup and cook it, or cook fruit down into a jam or jelly for bottling. Jellies require pectin to fully "gel" and sometimes it is wise to add lemon juice or sugar or salt or vinegar to your hot pack or juices for the best outcome. Consult recipes, and keep track of your own inventions by writing down your ingredients and process. Every batch is a learning experience!

4. **FILL JARS TO ½-1 INCH BELOW FULL** - You can "hot pack" with a heated product, or "raw pack" with just the heated juices or syrups or brines you add on top of your raw items. Cooking destroys bacteria so it is a wise step sometimes especially with produce that is less acidic. After filling, pack well, remove air bubbles and push food into empty spaces with a chopstick. Tap on the counter to remove bubbles and settle the product. MAKE SURE there is headroom at the top of at least ½ to 1 full inch. MAKE SURE any plant product is covered with sauce or juices by that much as well. Some jellies and jams can be topped off with Beeswax or Coconut Oil to preserve them for longer. In the old days they used paraffin - but that is a petroleum product and has no place in my kitchen.

5. **WIPE CLEAN AND LID** - Hold the hot jar with a kitchen towel or oven mitt. Carefully wipe the inside of the jar and lid with a clean cloth before combining to seal tightly. There can be absolutely no residue on the jar, rim or lid, or the seal will   fail.

6. **PROCESS IN BOILING WATER BATH or PRESSURE CANNER** - After the jars are filled and closed, place them into your large pot of boiling water or a pressure cooker/canner for heat processing. This essential step will kill bacteria and create a vacuum seal with the lid for air-tightness and best preservation.

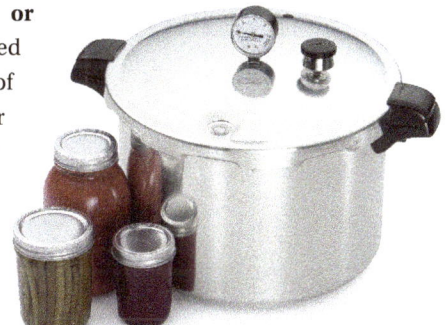

7. **TIMES FOR PROCESSING - FRUITS:** 10-25 minutes, more time if less acidic; **JUICES:** 3-10 minutes; **SOUPS & STOCK:** 3 hours or pressure canner; **TOMATOES, SALSA & SAUCES:** 35 minutes; **MEATS, THICK VEGETABLES, LOW-ACID FOODS & WHOLE MEALS:** several hours in a boiling water bath, which takes a lot of supervision, better to process with a pressure-canner or pressure cooker for higher temperatures/lower process times. **PICKLES & PRESERVES NEED NO PROCESSING:** just make sure liquid is above fruits or vegetables.

8. **CHECK LIDS AND STORE** - After processing, the lids should be tightly sealed to the jar with an airtight, concave, solid fit. Wipe jars completely dry. Label with contents and date and ingredients if you so desire. Store upright away from light and heat. Properly sterilized canned food will be free of spoilage when intact seal and jars are stored below 95°F. Keep them cool, as storing jars at 50° to 70°F enhances retention of food quality for a good long time.

Light and heat will destroy the valuable Antioxidant power of your precious preserved foods. If you store your canned goods on shelves in a kitchen, root cellar or pantry, have a drop cloth or some burlap bags that you can hang or drape over the jars to keep out light. A roll-up drape with a dowel in the bottom, affixed to the top of the shelving unit would be ideal and easy to pull aside for swift access to your goods. Plan to make some extra jars to decorate as gifts for the Holidays. Take some of your surplus jars over to surprise a neighbor or drop off at a homeless shelter.

Time Tables below are from the vintage *Home Canning Guide* by Kerr, published in 1941. Note the times for heating fruit products in the oven as an alternative as well. I remember tables just like this that came with the pectin my Mom used to make jelly. This old standard table has helpful information, which is also important to preserve!

TIME TABLES
(Time in Minutes)

VEGETABLES	Precook (Boil)	Hot Water Bath	Pressure Cooker Min.	Lbs.
Artichokes	3	180	40	10
Asparagus	3	180	40	10
Beans, Lima	3	180	55	10
Beans, String, Wax	3	180	40	10
Beets	15	120	40	10
Brussels Sprouts	5	120	35	10
Cabbage, Carrots	5	120	35	10
Cauliflower, Broccoli	4	150	35	10
Corn	3-5	210	80	10
Eggplant	5	120	40	10
Greens	Wilt	180	60	10
Hominy	3	120	40	10
Kohlrabi	5	120	35	10
Mushrooms	3	180	60	10
Okra	3	180	40	10
Onions	5	180	40	10
Parsnips	5	90	35	10
Peas	3-7	180	60	10
Peppers	3-8	120	35	5
Pumpkin		180	60	10
Rutabagas	5	90	35	10
Sauerkraut	—	15	—	—
Spinach	Wilt	180	60	10
Squash	*	180	60	10
Sweet Potatoes	20	180	60	10
Tomatoes	— (See Tomatoes under Fruits)			
Tomato Juice	5	5	—	—
Turnips	5	90	35	10

SOUPS

	Precook (Boil)	Hot Water Bath	Pressure Cooker Min.	Lbs.
Asparagus	*	180	40	10
Clam Chowder	*	240	90	15
Fish Chowder	*	240	90	15
Pea Soup	*	180	60	10
Soup Stock	*	180	45	15
Tomato Puree	* (See Tomatoes under Fruits)			
* See individual recipe.				

IMPORTANT...All vegetables and meats canned at home should be boiled in an open vessel 10 to 15 minutes before tasting or using.

TIME TABLES
(Time in Minutes)

FRUITS	Precook (Boil)	Hot Water Bath	Pressure Cooker 5 Lbs.	Oven 250°
Apples	3	25	10	75
Apricots	—	20	10	68
Berries	—	20	8	68
Cherries	—	20	10	68
Cranberries	3	10	—	—
Currants	—	20	10	68
Figs	5	30	10	90
Fruit Juices	—	30 (180°-simmering)		—
Grapes	—	20	8	68
Peaches	—	20	10	68
Pears	3-5	25	10	75
Pineapple	5-10	30	15	90
Plums	—	20	10	68
Preserves	*	20 (180°-simmering)		—
Quinces	3	35	15	75
Rhubarb	—	10	5	68
Tomatoes	—	35	10	75

Walnuts at 225° for 45 minutes any size jar (Oven).

MEATS	Precook (Boil)	Hot Water Bath	Pressure Cooker 15 Lbs.
Lamb, Veal, Beef, Pork	*	180	60
Chicken	*	180	60
			or 90 min. at 10 lbs.
Fish—all kinds	*	240	90

* See individual recipe.

(Meats packed raw do not require addition of liquid.)

NOTE—If canning fruit in water bath in half-gallon jars add 10 minutes to time given. If canning fruit in oven, for pints reduce time one-third. Half-gallon jars increase time one-third. When canning vegetables and meats, for half-gallons in pressure cooker or water bath, increase time 20%.

The time given in the time tables is based on the one-quart pack (except as per note above) and on fresh products at altitudes up to 1000 feet. For higher altitudes increase the time 10% for each additional 500 feet, except for pressure cooker canning. For elevation up to 2000 feet use pressure given in time tables. After first 2000 feet one pound of pressure should be added for each additional 2000 feet of elevation.

~ the garden of earth ~

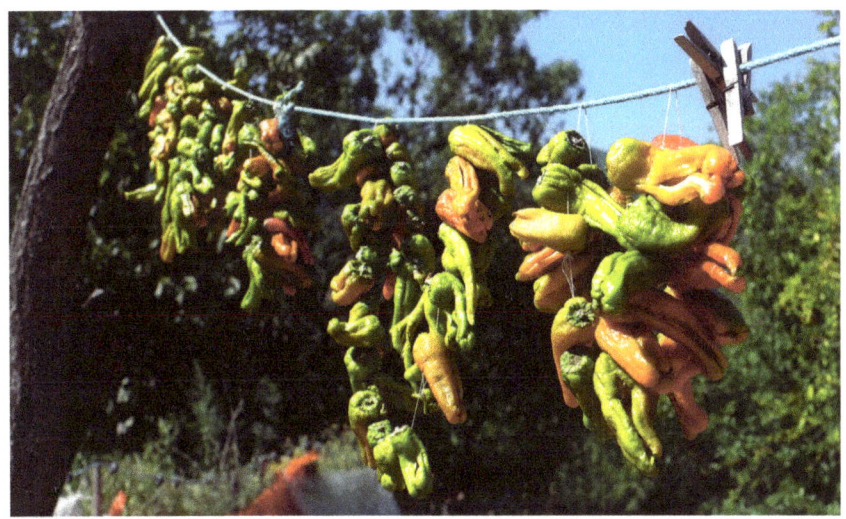

DRYING

herb preserving and food dehydrating

Oh, to be somewhere in a hammock on a Greek Island, drying Olives and Apricots in the baking hot Sun! Nature offers many delightful ways to DRY and preserve your food. Water, and the spores and bacteria in water, are the main culprits of mold and the early decay of stored food. Dehydrating the food *first* removes this possibility, and offers you another way to make stores of your garden bounty. **Not only does dried food keep longer, it weighs much less if you are backpacking or traveling.**

Always remember to drink extra water when using dehydrated foods, since you will use a lot of your own internal water to rehydrate them for digestion.

There are various methods used to dry food, but using the **amazing power of the Sun** is a natural and free one! Using this method you must keep a sharp eye on your wares as animals, birds and bugs can be interested in the food, too! I like to place a thin layer of cheesecloth over my drying food, and I try to do it on a day when I am out in the yard to keep watch, and to keep moving the trays into the Sun. **This method may take 2 days, remember to bring your food in overnight.**

Commercial grade dehydrators and even small freeze-driers are not very expensive anymore, and make a great investment if you become an avid food-drier. When Dave Allen had his Olive Jerky business, we had 5 dehydrators running most of the day, every day (in rooms we didn't hang out in, because they do make a droneful noise).

Kids love dehydrated fruits and veggies as snacks. Many of the vital nutrients are preserved in drying slowly, so you have a super healthy, homemade food option. Drying makes food nearly weightless, so you can even keep snacks in a pocket!

Your Oven can serve as a great dehydrator once you get the hang of keeping the temperature low enough. If you can get the dial to go to the lowest setting below 150 degrees, that would be best. This will take a few hours at least so try to plan for a time when you don't need the oven for anything else, or after you have already cooked something and the oven is still warm.

A Barbeque grill can also work for drying food. The key is LOW and SLOW, and this can be a great use of the last vestiges of the coals. Obviously meats are better done in a barbeque. Always use natural charcoal and woods that have not been treated with lighter fluid or accelerants. Here are a few specific suggestions for best results.

HERBS: You should dry herbs upside down, stems up, so the goodness can be pulled by gravity back down into the flower or leaves as they dry. Best idea is to make a loosely-bound, small bunch with a string or clothespin, and hang it in a cool dry place with good airflow. When the herb becomes brittle, strip it off the stems and place in a glass jar. Label and date for use in teas, baths, sauces, extracts or cooking.

FRUITS AND VEGGIES: It is most important to cut the produce into fairly thin but very uniformly-sized, small pieces so they all dry equally. Place on screens in the Sun with a piece of cheesecloth over the top to detract pests, keep moving into the sun as it moves across the yard if you have shade trees. Or place into a food dehydrator at low temperature (**below 115 degrees to preserve enzymes, vitamins and rawness**) checking and turning at least once. Also, drying on parchment paper in a very low-temperature oven with the door cracked works great too - all methods take a good few hours and do need to be watched carefully. Dry to a good crispness so your stored food does not contain enough water to mold. Some produce like apples tend to brown, so before drying, dip into a weak solution of citric acid or lemon juice in water.

MEATS: Cooked meats can be dried. Ground beef or vegan beef substitute can be browned and then put on trays to dehydrate, as well as small slices of poultry, beef or fish. Tofu can be preserved in the same way. Smoking in this case is a great method because the smoke kills bacteria, flavors the meat or tofu, and dries the product at the same time. A backyard grill can be used to smoke food with old pie plates of dampened mesquite or hickory set onto the coals. This is essentially the way you make jerky, and can be done around a campfire as well. Experiment with herbs and woods to flavor your products.

FRUIT LEATHERS AND SAUCES: Puree-ing fruits makes them perfect for fruit leather. Spread on parchment paper or dehydrator sheets at about ¼ of an inch thick. You can do this with tomatoes and vegetable sauces as well, adding seasonings and herbs, blending quickly before spreading out. After the first round of drying, peel off paper or sheet and turn over to dry the underside fully. These can be rolled with waxed paper or stored flat in plastic bags.

Easiest Fruit Roll-Ups Ever

No need to measure with this simple recipe, just add whatever needs to be used up from the refrigerator! Experiment with fruit combos, add adventurous spices like Cinnamon, Ginger, Nutmeg, Cayenne or Turmeric for added nutritional punch.

Combine 1 or 2 **Bananas** with 2-4 cups of whatever **Fruit** you have. **Berries** work great. You could even blend in some **Spinach** or **Arugula** to hide veggies in the mix!

Whip up in the blender, or use an immersion blender until quite smooth.

Spread evenly (and very thinly) on parchment paper or a silicone pad. Place in dehydrator at low heat, below 115 degrees, until dry and pliable. If you don't have a dehydrator, use a super low setting on the oven (below 150 degrees) and check often.

At some point it is helpful to turn the fruit leather to fully dry both sides.

You can cut right through the parchment paper, making the yummy Fruit Leather into strips that can be rolled or stored flat.

TIPS FOR DOING MORE WITH LESS:

<u>**WHOLE MEALS**</u> - Once you have dehydrated several items, you can combine them with condiments into freezer bags, to be rehydrated on the trip or the trail. **Add spices, dried herbs, salt & pepper, coconut milk powder, broth cubes, dried cheese shreds,** anything you would want in the dish, to be reconstituted later with hot water alone. Season well for best flavor results later. These make perfect, lightweight, super easy meal preparations for camping, rafting and backpacking.

<u>**KEEP HIGH AND DRY**</u> - Do not place in your home-dried items in an airtight jar or package until you are **sure the product is fully dried**. Residual moisture can cause mold and spoilage. I always save my ***desiccant silica packs*** (the little drying squares that say 'do not eat!') from vitamins and dry goods. Store your dried herbs and foods with some of these desiccant packs to absorb excess moisture. Check your dried food stores often to make sure there is no spoilage.

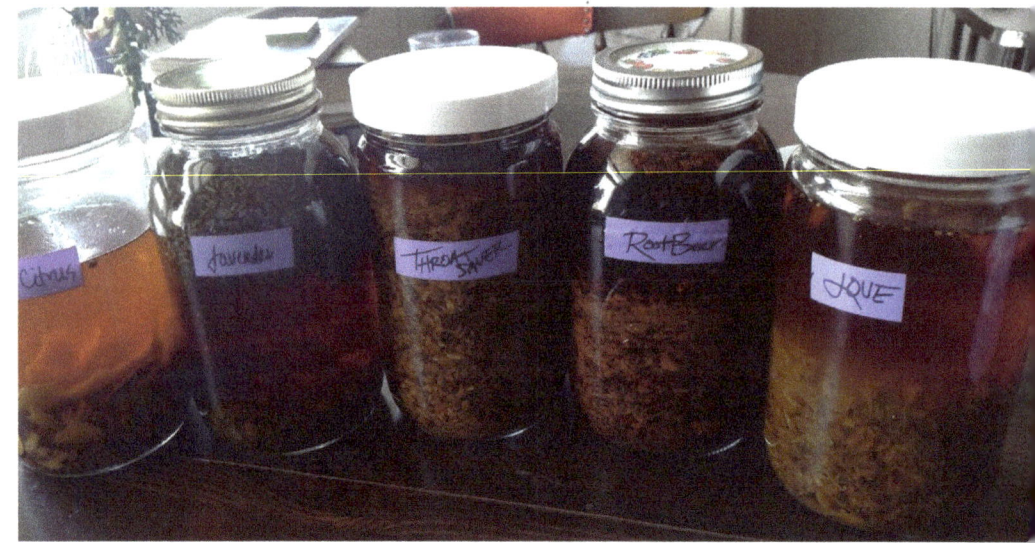

EXTRACTING
valuable medicine-making skills

HERBAL REMEDIES MADE EASY

With a few basic techniques in mind, you can make your own medicinal extracts (also called herbal tinctures) and herbal-infused oils. These extracts can be taken on their own, added to hot water to make tea, used for enhancing soups and smoothies, or as a base for something even more wonderful like a medicinal syrup, massage oil or oxymel. My favorite use of herbal alcohol extracts is to add them to sparkling water as a cocktail. With each sip I am giving my body vital nutrition and supporting my health.

Herbal Extraction is the way we draw out the Medicine from plants. To do this requires the **assistance of the Moon**, if you can believe that! The magnetic power of the Moon is so strong it creates the tides on this Planet, and affects your Body and the Plants as well. This is another great example of how we are all cosmically connected and interdependent and part of the design. Between the **New Moon** and the **Full Moon** there is a particularly strong magnetic pulling action, which we utilize to extract the potent natural chemicals from plants into our medium. The Moon makes it all possible and potentizes the result.

It can take at least two weeks, and sometimes many more, to get a good strong extract, depending on the desired strength of your remedy. You should taste your extract to determine its relative potency and make an innate decision about whether to let it soak for longer or not. I confess I have 3 and 4-year old tinctures lying around with the herbs still in them and they are amazing! In general, during that "cooking" time it is wise to visit and shake your herbal extracts at least once a day, and when you do, take a second to imbue your creation with positive energy and the Love Vibration. Once you have determined it is done, your remedy may be strained and filtered to remove any plant material, and then naturally preserved if you like for greater shelf-life.

Filtering and bottling are always done after the Full Moon has peaked. This is because of another strong Lunar quality - **EXPANSION**. This energy makes liquids dramatically expand, and literally pop their cork! Vintners know they cannot bottle just before a Full Moon or their wines will all be spilling out onto the floor, following all the popped corks!

Once you learn the principles of extracting medicinal qualities from Plants, you can use this skill to make MANY THINGS for your household, medicine cabinet, liquor cabinet and pantry. This is yet another amazing way of preserving the vitality and quality of living foods and medicines, so they may be stored and utilized in any season. Usually Spring and Summer yield the best living sources for extraction, but dried herbs and foods can also be used all year long, and still make strong remedies.

Here are some of the very cool things you can create, once you know the basic Extraction Process:

MEDICINAL EXTRACTS - with Alcohol, Water, Glycerine, Vinegar, Honey, or Oil for the base

BITTERS - Alcohol with added Gentian or Wormwood, other bitter herbs

HERBAL BEAUTY OILS - with liquid base oils, solid oils like Coconut & Shea

FLAVORING EXTRACTS - use Alcohol or Glycerine, Vanilla, Citrus Peels, Nuts, Fruits, Seeds & Spices

FLAVORED VODKAS & VERMOUTH - "herbally-enhanced" Wines & Spirits

FLAVORED OILS & VINEGARS - many different possible Oil or Vinegar bases

TOPICAL LINIMENTS - Alcohol, Vinegar, or Witch Hazel-based, topical pain liquids, for large area massage

HERB-INFUSED BASE OILS - medicinal oils to be further used in salves. balms & creams. A good medicated base oil already has prime herbal value before anything is added.

CLEANERS & SANITIZERS - make All-Natural Household Cleaners with this process, using Alcohol, Witch Hazel, Vinegar with Herbs, Essential Oils & Citrus Peels.

BASIC EXTRACTION PROCESS

FIRST, CHECK THE CALENDAR and plan ahead to **set your extracts up on the next New Moon**. Buy or harvest your herbs, research your ingredients, and work on your recipe in the weeks prior. Especially for Holiday gifts, make sure have a Full Moon in your preparation time before you need to give the gift! Or "force" at the last minute.

ALWAYS WRITE DOWN WHAT YOU CREATE. I have a Plan, and then sometimes inspiration strikes, or most times, other herbs call to me. Make sure to note this in your recipe. You think you will remember, but sometimes your memory fades if you make several extracts at a time. Document your brilliant recipe ideas every time.

HERBAL SOAKING TIME varies according to taste. Once everything is put together, let your jars sit for **at least 2 weeks** so you can strain and bottle **after the Full Moon**.

If for any reason you can't time your medicine-making with the Moon, or you are a in an urgent need, you can **"Force" the Extraction** using super low heat on the stove (or in the Sun) for a few hours, or up to a few days. If time permits, still allow your extract to sit for at least a week or two - or better yet beyond **the next full Moon** - for strongest medicinal quality. But if there's not time, you can proceed after a nice long, heating.

1. PREPARE YOUR SOAKING JAR: Sterilize your large Mason jar and lid in the dishwasher, hot water bath, or use rubbing alcohol or vodka for a quick sterilization. Dry and set aside with your herbs. The extracting process should be done **on or near the New Moon.**

2. PREPARE YOUR MEDIUM (also known as the *Menstruum*) - the base:

- *Alcohol:* Use an **edible drinking alcohol only**, with at least 50 proof, better at 80-190 proof. Organic Spirits Vodka, Gin, White Wine and Brandy work really well.

   DO NOT HEAT -always keep alcohol far away from the stove.

- *Oils/Honey/Vinegar/Glycerine:* Warm on low heat first. Sometimes I will put the herbs directly into the pan, cover it and let the whole thing *gently* heat on the stove. A crockpot works great for an all-day low heat simmer.

3. PREPARE THE HERBS (also known as the *Mark*): Grind, chop, pound, blend or even crush your herbs with a mortar and pestle or a rolling pin. This is called *maceration*, and it is done in order to release more essential oils and provide a greater herbal surface area for the extraction. Place the herbs inside your clean jar. You want to estimate the amount of herbs to match about how much extract you are looking to make - and take into consideration the jar size. I usually fill the jar about half full with herbs, and remember there must be Medium enough to cover them with close to an inch of liquid on top.

If you are using **fresh, just-picked plant material** - remember it contains a lot of water. I like to let leaves wilt a bit to dry. Water can cause mold and contaminants to wreck your extract. When you use fresh plants, many Herbalists including James Green recommend using a 190 proof alcohol (like Everclear) and blending it with the mark in a blender or Vita-Mix

> { For many years I have used Organic Grape Spirits from a company called Alchemical Solutions to make my extracts. They have an AWESOME selection of wild organic Alcohols and specialty Spirits (Coconut, Cane, Corn, Lychee, Pear, Grape and Wheat) for all of your extracting adventures. https://organicalcohol.com/ }

4. COMBINE HERBS & MEDIUM (Mark + Menstruum): Add the desired medium on top of the herbs, using a chopstick or spoon to assure you are wetting all the plant matter. Fill the jar to at least 1 inch above your herbs. It is essential that there is no matter sticking up into the air to spoil. Put on and tighten the lid.

5. SHAKE 100 TIMES: This is called *Succussion*, and is a vital part of coaxing the medicine out of your macerated herbs. This method is used in Homeopathy potentizing and the making of flower essences. This is the time to imprint your medicine with the needs you and your Family have. Add energetic input and LOVE.

6. STORE: In a cool dark place and shake everyday. I put a piece of tape on the jar with the name of the recipe and the date. After 14 days at least, spoon out a small amount of the liquid to taste and evaluate. Mmm, yummy. Choose whether it is done, or you want to continue the extraction for additional moons. If you want to let it steep for longer, try to make sure you choose a date AFTER the Full Moon by at least one day for bottling.

7. STRAIN & FILTER YOUR EXTRACT: Once you like the strength of your extract, strain through a wire strainer lined with cheesecloth. Gather the cheesecloth into a bundle and squeeze out the remaining liquid. There are hydraulic presses that assist this. If you make a lot of extracts they are worth it. If you like, you can further filter this extract through a coffee filter.

8. PRESERVE and LABEL: If shelf-life is an issue, you used *fresh* plant material, or you want to be extra careful, you can use a small amount of **Vitamin E Oil, Rosemary Extract, Benzoin Extract, Grapefruit Seed Extract or Vitamin C Powder** as a natural antioxidant preservative. Unless I am making a large amount of bottles for the marketplace, I usually skip this. Place into clean, sterilized dark bottles, and immediately label each one with the name and date with masking tape so you can identify in order to make a proper label or gift label later. You want to believe that you will be able to properly identify each product later, but chances are very great that you will not be able to accurately tell which product is which, in dark bottles or by taste alone. Trust me.

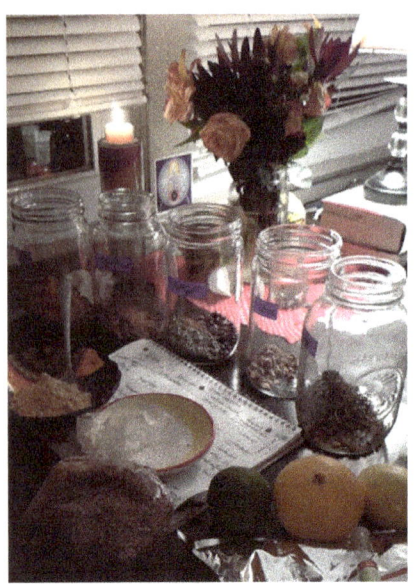

I make a big, sacred production out of my New Moon extract-making. I get ALL of my herbs out, in case something unforeseen calls out to me to be used. I light the candles and say a few words and connect with the Nature Spirits. I like to set up a few Extracts or flavors of Bitters, since it is a bit of a process. I usually have about 2-5 jars in the cupboard "cooking" at a time. I fully admit that sometimes I make extracts or bitters from which I have **never** strained out the herbs, and these "many-year infusions" are insanely potent and delicious. The most important point is to make sure to add enough alcohol to cover the herbs to keep them away from air and spoilage. When I remove some extract to bottle or use, I will add more vodka or alcohol to make sure the herbs stay covered.

HERBAL INFUSIONS

The simplest form of Extractions are made with **Hot Water**. Most people experience this process in their daily ritual of making Tea or Coffee. Herbalists call these **Infusions or Decoctions**, which refer to *medicinal extracts* that can be made simply with Water. You will find this method perfect for the water-soluble medicines contained in each plant or herb, and as a very useful method when time is a factor. A good Infusion will be made with water that has just been boiled, poured over crushed herbs or tea bags, and allowed to steep for at least 5 minutes before starting to drink. Tea is a great way to make a strong herbal remedy RIGHT AWAY when you need it in an urgent situation. Use 2 tea bags to make your Infusion stronger, or combine 2 different tea blends you may need at the moment. Leave the tea bags in the cup (unless it is a strong black tea) so the infused remedy can get more potent with each sip. The longer it infuses the stronger the medicinal action and flavor. Just remember, herbal matter will begin to decompose in water and ferment very quickly, so don't leave herbs or tea bags infusing in water for more than 24 hours. You can taste it turning sour and you'll know right away how long is too long.

- CELESTIAL HERBAL INFUSION: You can use the **Sun** to enhance the process by making a **Sun Tea**, with many tea bags in a large jar of Water sitting in the Sun all day. Or make a **Lunar Tea** - place your Herbal Infusion under the **Full Moon** overnight to add mystery, expansion, feminine energy and enhanced intuition to your remedy.

- GEM ELIXIR INFUSION: Add an extra dimension to your drinking water by adding Shungite for purifying, Amethyst, Rose Quartz, and other crystals for their properties. See an extensive list of Earthen Mineral Remedies in Volume Three.

Aromatic Vinegars, Flavored Vodkas, & Fancy Oils

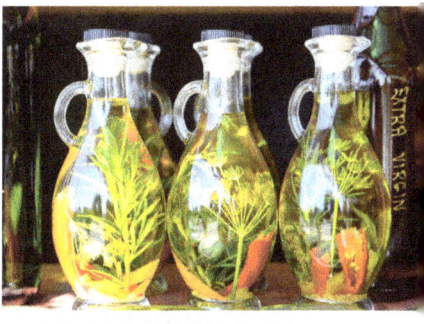

Makes 6-8oz. bottles, 12-4 oz. bottles, or several large bottles.

Prepare: Sterilize in the dishwasher a large glass jar, half-gallon or larger (64 oz.) with the lid, as well as your decorative gift bottles and their lids.

You'll also need:
- **Herbs of Your Choice** - Rosemary, Tarragon, Thyme, Fennel, Fruit Peels, Nuts, Spices, Seeds, Pink Peppercorns, Pepper Slices, Garlic, whatever you like
- **Vodka, Vinegar or Oil** of your choice, 6 cups (48 oz.) - I like W**hite Champagne Vinegar** and **Extra Virgin Olive Oil** for their clarity, so you can see the herbs. Any strong **Spirit** can be used and flavored, but the clear ones are the most attractive.
- **Ribbon, Labels, Stickers or Tie-on Cards**

Extraction Process: On the New Moon, place dry, slightly bruised or macerated herbs into the large, sterilized half gallon jar. Remember to notate your recipe as you go, so you will be able to duplicate it next time! Carefully add the Vinegar or Oil or Vodka until all the herbs are covered - add extra if needed to do so - measurements are not exact or necessary. Shake and set in a cool dry spot for 2 weeks. Check on it, and shake daily if possible, give it lots of Love. Place the nicest-looking clean, dry herbs stalks, peppercorns, citrus peels, seeds or nuts in the decorative jars.

After the Full Moon, strain the wonderfully-scented Oil, Vinegar or Vodka through cheesecloth into a measuring cup with a pour spout. Carefully pour your strained, extracted herbal medium into each of the bottles. Tightly cap and place a strip of colored electrical tape around the lid as a reuseable seal. You could also drip candle wax around the top to make a spill-proof seal for shipping.

Print or draw a pretty label on full sheet Avery label paper, cut to size or shape desired and stick on the jar. Or use a hanging tag on a string around the neck of the bottle. Label your creation with some fabulous name you come up with, and include "Handmade Especially For You" or some nice, personalized sentiment on the label or card.

> **QUICK RECIPE:** Simply add **Whole Herb Stalks, Seeds, Spices, Citrus Peels or Nuts** to a nice looking bottle of store-bought **Vinegar or Oil or Spirit** from which you have removed the manufacturer's label. Decorate and personalize. It will get stronger as it sits on the recipient's shelf, and makes a really fast and easy (but thoughtful and beautiful) gift.

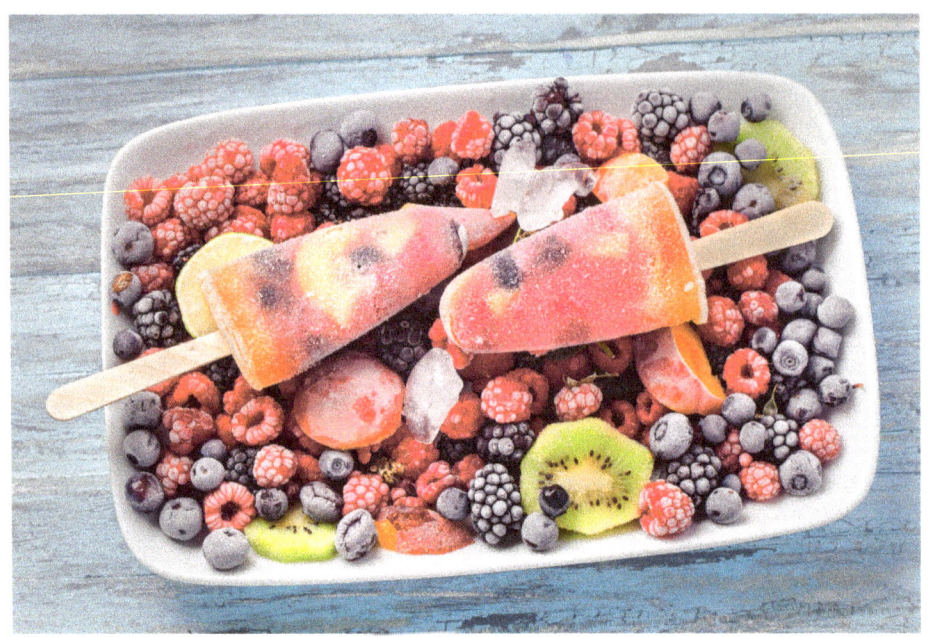

FREEZING

long-term storage / electricity required

Freezing is one of the EASIEST methods of preserving food. Stock up on foods when they are on sale and freeze them. Lately we have been toying with the idea of purchasing an additional chest freezer for supplies and supplemental food stores. As it turns out, there are many affordable small freezers for just this kind of storage, and the chest freezers are more efficient and better at conserving energy and cold. Much of our food supply can be stored for long periods of time in freezers, but again it is important to remember this requires additional electricity and can contribute to a higher electrical bill. And if it should become an issue, any food stored in a freezer if the power FAILS will only last for so long.

Because this is a solution that requires electricity, it would be wise to know about several other options for cold storage, just in case. Read on - **the next section gives you tips about how to do the same preparation but with systems that do NOT require electricity.** Hopefully we will never have to live without our modern conveniences, but it sure is wise to know some alternatives!

Over-filling your regular freezer can cause airflow problems and can ultimately burn out the freezer's motor. It is not wise to fill every space all the way to the top, be especially careful about keeping the air intake fan unobstructed. Also if you do add an extra freezer, keep it outdoors in the winter to utilize the temperature drops. Freezers kept in cold rooms or basements hold temperature 25% better than in warm rooms. You may even be able to keep one unplugged for the Winter in cold climates.

Make a **location map** to keep your foods and their positions in the freezer straight, and organize the food within according to the frequency you use it and the items to which you want top access. Using rigid glass or plastic containers that can be moved easily in searching for items helps, and making neat stacks of flat items can be beneficial. You might keep an inventory sheet on the freezer so you can keep track of what goes in and out.

If for any reason the electricity goes out, keep the doors and lids to the freezer CLOSED, and pile on quilts or blankets to keep the cold in. Food will stay frozen especially if it is well-packed for between 2-4 days. A general rule is that if there are still ice crystals in the food it can be refrozen safely. If food has completely thawed, it must be prepared and eaten, or cooked before freezing again.

Food can be stored in freezer bags, rigid containers, and also heat-sealed and vacuum-packed with the relatively inexpensive devices on the market these days. Generally food you freeze yourself may last for up to a year. I do like to put the date on things I freeze for this reason. Make sure to seal all containers and bags especially tightly to avoid "freezer burn" - which is actually an oxidation and dehydration of food that gets exposed to air. Freezer burn does not damage the edibility of the food, but will result in dry places and inconsistency of taste and texture.

With that being said, there are MANY ways to make the most of your space, and new ideas for preserving unique freezer items can be found below.

BEST FOODS TO FREEZE AND HOW

EGGS - Whites and yolks can be blended and frozen in ice cube trays. Or separate eggs & freeze and bag as well, freezing in muffin tins or paper cups first. Some recommend adding 1/8 tsp of salt or sugar per egg before freezing to preserve better texture. Eggs will keep for up to a year. If you do add salt or sugar note it on the storage container for different uses later

FISH - You can order fish in bulk from mail-order companies and freeze it into cooking portions. Fish freezes well and will defrost very quickly in a bowl of cool water.

COOKED RICE & QUINOA - With or without vegetables, slightly undercook & freeze into portion sizes. Use larger bags you can flatten easily for bulk storage.

AVOCADOS - The ripe ones don't last long - preserve them! Scoop out with an ice cream scoop or large spoon and place on trays to freeze. Place into bags when solid. They freeze really well, still taste perfect, and don't get brown or weird when they thaw!

NUTS & SEEDS - No special prep needed. Consider double-bagging. Most seeds and nuts stay good for up to 2 years. Buy in bulk, or stock up at holidays when there are super sales on nuts. Freezing keeps seeds and nuts from going rancid.

BUTTER - Buy an extra box each shopping trip and store in the freezer. Butter can pick up "freezer smells" if stored for too long. Salted Butter stores better, and for up to about 12 months.

GARLIC - Place whole unpeeled garlic cloves in a Mason jar and freeze. Or peel many cloves and smash into a pulp with a little olive oil, freeze it solid & flat in a ziploc bag. A small amount can be broken off when needed. This can make the other freezer food smell garlicky, so store in a glass jar or double-bag it!

PEPPERS - Cut in half, de-seed, stack and freeze

GRAPES - Freeze about 2 hours on a tray after washing and drying, bag up. Frozen grapes are a great hot weather snack, and make an exceptional sorbet when blended!

FLOUR - Freezes really well. Freezing kills and prevents any pests, and keeps flour from going rancid when stored for long periods. This is a great choice for preserving specialty flours you use less often.

HERBS AND EDIBLE FLOWERS - Submerge items completely in ice cube trays using water, juice. wine, or olive oil, to make herbal treats for adding to sauces or fancy drinks. These can also be popped out of the trays and put into baggies or containers to save space. Silicone ice cube trays with lids are great for easy storage.

BANANAS - Peel and freeze whole, or sliced for smoothies or chocolate-covered bananas

CORN ON THE COB - Best to blanch about 3 minutes first. Can be frozen on the cob or sliced off to freeze flat in a bag. Corn is one of the best harvest foods to stock up on in summer.

COOKIE DOUGH and PIE CRUSTS - Next time you make some, double the batch and freeze into flat pie plate shells and pre-formed cookies for cooking just a few at a time!

CITRUS FRUITS - LEMONS, LIMES, ORANGES - Peel & slice citrus rinds and freeze, add juice to ice cube trays or small ziploc bags. BERRIES - dry pack with no extra process, ideal for freezing, better than canning, preserving taste and texture and the ability to use just what you need. STRAWBERRIES seem to freeze better with a sugar syrup, called a wet-pack, which is why you often see them like this at the grocery store.

ANIMAL PROTEINS - Vacuum-seal with veggies for easy meal prep in boiling water. Double-bag for odor prevention.

BALLS of GREENS - In Bon Appetit I found a great tip about making balls from greens like kale, chard, basil and spinach. Blanch the whole leaf greens super quickly, about 10 seconds max, then cool, chop and season if you like. Take a small amount into your clean hands and squeeze them to remove as much water as possible, then roll into small balls and freeze on a baking tray. When fully frozen, balls can be transferred to glass storage or ziploc bags and placed back in the freezer. You can add a ball or two for flavor to omelets, sauces, pastas and soups.

VEGETABLES - Quick Blanch first by putting your veggies very quickly in boiling water for 1-5 minutes, remove and then allow to cool. Blanching stops the enzyme action of decay and will preserve flavors and vitamins. You can google specific times for each kind of veggie, but in general about 3 minutes is quite enough. You want the color to brighten, not begin to fade, and you want the shortest amount of time for preserving nutrient value, sometimes just seconds for greens. After completely cooled, put loosely into ziploc bags and freeze flat for ease of storing.

BROCCOLI & CAULIFLOWER - Perfect for freezing, quick blanch or steam to reheat.

CHEESE & MILK - Dairy and plant-based milks freeze well, so do cottage cheese, cream, and all cheeses. Double-bag the smellier varieties!

FULL MEALS - Pot pies, meatballs or faux meatloaf, braised protein & vegetables, poultry (but not in cream-based sauces - will break), pasta in sauce if slightly undercooked, casseroles all freeze really well.

FLAVOR CUBES - You can buy special small-celled ice cube trays, use your old ice cube trays, or even small ziploc bags to freeze extra Coconut Milk, old Wine, Juice, Pesto, extra Pasta sauce, Curry sauce, leftover Soup, Pasta Water and the last of the Stock. Cream-based sauces are not recommended, as freezing causes sauces to "break."

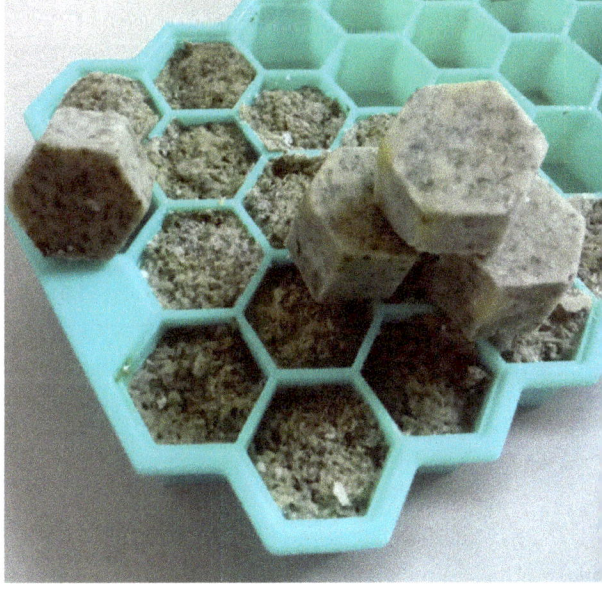

Flavor Cubes can be thawed quickly to make a sauce or just thrown into whatever you are making. They are the perfect thing to grab when you need to add instant flavor mojo and a punch of umami to anything.

~ the garden of earth ~

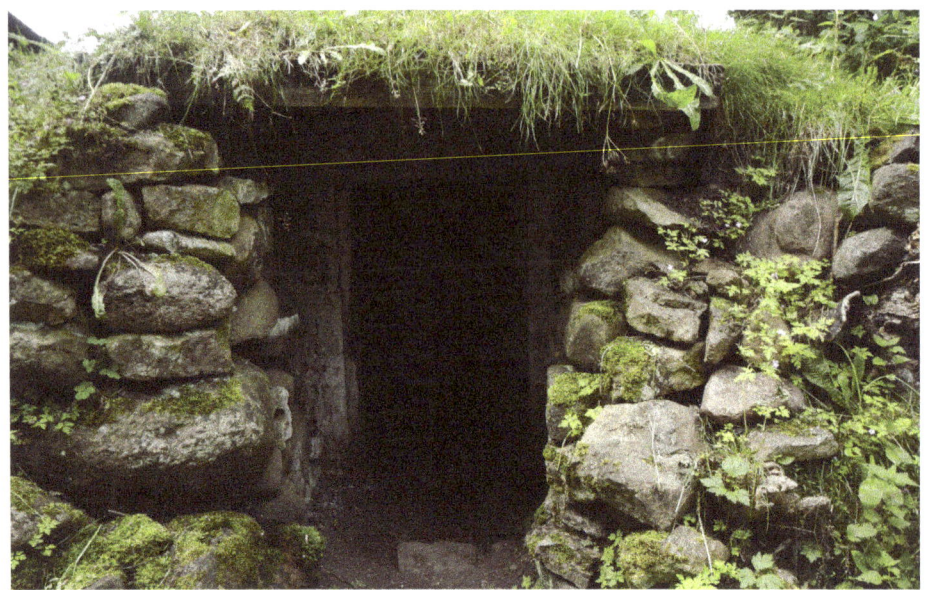

ROOT CELLARS & FRIDGE HOLES

utilizing the Earth alone to preserve food year-round

Archeologists have found evidence of Root Cellars in ancient digs around the World, some from **40,000** years ago! Australians were some of the first to invent these techniques out of necessity in their hot climate. They discovered they could store food deep into the ground and keep it much cooler, preserving their food sources for many months longer. Primitive holes evolved into full-scale underground buildings for the earliest version of refrigeration. Europeans also had an historic love of Root Cellars and likely brought this "technology" with them to the US. These "new" ways of storing food were the inspiration for the invention of electrical refrigerators. While this type of Root Cellar may have fallen out of fashion with all our modern conveniences, they are nevertheless an ingenious method for extending the life of fresh food. With no expensive power needed, underground storage could come in handy in an electricity crisis. Let's all start building Root Cellars again.

Homes in the Northeast are equipped with Root Cellars, but it is difficult in some geographical areas, especially in the Rocky Mountains (too rocky) or Florida (too wet), to dig them. Some places simply have weather that is too extreme. If you can't build one, it is time to look for cool, dark places in your house that might work. Wine Cellars could double as a wonderful food storage area. Basement rooms that can be kept dry, or downstairs closets would work as well. Make sure if there are any exposed water pipes in your cellar that you insulate them so they will not sweat and leak moisture onto your stores. Find a space you can dedicate to food storage and preservation.

From what I can glean from experts, keeping the temperature stable and at about **32-40 degrees Fahrenheit** is the most important thing. Size matters, and roughly 60 bushels of food can be stored in a space 8' x 10.' Many sources suggest you check your food stores as often as once a week to confirm their condition. Keeping the cellar or store **dark and cold and dry** is key, but if it freezes, the food will likely be mushy and spoil. Open the root cellar as little as possible beyond checking your stores. An ideal cellar is **NOT airtight** - the ethylene gas released by fruits and veggies needs to escape, and humidity and evaporation need to be cleared to prevent mold. Keeping everything **in the dark** is key to avoiding spoilage, as light can reduce the antioxidant power of canned fruits and veggies. If items in your cellar start to shrivel and dry, there is not enough **humidity**. Mist them, keep a shallow pan of water in the corner, or cover produce with some wet washcloths, burlap or sand to keep a damper atmosphere.

When preparing to store fruits and veggies, pick only the very best unblemished and complete pieces. Any scratches, bruises, rotten spots or nicks will encourage spoiling (the old "one bad apple spoils the whole bushel" thing is real). Handle produce very carefully. Pickle or Ferment any lesser quality veggies, and Can or Jam up the fruits that have bruises or bad spots. Do not cut into anything you intend to store, choose only the best of your crop. It is best NOT to wash anything. You don't want to encourage any moisture that later would turn to mold. You can pack the product in leaves, straw, peat moss, sand, burlap from old coffee bean sacks (which your local coffee bean roaster would love to give you), sawdust, or layers of kraft (not colored) spring fill packaging or kraft paper. Late-maturing crops are better for storage. Many seed varieties will indicate on the package if they are more or less appropriate for cold storage.

Make sure your cellar is designed for maximum air flow, with shelves an inch or so from the walls, and enough space so no item is crowded or touching. Ideally, your shelves could be slatted wood or metro racks for even more airflow. Some cellars have fans and ventilation which is ideal. It is wise to invest in a thermometer with an humidity gauge so you can understand the varying conditions inside and keep them ideal.

THE BEST FOODS FOR ROOT CELLARING:

ROOT VEGETABLES - Carrots, Turnips, Rutabagas, Beets & Parsnips, leave in the ground as long as possible, mulching with straw, and they will be sweeter after a frost. Cut off leafy tops, cover with moist sand. Keep Potatoes in the full dark or they will sprout. With Beets and Carrots keep the little root at the bottom intact, and keep each root separated with sand, as they spoil faster if touching. Rutabaga gives off a strong smell when stored, and would be better for a 'fridge hole in the yard. Ideal storage time for Roots: 3-5 months.

POTATOES - After harvesting, cure away from sun and light, in a dark cupboard or closet for up to 2 weeks to toughen skin for storage. Potatoes are better stored in a less cool environment, 40-45 degrees F, and can store for 4-6 months.

WHOLE GRAINS - In Mason jars or tupperware to stay dry - desiccant packages help.

CURED MEATS - Hang these up high if possible, to avoid animals and pests getting to them. Some people store in old nylon pantyhose or netting from fruit bags.

BRUSSEL SPROUTS & CABBAGES - Dig up with roots still on, and replant in Root Cellar in boxes of soil or sand, or just store in buckets with straw between layers. Hang Brussels stalks to store. Red cabbages seem to store better than green. Stored Cabbages **do smell** - so they are also a great candidate to store *by themselves* in a 'Fridge Hole in the yard, in which they will last 3-4 months and longer.

ONIONS & GARLIC - Cure after harvesting by exposing to the warm weather but NO SUN for 1 week first. They are best replanted or covered in straw or soil. Sometimes it helps to store in mesh bags or hanging in old pantyhose to keep pests away and to keep them dry to prevent sprouting. Can last 5-8 months

BROCCOLI - Can be stored for a while in mesh bags, but keep away from other veggies and fruits as it releases ethylene gas which encourages ripening.

PEARS & APPLES - Best to store individually wrapped in kraft paper to reduce the ethylene gas emissions, in boxes or wooden crates. Store only *unblemished* fruits at very low temperatures. Can last 2 to 7 months. The tart Apple varieties like Granny Smith & Pink Lady store the best.

DRIED BEANS - These store well anyway, but have much longer shelf life if stored cold and dark in a Root Cellar. Best to freeze them overnight *before* storing, to kill weevils, and place in airtight containers or jars.

SQUASH & PUMPKINS - Harvest before the first frost and keep stems intact. Most people recommend **curing pumpkins outdoors in the Sun** for 5-10 days first before storing. Can be stored for up to 6 months. Some squash store better - mainly the very hard-skinned varieties.

TOMATOES - Pull up the entire plant and store it hanging upside down in the cellar, or paper-treat like pears. Best done with still-green tomatoes, can last 1-5 months.

SWEET POTATOES - Cure like pumpkins, but in a warm damp place to toughen skin before storing. Best to wrap in paper individually for storing.

LEAFY VEGETABLES - Kale, spinach, escarole and leeks can be replanted in sand or soil, and even if they shrivel & dry on the outside, the inner leaves will be quite edible.

FRIDGE HOLES - COLD STORAGE HOLES

What happens if the electricity has failed and may be off for several weeks, but you have no Root Cellar? How could you preserve some of your perishable food before it goes bad? **The deep-down ground temperature usually stays at around 40 degrees Fahrenheit** and is perfect for cold storage. You can make your own refrigerating 'fridge holes in the ground in your yard.

Some of you may remember your Grandparents doing things like this. I've read some interesting stories from people who have vivid memories of their families participating in this lost art and they recall trying to locate their stashes in deep snow! You could repurpose ratty old coolers reclaimed from too many camping trips, and bury them in the yard to initiate new underground cellaring.

MAKE YOUR OWN COLD STORAGE

Find a large container like an old cooler, a 5 gallon bucket, large trash can, rectangular storage bucket or wooden barrel. Drill drainage holes in the bottom.

Dig a hole in the yard that is an inch or two deeper than your container (with lid on). Line the bottom of the hole with sand and gravel to make a drain.

Sink your container fully into the ground. Pack the dirt firmly around it until its top is even with surroundings, leaving room for the lid to easily be pulled on and off. You may need a bigger hole with more gravel if your soil does not drain well. If you use a very large vessel, you can put smaller buckets inside it to assure your food is easier to access and stays drier.

Line the bottom of the vessel with a little gravel to promote humidity and airflow. Carefully add your produce with layers of straw or leaves to keep each item from touching or bruising, and follow with a layer of straw on top and add the lid, which should also be drilled with a few air holes. You can fill your main container with cardboard boxes or other smaller buckets or crates, for ease of separation of items.

Once your 'fridge hole is dug and filled with your produce, put the lid on securely, and then pile hay, leaves, old blankets or burlap bags to keep the bucket fully covered and insulated. This also lowers water flow but is mainly to keep the whole system from freezing, which is beyond the refrigeration we hope to attain. I think it is a good idea to MARK your bins with a flag, cement blocks or a stake, just in case snow or leaves make it difficult to pinpoint in the yard.

Just as you would with your cellar, check the items within your cold storage regularly for spoilage, though there's no need to check your food as often as you would if it was stored inside. Depending on the variety, food can be kept cold this way through the entire winter and still be edible and usable.

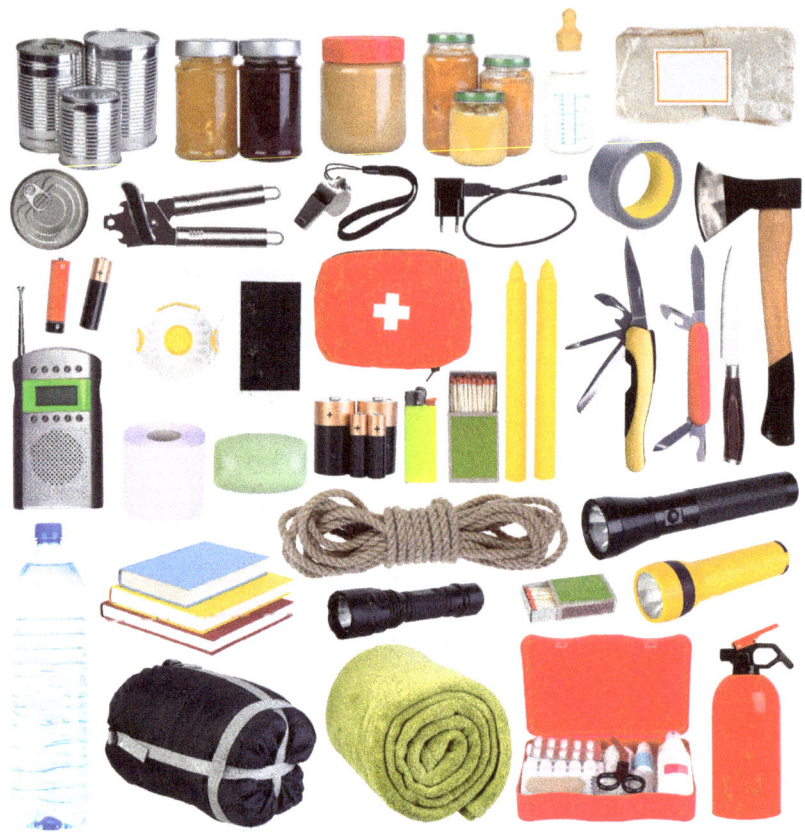

PREPARING

"Always Be Prepared."

I have seen proof that this famous motto has it right! **Being Prepared** is a way of life - one of the many valuable *Systems* my husband has taught me. Dave Allen sees to it that we keep our house and vehicles "stocked and ready to rock." This has come in handy more than a few times, and probably saved our lives, too. Being prepared for anything is essential in these strange times, when gas shortages and food shortages are happening more often. At our house, we seek to never run out of anything we need, and can shop much less because of our well-stocked pantry, homemade food stores and prepped supplies. A whole year went by when you couldn't get rubbing alcohol AT ALL in the stores, but we still had some. The toilet paper scare didn't faze us, totally prepared for that, and our food stores grew each trip to the store. That's us - just a couple of pioneers out in the country making sure we are good to go! In reality, these days we live in a small bustling neighborhood, but we prepare and preserve as if the stores are fifty miles away.

ALL OF THE METHODS IN THIS BOOK LEAD TO THIS

Preparing places the power of the Earth's bounty in your hands. Assuring you have a robust store of freshly-preserved garden food and dried herbs and medicines for supporting your family's Food Supply is the goal. Creating a more solid and reliable ability to feed yourself is the key. Think of the many advantages you create with your pantry preparations. Now, *before you are in need*, is the best time to make sure you have a few more essential items on hand, and that you have solid goals for readiness.

You can find shows and podcasts and posts about "Prepping" that actually have some brilliant ideas about what to keep in your home, pantry or storm cellar. This concept has risen beyond the level of mere trend, now that more people have lost power in storms, or had to stay home in lockdowns, or evacuate at a moment's notice. Wouldn't it be important to make sure you could feed your family, or heat your home, if there was no power for weeks in the winter? If you had to jump in the car to save your life what would you take with you? If the stores closed down for weeks could you still eat? What if you needed water or had to build a fire? Any of these scenarios could be a matter of life or death, so let's all just be prepared in case.

There are certainly preppers who take it to the extreme, stocking elaborate underground bunkers with 10 years of food and water and ammo and all the rest. I am not advocating that you must become like that (unless you feel so guided!). But those people *know they will have what they need* no matter what happens, and that can be a great comfort. I just try to learn from people who have progressive ideas, and see what kinds of things they have thought to do. At our house, our mission is to act not out of FEAR, but out of **READINESS FOR ANYTHING.**

> "Better to have it and not need it,
> than to need it and not have it."
>
> *- Woodrow Call, Lonesome Dove*

A lot of the things on the Prepping List are the same items we take with us when we camp, too! All of it is great stuff to have in your car, in your emergency shelter, or stashed in buckets with your back-up supplies. Having any of these items readily on hand will assure you can handle a variety of challenges with ease.

In addition to the items here, keep good quality **all-weather gear** in readiness (**waterproof top layers, insulating under-layers, boots, gloves and hats**) regardless of where you live. In your vehicle, make sure you always stock rain gear, boots, cash, food and water when you travel even short distances.

~ the garden of earth ~

PREPARING ESSENTIALS

smart items to have conveniently stored for all kinds of conditions

2-4 Weeks Emergency Food	**Flashlights Everywhere**
2-4 Weeks of Water (1 gallon/person/day)	**Food For Pets**
All-Purpose Knife & Sharpener	**Honey** (energy food & for disinfecting wounds)
Back-Packs & Knapsacks	**Hydrogen Peroxide**
Batteries of All Sizes	**Jars & Water Bottles**
Battery-Powered or Crank Radio	**Local Maps & Topography Charts**
Blankets & Hats & Boots	**Matches & Lighters**
Camp Stove	**Medicines & Supplements**
Candles in Each Room	**Portable Small Tools**
Can Openers, Utensils, Pots	**Rubbing Alcohol / Liquid Fuels**
CASH on Hand	**Solar Lamps, Lanterns, & Chargers**
Duct Tape, String & Rope	**Spare Liquor, Coffee, Chocolate**
Empty Buckets & Boxes	**Sprouting Seeds, Trays or Jars**
Extra Toilet Paper	**Survival Books/Wild Plant Guides**
Firestarter: Tinder, Sticks & Striker	**Tarps & Bungee Cords**
Firewood	**Walkie-Talkies**
First Aid Kit & Medical Supplies	**Water Purifying Methods**

Someday, due to unforeseen circumstances, you might have to quickly evacuate, prepare to travel a long distance, leave for a hotel temporarily, or need to go stay with relatives. Keep a couple of large **EMPTY storage buckets, boxes and back-packs** on hand that can be easily filled with your supplies. It is smart to **make a list** of the most important things you wouldn't want to accidentally leave behind, and stash it with your buckets and bags. Remember how hard it is to think when in a crisis, and prepare yourself accordingly for future success. An "Evacuation Essentials List" would be so helpful, just in case.

What you take with you is in direct proportion to the severity of your event. If the house is at risk of damage, you will be grateful for those big, easy-to-carry empty buckets and bags into which you could place your priceless things. Remember **MEDICATIONS, MONEY, IMPORTANT DOCUMENTS, BIRTH CERTIFICATES, JEWELRY, ARTWORK, VALUABLES, GOLD & SILVER, KEYS, PHOTO ALBUMS, LAPTOPS, PHONES, CORDS & DEVICES.**

ADDITIONAL SOURCES

Keep in mind that the successful military concept of **redundancy** - having BACK-UPS for everything - saves lives! While being civil and not hoarding, you can provide your home with extra stores and additional sources of necessities. We started our Emergency Food Supply with one large-size storage bucket. We added items until it got full, and then we started a new bucket. Sometimes we double-up on buying items when we shop. If you buy two bags of rice just 2 weeks in a row, you have the beginnings of an "Emergency Food Supply Stash" for yourself! Get one extra item each time you visit a health food store and stick it in the box. Buy grains and beans in bulk at your local health food co-op. Remember to stock extra condiments, salt and spices, and grab that "10 cans of tuna fish" the next time it is on sale. You might be called on to share the food you have someday, or possibly use it to barter for something you need.

Stock high-quality, low maintenance, low preparation foods. **Chia Seeds** are great to prep because they do not have to be cooked to be eaten. Chia can be sprouted for healthy microgreens, soaked in water or juice to make a pudding or porridge both sweet and savory, or combined with fruit, avocados, or blended into smoothies. Chia provides tons of energy, protein and superior nutrition, perfect for survival.

We try to rotate food out of the boxes to keep the stores fresh. This is a food resource BEYOND our pantry as a back-up store if needed, and it is incidentally totally portable as well. We have found it is really helpful to make an Inventory List of what items you have, and to keep track of foods you use from the stash.

In terms of **Drinking Water**, you need to plan for **1 gallon per person, per day.** You also need some water for cooking, washing hands and dishes, and possibly in the bathroom as well. You can re-use your dish and washing water (grey water) for filling the tank and flushing the toilet. You can set up bowls and buckets and jars to catch rain water. You never realize the convenience of running water until it is gone!

Make sure in addition to stored emergency water, you ALSO know where the nearest **drinkable Water Wild Spring** is located. This is also called "potable water" from the Latin word *potare* which means "to drink." And it also follows, never drink from a source that says it is "non-potable" no matter how thirsty you are - this would mean it is contaminated in some way and not safe. **Always make sure you have a back-up source for Fresh Water.** Can you purify water if you find some? Where is the nearest stream or lake or river to find water, and maybe even to fish? Visit the cool site **www.findaspring.com** for springs and potable water sources in your area. I have a whole section on Water and dowsing for it in The Elements in *Volume Three*. Consult local area experts, and ask the old-timers of the town where the water is - do it now, so you have water back-up plans, before you may need it later. Locate physical maps of your area and keep some on hand. Stock water filters, filtering water bottles, or the handy water-filtering straws to make the purifying of any water source safe and easy.

Energy is a concern if you are in a storm or lose power. Make sure you have some **ALTERNATE SOURCES** of the following:

> **POWER** - solar chargers, generators & extra fuel
>
> **HEAT** - firewood, ceramic candle heaters, firestarters, warm clothes
>
> **LIGHT** - candles, flashlights, solar lanterns, battery-operated lights, camping lanterns
>
> **ALTERNATE COOKING METHODS** - Small propane cook stove, grill with charcoal, liquid fuel, sterno, candle stoves. Find pots, pans & utensils that fit these smaller stoves, and store with them.
>
> **EXTRA FUEL** - Charcoal, wood chips, firewood, propane canisters, cooking fuels, old paper, sticks from the yard, construction scraps

*CAUTION! Keep in mind any flame consumes oxygen and if you are in a closed space with no ventilation like a vehicle, even just one candle can exhaust your oxygen supply and lead to death. Cookstoves and gas lanterns should never be used inside unless it is with VERY adequate ventilation. Never fall asleep with candles burning.

Remember always "**FIRE FIRST**" - put out the flame, blow out the candle, put the screen in front of the fireplace, turn off the burner or stove *first* before you do anything else. Think of flames as though they are alive - the Element of Fire is very much a vital and dangerous thing and deserves your undivided attention! Much more about FIRE in Volume Three where we break down everything about The Elements and how they are reflected in our Health, our Moods, our Energy and our very Lives.

WHAT IS ALREADY THERE IS EASY TO OVERLOOK

Oftentimes, there are abundant resources we don't even think about, all around us - just like the **WEEDS!** Start your education by finding all the Wild Food growing around you. Go further to find where the Water flows nearby and confirm for yourself a good source of spring-fed drinking water. Then look around the yard for what else you nave been provided - sticks and leaves and old bricks and many things you already have could be repurposed in a time of need.

NATURE PROVIDES, but we must notice what She offers! Remember to seek out the many **natural sources** in your yard and neighborhood for your Supplies, and make use of what you find nearby. We use the many twigs and branches from all of our trees for abundant year-round firewood. Before I plant the garden I dig for the clay in the yard to mix in with the soil for aeration. I use the sod I dig up for shoring up a fence or making a water barrier for a new tree. We use our leaves as protective mulch for the flower bushes, and support for the compost. We eat the Weeds we pull, and go outside to find food all the time! We work *with the land*, even on our little lot in our little residential neighborhood, as if we lived on abundant acres. We seek to utilize what we have been offered by Mother Nature and she always keeps us well stocked!

You never know when a little good Preparing and Pantry Stocking will come in handy. I sure hope you won't need it, but I will say it again - if just one thing you learn in this book helps you someday, I will have done my job.

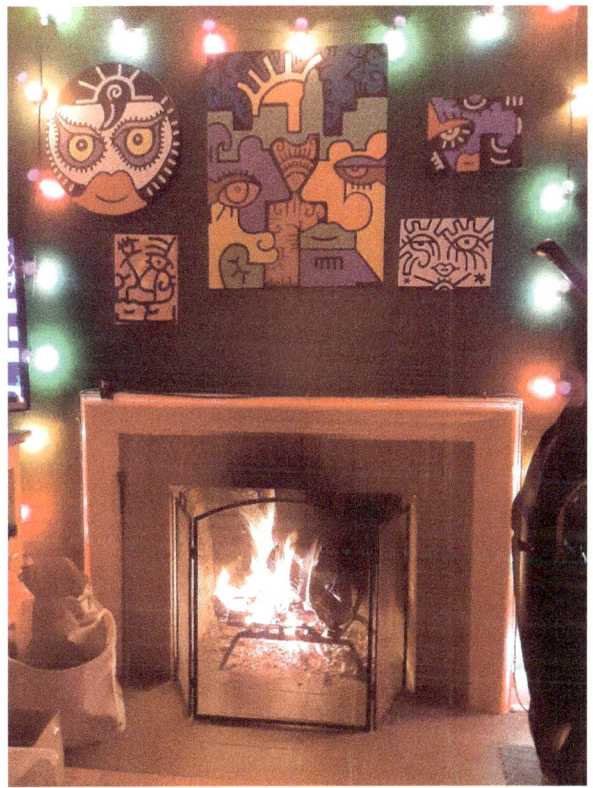

May you always have All you need, and Extra for others!

*****

In the next section we get to hear from our heroine, our Mother, the energy of **GAIA**, the One True Mother Earth. She has a lot to say! I hope you can take comfort in her message, and rest more easily knowing a bit more about her love for YOU, and for all of Humanity.

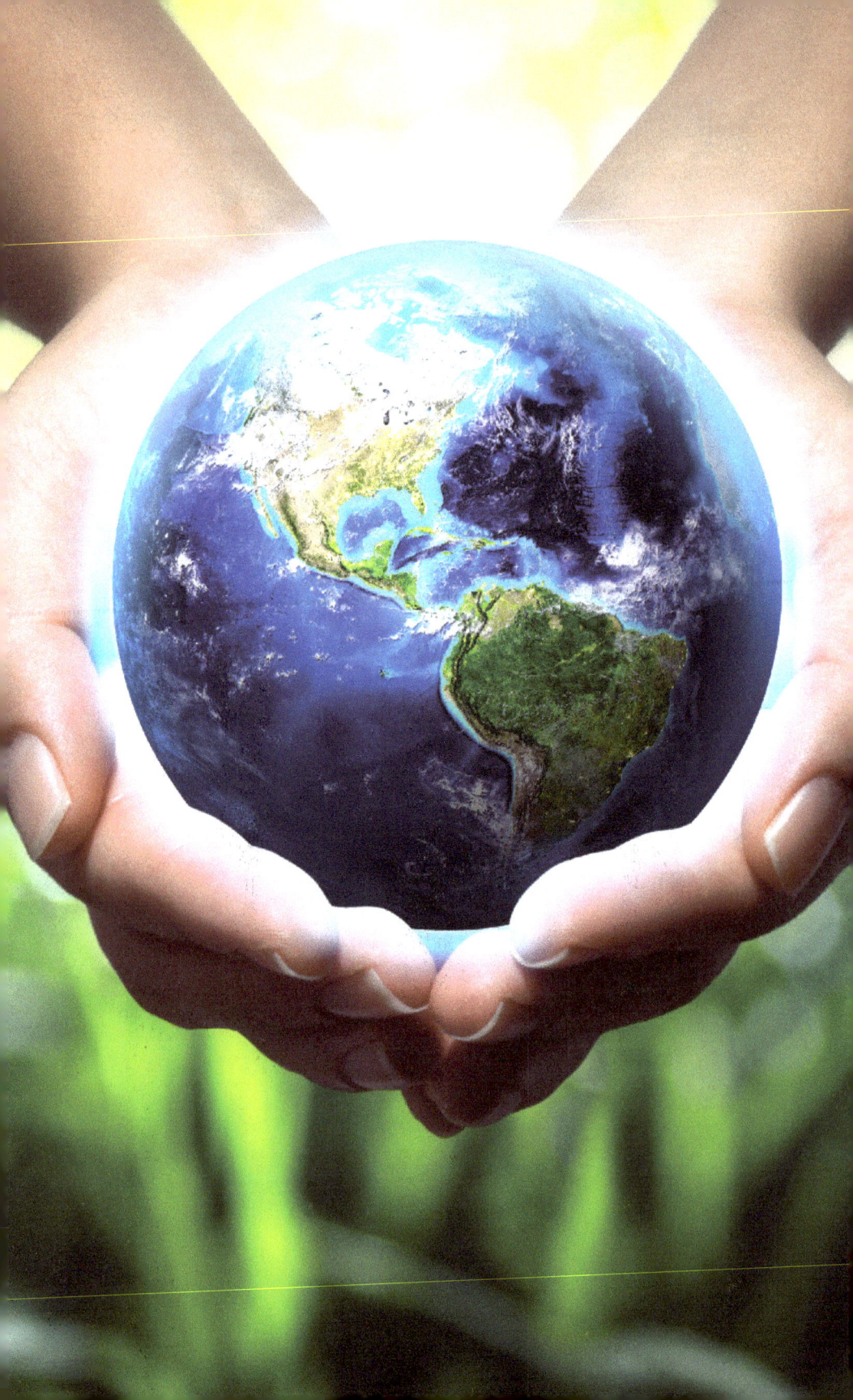

~ the garden of earth ~

~ Chapter 6 ~

MOTHER OF THE GARDEN

> "We call the Earth Gaia, a poetical form of "land" or "earth," and a common alternative for Mother Earth or Mother Nature. In Greek mythology, Gaia was the ancestral Mother of all Life. Gaia is the Sentience of the Earth, the intrinsic connection between all living things on the Planet. Another word for Gaia is Anima Mundi, or World Soul, the *vital force* of the Earth. Anima Mundi is related to the World in much the same way as the Soul is connected to the Human Body."[23]
>
> *~Pepper Keen Lewis, channel for Gaia*

IN HER WORDS

If you had the opportunity to speak with the Soul of Planet Earth, Gaia, your Truest Mother Earth, and could ask her ANYTHING - **what would you ask?** It's funny, we all think we want to dialogue with Deities, or meet Higher Realm Entities, but the first problem you encounter is exactly what to ask about! It's hard to boil your entire Life down to just a few questions, and you don't want to waste their time or be foolish with the opportunity. It can be a little intimidating! But the best thing to do is ask what is on your heart. I spoke with Gaia when were in the midst of the recent health crisis on Earth. I was intrigued to see (in almost time-loop fashion) how her guidance while helpful then, is still perfectly appropriate for the situations we face today.

In this chapter, I get the chance to ask many questions of Gaia, and her answers come through world-renowned spiritual expert and channeler, **Pepper Keen Lewis**. I have personally known Pepper since 1994, and have lovingly experienced Gaia through her sessions and events all over the country. I cherish her, hold her in the absolute highest regard, and have always felt the truth in her transmissions. I know some people may not understand or trust channeled material, but this is one of the ways Humans have always received guidance from the Divine. I advise you to run the information through your own heart to see how it **feels**. Take what resonates now, and read it again later to see what may be revealed to you when you are ready to learn more.

In this interview, I sought to ask topical questions that I felt might matter most to all of us at the moment. I also asked her to shed her Light on what I have been exploring in this book. I made every effort to preserve what she said faithfully word-for-word, for it is in the crafty language of her perspective that Gaia reveals so much. She sounds old-fashioned, or almost from a different time. She's speaks metaphorically often, and can be very serious, but also quite hilarious. You might be surprised to learn of her Deep Love for Humans. Her tolerance of us is Unlimited, *even though we are such a handful!* She is our Mother, and offers us patience and perseverance the same way our own Mothers did. Her unmistakably high-vibrational, true essence is **Unconditional Love.**

She does not love the wicked any less for the part they play. She does not love the perfect any more, for they also play their part. She exists beyond the polarity and duality of good and bad.

And so you know - **She is NOT angry at us. She is** not **seeking her revenge with hurricanes and earthquakes. It's not personal, it is BIOLOGICAL!** She is *working* on a physical, biological level, just as we work through toxins within our own bodies. The Earth needs to process and digest, to utilize and release. She demonstrates a fractal Macrocosm of our Microcosmic lives, going through much of the same stuff we do. And she is WELL - the Earth is Well. She has a lot to say, so I'll let her speak.

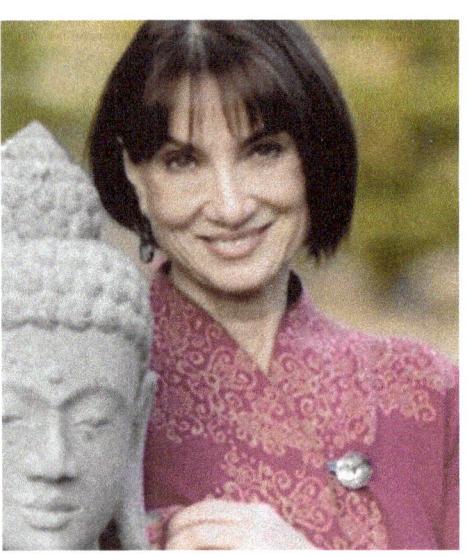

INTERVIEW WITH GAIA

Invocation by Pepper Keen Lewis: "We make ourselves One with the Moment. One with All That Is. And we draw it all to ourselves, even with the Simplicity of the in-breath and the out-breath. We are One with the Stars and the Stardust, the Earth and the Clay of the Earth. Inseparable from all that has ever been. Timeless. Accomplished. With memories that nurture what has been and what will be.

And yet in this moment, we make ourselves One with the Present moment, allowing all things to easily be drawn to us, from the Kingdoms and the Elements, from our Teachers, from all that which guides us from within and beyond the Earth. We allow all things to settle within us. We ask for our Health to be maintained, to be uplifted. We ask for our emotions, and All that we are, be balanced for the time period in which we find ourselves in. We ask for Kindness to be extended to us. So that we can see and that we can vision further, so that we can hear, so we can know, and that we can share.

And in this experience, we ask for Mother Earth, Gaia, Anima Mundi. We ask for the Wisdom of the Earth, and we ask it to become Ours. Not just now, but forevermore.

We ask for the accompaniment, the companionship, the partnership of the Earth in all that we think and say and do, and so it is."

GAIA: *(there is a distinct change in voice and cadence)* Indeed, Sweet One! All Words are welcome, all Wisdom is welcome! And so much better it is when these two are blended together! When words and wisdom are as one, it would seem that one could hear the birds singing. When words and wisdom are one, it would seem that one can imagine oneself swimming like a fish without needing to come up for air. When all of this is blended in the way that it can be and sometimes is, there is less hesitation in one's speech! There is less pause to consider a thought, because it has already become part of One. So this is what we will endeavor for our time period here. For all things between us to be so natural that there is no division, that there need be no time to consider the next question or how it will fit with the last, because already it dovetails, because that is how Nature is! That is how Nature IS.

Even between Predator and Prey there is not the separation, there is simply a knowing that one is Predator and the other is Prey and that the tables can be turned when the circumstances change. There's no separation between Light and Dark because it is understood that Dusk and Dawn link these. So why look for the moment or the time that says, "Oh now it is day, or now it is night," when it need be neither. So again this is what we endeavor to do - and to be with one another, to **erase the lines of separation**. To erase the Borderlands, the Badlands, that would say, "You cannot go there," or "to go there is dangerous," or "to go there is the wrong direction, or the wrong way." We would endeavor to erase these, and to **make all paths equal**. All paths as One. So that whatever direction you are to aim your compass, you will be guided on how to get there. For why should you not move in any direction that you choose? Why should there be only front and back and sideways, or the right way or the wrong way or the future or the past? So let us see together what we can do to erase some of these Knowings and to free these Energies, not only for your sake, but the sake of others, and those whom you speak to, as well. And now that I have presented myself in this way, I will make myself Yours, as always, Completely Yours, for you to direct or for you to call upon. And you will see that I will Bless You, as easily and as well as I am able.

LAURA (L) : Oh Gaia....It is such a JOY to speak with You! I'm so happy to have this time to talk to you. You know that I talk with you often, you know that you ride shotgun in my car all the time, you know that you're always with me. But it's just a joy to speak with you through Pepper today, thank-you SO much for coming.

GAIA (G) : That is interesting, and I had imagined that I was the one in the driver's seat!

L: *(loud laughing)* Well, indeed, you probably are! You probably are.

G: Well then, as you wish to be the driver, I will also then allow you to guide this session as you wish.

L: Well, you know, you can take the wheel, that's okay! But yes, I wanted to have an interview with you for this book, like I did in the first one. I want us to express, and teach as many things as we can that might be important for people right now. I have some questions, but I want you to drive as well because you may have a greater perspective about what we need to know. I want your support, I want your help, I want to understand what we can do, how we can manage to live through these strange and weird times.

G: And you wish my commentary upon this strange and unique time?

L: Yes, I do, I would like to know what you think.

G: I will say to you that it is not as strange or as unique as you might imagine, though it is perceived that way by the generations upon the Earth now. Each generation has, in its own way, seen things or seen life that they imagined no one has seen before them, and no one has lived through before them. So I will draw your attention, for instance, to those who have endured the last World War, the Second World War. Imagine these individuals going to work and carrying again a face mask, a GAS mask to work and what that might have been like, you see? Or to wonder what it might be like to imagine that, very possibly, truly, it could be bombed, a city in which they live - or to live through the aftermath of that, or to live through loss of relatives and friends and such. Certainly these individuals could not have imagined a worse Fate or a worse Time, or that any others had lived through something so terrible such as that. Similarly those of the First War. Similarly those of other Apocalyptic Events in Life, as well.

And so yes, this is unique to this moment, and it is, as you say, as strange as strange can be. But what will come of it - THAT is what is the most important. What is to be seen. What it will YIELD. What kind of individuals will this yield? What kind of individuals will this make? Is it in fact, apocalyptic or is it only in fact something that is fear-driven? A Calamity of sorts, or is it a true apocalypse? You see? These are the things that one must consider.

So for now, it is better to consider that Yes, it is a Calamity of sorts. A mishandled, poor-judge-of-characteristics-Calamity that has befallen All, and it will make its way into the History Books, as well.

But this is only one aspect of these times, of these times that are currently being lived. And so there are yet to be more discovered aspects of it. So the most important thing of all is Who Am I in this process? I'm going to find myself through this process. Through my Culture. Through my Understanding. What is the Unfoldment of My Life? What can this mean to the smaller picture or the larger picture, and how is it that I can help myself and my Earth and my fellow CLASSMATES, as it were, through this experience as well? And this is the best way to view it.

L: What can I offer my readers to help combat the fear they may feel sometimes?

G: I will say to you that THIS FEAR IS MISPLACED. It is not misguided, it is simply misplaced. And that when fear surrounds an issue such as this, well, it somewhat diminishes the PROPERTIES of the Solution, because the fear is so guarded, you see, that even the solution itself is put off a bit, or becomes a little bit less POTENT.

So when we're surrounded by a great deal of fear, the potency of ANYTHING becomes less! The potency of creativity - if one is guided by fear, creativity is less. Guided by fear, solutions are less, sleep is less, adventures are less. (**L:** Wow.) And so to educate others would be to say that **Fear - not only is it limiting, but it diminishes the entire Being, it can shorten a lifespan!**

And so HOW to reduce Fear, well in some ways is by education, in some ways is by asserting one's IMMUNOLOGY if you like, one's own immune abilities. To strengthen these whenever possible. To reduce the stresses inside one's life, or inside one's body as it can be, and to share in all of this, will then make better even this virus.

L: Okay. Great advice. You know I completely agree about Natural Immunity. I found a weird coincidence with something you used to teach about the "Ring Pass Not" and how we would come to a time when we would have to go through something we could not avoid. This "corona" even looks like a ring - I don't know it seemed very weird. This time now seems like the Ring Pass Not?

G: Yes, in some ways, you see because it will come back - one cannot then make it past this borderland, this border, what it would be - this boundary, yes, the boundary. One cannot make it past the boundary without UNDERSTANDING, it will push one back to it, to understand it, you see? So yes, it is.

L: So at the root, what do you believe we are trying to understand by experiencing this situation now ? What must we understand?

G: I will tell you that the situation itself is not the true understanding, it is to understand "Human." And the part that Humanity, the Being that Humanity is, the physical being, the evolutionary being that is Humanity, MUST in its own way become MORE than this type of Human. So here I will tell you that some WILL and some WILL NOT. So this is the opportunity! The opportunity is, yes, to expand out beyond this boundary, to push beyond it, to become something ELSE and something MORE. But not all will be able to. And so the Fear will hold some back, the very evolution will hold others back. The physical constraints, whether it be of age or understanding or what one truly believes in, what reality one believes in.

So one must be able to push BEYOND these boundaries, to make of them invisible, to make themselves resilient, in order to pass something that is well, with non-form, through something that is material. Literally to pass through the walls, as it would be, into becoming the next "Essential Human Being." So this is part of that, it is part of an evolutionary TACTIC, if you like. And there will be much more to contribute to this, to add to it, or understand. But yes, this is the time for the unleashing or the letting go, or the opening of what has been stored, or like that. The Opening of the Pandora's Box, like that, we will call it that, it is that time. Pandora's Box is now open, and all manner of interesting phenomena will come from that box, this being one.

L: Okay - that's very, very interesting. Do you have any other suggestions for upgrading our Immunity so we can stay well?

G: Simply to understand oneself, the organic nature of one's being, all of the processes of the body. How FOOD, literally, is taken in, how it is processed, how the digestion works. How the FOOD becomes something else other than food, becomes ENERGY, becomes that which must be expelled in the body. And to see that this takes place in every organism upon the Earth, whether it is the trees that will take in the moisture and the air to combine and make sugar & proteins for the tree itself. To see that every living organism undergoes the same process, and in that way truly understanding what Humanity is, what a Human Being is, what a Human organism is.

L: Right. So the health crisis and so many people in all this Fear, that hasn't really affected you too much?

G: No, not at all.

L: Okay, good!! I know we always talk about how Humans think they are so powerful, right, Humans are sure that they can destroy Earth, end Gaia. And it is always so funny to know that we think that way, ***but you don't!*** It's beyond good to know you are not too affected.

G: Certainly all that Humanity does affects the Earth, but it is not **potent** enough to destroy it. It is one of the organisms upon the Earth that should be known. Now the consciousness, certainly, that can be raised.

L: What about all the medical waste - how are we going to resolve all that?

G: It will be absorbed into the Earth as well.

L: Yeah? It just seems like a lot of gloves, a lot of masks, a lot of antibacterial soaps -

G: Yes.... but it is not different than incinerating a body, cremating a body, you see? And all that the body has ingested throughout its entire life, whether it is in its nerves or in its body and such, you see? It is all held there in the body and that also is returned to the Earth. But you see also when something is returned to the Earth in that way, then it can also become INERT. Then it can be managed differently, then it can be reduced in its energetic size you see, and then it is absorbed by the Earth as an inert product.

L: I see. Well that makes me feel a little bit better! I guess it is like the toxic things we sometimes take into our bodies that become changed and resolved by the processes our body performs. Okay, wow. Now, do you think that we on Earth are going to see a Solar Flash that will create a consciousness shift, is that something that we will see?

G: No, it does not appear so, not in the way that you are describing it, but do make your questions more specific so we can explore the topic to your heart's delight.

L: Okay, well it is something that many truthers are talking about, that the Sun will give off a major Solar Flash, as it may have done every 26,000 years or more frequently, and that will help change the consciousness of the Planet. Is that something that is really going to happen with the Sun? Or how are we going to shift our consciousness?

G: The consciousness will continue to evolve and shift, as you say, according to how one IS, according to Being. Here, I will say this: there is Being and there is Becoming. Becoming leads to ideas such as flashes of light or enlightening or consciousness shifts and such, something happening - something external happening that will then trigger some internal growth or evolution or understanding or movement into a next cycle. That is the process of Becoming.

When one enters instead through Being, Being automatically calls upon Wisdom. One does not need an external Source in order to cause that Wisdom to exist, or to rise. So one is not looking for the cause and effect. In Becoming, one needs cause - an external cause - in order that there be an internal effect, so that then there can be another external movement into a different Consciousness. In Being, all of this takes place in the moment, in the ever-present Now, so there is no need to summon something or someone, or a God or a Sun in order to have this experience. It is already naturally in the Now. You do not need to notice, "Oh, that was the Flash we were waiting for, NOW we are moving into the next New Age." You see? Again, this is a human understanding of needing to call upon something or someone, a God, an angel, a teaching, a Buddha, what it will be.

And that is not to say that there cannot be differences in unique Sunspots and energies and what it will be. All of this can certainly come about. But to ASSIGN to it ALL of the responsibility for all of the movement of Humanity into the Next Age, that is perhaps a little bit too much to give, a little bit more responsibility to give to one Flash. But it does give many teachers, or evolutionaries, something to talk about or write about, certainly!

L: Right. So is there a Consciousness Shift happening now?

G: YES. It is happening now, and it is happening for some. Rather, it's happening for ALL, but it is not very noticeable in many. And this is important to note as well. And it is not to separate Humanity, it is simply that some will recognize this because they have already lived through it for eons of time, not simply this little time period now.

It is eons and eons of Time. The Buddha who found Enlightenment also so long ago, did not find it only in one lifetime. It was simultaneous lifetimes in other experiences that facilitated that event. But Humanity is accustomed to seeing, "Oh, here comes this Great Being and this is what they did in a few short years. And so I must aspire to something similar." So, what is taking place is more all around, and all the time, if you like, and it is movement, it is the movement of energy knowing itself.

L: And is this movement, is this a dimensional shift? Are we moving out of 3D into Higher Dimensions?

G: Not HIGHER, not in that way again. Perhaps it is better to say INNER, or perhaps it is better to say DEEPER. The "higher" then, that higher/lower, better/worse perspective is not as helpful. But if we were to say "INNER REACHES" - movement toward the Center, that is perhaps a better way to put it. The movement is toward the Center. And toward the Center of Being.

Now using the same measure-board or description as moments ago, the Center is Being, and as you move outward to the outer, or to the circumference or what it will be, that is Becoming. The Center is Being, Being is Stillness. Being is Wisdom. Being is All That Already Is, because there is nothing else to "get." There is nowhere to go. This is Being. But as one moves out from the Center to the circumference, out toward the Human life - and the circumference of the circle being a human life or the cycles of Becoming then - one moves out through the different spokes in the wheel, or rays of the Sun or however it will be considered in this way, that is then movement toward Becoming. Movement towards cause and effect. Movement toward knowledge, information, growth - again by something EXTERNAL affecting something INTERNAL.

L: Right - this gives me a whole new way of thinking about it. Instead of thinking we are trying to ARRIVE somewhere, we are " being there" now, right? We're Here?

G: Yes, that is correct.

L: Now does the Earth shift as well? Is the Earth shifting consciousness as well?

G: The Earth shifts consciousness. That which is Gaia essence, then, simply shifts to more Wisdom, or Being Wisdom. That is what is *exuded*, is better put, see? In the Earth itself, there is movement in the Earth, then, because the Earth is the physicalness, the Earth is the external quality of that which is Gaia. So yes, it will undergo changes and movements and understandings that affect the OUTER World.

L: Are you going to experience a Pole Shift?

G: Yes. Yes. At some point yes, and that is already underway, the movement is already underway. The magnetics of the Earth, like a current, is always, always moving and that shifting is taking place. But it is not yet near the point at which you will say the

Poles will tip, but certainly there will be an occasion of that, absolutely yes.

L: And is that something we will see in our lifetime?

G: It is possible, not likely, but possible. Only because of how you measure time you see - the way in which time is measured now does not make it likely. It is not easily placed upon a calendar! And so more than likely not, but certainly you will undergo the anomalies that will confirm that it is underway. It is underway, and it is shifting. Gravitational changes, shifts in how the different metals and such respond within the Earth, much of this, yes.

L: Yes, I see. And you have obviously shifted your Poles many times before?

G: Yes, yes.

L: Yes. There are scientists who talk about how the North Pole used to be at this location and then this location and then this location...

G: Yes, this is correct, this is accurate.

L: Right. I am happy we can help Humanity learn some things that might be important for them. Because of you I understand more about Being than Doing now. Are there more things you would like us to help teach Humanity?

G: Perhaps it would be wise for Humanity to know they cannot truly destroy the Earth. But it (Humanity) can certainly destroy itself! But even that will be remade and Humanity would return again, but with a different Purpose, with a different Understanding, in a different way. It can destroy itself, it cannot destroy the Earth. And yet, yes - it must look about and see what its carelessness has caused.

Its carelessness has caused the potential destruction, not of the Earth, but of Humanity's own World, that is what can be destroyed. Humanity's own world that it has created, and each other, certainly, you see? And for this, then, is not to say there is a "price to pay" and such - there is simply the next evolutionary moment. But a great many steps would need to be repeated or reinvented, it would be a SETBACK in many ways for this experience to take place. But the Earth will not come into any great harm, even though it appears to be. It can sustain this, you see? But Humanity may not be able to sustain it.

L: I do see. And I think this was one of my favorite things you talked about in our interview in the last book, you expressed that you are well. Are you still in that same situation, it was 15 years ago, are you still well?

G: Yes, that is correct.

L: And of course all the things Humanity is doing to contribute to the degradation of the Planet are not things you are in favor of, but you had told me before that we are too arrogant to think we could destroy YOU.

G: That is correct.

L: How about a question about the "**All Is In Plenty**" attitude? We talked about this the last time that I interviewed you. You said that once Humanity would realize that *All is in Plenty* that we would be doing much better. I just don't think people understand the attitude, and it's especially hard because we live in a money structure. Many things have happened recently to destroy people's businesses, groceries and gas are so expensive. I'm going to be speaking to a lot of people who may be close to giving up because their worlds do not appear to be "all in plenty." Can you offer any advice?

G: Sometimes it is appropriate to give up. And what happens when one gives up? What happens when one gives up everything? Well, there is an ending of sorts. In the giving up, there is a letting go. Sometimes it is appropriate to do that. What is the difference between giving up and letting go? The difference is in what the *next beginning* will look like. There will always be a next beginning, because time is not truly measured by beginnings and endings, but is truly a continuity.

But in the perception of things, the difference between giving up and letting go is what the next moment will look like - or what abilities or what strength one has to create the next beginning. Just as in a poor birth or a rich birth, or what it will be, the health of one's being is at stake. So even when one is considering giving up, considering it is the ending, or the end of all things, the end of all, one does not see that all one is doing in essence is making for themselves a poor birth, or a poor re-birth, or a poor next beginning with less resources.

So better it is, the letting go, to say, "*Well I tried that and that did not work, obviously does not work, I am in poor straits or conditions and so I have no better choice* (not no choice, but no better choice) *than to let go of what did not work so I can then invite another possibility.*" And of course this is not always a party, is not always a grand becoming, and a celebration of what will be in the next movement. Sometimes it is quite difficult, quite challenging, and one must BE in that moment, exist in that moment, come to know its depth. But if one comes to know it's DEPTH, one will also come to know GREAT HEIGHTS as well.

So, it is more the understanding of the movement of all things, that indeed **the depth of something is the rise of something else!** It is understanding the cosmology of even being Human, or of a Human life as it will be, and not rather the simple circumstances of "I like this, or I do not like, or this was easier, that was hard." Now the "**All in the Plenty**" is that as well. It is to see that some things are sufficient, some things are enough. And it is, as you say, the culture in which you live is based upon a system in which this makes it very difficult to understand this lesson, or this teaching. That the All is IN the Plenty, and the Plenty is IN the All. And that there is in fact *enough* or *sufficient* or even at times *a great deal* - but that it is not being **shared or distributed correctly**. But that again is not the fault of the system itself, but the fault of those that create it, abide it, or force others to fall under it as well.

L: That kind of brings me to a question about the fact that some Humans feel like we have been enslaved, they feel we are NOW experiencing a form of slavery. Is this true?

G: It is not necessarily true, but it is fair for Humanity to look to those who have oppressed it, and not wish to look at itself as its own oppressor, you see? It is safer, if you like, more valuable, more interesting to the story to say. *"Oh it was a long, long time ago, from this other world and that other being and they monkeyed about and... and nixed our ability to grow at our own rate,"* and such. But it is only because Humanity does not have its own memories of so many times ago, and some of these times were so completely different - the world was so completely different than it is now - that it is easy to consider it a complete Other-world or complete Other beings, you see? Because oh-so-foreign it is to the Now.

Now, **YES. Humanity is oppressed**, **it is enslaved,** if you like. But for the most part, Humanity does not know what freedom is! If one goes about blindfolded, one does not know what it is like to see the light. But in this case, one has not removed the blindfold because they do not yet wish to see the truth. Truly it is that one could say, "I wish to see the Truth, certainly I could handle it, I could know it!" or what it would be. But the blindfold stays on - and the cell door, unlocked, remains open.

L: I seeeeeee. Okay, that surely gives us something to think about. And that leads me to something I am talking about in the book, about **Assuring our Food Supply**. I have been wondering how to support people if the food supply becomes diminished or challenged for any reason. I want to offer my readers some suggestions, what kinds of hope can we offer them about the food supply?

G: Best it would be, to **not become accustomed to what is available now**. And to truly become accustomed, then, to what is Food and what is Not Food, for this is truly not known. **If something comes in a box, it is not Food, it is very simple**. You see, if it is grown, and truly grown and out of the ground, or with the water hydroponically, or with the natural elements, it is Food. If it is brought about by seed or plant or elemental proportion or such, by what means it is grown that can be debatable, but that is food. **Once it is combined with either inert elements or those that are truly chemicalized, or human-made, it is not truly Food**. That does not mean that it is not edible, it simply means it is not a Food of the Earth. And so that is how to consider it: Is it a Food of the Earth? Will it then benefit my Body?

Now, much and longer time ago, I gave a simple statement that All Things that are Natural in their own way, all things that are grown or such, must have at least **Seven**

Different Purposes. So let us imagine then, that there is an herb then, and this herb you see, well yes it is edible, it is a condiment, well yes perhaps it can be made into a salve, yes, to some individuals it may be a poison as well. Even a poison then is a PURPOSE, you see. So all things must have then, at least you see, their Seven Purposes. And this is how to begin to understand Food as well.

Next, it would behoove most people to truly see for themselves, if it is at all possible, how Food is grown. For the most part, most beings will see little pictures, here is a farm animal and here is a little corral, and there is a little garden with the Sunshine behind it, and Lo, look, there is an image of Corn growing, 8 and 10 and 12 feet tall, just as your ancestors would do. And so in your mind you say, "Oh, look what I am eating as my ancestors did!" or such, you see? But that is not the case today, it would be important to truly see what is it that is grown, where and how it is grown, and by whom is it grown, to truly know. For even those things that are brought to market, even to Farmer's Market, are sometimes deceptions as well. So this must be understood.

It is important to see how it is that *animals* are grown, and how is it that they are slaughtered, and how it is that they come to be considered food, or such, you see? So this knowing will be of benefit to Humanity (who does not truly wish to know these things). They wish to know, but not truly! They wish to know what is the healthiest version of that, that they can do, but they do not wish to know what is the version of that, that they cannot do, or what else they can do. For the most part, Humanity still wishes the status quo on this, "Just give me what I am most comfortable with, and yes I know that I have lessons to learn, and certainly I will get to that, and yes, I am deeply committed to the environment and such, but maybe not today." *(Laura laughing)* It is like that. But so that is the average person that we are speaking to, in that way. See, and so this must be understood as well.

And so an education then, must be a TRUE education. With open eyes, and with open minds, and THEN open mouths! The mouth should be the last to open, you see, as one discovers what to do, and then how to move beyond that as well. For not all things that are considered Food will be available. Some things will be available off and on, it will come a time when foods will truly be considered seasonal as they once were, you see. It is available now, it is not available until next season. For now, all is well, it can be shipped or brought or unpacked or traded, or what it will be, so much that one considers that everything is available in all moments and at all times! So it is better to think, then, in terms of that it is not ALL available, and such, see?

L: Yes I do, I do. And then some of the ideas about growing our own food, is that where we need to go next?

G: It can be. Certainly it is an appropriate idea to grow one's own, to see the growing, and to do so. But I do not see that, given the population of Humanity, that this will take in other areas, certainly it will not take in urban areas. So, if you are speaking then, or writing then for those that are in the agricultural areas, certainly then it would hit home, "Well of course we need to grow our own, or provide for ourselves, or provide somewhat." But if you are speaking to those in urban environments, they will say "Well that is fine for others but what are WE to do," you see?

L: I do see, and what *about* those urban areas, what are they to do?

G: They are to come together in the ways that are **Cooperative**, if at all possible. **Cooperative ways of purchasing, or sharing, or inviting, or trading for**, or in such ways - in smaller communities, and yes, perhaps even on rooftops and such! But particularly in those areas, and particularly for those I will say of the lower-income variety as well. They must begin to think for themselves and not in terms of what either governments can provide, or others will provide for them. They must begin to think as a Cooperative system, as a community, as neighborhood, as neighbors - to begin to *share together*. Even if it is to purchase at wholesale or the quantities, and then to share or divvy into smaller amounts. Truly to begin to say, "If I provide for myself, I *must* begin to provide for my neighbor, as well!" When one has a mindset that is open and expanded to **share**, then more will come to them as well! It is an old concept, but one for the most part that lies forgotten, now that one barely knows who one's neighbor is.

L: Right, right, right - yes, you are so completely and totally right.

G: In olden times, everyone had something to contribute, you see! So it was not that everyone MUST grow their own food or they will starve. In olden times it was not that everyone grew food, but they were able to exchange or purchase what one needed, you see, and it may be that way now. It may be that one will need assistance with the technology project that others will know so much more, but they do not know how to feed themselves.

L: Yes, the Barter System!

G: Yes or some method of exchange or coming together, see?!

L: It's great to tell people that, so that they remember, and realize that those old ways were there for a reason, because they worked! Yes!

G: But the difficulty now is that some things are seen as more valuable than others. **FOOD is not yet seen as truly valuable, because it is so available, you see?** So it is not seen as such a valuable commodity. Technology, however, is high now, the ability to give transportation, for instance, is a high-value item now. If that changes, then a different value system must come about.

There will come a time, however, where the ability, or the want to exchange in some other ways will erase one fear, or replace it with another, or there will be a fear of something else. But you see, Humanity is now in a time of Fear, it is in a time of Crisis, and in some ways Fear will propel it forward as well. In the same way that Knowledge propels one forward, Fear can as well. But Fear will cause one to must take a step, where they would not otherwise, you see? It is not necessarily the best of all motivators, but it is a motivator.

L: Is there anything we can offer Hope about, any other things you think are important for Humans to know about today?

G: What if there was something between Hope and Hopeless? What if there is a midpoint? Because at times when one is Hopeful, one is hopeful, yes, that this must be better, or that must be over, or this will be normal again, or better than it was. And so at times, Hope becomes somewhat of a fantasy. And it is not the true nature of Hope. But the True Nature of Hope is a little bit more like Faith in Oneself, or Faith in the Process. Faith in the Next Coming Forward. Faith in the ability to get through something, faith in the uncovering of Knowledge or Guidance.

It is not simply, "Make it better, or take the pain away." It is the *discovery* of how things will come to be, and that they will come together in ways that may not yet be known. And so that understanding, we do not know everything. There are so many things we have not thought of yet! We are a generation of curiosity seekers. We are Explorers. We are ones who have sought and come from other difficult moments, and understand these, you see? So what I say, then, is that here is a place that is before or beyond Hope, and it is not to say that it is Hopeless or that Hope does not exist. It is more of a Knowing that we are Here, and purposeful as we have said, and we will figure this out! We will find a way through. And that is not the same as Hope, which in some ways has been put forward in a very juvenile way. And so it is a more mature version of Hope, perhaps, that is better put forth.

L: Yes, I agree. And that is your belief, that we will move forward and we will move through our challenges, right?

G: YES! Because that is what Humanity is here to discover, you see? The process is Life Itself. The process is what Life will deliver to your table, or to your day. And the process is also not to become too attached to the process! Or the lesson, or what one believes Life is about, or what one was told or promised years ago - that is also part of the lesson! For Life itself is a discovery that Life simply Is. Life Simply Is. The meaning of Life Simply Is. The Purpose of Life is What One Will Give To It. It is what one will discover, it is what one will allow, or invite, or share in that is what makes a Life both more interesting and delved into deeper, and like that.

L: *(I asked a personal question about my health, but since Gaia said some amazing stuff about Fear and how to deal with it, I will share some of it here.)*

G: Your health is Well. There is no grand consideration in this area. Now in terms of

FEAR, does it get IN you, as you have said? Oh, Yes! Fear can enter through the pores of the skin, through the mind and the brain, through the eyes and what one takes in visually, and through the mouth - and when one speaks one's fears, well, there they go, gathering inside the mouth and you swallow them up, you see? So Fear does, indeed, get inside!

Now, in the same way, Fear can also be purged, you see, just as all things are purged from the body. Liquids are purged from the body and out they go in the urine, you see? The body knows how to purge itself. So simply because Fear enters the body, does not mean that it becomes lodged there forever. And so if you like, you may give yourself the daily directive as well, that **"Fear that enters in the morning, out it goes in the evening."** You see? Or you may give yourself this directive as you sleep, that while you sleep and you dream, that your body is then *purged* of these daily difficulties.

And that is not to say that you will arise the next moment in very perfect health and that all things will be well and you will no longer be subject to any toxins. But certainly you are capable of purging yourself from daily fears, and daily toxins, and the dust that settles upon you, that is then rinsed away in the shower, and like that.

L: So I understand there is a lesson to be found in taking too many supplements out of Fear, and how that can be toxic as well?

G: Yes, that is correct. So again, take those things that will simply enhance the balance that is already there. You are not looking to *correct*, you are looking to simply enhance the balance and the health that is already there. So that you do not communicate to yourself or to others that there is something *wrong that must be fixed*! Now, if there IS something wrong that needs to be fixed, your body will communicate it to you, just as your customers communicate it to you, *"I do not feel well, I feel this or I feel that, I need help, I need a great deal of help,"* and they will tell you what has been tried or not tried and like that, this you understand already.

Simply be very, very gentle and kind to your body as well. Not as if you are unwell or sick, but *"There there, Body,"* you wrap your arms around your body, *"There there."* You know, not so much *"We are this..., we are this...."* But **"We are HERE - We Are One."** You see? Be very kind to your Body.

L: Oh Gaia, your wisdom is so timely and so perfect. I am so grateful for you. And I look forward to all our engagements out and into the Wild.

G: Indeed, Sweet. It will be so. It will be so.

L: I love you very much, and I thank you SO much.

G: I bid you Good Day.

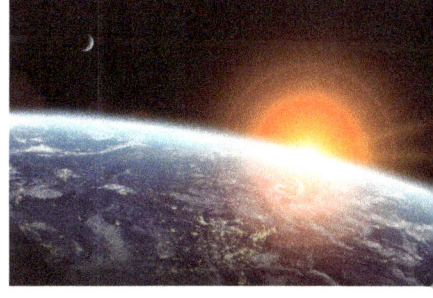

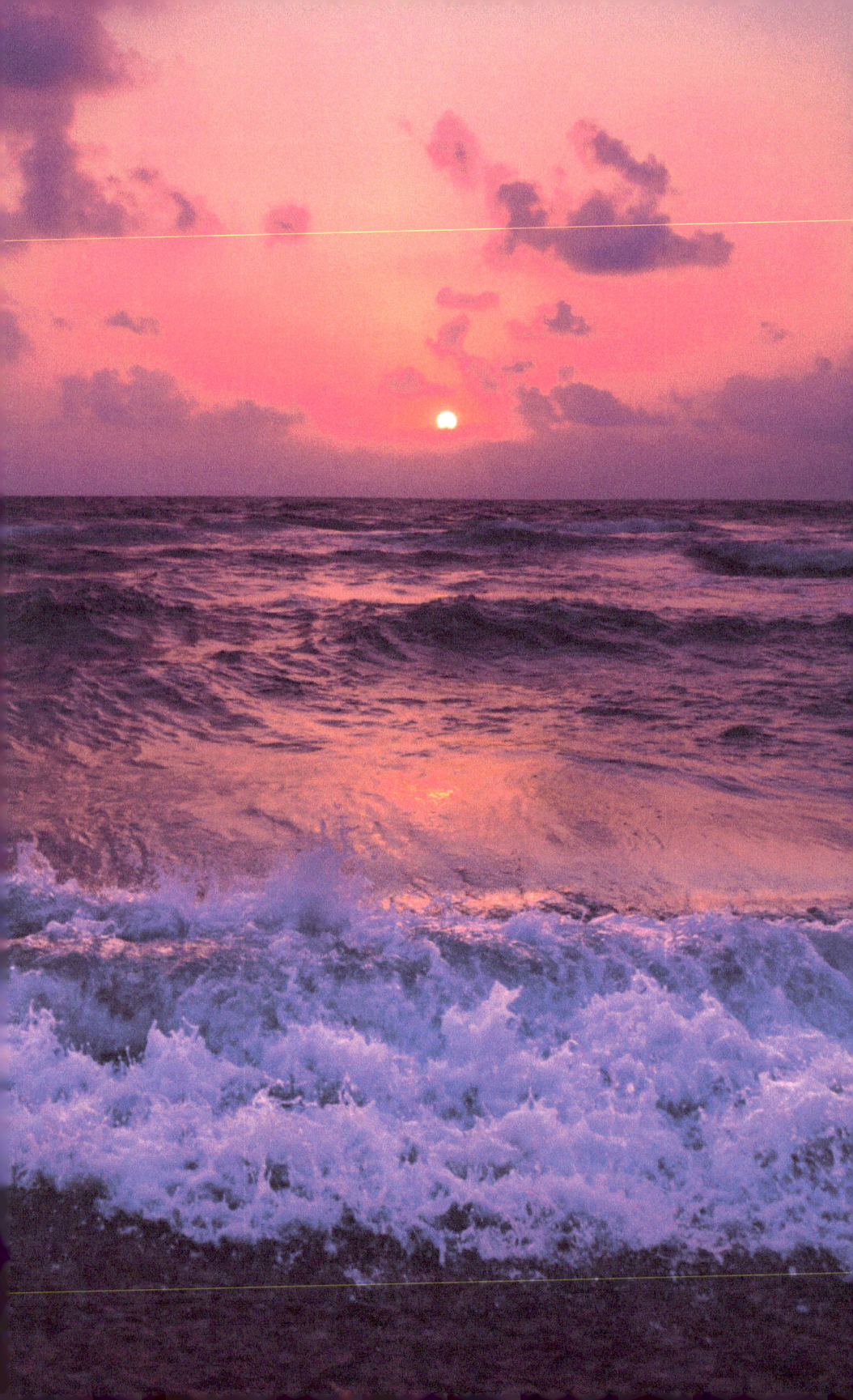

~ Chapter 7 ~
WISDOM OF THE GARDEN

> "Forget not that the Earth delights to feel your bare feet and the Winds long to play with your hair."
>
> ~ Khalil Gibran

WHAT A JOURNEY

If you have made it this far, thank-you! You are now in possession of an encyclopedic amount of natural information you can reference for the rest of your life. You and I have both grown on this journey. It has been easy to become more connected to our beloved Planet Earth, and along the way learn details and recover skills we can all really use. What else is there to say after 365 pages? Maybe you would indulge me just a few more words of encouragement, a couple more techniques I use to **Stay Happy.** I believe the best use of your precious time is to seek and be in Happiness, keeping the vibe high, and your intentions positive. But sometimes, Happiness is the least accessible feeling, there seems no light at the end of these tunnels. YOU can alter that. And I want to encourage you to **LIVE** your special brand of magic more fully, so you can get *your* gifts out into this Beautiful New World.

We each contribute to this Garden, every single moment.

YOUR VIBRATION MATTERS

Everyday, you offer your own personal **Vital Force Emanation** to the people of this Earth. Your energy radiates out, to every being, every plant, and every thing you see - and they can feel you! We each broadcast our own Superstar Frequency on this "Gaian Radio." **Will your vibration and your contribution be High and Joyous?** Or is your signal spotty, unreliable and drops out? Do you have a pure, optimistic outlook that warms every room you enter, or are you the reason it drops cold? Keep in mind that you can *alter* your emanation and your **broadcast** at any moment. It's your energy and your personal devotion that will show.

Your ENERGY creates through your thoughts, your dreams, ideas and inventions, lessons, wisdom, social actions (and descendants!). These will become chapters in the story of this Garden, all with *your* individual energy signature attached. What have you come to create? What **Energy Legacy** are you leaving as a result of living Your Life? What frequency are *you* passing on?

TUNE YOUR DIAL TO THE GOOD NEWS CHANNEL

When you feel low, as Abraham instructs, concentrate on the **next better thought**. Imagine how it would *feel* to feel better, until you find your way up into the positive spectrum. Remember, you cannot be in Love and be in Fear at the same time, because they are polar opposite frequencies. **Concentrating on Love makes the Fear vibrationally disappear**. Maintaining a Loving State of Mind is a constant effort that eventually becomes a habit, a really GREAT habit. And it is the *secret* of successful people who broadcast the most positive energy available.

Another one of my favorite phrases of Abraham's, that I love to say and to live by is,

"Everything Always Works Out For Me."

When you live with this in your mind, you find yourself creating it! As Humans, our sacred task is to monitor what kind of Show we are putting out on the airwaves, what we are creating, what energy we are broadcasting, what culture we are promoting - and to seek to raise the energy higher if we can. Like switching a channel on the television from a cop show murderfest to a beautiful Nature show! There is another frequency that is always available to be tuned-in to, to be joined, and you have free will at all times to change the channel. Make a shift in your messaging. I wrote a song about this for our album in 2015, and the lyrics say it well:

> "It's not nearly too late - to set this world straight
> All you gotta do is make up your mind.
> See you've got a power that can move mountains -
> Playing Good News inside of you, both day and night.
> SO - just move the dial - play it for awhile
> You've got a Good News Channel in You....
> It's true what you say can make the world change.
> Your very thoughts can light the way, soooo -
> You write the story - Chaos or Glory -
> Be a Good News Channel today."

Lighten your load! Lift yourself up higher! While it can be a challenge to break out of a bad mood or a negative way of thinking, it is part of the responsibility of living. You must simply find techniques to do it. When you remember that **the energy you broadcast is the energy you receive** - it makes it easier to change your output because you know it will change your input. Whatever approach works for you, **even imagining a shift in your mood can literally create one!** It is in your control, so you can make the difference by doing something about it. Visualize your own little dials in your imagination and literally just change the channel! Use the "dial" imagery to tune in to a better feeling, a higher frequency. This is a powerful way to change many things within your mind and body. I have used the dial visualization when I needed to turn up an increase in serotonin, or raise my blood sugar when I couldn't eat, or to bring my spiritual vibration DOWN low enough to drive safely. Visualize it, see it done, and that energy will be created and will affect you.

Knowingly broadcast an extra high vibration that raises people up. Create the kind of positive energy that keeps OTHER people going. **High Frequency Vibrations Are ABSOLUTE Medicine**. They are the antidote to fear, hate, and bitterness, and you can use them like a remedy when you feel low. The lightest emotions of **Joy, Gratitude** and **Love** can be sought on purpose, you can call these frequencies (Angels) in, and seek to be a Beacon of their Light.

THE MAGICAL FLOW

Positive thinkers agree it is helpful to stay "in the flow" instead of struggling against the River of Life, fighting and overdoing it to achieve greatness. Many of us (especially the short ones or the different ones) grew up believing we had to push the river, stay active, bulldoze harder, hammer everybody in order to be noticed or move forward. Sometimes we'd overdo it, over-achieve, over-stress, and push ourselves too far, even to the detriment of our health or relationships.

All along there was a secret we didn't learn in school (although the Buddhists and Taoists teach it). **You CAN LET GO, and allow the River to float you TO what you need** without striving so hard to get there. Taking a few good river trips will help you understand this one! You learn right away to let the River do the work, and to gently ease yourself into the best flow, positioning for the least resistance and most effortless forward motion. I have been working with this concept for awhile, seeking NOT to push the river, trying not to push the outcome, not to push myself onto everyone and into everything. **Just like changing your Food habits, seek that which is more NATURAL and AUTHENTIC, ORGANIC and REAL.**

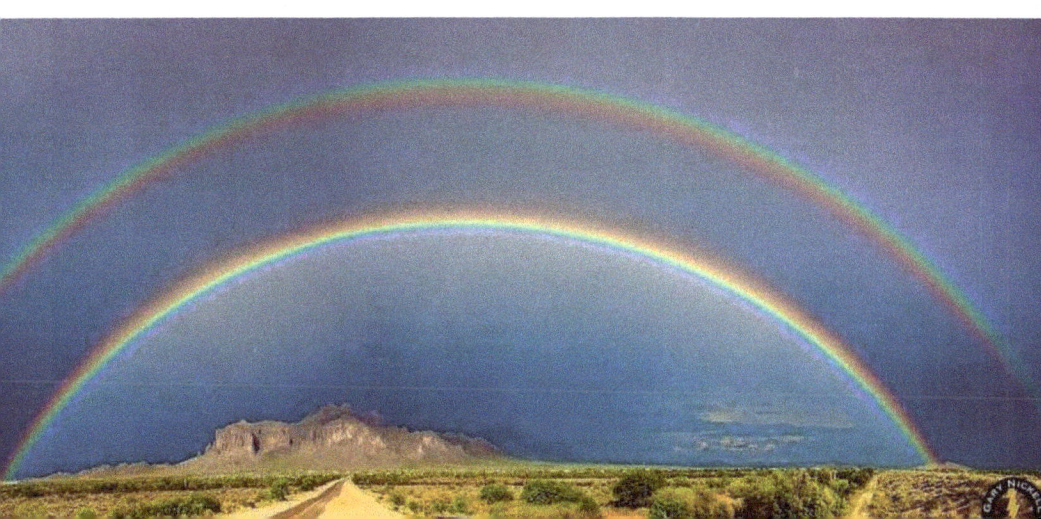

This is a mature teaching (that I am totally still working on). It dovetails perfectly with Dave Allen's counsel, that you should allow things and people to come to YOU. Let it be *their* idea. Utilize your magnetic heart to draw to you what you desire. While contemplating this in meditation one day, I distinctly heard the words, "**I Let Go, I Am In the Magical Flow.**"

"**I Let Go, I Am In the Magical Flow**." I feel amazing when I say this! I think it is a mantra for freedom, for re-lease, and a reminder that what you need will **magically flow right toward you.** You may think this is simplistic, too good to be true or maybe even impossible. But try saying this for a few days and see what happens!

As a wise man once told me, *"If you don't like how things are, just wait."* Ironically, this is perfect Magical Flow advice, because things are always changing so quickly! What triggers you today may no longer be in effect tomorrow. People move on and situations can change in a moment. It takes patience and perseverance to calmly watch the flow of the River in your life, and be open to what it brings in its own timing.

> **"Adopt the pace of Nature; her secret is Patience."**
> *~ Ralph Waldo Emerson*

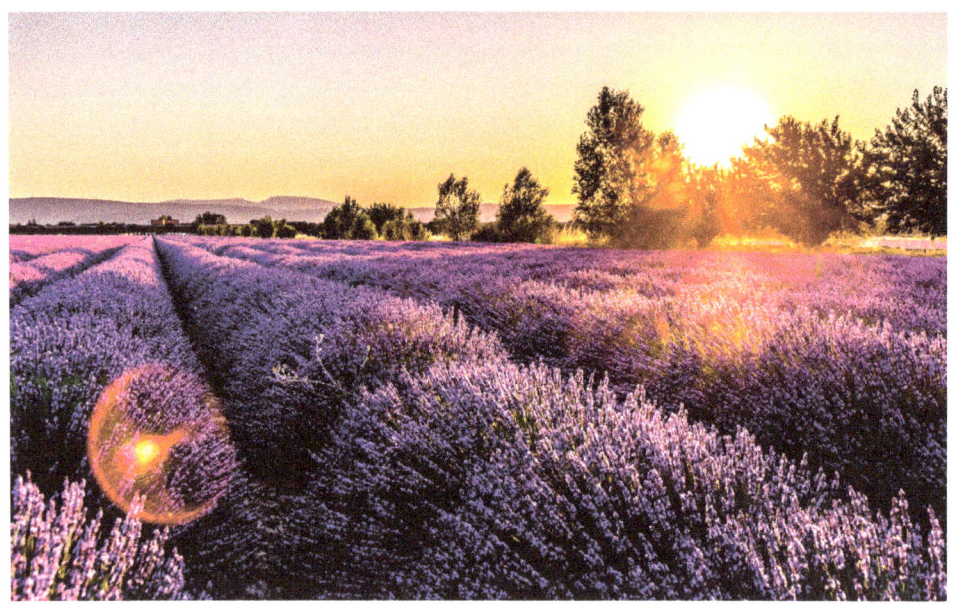

ALL TASKS ARE SPIRITUAL

A good way to remain in the Present Moment, in the Magical Flow, is to perform your actions and tasks more SLOWLY and with an intention of Grace and Harmony. If we make our efforts more purposeful and mindful, honoring them with our **complete attention**, each individual task has an extra available energy, that may actually help us to perform it better. Like the Buddhists say, *"If you are cutting an apple, just cut the apple."* I realize this implies that we drop our famous addiction to Multi-Tasking. Oh, how we love to prove how many things we can do at once! And we love to do everything *super quickly* to prove our brilliance and efficiency. WHY? This notion we all just accept is ridiculous, that working a million miles a minute, and doing twenty-seven things at once, is a virtue. That's just plain brainwashing for better productivity.

This morning when I heard the words, "**All Tasks Are Spiritual**," it dawned on me that if you live that way, a beautiful Spiritual Life is yours! You do not work on your Spirit only at church or temple or meditation time. THIS IS A FULL-TIME OCCUPATION, moment by moment. So it follows that *everything* can be done with this in mind, every little task becomes a spiritual opportunity. I want to live a Life that makes *all moments* more special and Spiritual. That is a virtue, making what I do intentionally special and immensely Spiritual.

SEVEN GENERATIONS

Let's expand a moment on the idea that everyone is working hard on their own stuff. You have your own personal floods and cataclysms - and YOU are also their solution! Face it, the best thing to do right now is to FACE IT. We are all being impulsed and compelled to look directly at our own imperfections - some call this doing "shadow work," - and to improve upon them. You could also call it processing "challenges" or "blocks" or "baggage." Each of us have come to this Life with certain things to work through (karma + desires + contracts). What is challenging to you is the very stuff that will help you to grow. It's all an enormous set-up! All of your *stuff* is coming up to be **healed**, so that you can Evolve. Your Soul is crafting many ways for you to practice this kind of **Overcoming** and **Mastery**.

An interesting fact is that your composite personality contains **Beliefs** you operate within that have likely come NOT ONLY from your own choices, but the **Ancestral Choices of Seven Generations**. Yes. Many of my teachers confirm that our DNA contains programs that are Signature Core Beliefs from our genetic ancestors, going back *(at least)* seven generations. That would be beliefs and ideals formed somewhere around the 1850's! This means that you will find Beliefs that you are operating within, that are not necessarily your own style. Like having to be the Overachiever - that may exist in you because your Italian immigrant Great Grandfather had to scrape and scrap to be noticed and accepted and be the best, because HE was the one who got to go to America to live the American Dream. So, he had to overachieve to survive and YOU are doing it still. WHO KNOWS? You get to choose if this is the way you want to continue on - if this is your most truthful, **present** and **authentic** way to live.

When you find yourself believing and acting in a manner that doesn't seem like your own, you can ask to clear this old belief, tell the Universe it no longer serves you and ask to replace it with a better one. Reprogram your operating system and do an update! I remind you again about what Louise Hay always says, "**Your Point of Power is In the Present Moment.**" I find it comforting that we are able to choose, right now, whether or not we want to "BE" and embody a certain quality or energy. It only takes a second - AND a better thought - to change who we are.

In these revolutionary times, that Pioneering Spirit of yours wants to move beyond your old limitations, to break ground and Become More! Keep in mind that **Your Life Has a Mission.** You are supposed to be discovering things about yourself and changing for the better. You are supposed to be discerning what you love and don't love and making choices with that sense of contrast. You are supposed to be choosing, "I am THAT. I am NOT THAT." So, continue to discern and change and be true to your evolving self. I know it does feel weird and hard sometimes, but I believe you will be happy with the result. The best part is that every time we **improve ourselves, we change the energy of this Garden a little bit more toward Peace, Happiness and Harmony.** It is in fact the only way to do it.

NOTHING IS MISSING

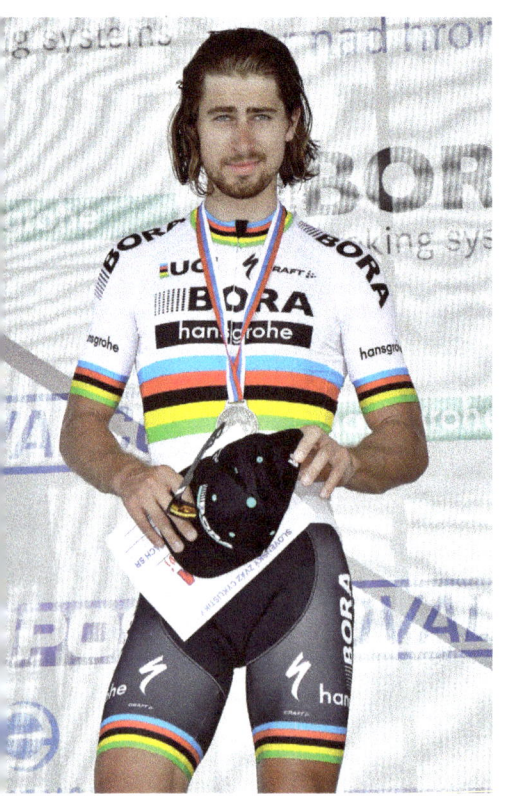

Peter Sagan, legendary three-time World Road Cycling Champion, has a famous quote for the media, "**Nothing Is Missing.**" He uses it when the critics demand to know why he hasn't done this or won that. He would always smile a sneaky little smile when he said it - and then go off and win another major race! His simple phrase has really changed my life. I have it posted in the kitchen where I see it everyday to remind myself.

Nothing Is Missing. When we realize **we are always given everything we need**, when we live from the perspective that we **ALREADY HAVE** what it takes, we begin to act stronger and feel empowered *as we are right now*. We begin to believe in ourselves, our preparation, and our Spiritual support, and we can find strength because this is so. This is a prayer, this is a mantra, this is an affirmation, this is a Self-Fulfilling Prophecy. And when it is directed to create positive outcomes, it is highly effective. This is a tried and true practice of Winners. Like Peter.

GOLDEN LININGS

My Daddy was the Wisest of Men. When I would get down, he would speak to me his often-repeated and classic motto: *"Do the Best You Can with What You've Got."* Which would actually help a lot. It gave me something to do, to actively make the best of every situation, making it succeed in *all* the ways possible, because that was what I had to work with. **Finding the Gold in WHAT IS, what is given in each moment, instead of fighting it, defending it, excusing it, or wishing it was different.** Ironically, it helps to think this way, and I continue to pass on his simple but helpful phrase for inspiration. Just Do the Best You Can With What You've Got. There's always more Gold in the moment than you can initially see.

We are all given a series of events to work with everyday. My purpose is to respond to what I am given, in the best possible way I can, with my actions, my faith in the process, my patience, and my Overcoming Spirit. My journey is to accept that even the challenges make me more beautiful.

> "Should you shield the canyons from the windstorms you would never see the true beauty of their carvings."
>
> ~Elisabeth Kübler-Ross

FIRM FABULOUS PROGRESS

Another of my Father's mottos that encourages me, is to strive for "**Constant Daily Improvements.**" He would remind me that working on myself, being humble and striving to be KIND were the hallmarks of being a good person. The key is to work on doing something every day that makes an Improvement in the World. Whether that means exercising, or teaching, or campaigning, or taking your vitamins, or being nice to the waitress, or putting your clothes away, or calling your Family. Just making any small Improvement sends a signal of purpose and intent into the Field. You keep doing this good work everyday, intending, progressing and striving to be a Person of Excellence, and the results are palpable.

My Father would astonish me the way he could make a total stranger feel comfortable, simply by being kind to them, smiling and taking an interest, listening and being genuine in return. This netted him results everywhere from restaurants to the General Motors/Labor Union bargaining table. Treat all people as your Family and you can't help but create Happiness and Peace everywhere you go, like he did. Be extra KIND to everyone you meet and see where that leads! Everybody really is going through something we can't see or understand. Smile and make someone's day BETTER. Recognizing we are All One and treating others the way you want to be treated really is a healing Life practice.

> "All Things are our Relatives. What we do to anything we do to ourselves. All is really One."
>
> ~ Black Elk

My Daddy had a ridiculous and brilliant sense of humor, and a very loud laugh. *"If all else fails,"* he would say, *"You gotta just laugh about it!"* and then he'd belly laugh until it echoed! How true, what else can you do? There really is no situation that can't be improved with laughter and a lighter attitude. Yes, LAUGHTER definitely is a potent MEDICINE. Staying light and maintaining your sense of humor is some of the best advice, and medication, ever. Making a conscious choice to step back and not take everything so seriously will serve you and your health so well. Lighten up, it works.

Just like him, I have adopted the tendency to REALLY laugh loudly when something is funny - I mean, I can't even help it, I shout it out! The irrepressible joy released when you belly laugh is immense and truly healing. And yes, like my Daddy, I have become famous for my laugh. What a wonderful legacy.

SHARING YOUR BOUNTY

Most of us know the value in doing good deeds, in being of service to others. But I hope we could revisit this concept and all of us could ramp it up a bit. This is the perfect time to **share what surplus you have** from your Garden and your Life. Give your old clothes to thrift stores, tip a little more generously, give your time to the needy, seek out people you could help, volunteer for some cause which you always wanted to support. Check out the many things going on in your community, or start something brand new! The cure for loneliness could be in reaching out and giving to others in brand new ways. You may invent a new way to connect your neighborhood! During the pandemic, my dear, sweet Mother painted rocks with colorful and positive

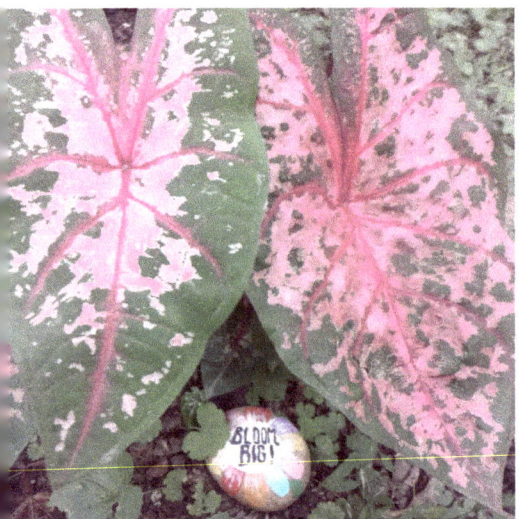

messages, and clandestinely placed them in her neighbor's flowerbeds at night. The joy this simple small act gave *her* was wonderful, but it spread beauty to so many! Other people in the neighborhood noticed, I am sure they smiled deeply, and dreamt up their own ways to do things to spread Love. People started sharing jigsaw puzzles and old novels in the Little Small Library at her corner, and many people put up holiday lights to create a more joyous atmosphere in the midsummer. One small act of kindness created the joy in people's hearts to do more. **Magic Spreads!**

What I believe matters most is that you **use your Life to be a Blessing**, in your own unique and very special way. You can count on support from your Planet, your Plants, your Plant Heroes, and all your People in this mission. And sometimes it will be harder than other times. But even in personal hardship, it is so easy and so healing to simply offer silent blessings to others, while you ask for some of your own. *Just Keep Going*, and know there's a whole host of energies working with you. Know that everything you do to bring positive returns for others, is also for you. That IS the Law of Karma - what you give is returned to you, and often many times multiplied. So, pay it forward first, by continually finding ways to nurture and support others.

> **"By practicing Kindness all over with everyone you will soon come into the Holy Trance, definite distinctions of personalities will become what they really mysteriously are, our common and eternal Bliss stuff, the pureness of everything forever, the great bright essence of mind, even and one thing everywhere, the holy eternal milky love, the White Light everywhere everything, empty bliss, svaha, shining, ready, and awake, the compassion in the sound of silence, the swarming myriad trillionaire you are."[2]**
>
> ~ Jack Kerouac

Yes. That is what I wish for you. The shining brilliance of the very best of this Garden.

THE POWER OF "I AM"

It is said that whatever follows the phrase "**I AM**" is looking for you, and will hunt you down. Speaking the "I AM" is a moment of definition, a moment of **choice for your future.** What truth are you speaking about yourself, drawing to yourself, with each use of the "I AM?" Take care with this powerful prophecy, and assure yourself that each statement you make from a position of "I Am" is aligned with what you truly desire for yourself. Languaging matters; what you speak of, you offer power to bring into being. Your use of the word, and being impeccable with your word, is a skill best developed. Do not EVER berate yourself and speak negatively of yourself, it is not funny or necessary. Do not say things you don't mean. There is a potency to your words, a spell-casting, and a Sovereignty they create that is your birthright. This power and ability is your God-given legacy, and THE WORD is your choice and your tool to utilize. Use correct languaging about yourself and your situation. Speak Peace and your Future into being: **I AM CREATING PEACE. I AM WELL ABLE. I AM GRATEFUL FOR MY BOUNTY. I AM LIVING IT PERFECTLY. I AM ENJOYING MY EXCELLENT LIFE. I AM MORE THAN ENOUGH. I AM A SUCCESS. I AM PERFECTLY MADE. I AM.....**

DO YOUR THING

Find what makes you feel fulfilled and joyful and excited, and just keep doing it! *Explore* your wildest dreams for they were put *in you* for a reason. Even when the odds may be stacked against you, or the future looks dim, keep working with your gifts and desires. What you feel hopelessly drawn to do is most likely where you will find success. What comes **fairly easy and effortlessly** to you is a hint (though you still have to do the work) - and if it keeps you up all night ,that is a big clue. Usually, your mission is something you *"have to do."* Or something to which you just keep finding yourself naturally dedicating time to, the thing that creates the MOST EXCITEMENT in you, what you can't stop thinking about. Your true desires are like rockets out into the Universe that draw the Ether and the Power of Creation to assemble your dreams. Spending time perfecting the vision of your desires is time well-spent for creating them. In fact, it is verifiably the **emotions of living as if your dreams had already come true that makes them happen**, alters the Universe on your behalf.

Not to mention that **YOUR THING** is the reason why **YOU'RE HERE**. No one can do what you can do. You made a deal to come back to Earth at exactly this time to do your best work yet, to be a part of Radical Transformative Change. You returned now to move *through* all your worst challenges and create your most magnificent results! You planned this, you chose the circumstances, and the timing, chose your parents and your loved ones, and when to meet them. You chose the many hardships that will prepare you to ultimately make it through anything. You chose which problems to solve and endowed yourself with the ability to do so. You chose both the successes and the lessons. The stress stimulates extreme growth, just like with the Plants.

I am excited about the many new ways you will make your **own blossoming happen,** together with the help of the Garden. There's just no more time to waste, we all need to be running at peak performance! *Make all the difference you can.* Work joyfully on your Personal and Planetary Broadcast. Make the most of all the Natural Foods and Wild Medicines we have here. Gaia offers you all her Bounty, which is Limitless, so support her and her creatures back, in every way you can. From me, Gaia, and on behalf of all the other helpful energies on and around our Beautiful Planet Earth - let us just say to you,

> "WE LOVE YOU, we support you and we thank YOU for all the impressive Good Work you do here. **You are greatly appreciated, and YOU make a great difference to our Earth.** Thank-you, Dear Friend."

~ The End ~

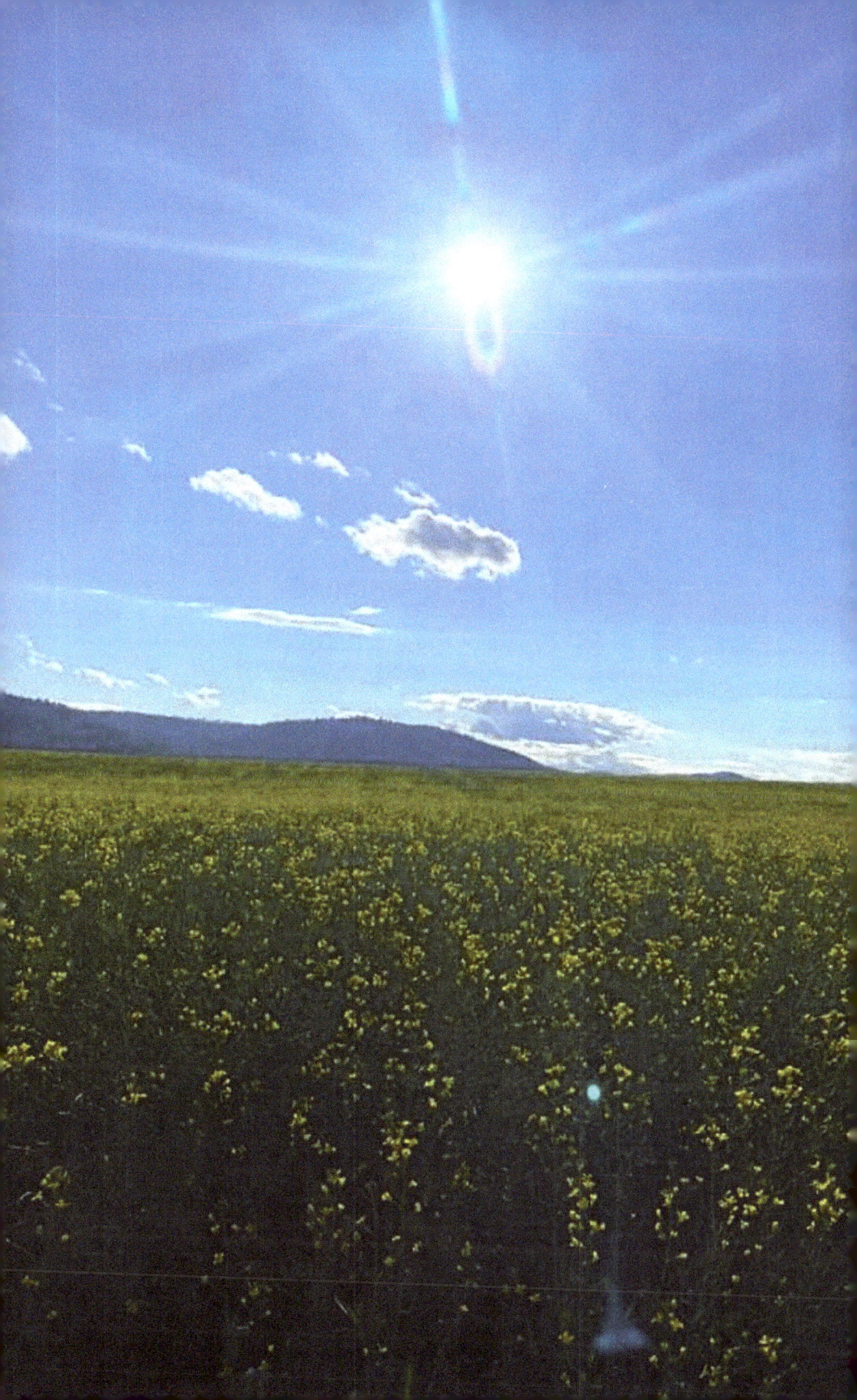

Heartfelt Acknowledgments

Thank-you, **Dear Reader,** for engaging with me and exploring the Secrets of Nature! I do hope you will look for **Volume Three** - because it is the perfect companion to this book! Originally, I wrote one enormous book and really still wish I could have presented it that way. But I think it worked better to split it into two volumes, so stay tuned for the release of *The Garden of Earth Volume Three - Elemental Remedies and Planetary Magic!* You will love the exceptional, out-of-this-World information.

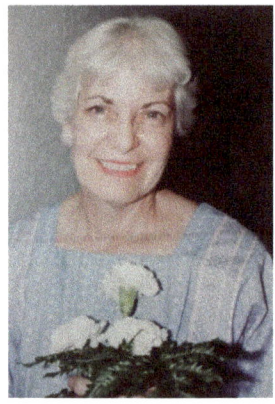

I dedicate this book to My Sweet Mother, **JoAnne Lamun** - Dearest Mommy - the Great Solver of Problems, Brilliant Director of Everything, Keeper of the Family, and Inspiration to Millions of Children. Your love and support created this craziness we call me, and your friendship nourishes me still. Loving you is a blessing I count every single day. Mommy, I want to thank you for inspiring me to sing, to teach, to write, to paint, to laugh and to LIVE. You taught me how to create - how to put my whole heart into my creations and make *special stuff that matters.* Thank-you Mommy, You are never far from me now. I can only imagine what you are directing in Heaven. Thanks for your continuing support and all the Butterflies. I love you so much.

To my Sweet Suorella, **Lisa "LeeLee" Lamun** - you are a True-Blue Sister and Friend, Unique & Wonderful, Brilliant Spontaneous Musical Creator & Performer, AKA the Great Reformer, Personal Assistant to the World, Best Clinical Research Subject, and Supreme Caretaker of Everyone, ever. LEELEE, thank-you for always giving me something to laugh about and learn about! My sweet Sister - all these years of trying to crack you up, driving Mom crazy, knowing you are always there knowing me so well, are priceless. Your support and strength and advice is always greatly appreciated, and I am so proud of your personal progress. I guess we might be growing up (just a little bit)! I am so glad Mommy made you for me to play with. I am honored to be your Sister for this Great Journey. You just keep getting BETTER and BETTER. I love watching you remake your Life and I find it quite inspirational.

Everything I do is in honor of my Beloved Husband, **Dave Allen** - Keeper of the Love Flame, King of the House, Musical Partner Supreme, Systems Crystallizer - without whom there would never have been a *Volume 1,* let alone a *Volume 2* and *3* today. You make it possible for me to BE, for me to enjoy my life, and do everything my heart desires! The many things you accomplish everyday to keep our Forest House running, dinners on long days, your constant seeking and researching, the hilarious jokes and all the laughing, your amazing singing voice and stacks of harmonies, multi

~ the garden of earth ~

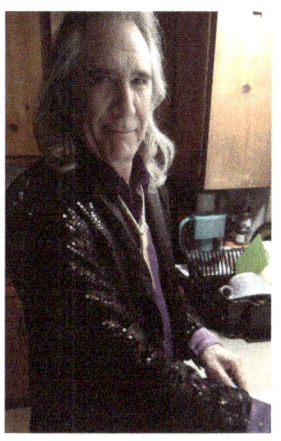

instrumentalism and studio wizardry... seriously the list goes on and on. BABE, you are the LOVE and LIGHT that makes me shine. You complete my life, and I want to be alive simply to be with you more & more. Here's to Playing Music, Creating Daily Everlasting Love, Our Ranch, Our Animals, and Ascending Together!

I also want to acknowledge your amazing Sons, **Tucker** and **Gus Allen**. I love you guys, and have since you were tiny children, when I would sneak you chocolates at Healthy Solutions. It has been a privilege to watch you become outstanding men.

To the Best Daddy Ever, **Big John Lamun** - DADDY your light shines even brighter in me now since you have moved to your New Plane of Unlimited Existence. I can always count on you to be right here, whenever I need you, and it is my Joy to still be connected with you completely. I know you are watching me even as I write this, and I want you to know that your wisdom lives on in my valiant attempt to write these books and live your mottos. I feel your Unlimited Love, and just like you, I remain always *"Just So Proud To Be Here."* You encourage me to always be kind, and your words, loving influence, and wise teachings fill these pages and my life. I know I am a good person because of you. I love you so much. "*Do it, do it, do it!*"

To a Brother from Another Mother, who inspires me from afar with his photos and awe of Nature, **Johnny Rigg**, you are a delightfully wild Angel-In-All-Clothing. Thanks for all the help and love you gave our Mother, being a real part of our Family, and for the Light you share with everyone. Good Job, dear Friend; your excellent, Rainbow Living is being noticed and appreciated. And to our dearly everpresent neighbor and Sister **PUA**, and **Trudy Cronan** and **Tsunemi**, thanks for everything, you are true Angels!

A Soul Sister who continues to change my life for the better is **Paula Kalustian** - my Best Director Ever, and Ongoing Personal Life Supporter. Thanks for always checking on me and keeping me Center Stage, Brightly Lit! Your help with this book was paramount to it becoming what it is today, I truly cannot thank YOU enough for reading and critiquing the whole thing. I love discovering the magic of Life with you. And thanks for all the clothes all these years - if I look good, it is because I am wearing Paula's clothes. It is awesome to be with you and the following California Angels in this Second Family. Thanks for bringing us all together.

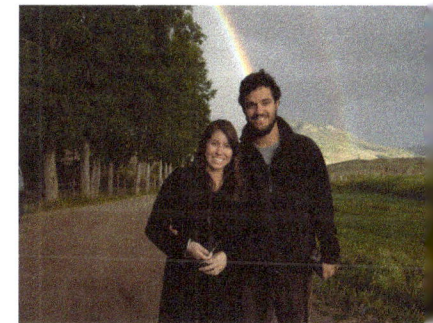

While I never had kids of my own, I got to experience the joy of parenting as a gift from Living Legend **Steve Anthony Mesaros and Jill Anthony**, the Mommy and Daddy of that Second Earth Family. Along with Paula, they welcomed me to live in their home many times over the years. We all helped care for their daughter **Aleka** (whom I always considered to be my surrogate

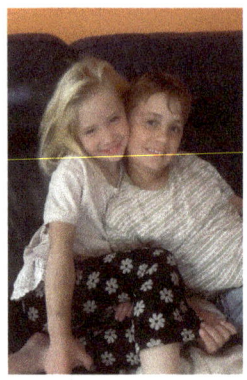
daughter). Now Aleka has rewarded us by marrying an astonishing wizard (and actual know-it-all), **Sean Ballard Bruce**, and their magical union brought into the world two tear-jerkingly perfect "grandchildren" for me. The irrepressible, brilliant farmer and baseball player at 9, **Rowan Bruce** and the zen-smiling (tiny dancer, wise-old-woman at 5) **Maven Bruce**. Watching these children grow up is one of the true highlights of my life. Thanks so much for letting OE and D'Annen be a part of your Family circle. We love you all beyond words on a page. We must get closer and play more often!

To my (questionably) adult Best Friend, Bestie **Gardner Orton**, for all the adventures and meditations and vortexes and a true Friendship of the Ages. Watching you become a Daddy has been a miracle and I am so stoked for your pride, Ashley, Augie, (plus Spirit Kaya and the additions to come). Love you, dude, here's to more.

To my lifelong Best Friend **Kathryn Wadsworth** - you know me better than anyone on Earth, and I am so grateful we are so totally close after all these years. I love you so much, Pearly Shells forever! Thanks for sharing George and Susan, too. And cheers and New Years forever to our fellow Interlochen Girls: **Essie Commers, Jennifer (Grover) Wedgwood, Pammie (French) Blaine, Shannon (McGinley) Woods, Melanie Drane,** and **Nancy Stone** - you will make me laugh until I pee, forever!

I am so lucky to still be in touch with my elementary school Best Friend, **Carole Gleeson Descheemaker**. I love laughing and reminiscing with you after all these years. Your Life and your Family is (always and as ever) beautiful and inspiring.

Great Love, and thanks for the Beautiful Music, to a Musical Spiritual Partner and his partner, **John Hegner & Rebecca Hegner**. You are always the Definition of Love.

Little Mooners Unite - to all the Little Moon Essentials Goons, I love you so much still! Dearest **Catay Jasper, Meghan Hanson Peters, Alison Gianfagna, Charlotte Echo Ernst, Nora Felix, Emily Rosenkranz, Deelicious Denise Barry, Dianne Gentry, Athena Dawson, Liz Hicks, Jenn Stone, Haven Thomas, Ange Young, Kristin Vortex, Anita Hartley, Courtney Van Tubbergen, Meghan Jezo, Chloe Marcellus, Mark Lehman, Reese Morter, Paulie Anderson,** plus any Moon-angels I have forgotten, (Dave Allen and LeeLee, too)!

Love to all of our inspirational Steamboat Pals (especially "The Girls" **Colleen Boynton, Ann Halloran, Jill Elaine, Bernadette Murray** & **Jill Asmus Leeson**), Soulspeakers and Sister Priestesses **Megan Sisk & Samantha Caparrelli, Kristi & Jimmy Neal, Annie & Greg Dore, Randy & Mary Kelley**, and the best Bandmates - **Steve Boynton, Willie Samuelson, Kip Strean, Jon Gibbs, Paul Potyen, Timmy**

Cunningham, Neil Summerfield Marchman, Graham Waters, Dank Oebnick, Pat Waters, Skip Warneke, Todd Intergalactic, Pilgrim....

I'd like to make a special dispensation, **Best Ever Special Thanks** to a dear friend who, through complete typographical error, was left out of the dedication in my first book. Her name is **Joy Love Light (Good Medicine Mama, Honeybee, Deliciousness, Joyful) Winkelman** - and I have known her in this life for over 20 years. She was absolutely instrumental in welcoming me into the Raw Family. I watched her Goddessness dance around and eventually marry another dear friend, **Geronimo Joe Kent Zapf**, in order to create some special new Beings - their two wild and gorgeous children **Hunter & Aiden**. I am in awe of the Mother/Tigress/Goddess you have become. JOY - you were always in the first book and it broke my heart you were left off the page. Please feel what amazing love I have for you, and your Beautiful Family! Whatever changes and growth that come will be directed by your heart, so we will always support you in Everything you Both do.

The influence of the Raw Family remains so strong - you know who you all are and we all changed the world together! To name a few, I continue to be inspired by **Steve "Love In Action" Adler of Sacred Chocolate, Kimberly Reschke, Kerry "Dancing Butterfly" Anahata Ananda, Elaina Love, Jerry Fun Yung Moon Murtagh, Jahsah, Laura Fox, Wild Food Cafe and Rainbow Wild Fooder Joel Gazdar and Aiste, Bliss Crusaders Happy Oasis and Johnny Lightning, Juliano (my original Raw WayShower), Good Medicine Geronimo & Family, Camille "GojiGirl" Rose Fields, Chef Gabrielle Twin-Angel-Mom-Cacao-Creatrix-Brick, Daniel Surthrival Vitalis, Rainbeau Spiritual Entrepreneur Mars, Brigitte Herbal Wonder Mars, Jeff Boticelli Astrological Angel Annie Boticelli, Puma St. Angel and Morgan Langan**...and every retreater ever.

To My MANY Teachers - First, the *Sacred David Triangle* - all Davids, all drummers, all brilliant, all highly influential mentors in my life:

David Avocado Noni Cacao Wolfe - Father of the Raw Food Lifestyle and Beloved Brother Avo to all of us, you opened the Garden up for me so many years ago and changed my life with your true original thoughts. I am literally the healthy person I am today because of you, and you set me on my Living Food quest. Watching your Telegram, livestreams and videos during the Plandemic were light-filled moments in deep darkness. Thank-you for your humor, your knowledge, your memes of life, and your deep-hearted spirit. I will love you forever for opening my eyes.

David Wilcock - I see you as a brilliant archivist and fellow Pisces dreamer. I have learned so much exploring the magic geometry of Nature revealed by your researching. I Honor you as a Co-Conspirator for Goodness on Earth, and thank you ON BEHALF of the Earth and her Peaceful People. You are a true inspiration for my writing and our Garden's mission to Ascend in Light.

~ the garden of earth ~

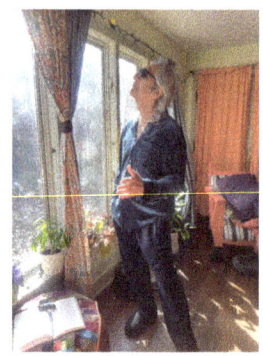

David Allen - my Husband, Witness and Spiritual Teacher of Systems & Blues & Life. I thanked you already - but here I must relate to you as my Teacher. I can't even count the ways your systems and methodology and your influence have changed me for the better (I never lose my key anymore, it goes in the bowl, my "system," every time). I learn something new from you everyday and you are an entertaining and hilarious mentor. Making music with you is such a natural joy, one of my most favorite things to do with my favorite person. Singing with you changes the air. You are my Rainbow.

Balancing them - ***The Sacred Goddess Triangle***:

Brigitte Mars - World-Renowned Herbalist & Activist. Meeting you in 1988 changed my life for the Divine Best!! Your continuing teachings and joyful knowledge helped create the person I am today. I credit you with the inspiration for my body care company Little Moon Essentials. Since you created a tea for every reason with Unitea Herbs and your Remarkable Rainbow of Tea Remedies, I sought to do the same with my body remedies and Life-Altering Baths!! Thanks for the raw inspiration of Love every time I see you, especially helping with Mother's passing. Adding **BethyLove Light** to our lives is a Magical Musical Rainbow Gift - thanks to both of you angels!!!

Pepper Keen Lewis - in every form, you are a great inspiration, and I count you as one of the most influential people of my life. I love how our lives and life choices have paralleled. I think of you all the time, and helping me to learn to feel my connection to Gaia is a gift for which I will never stop thanking you. Thanks for all these many years of Friendship, Gaian and Specially-Peppered Guidance, and Real Love. It has been great to walk beside you in Life.

Lee Cook - your magical support has been the main source of Spiritual Assistance that I have counted on for more than 36 years now!!! Wow! You are my Faerie GuideMother! I am so grateful for you. Thanks for keeping me hopeful and giving me visions of possibilities I can create. Your guidance has kept me going and helped me create my wildest dreams, and BEST OF ALL helped me FINISH THE BOOK! Thanks so much for that latest perfect push. "*Oh, Sweetie....*"

Thank-you **George Washington Carver** for your very special life. "*I don't know when I have ever been so inspired by a Human,*" Laura said, crying her eyes out. Researching you, I simply fell in love with you, and I now feel bold enough to call on you to assist me. I seek to remind people of your good work and perfected connection with Nature.

Written here as a group, but each SO SPECIAL to me, I Love You ~
Dear Roy Upton, Chad Atkins, Randal Turner, Jasper Grant, Joseph Schuster, Mike Cimino, Meg Lewis, Colleen Sudduth Buchmeier, Jenn Grinels, Merideth Kaye Clark, Sylvia Pelcz-Larsen, Cynthia Pileggi, Mindy Green, Debra St. Clair,

~ the garden of earth ~

Feather Jones, Esther Hicks, David Icke, Sacha Stone, Emery Smith, Randy Veitenheimer, Giorgio Tsoukalos, Janine Morigeau & Jean-Claude of Beyond Mystic, Meg Moonbeam, Clif High, Shirley MacLaine, Laura Eisenhower, Julie & Sophie of Maison Jupiter, Terrence Howard, Lee Carroll & Kryon, Barbara Hand Clow, Barbara Marciniak, James Tyberonn & Metatron, Anthony William, Lalitha Thomas, Debra Craydon, Jeanne Michaels & Jaap Van Etten, Michael & Amayra Hamilton at Angel Valley, Diana Gabaldon, St. Germain, Natalie Kalustian, Allison Coe, Molly McCord, Susan Miller. I have enjoyed learning from you ALL through your classes, our personal experiences, your books, posts, livestreams and videos! You are all Mind-Opening Agents of Positive Change, I owe my positive attitude, radical information overload, and creative abilities to your teaching, support and guidance. I am grateful to you all!

To my Blues Family, I LOVE YOU: **Shaun Murphy & TC Davis, Brad Webb, JD Taylor & Little Boys Blue, Pops Fountaine, Dan Cochran, Jack Rowell & Sweet T, David Hudson, Reba & David "BigBit" Daniels, David Pierce, Russell Lee Wheeler, Donnie Miller** (and always **Deanne Miller**), **Jeff Jensen, Jimmie Jones, Bill Ruffino, Willie Hall, Peter "Blewzzman" and Rose Madonna Lauro, Randy Coleman, Kenne Cramer, Shakey Fowlkes, Grady Clark, G. Lee Worden, Doug Siebert, Tommy Stilwell, Moe Denham, Larry Van Loon, Lee Shropshire and Andy Scheinman, Roguie Ray LaMontagne, Markey Blue and Ric Latina, Geoff & Karen Newhall, Johnny "Kid Memphis" Holiday, Tom & Melissa DelRossi, Leo Goff, Gina Hughes, Miranda Louise, Cara Lippman,** my Memphis Jam Best Friend **Jackie Flora & John Flora, Patrich Platt, Andrew Durham, Jeff & Kim Smith**, luncheon-mates **Janice & Tony Negri, Melanie Mangum**. Great thanks to all the Blues DJ's who played our music all over the World: **Gil Anthony, Kev"Legs" Walker, John van Lent, Leen Velthius, Kevin Hardy, Cleve Baker, Vinnie Marini, Kevin Beale, "Sunshine" Sonny Payne, Marc Applegate, Irene Barrett,** and more!

To my New Family of Jackson Friends - wow, too many to list (and bold), including my Spiritual Family Rachel Cathey, Best Friend Cruz (Twin) and Josh Cathey; Super Best Friend Sarah Jones plus Josh and Boone Jones; Dearest Sisters Nancy Nanney, Lori Weir, Paige Keith (& Erik Klasa), Holly Reeves & Chris Reeves, Diana Cotten, Kindra Colling, Ashley Pope, April Horn, Chasity Cavote and Kati Ivy Newton (and Clara, Christina & Hayden, et al), Yogini Erin Nerren, Terri (The HipBee Framer) Downey, Kindall Thomas of Dragonfly Hemp & 420 HempFestival, Healer Hashakar & Tommy Hobbs & Fam, Tiffany Purnell, Addie Ruth Carter, Nicci Gano, Donna Thomas, Chris Smith and Dale, Leesa Taylor Smith, Tanya Kelsey Wright, Ray Carter, Lily and DJ, Kim Everett, Kim Laakso, Cassie Brisentine, Jordan Reaves (+ Devan & Octavia); Beauties and beloved friends Rebekah & Macey Jones, Joy Yeh, Wendy Lee Googe, Anna Durrance, Amy Flippen Ross, Bookini Lauren Smothers, LOLO & Eve Pritchard, Hickerson & Rachel, Dustin Lee, Everybody from The Tavern, Melanie Lupino, Peter Thomas, Mirza Babic & Alex, Mitch Carter, Amber Owens, Toni & Chris, Shekinah,

~ the garden of earth ~

Summer & Mr. Sparkly, Chrystal & Robert Montgomery, Margaret & John Fiddler, Chris Felder & the whole Grubb's Grocery crew - Keiti Robertson, Dennis Sullivan & PJ, Amy Moore Brewer & Colby, Steven Heit, Alan Patterson, Jeff, Madison Holt, Bo & Noah, Little Bryan, Rio, Frank and Jesse James, Judy Ellis, Michelle & Walt James, John & Debra Phillips, & Debra Lewis. Plus awesome friends Kaden Kado, Stormy & Bev (& Junior, too); musicians Brother Ben T. Colling, Ben Jessie (Best Mechanic Ever, too), wailers and dear friends Sarah and Anna Lee Johnson of Herz, Tyler Goodson & Shine, Mike Mayes, Justin White, legend David Michael Thomas, and the late great Jimmie Morris, Sr. (our bass hero, and his amazing sons, brainiac Jimmie Morris, Jr. and Clifford, too).

Talk Radio Family - To my Dear Dan Reaves, SeaBass "my Boo," Chuck Walker, Brother Keith Sherley, Melissa Rhodes, Mike Doles, Gina Langley, Pastor JP, the dearly missed Miss Rosie Robinson, Earth Angel Cyndi Springer, Big Rick, and The Infamous Bull - thanks for all the talking, and the work when I needed it most.

Great Thanks to **The Broom Closet** in Jackson, my dearest Soul Sister **Rachel Frye**, and our leaders Stephen & Emily Guenther for all the time and understanding it took to deal with me finishing this work. And to my **Tarot Tribe** (truly blessed that there are too many to name) thanks for teaching me this craft and supporting me to let it all out.

Yep, ironically I said the Book was done on Earth Day 2022, and done again Fall 2023 and Fall 2024. But this is the day I am truly calling it! CHEERS! Let's just say, it takes **awhile** - and a village - to get it right. Thanks to everyone, especially the Garden, for your patience, friendship, and synchronistic, divine influence on this book.

With genuine Gratitude and Love, I have had so much fun,

LAURA

Earth Day 04/22/2025
In the Big Trees of Jackson, Tennessee

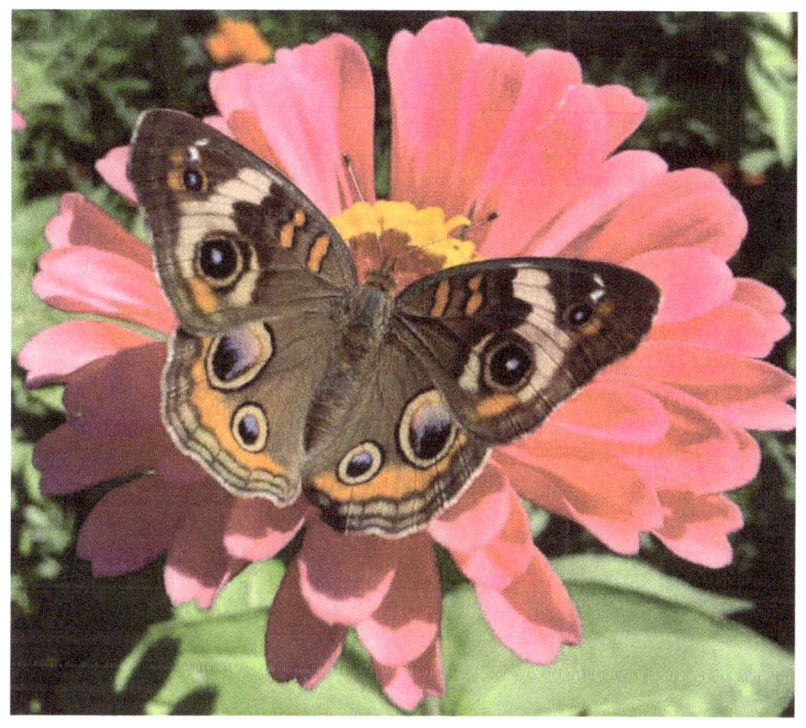

"Just living is not enough...
One must have Sunshine, Freedom, and a little Flower."

~ Hans Christian Andersen

FOOTNOTES

1 Fact Checkers pg. 20
https://www.forbes.com/sites/kalevleetaru/2016/12/22/the-daily-mail-snopes-story-and-fact-checking-the-fact-checkers/?sh=5e574822227f
https://foodbabe.com/do-you-trust-snopes-you-wont-after-reading-how-they-work-with-monsanto-operatives/
https://www.buzzfeednews.com/article/deansterlingjones/snopes-cofounder-plagiarism-mikkelson
https://www.acsh.org/news/2019/11/04/debunkers-debunked-who-fact-checks-fact-checkers-14378

2 Maharishi Effect pg. 30
https://tmhome.com/benefits/study-maharishi-effect-group-meditation-crime-rate/

3 Clorox and Burt's Bees pg. 44
https://investors.thecloroxcompany.com/investors/news-and-events/press-releases/press-release-details/2007/Clorox-to-Acquire-Burts-Bees-Expands-Into-Fast-Growing-Natural-Personal-Care/default.aspx

4 Bites of Food Pollinators Guarantee pg. 55
https://downeast.com/sponsored-content/how-wild-blueberries-give-a-lift-to-the-land-we-love/

5 Butterfly Highways pg. 57
https://davidsuzuki.org/take-action/act-locally/butterflyway/
https://ncwf.org/habitat/butterfly-highway/
https://monarchjointventure.org/get-involved/i-am-a/department-of-transportation

6 Frank Cook pg. 63
https://www.eatweeds.co.uk/frank-cook-remembered

7 Mark's Teaching Gardens pg. 72
https://kckorganicteachinggardens.org/author/marktmanning/

8 Cancer Risk Lowers with Fruits and Veggies pg. 91
C.X. Zhang, S. C. Ho, Y.M. Chen, et al "Greater Vegetable and Fruit Intake Is Associated With a Lower Risk of Breast Cancer Among Chinese Women," *International Journal of Cancer* 125, no. 1 (2009) 181-188

9 Bread Waste Solutions pg. 104
https://www.theguardian.com/food/2018/oct/05/using-their-loaf-baker-reuses-leftovers-to--waste-bread
https://www.ecoandbeyond.com/articles/much-bread-waste-uk/www.toastale.com

10 Chris McCandless and Foraging Safely pg. 119
https://www.newyorker.com/books/page-turner/chris-mccandless-died-update

11 King Clone pg. 139
Directions and details, should you want to travel to check out the protected rings, or simply look at the photo tour.
http://www.lucernevalley.net/creosote/index.htm
http://www.lucernevalley.net/creosote/photo_tour.htm

12 Harvard Study Reveals Cannabis Is Helpful pg. 148 **CANNABIS**
https://www.health.harvard.edu/newsletter_article/pot-smokers-can-maybe-breathe-a-little-easier

13 Weight Loss Herb pg. 169 **DANDELION**
Racz-Kotilla, Elizabeth and Gabriel. 1974 *Planta Medica* pg. 26

14 Daniel Vitalis Research pg. 175 **FIREWEED**
https://www.researchgate.net. Publication/337604020_Fireweed_Epilobium
      angustifolium_L_botany_phytochemistry_and_traditional_uses_A_review
https://www.researchgate.net/publication/341822826_Pharmacological_properties of_fire
      weed_pilobium_angustifolium_L_and_bioavailability_of_ellagitannins_A_review
https://www.fs.fed.us/wildflowers/plant-of-the-week/chamerion_angustifolium.html

15 Prehistoric OG Plant pg. 180 **HORSETAIL**
https://www.gaiaherbs.com/blogs/herbs/horsetail
https://www.extension.purdue.edu/extmedia/ws/ws-29-w.pdf *The Ancient Horsetail*

16 Remarkable Remedy pg. 192 **MOTHERWORT**
"Demonstrated various bioactivities for the treatment of fibrosis, cardiovascular diseases,
      cancers,uterine diseases, brain injuries, and inflammation" Cheng, F.; Zhou, Y.;
      Wang, M.; Guo, C.; Cao, Z.; Zhang, R.; Peng, C. (2020).
"A review of pharmacological and pharmacokinetic properties of stachydrine."
Pharmacological Research. 155: 104755. doi:10.1016/j.phrs.2020.104755. PMID 32173585.

17 Pollution Remediator pg. 225 **SUNFLOWER**
https://pharmeasy.in/blog/health-benefits-of-sunflower-seeds/
      Adler, Tina (July 20, 1996). "Botanical cleanup crews: using plants to tackle polluted
      water and soil."*Science News*. Archived from the original on July 15, 2011.
AFP (June 24, 2011). "Sunflowers to clean radioactive soil in Japan". Yahoo News
Antoni Slodkowski; Yuriko Nakao (19 August 2011). "Sunflowers melt Fukushima's nuclear
      "snow." Reuters.

10 Vitamin D Deficiancy Season pg. 262
https://rumble.com/vfbdc7-dr.-ryan-cole-ceo-and-medical-director-of-cole-diagnostics-
      on-vitamin-d-ive.html

19 Pottenger's Raw Food Cats pg. 274
https://www.trueleafmarket.com/blogs/articles/raw-foods-health-pioneers?source=pepp
      erjam&publisherId=96525&clickId=3512441290&utm_source=PepperJam&utm_
      campaign=affiliate

20 Viruses pg. 287
https://www.coursehero.com/file/80569494/Viruses-docx/

21 James Lovelock pg. 306
http://www.jameslovelock.org/ *Climate Change on a Living Earth*, public lecture given at the
      Royal Society, 29 October 2007

22 Monica Gagliano pg. 318
https://nautil.us/issue/84/outbreak/guided-by-plant-voices

23 Pepper Lewis pg. 355
https://pepperlewis.com/articles/is-gaia-leaving-her-own-planet-earth/1505/

24 Jack Kerouac pg. 383
Jack Kerouac Original Poetry, quoted in *365 Ways to Find Peace: Meditations & Inspirations*
      by Marcus Braybrooke

~ the garden of earth ~

SOURCES & RESOURCES

I have prepared an Extensive Bibliography, plus some great Resource & Publication Lists which are available online at :

https://www.lauralamun.com/vol2extras

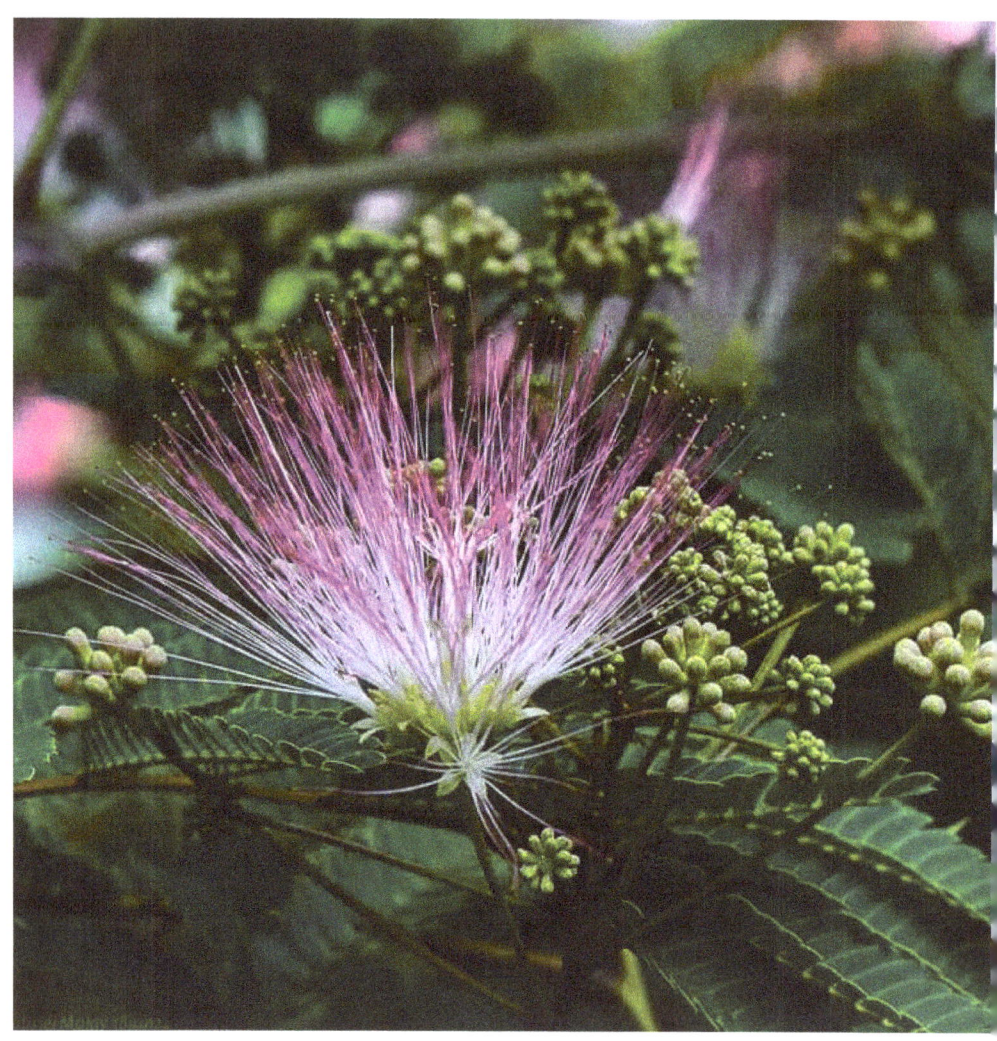

"Somewhere between right
and wrong
there is a Garden.

I will meet you there."

~ *Rumi*

~ the garden of earth ~

IMAGE AND ILLUSTRATION GUIDE

Page	Image	Photographer	Locale
ii	**Sunflower Sunshine** - Laura Lamun, Jackson, Tennessee		
vi	**Brigitte Mars** - dress and photo by Donna Eagle, Boulder, CO		
5	**Rainbows** - https://static.wixstatic.com/media/5ed8db_918646f4aa54903a4d40c1624e53cc8~mv2.jpg		
6	**Vienna Garden Gate** - Pixlr stock photo Victor Malyushev, Vienna, Austria		
13	**Peace Sign by Nature with Nature** - Raw Spirit Fest - Laura Lamun, Santa Barbara, CA		
19	**Donnie Miller & Little Laura** - Laughing Moon Photo, Debbie Green, Murfreesboro, TN		
21	**Press for Peace** - Bekky Bekks pixlr stock image		
24	**Milky Way Mountains** - Vincent Ledvina on unsplash		
27	**Dalai Lama** - https://www.seekpng.com/ipng/u2e6y3a9u2a9i1u2_his-holiness-		
28	**Emoto Crystals** - https://luminousoul.com/blogs/blog/hidden-messages-in-water		
29	**Monks** - https://dhammafootsteps.com/2014/02/14/magha-puja-day-2014/		
31	**Happy Oasis Meditation** - Facebook personal photo, Granite Dells, AZ		
34	**Big John Lamun** - Laura Lamun, Rainbow Circle House, Lathrup Village, MI		
37	**Little Moon Laura** - Corey Kopischke, Steamboat Springs, CO		
39	**Todd Rundgren @ Ryman Auditorium, 2016** - Laura Lamun, Nashville, TN		
40	**Wish You Were Pink Laura** - Todd Intergalactic, Steamboat Springs Ski Area, CO		
41	**"Sunshine" Sonny Payne & the Allen-Lamun Band** - Peter Blewzzman Lauro, Helena, AR		
42	**Letting Go Portrait** - Corey Kopischke, Steamboat Springs, CO		
43	**Labyrinth Laura** - Jill Anthony Mesaros, Leucadia, CA		
44	**NIMA Red Carpet** - Laura and Dave Allen, Blues Directors - unknown, Nashville, TN		
45	**MIAGT Album Cover 2015** - Laura Lamun and Dave Allen, Nashville, TN		
46	**Brad Webb Blues Note on Beale Street** - Facebook post image, Memphis, TN		
48	**Between the Trees** - Dave Hoefler on unsplash		
50	**Me and LeeLee** - some photographer in the 1900's took it, Lathrup Village, MI		
52	**Farm-Aid Logo** - https://www.farmaid.org/		
53	**Pollinators** - File ID 121795558	© Verastuchelova	**Dreamstime.com**		
54	**Monarch** - Sean Stratton on unsplash		
55	**Bee on Orange Coneflower** - istock photo		
57	**Bee at Sunset Magic** - Simon Berger - Pixlr stock photo		
58	**Honey Pot** - **Honey.com** promotional image source		
62	**Garden Party** - istock photo		
63	**Vegan Sammy Supreme** - pRKDJZWNUvY Pixlr stock photo		
66	**Resistance is Fertile** - Tim Glenn http://www.soulpurposereadings.com/		
67	**Vegetable Garden** - ID 25414035 © Laszlo Halasi Dreamstime		
69	**Backyard Garden** - Merideth Kaye Clark, Portland, OR		
69	**Rowan the Gardener** - Aleka & Sean Bruce, Encinitas, CA		
70	**Mark Manning and KCK Schools** - Facebook image, staff photo		

~ the garden of earth ~

71	**Grandchildren Rowan & Maven & Peaches, Encinitas, CA** - Aleka & Sean Bruce
71	**Favorite Grubb's Customer & Organic Angel** - Laura Lamun photo
72	**Little Seed Library** - The Heirloom John Forti - **jforti.com**
73	**Fruit Tree Planting Foundation** -ftpf.org, staff photo
74	**Moon Phases** - https://pixabay.com/photos/landscape-night-star-phases-5186058
75	**Undefined Moonbow** - FB_IMG_1650830109755/ Picabuzz
76-78	**Findhorn Gardens** - Findhorn.org, Lauren Berrizbeitia, Ecovillage Northern Scotland https://www.slideshare.net/FindhornFoundation/findhorn-foundation-powerpoint-presention.jpg
79-80	**Perelandra Gardens** - https://www.perelandra-ltd.com/Photo-Gallery-C49.aspx, VA
81	**Luther Burbank Thornless Cactus** - 1916 postcard https://digital.sonomalibrary.org/
87	**Swallowtail Butterfly** - Dulcey Lima on unsplash
88, 90	**Rainbow Radish Sprouts** - Laura Lamun, Forest House, Jackson, TN
92	**Sprouting Jars** - ID 39023981 © Benoit Daoust	Dreamstime
97	**Fermented Beets** - The Matter of Food, Pixlr stock photo
100	**Sourdough Kid / Little Baker** - Artur Rutkowski on unsplash
101	**Sourdough Starter** - ID 60579955 © Sohadiszno Dreamstime
105	**Blueberry Sourdough Buns** - Pixlr stock photo UGIJrLHWvp4.png
106	**Compost Bin** - ID 59118581 © Airborne77	**Dreamstime.com**
108	**Compost Pile** - ID 15886666 © Darko Plohl	**Dreamstime.com**
112	**Dandelion Field - View from Braunwald** - ID 9557540 © Peter.wey	**Dreamstime.com**
113	**Gonzo at Clark Mansion 2006** - Laura Lamun, Clark, CO
114	**Gonzo Forever Memorial Bath-Of-The-Month 2007,** LL, Steamboat Springs, CO
118	**Brigitte Mars** - Facebook post, unknown photographer, Boulder, CO
119	**Alicia Bay Laurel Book Signed** - Laura Lamun, Breezy's Dream House, Boulder, CO
121	**Mango Tree** - Photo 9742865 © Vladimir Melnik	**Dreamstime.com**
124	**Forget-Me-Not Laura** - Joebob Graham, Flattops Wilderness, CO
125	**Broccoli Flower** - File ID 49219396	© Hse0193	**Dreamstime.com**
126	**Soapwort** -File ID 194409259	© Robkna	**Dreamstime.com**
127	**Indian Pipe** - Photo/Source: Nance Noel / Gardening Know How
127	**Peanut Family Enormous Plant** - Licensed Adobe Stock 418041157
129	**Mint Family** - File ID 153437729	© Marazem	**Dreamstime.com**
131	**Cacao Flower** - Creator: Andreas Kay Copyright: © 2017 Andreas Kay
132	**Passion Flower Sarah Gave Me** - Laura Lamun, Jackson, TN
134	**Crab Apple Blossoms** - File ID 14658544	© Kenneth Keifer	**Dreamstime.com**
136	**Perfect Pansy** - Laura Lamun, Jackson, TN
137	**King Clone** -Frank Rodrigue, http://www.lucernevalley.net/creosote/photo_tour.htm
139	**Gardner & Son Augie Foraging** - Ashley Orton, Jericho, VT
140	**Dandelion Splendor** - ID 04Nh3LC_EwM.png **Dreamstime.com**
141	**Burdock** - shutterstock image
143	**Burdock** - Christian Fischer, own work, North-eastern Lower Saxony, Germany

145	**Purple Cannabis**	- iStock photo ID:1189375554 Yarygin
148	**Happy Medical Marijuana Warehouse Worker**	- Laura Lamun, Steamboat Springs, CO
150	**Cannabis Microscopy**	- FB_IMG_1584128828135.jpg
151	**Cattail**	- ID 2879491 © Chris Rokitski	**Dreamstime.com**
154	**Cattail Pollen**	- http://hungerandthirstforlife.blogspot.com/2010/06/wild-about-cattail-pollen.html
155	**Chaparral**	- Laura Lamun, off I-70 just in California
156	**Tall Chaparral and DA**	- Laura Lamun, off I-70 just in California
157	**Chaparral Flower**	- https://www.utep.edu/herbal-safety/herbal-facts/herbal%20facts%20sheet/creosote-bush-chaparral.html
159	**Chicory**	- iStock photo ID:499293650 by Ailime, Paisley, Canada
160	**Chicory Flower**	- ID 14103420 © Dink101	**Dreamstime.com**
161	**Chicory Root**	- https://i.pinimg.com/originals/2f/19/c5/2f19c5224222c578c4d10993095bc4ef.jpg
162	**Comfrey**	- Hans, https://pixabay.com/photos/rough-comfrey-flower-blue-115165/
163	**Comfrey Leaves**	- Lynn Greyling License: CC0 Public Domain
164	**Comfrey Flower**	- © Peter M. Dziuk, 2004
166	**Dandelion Bunch**	- Laura Lamun, FRont Yard, Jackson, TN
168	**Dandelion Macro Flower**	- Don Kinney **https://www.motherearthimages.com/**
171	**Dandelion Sphere**	- Greg Hume - Own work, CC BY-SA 3.0, **commons.wikimedia.org/17890537**
172	**Fireweed**	- Adobe Stock FILE #: 361595931 by Brad
172	**Fireweed Leaf**	- detail http://wildernessarena.com/food-water-shelter/food-food-water-shelter/food-procurement/edible-wild-plants/fireweed
174	**Fireweed Flower**	- Jason Moore **pixabay.com/photos** /fireweed-flower-blue-sky-plant-1359520/
175	**Fireweed In Alaska**	- © Betsey Crawford **https://thesouloftheearth.com/** Alaska
176	**Horsetail**	- **https://ruibals.com/all_plants/equisetum-hyemale-horsetail-reed/**
176	**Horsetail Young**	- By Rror - Own work,CC BY-SA 3.0, commons.wikimedia.org/w/index.php?curid=4077821
178	**Horsetail Flower**	Pixabay **https://plants.ces.ncsu.edu/plants/equisetum-arvense/**
179	**Lamb's Quarters**	- Harry Rose CC BY 2.0 **plants.ces.ncsu.edu**/plants/chenopodium-album/
180	**Lamb's Quarters Flower**	- Image by WikimediaImages from Pixabay
184	**LemonBalm**	- **Homedepot.com/p/Gurney-s-Herb**-Lemon-Balm-250-Seed-Packet-61669/308621863
186	**LemonBalm Flower**	- Cbaile19 CC0 1.0 Universal Public Domain Dedication
188	**Lemon Balm Botanical Print**	- By Otto Wilhelm Thomé (1885)biolib.de/thome/band4/tafel_058.html
189	**Motherwort**	- **https://www.adaptiveseeds.com/product/herbs/motherwort-organic/**
191	**Motherwort Flower detail**	- **steemit.com/life**/@noblecentury/the-healing-properties-of-motherwort-
191	**Motherwort (Leonurus cardiaca)**	, D. Gordon E. Robertson, Ottawa, Ontario, Canada CC Attribution-Share Alike 3.0
192	**Mullein**	- Adobe stock image by travelpeter 754440330
194	**Mullein Flower**	- Max Licher, **swbiodiversity.org/seinet nazinvasiveplants.org/mullein**
194-5	**Mullein Plant and Rosette**	- Laura Lamun, Jackson, Tennessee and Walden, Colorado
196	**Nettle**	- Uwe H. Friese, Bremerhaven 2003 / Wikipedia. Stinging nettles, CC SA 3.0
198	**Nettle Flower**	- © Roger Darlington, **https://wildflowerfinder.org.uk**
199	**Henbit DeadNettle Macro Flower**	- Don Kinney, **www.motherearthimages.com/**

199	**Purple Archangel DeadNettle** - Laura Lamun, Jackson, TN
200	**Osha** - Jerry Friedman, Own work, CC BY-SA 3.0, commons.wikimedia.org/w/index.php?curid=25085911
201	**Osha Clinical Sample**- S. Rhodes, P. Smolenyak, 1999, Northern Arizona University
202	**Osha Flower** - Shawn Sigstedt wishgardenherbs.com/blogs/wishgarden/day-bear-root
203	**Living Love Root Candy** - Product by Joe (Geronimo) Zapf-Kent, Laura Lamun @home
203	**Osha and Shawn Sigstedt** - same as pg. 202
204	**Plantain** - Robert Flogaus-Faust, CC Attribution 4.0, Upper Engadine, Switzerland
206	**Plantain Closeup** - taken by Rasbak, (nl: Grote weegbree bloeiwijze) {{GFDL}}
207	**Plantain** - AdobeStock_558075776 J
208	**Purslane Grows Everywhere** - Laura Lamun, FirstBank parking lot, Bemis, TN
210	**Purslane Flower** - Adobe Stock #365684999
211	**Purslane Chimichurri** - Laura Lamun, Forest House Kitchen, Jackson, TN
212	**Red Clover** - H. Zell, own work, Karlsruhe, Germany {GFDL}
214	**Red Clover Botanical Drawing** - Prof. Dr. Otto Wilhelm Thomé Flora von Deutschland, Österreich und der Schweiz 1885, Gera, Germany, Public Domain
214	**Four Leaf Clover** - Laura Lamun, picked by DA in the front yard, Nashville, TN
215	**Shepherd's Purse Closeup** - Carl Axel Magnus Lindman, Bilder ur Nordens Flora
215	**Shepherd's Purse Basal Rosette**- dalgial GNU Free Documentation License, Version 1.2
217	**Shepherd's Purse Flower** - wildflowerwalker.com/2017/07/03/shepherds-purse-wisdom/
218	**Wild Mustards and Ocean** - Sam Sycamore, Brassicaeae, ediblewild.info, Big Sur, CA
219	**Sunflower** - https://golondrinas.org/tag/sunflower-sap/
220	**Sunflower Bee** - Don Kinney, https://www.motherearthimages.com/
221	**Sunflower Detail** - Laura Lamun, Farmer's Market bloom, Jackson, TN
222	**Sunflower Field at Sunset** - © Nikolay Dimitrov ID 5770923	**Dreamstime.com** 223
222	**Sunflower Laura** - Joebob Graham, Flattops Wilderness, Yampa, CO
223	**Violet Macro** - Don Kinney, https://www.motherearthimages.com/
225-7	**Violet Flower Essence, Field, Honey & Vodka** - Laura Lamun, Backyard, Jackson, TN
228	**Wild Asparagus** - norwoodcolorado.com/hunting-for-wild-asparagus-on-wrights-mesa/
230	**Euell Gibbons** - www.adventure-journal.com/2018/07/euell-gibbons-much-flakes/
231	**Asparagus Sprouting** - Adobe Stock by leopictures FILE #349357615
232	**Wild Blueberry** - KWJPHOTOART, Shutterstock image Stock Photo ID: 139755727
234	**Blueberry Flower** - Katy Chayka, minnesotawildflowers.info/shrub/lowbush-blueberry
235	**Blueberry Field** - How Wild Blueberries Give a Lift to the Land We Love	Down East Magazine, Photograph by: John Lane, Copyright: Evening Tide Photography
236	**Wild Blueberries** - Eric, blog eatlikenoone.com/when-are-wild-blueberries-in-season.htm
237	**Yarrow** - Joe Standaert, wcbotanicalclub.org/achillea-millefolium-common-yarrow-heintooga-spur/Heintooga Spur, NC
239	**Yarrow Flower** -Peter M. Dziuk, minnesotawildflowers.info/flower/common-yarrow
240	**Yarrow Botanical Drawing** - F.H. Wigg / processed by Thomas Schoepke plant-pictures.de
241	**Yellow Dock** - https://selfhealschool.com/whats-dock/
241	**Yellow Dock Seed Panicle** - By Stickpen / Own work, Public Domain

~ the garden of earth ~

243	**Yellow Dock Flower**	- ID 183086904 © Juan Francisco Moreno GÁmez, **Dreamstime.com**
244	**Deep Green Forest**	- by Aaron Katz on unsplash
246	**Yoga on the Beach**	- ID 39138627 © Martinmark, **Dreamstime.com**
247	**Gardner & 2 Avos**	- Gardner Orton made a living collage of Avo out of raw food!, Hawaii
250	**Rainbow Food Heart**	- iStock photo ID:526489895 Viktar
267	**Garden Gate**	- with Mommy, Laura Lamun, 2022 Glasey's Garden, Longmont, CO
268	**Good Food**	- 111062391 / Food © Sonyakamoz, **Dreamstime.com**
270	**Carrot Ginger Juice**	- Adobe Stock photo by alexandermils FILE #443876874
271	**Juices**	- Dhiren Maru - pixlr stock image
273	**Cayenne**	- Chamille White, iStock photo ID:1201298166
274-295	**Mudras**	- Dave Allen, Mudras Hand Model, Laura Lamun, backyard, Jackson, TN
275	**Book Workspace**	- Laura Lamun, White Room, Jackson, TN
278	**Bar Sign/Hangover Cures**	- Laura Lamun, Rural Juke Joint, Western TN
284	**Breastfeeding**	- Photo 31642608 / Breastfeeding © Evgenyatamanenko	**Dreamstime.com**
285	**LOLO and Xander**	- Facebook image used with her permission
286	**Meme for Love**	- Made by Laura Lamun, Jackson, TN
287	**Aleka Pregnant with Rowan**	- Laura Lamun, Encinitas, CA
289	**Happy Sleepy People**	- ID 64670295 © Syda Productions	**Dreamstime.com**
293	**Muscle Warrior**	- Photo 168695143 © Dragosh Cojocari	**Dreamstime.com**
296	**Sunshine Lupines**	- Happy Gardens Facebook image by @monzoon_k
298	**James Lovelock**	-2005 Bruno Comby of Association of Environmentalists For Nuclear Energy
300	**James Lovelock at 100**	- by Gareth Iwan Jones Chesil Beach on the Dorset South Coast. 6th June 2019
301	**George Washington Carver**	- http://encyclopediaofalabama.org/article/h-1064
305	**GeorgeWC in His Lab**	- Alabama Department of Archives and History
306	**Cleve Backster**	-his book and thesunmagazine.org/issues/259/the-plants-respond
308	**Cleve Backster**	-https://www.facebook.com/CleveBackster/Tribute Page
309	**Monica Gagliano**	- https://www.radiobue.it/study-reveals-that-plants-can-hear/
312	**Monica Gagliano**	- Plant Intelligence and the Importance of Imagination In Science	Bioneers
312	**Pink Sweet Pea Flower**	- by natalya2015 Adobe Stock FILE #444830803
313	**Bruce French**	- Mitchell Woolnough, Landline / Article By Margot Kelly
315	**Old Gospel Hall & Bruce French Archive**	- image: Brodie Weeding
316	**Blueberry in Hand**	- by Markus Spiske #jHrW-I7Nfw on unsplash
318	**Garden Bounty**	- Photo 117081162 © Andreaobzerova	**Dreamstime.com**
320	**Violets Drying**	- Laura Lamun, Forest House Kitchen, Jackson, TN
321	**Canning**	- Photo ID 42755188 © Monticelllo	**Dreamstime.com**
323	**Pressure Cooker**	- https://www.gopresto.com/product/presto-16-quart-pressure-canner-01750
324	**Canning Time Table**	- Home Canning Guide from Kerr, 1941
325	**Peppers Drying in the Sun**	- File ID 44715225	© Ufuk Uyanik	**Dreamstime.com**
328, 332	**Extract Making Process**	- Laura Lamun, Rosebank & Welcome Kitchen, Nashville, TN
333	**Oil 'n' Vinegar**	- Photo 44876485 © Renaud Philippe	**Dreamstime.com**

~ the garden of earth ~

334	**Frozen Delights**	- File ID 78121897 | © Yingko | **Dreamstime.com**
337	**Flavor Cubes**	- Laura Lamun, Wild Weed Chimichurri Recipe, frozen, Jackson, TN
338	**Root Cellar**	-Photo 74521089 © Barbro Rutgersson | **Dreamstime.com**
342	**Prepping Visual Aid**	- File ID 93395849 | © Photka | **Dreamstime.com**
347	**Fireplace Bliss**	- Laura Lamun, Jackson, TN (ART by our dear Billy the Artist)
348	**Earth in Hands**	- ID 38622929 © Romolo Tavani | **Dreamstime.com**
350	**Pepper Keen Lewis**	- her personal photo, photographer unknown
363	**Earth, Sun and Moon**	- by sdecoret Adobe Stock FILE # 106164892
364	**Ocean Purple Sunset**	- Pixlr stock photo, Yousef Espanioly
367	**Double Rainbow**	- by Gary Nickell, Superstition Mountains, AZ
368	**Lavender Field**	- by Leonard Cotte pixlr
370	**Peter Sagan Photo**	- 95422508 / Peter Sagan © Martin Surik | **Dreamstime.com**
372	**Bloom Big Mommy's Rock**	- Laura Lamun, Caladium Palladium, Jackson, TN IMAGE
375	**Field of Flowers and Sunlight**	- Megan Sisk, with Love, Ft. Collins, CO
viii	**Beloved Mommy**	- photographer unknown sometime in late 1980's?, MI
ix	**Dave "Sparkle" Allen**	- Laura Lamun, Rosebank & Welcome Kitchen, Nashville, TN
ix	**Aleka & Sean Double Rainbow**	- Laura Lamun, The Ranch, Oak Creek, CO
x	**Grandchildren Rowan and Maven**	- Jill Anthony Mesaros, Encinitas, CA
xii	**Dave The King and His Birthday Suit**	- Laura Lamun, Forest House Living Room
xv	**Butterfly & a Little Flower**	- Laura Lamun, Jackson, TN
xviii	**Mimosa Blossom**	- Laura Lamun, Jackson, TN
xxxiv	**Laura and DaveAllen**	- Some Blues Friend, Lafayette's, Memphis, TN
xxxv	**Tarot In My Rainbow Room**	, The Broom Closet - Rachel Frye, Jackson, TN

Index

A

abundance 1, 170, 172, 198, 199, 210, 221, 234, 249, 269, 275, 286
acne 59, 142, 160, 224, 242, 251
Allen-Lamun Band 41, 44, 45, xx
altar 153, 177, 217
Angel 2, 21, 23, 35, 78, 312, ix, xi, xiii, xiv, xxi
anxiety 95, 146, 147, 149, 164, 185, 190, 191, 209, 220, 252, 259, 260, 261, 273, 290
Aphrodisiac 229
aromatherapy 3, 37, 248, 289
asthma F, 58, 94, 146, 163, 177, 193, 197, 205, 213, 220, 224, 239, 242, 262

B

baby 43, 224, 240, 251, 271, 284, 285, 286, 287, 288
beans 64, 65, 74, 83, 84, 85, 95, 127, 131, 252, 253, 260, 261, 262, 263, 264, 266, 294
bees 42, 53, 54, 55, 56, 57, 58, 59, 60, 70, 85, 126, 172, 186, 199, 214, 234, xvi
birth 51, 128, 239, 252, 266, 358
bitter 94, 142, 156, 159, 160, 161, 166, 167, 169, 171, 172, 177, 180, 187, 190, 201, 205, 224, 229, 237, 238, 242, 329
blood-building 243
blood sugar 58, 59, 93, 94, 95, 177, 180, 209, 220, 238, 259, 271, 367
blues 19, 39, 41, 42, 43, 44, 45, 46, 47, xii, xiii, xx
breath 31, 168, 180, 193, 224, 350
breathing 202, 203, 224, 274, 275, 290, 291
Brigitte Mars vi, 1, 42, 68, 118, 119, 143, 170, 185, 193, 247, 269, 272, xii, xx, xxi
Burdock 123, 141, 142, 143, 144, 261, 264, 280, 282, xxi
burns 59, 131, 163, 174, 177, 205, 206, 209, 216, 267
butterfly 55, 234, xi, xvi, xxi

C

Cacao 130, 131, 264, 276, xi, xxi
Calcium 93, 94, 95, 107, 142, 146, 151, 155, 162, 167, 173, 176, 180, 184, 189, 192, 196, 205, 209, 212, 216, 219, 237, 241, 255, 260, 261, 262
cancer 19, 59, 61, 89, 90, 92, 93, 94, 95, 132, 133, 137, 142, 144, 152, 158, 167, 173, 177, 213, 220, 229, 233, 234, 236, 242, 251, 252, 253, 254, 255, 256, 257, 259, 265, 271
Cannabis 125, 145, 146, 147, 148, 150, xvi, xxii
Cattail 151, 152, 153, 154, xxii
CBD 126, 146, 147, 148, 149, 150, 258, 259, 290
chakras 201, 225
Chaparral 137, 155, 156, 157, 158, 272, xxii
Chicory 68, 123, 159, 160, 161, 169, 243, 263, 264, xxii

Chinese medicine 152, 201, 228, 289
cholesterol 93, 95, 130, 160, 167, 185, 209, 213, 220, 224, 230, 233, 254, 256, 271, 292
circulation 167, 173, 180, 199, 201, 216, 238, 273, 275, 279
colds 58, 130, 133, 156, 174, 177, 193, 216, 224, 230, 248, 254, 264, 266, 282
colors 255
Comfrey 124, 162, 163, 164, 165, 205, 272, 288, xxii
creativity 149, 353

D

Dandelion 54, 68, 119, 123, 140, 159, 166, 167, 168, 169, 170, 171, 215, 243, 264, 278, xxi, xxii
Dave Allen 2, 37, 38, 40, 44, 46, 47, 55, 60, 64, 148, 169, 201, 214, 325, 342, 368, viii, x, xx, xxiv, xxxiv
David Avocado Wolfe 37, 89, 147, 73, 247, 249, 258, 268, 269, 272, xi
Dead Nettle 199
decongestant 167, 197, 205
diarrhea 134, 180, 209, 216, 255, 262, 268
digestion 63, 65, 92, 94, 98, 160, 167, 168, 190, 193, 201, 216, 220, 242, 255, 259, 260, 262, 264, 273, 325, 354
divination 163, 168, 239
Doctrine of Signatures 293
Donnie Miller 19, 44, xiii, xx
Dorothy Maclean 76, 78
Dr. Masaru Emoto 28

E

Earth C, E, iii, v, 1, 3, 4, 5, 7, 8, 9, 11, 15, 16, 17, 18, 21, 22, 23, 24, 25, 26, 27, 28, 29, 30, 37, 47, 50, 73, 77, 78, 84, 86, 87, 89, 100, 113, 114, 116, 118, 119, 122, 125, 130, 135, 137, 156, 170, 174, 177, 178, 180, 206, 213, 232, 236, 246, 247, 261, 269, 272, 274, 282, 293, 297, 298, 299, 300, 307, 313, 314, 315, 338, 343, 347, 349, 350, 351, 352, 354, 355, 356, 357, 359, 365, 374, viii, ix, x, xi, xiv, xvii, xxv, xxxiv, xxxv
eczema 59, 137, 142, 144, 160, 175, 185, 197, 205, 213, 226, 242, 267
edible flowers 3, 118, 124, 126, 136, 183, 223
edible Weeds iii, 140
Eileen & Peter Caddy 76
elements 4, 67, 106, 191, 213, 346, 350, xxxiv
energy 12, 14, 16, 18, 21, 22, 24, 26, 27, 28, 29, 30, 31, 32, 34, 36, 58, 59, 63, 71, 74, 78, 80, 89, 90, 93, 95, 98, 133, 142, 146, 148, 149, 153, 160, 161, 163, 164, 168, 173, 174, 178, 186, 191, 198, 199, 201, 202, 203, 213, 215, 217, 220, 221, 225, 229, 231, 234, 236, 239, 242, 246, 247, 252, 254, 260, 261, 268, 269, 270, 271, 273, 274, 275, 276, 277, 279, 282, 287, 293, 295, 298, 319, 329, 332, 334, 344, 345, 347, 356, 365, 366, 367, 368, 370

Essential Oils 142, 146, 155, 165, 167, 173, 184, 189, 201, 213, 216, 272, 275, 276, 278, 283, 287, 289, 290, 294, 329

Ether 30, 374

extracts 118, 157, 169, 189, 207, 257, 259, 326, 328, 329, 330, 331, 332

F

feet 130, 137, 142, 154, 177, 180, 193, 197, 272, 278, 281, 290, 314, 365

fertility 59, 132, 177, 194, 197, 217, 221, 230

fever 57, 133, 156, 201, 205, 209, 216, 224, 238, 239

fire 115, 137, 144, 152, 153, 161, 174, 198, 205, 269, 343

Fireweed 86, 172, 173, 174, 175, xvii, xxii

first aid 142, 146, 152, 156, 160, 163, 168, 174, 177, 180, 185, 190, 193, 197, 201, 205, 209, 213, 216, 221, 224, 230, 234, 239, 242

flower essences 157, 331

flu 59, 156, 230, 238, 239, 251, 256, 263

folklore 142, 146, 152, 156, 160, 163, 167, 173, 177, 180, 185, 190, 193, 197, 202, 205, 209, 213, 216, 220, 224, 229, 233, 238, 242

frequency 5, 12, 14, 18, 22, 26, 27, 28, 78, 287, 335, 365, 366, 367

G

Gaia iii, iv, 3, 4, 5, 10, 21, 23, 24, 25, 29, 35, 60, 71, 116, 239, 247, 261, 269, 285, 298, 299, 300, 349, 350, 351, 354, 356, 362, 363, 374, xii

gardening iii, 54, 67, 69, 70, 71, 75, 76, 77, 78, 79, 80, 81, 82, 88, 89, xxi

gardens 50, 66, 67, 68, 70, 71, 75, 77, 79, 80, 105, 116, 118, xvi, xxi, xxiv, xxv

Gardner Orton 139, 247, x, xxiv

gifts 9, 64, 67, 72, 102, 227, 272, 322, 324, 330, 365, 374

goddess 118

gratitude 2, 23, 30, 144, 293

H

hair 96, 134, 136, 143, 173, 177, 178, 197, 199, 213, 251, 252, 254, 257, 261, 307, 365, xxxiv

hangover remedies iii, 278

happiness v, 14, 27, 146, 149, 210, 305, 365, 370, 371, xxxix

hay fever 57, 239

headaches 59, 132, 149, 173, 188, 190, 201, 224, 262, 274

heart F, 13, 19, 22, 24, 25, 27, 29, 30, 32, 35, 57, 61, 93, 94, 121, 129, 132, 147, 153, 161, 174, 176, 185, 186, 190, 202, 206, 209, 213, 217, 224, 229, 236, 254, 257, 258, 263, 265, 268, 273, 274

heart attack 209, 273, 274

Henbit 128, 199, xxii

hives 56, 58

homeopathic 128, 290

honey 56, 57, 58, 59, 97, 104, 130, 183, 185, 186, 187, 188, 207, 214, 225, 226, 227, 234,

235, 242, 243, 253, 264, 265, 276, 280, 285, 294, 329, 330, 344, xx, xxiii
Horsetail 114, 176, 177, 178, 213, 265, xvii, xxii
hypertension 167, 190, 253

I

immune system 11, 18, 57, 94, 136, 173, 209, 257, 271, 282
infection 152, 167, 193, 205, 206, 256
inflammation 93, 95, 143, 144, 149, 152, 175, 180, 190, 199, 205, 213, 224, 240, 254, 257, 259, 262, 265, 280, 282, 286, xvii
insect repelling 81, 82, 128, 129, 145, 152, 186, 303
Iron 93, 94, 95, 107, 132, 142, 151, 160, 162, 167, 180, 196, 205, 209, 212, 216, 219, 228, 241, 242, 254, 260, 261, 270
itching 144, 152, 164, 180, 206, 213, 216, 240, 251

J

Juliano 247, 269, xi
Jupiter 9, 160, 168, 185, 193, 201, 242, xiii

L

lactation 167, 229, 284, 285
laetrile 253
Lemon Balm 54, 81, 84, 128, 184, 185, 186, 187, 211, 276, 277, 280, 281, 288, 290, xxii
levitation 58, 59, 126, 230
Little Moon Essentials 37, 42, 290, x, xii
liver 19, 95, 124, 132, 136, 142, 157, 158, 167, 168, 169, 173, 180, 205, 233, 238, 251, 278
longevity 136, 191, 250, 254, 268
love v, 3, 21, 23, 25, 26, 34, 36, 39, 40, 41, 53, 60, 61, 69, 70, 71, 75, 78, 85, 87, 88, 91, 96, 100, 118, 119, 131, 138, 144, 154, 157, 158, 161, 169, 173, 174, 178, 179, 186, 187, 191, 193, 203, 207, 210, 213, 214, 222, 225, 231, 234, 239, 273, 278, 289, 297, 305, 312, 315, 318, 319, 326, 338, 339, 347, 350, 363, 366, 369, 370, 373, viii, ix, x, xi, xii, xvi, xxxiv
lungs 146, 162, 163, 190, 193, 224, 229, 259, 287
Luther Burbank 81, xxi

M

Machelle Small Wright 79, xiii, xxiii
Magnesium 89, 93, 94, 95, 107, 142, 146, 151, 155, 173, 176, 180, 184, 192, 196, 205, 209, 212, 219, 220, 228, 238, 241, 249, 255, 259, 260, 261, 262, 263, 290
marijuana 114, 125, 126, 128, 146, 147, 148, 259, xxii
Mark Manning 70, xx
Mars 153, 198, 201, 242, 300
Maven 71, x, xxi, xxv

Maybe It's A Good Thing 45
Meditation 14, 21, 28, 59, xx
memory 59, 146, 149, 198, 209, 229, 233, 275, 277, 307, 310, 330
menopause 95, 136, 144, 190, 213
mental health 209, 233, 264
Mercury 160, 174, 213
moisture 108, 111, 155, 210, 286, 306, 327, 339, 354
mood-elevating 279
Moon 74, 75, 84, 85, 142, 164, 165, 168, 185, 187, 209, 221, 227, 234, 268, 328, 329, 330, 331, 332, 333, xxi, xxv
Moon Gardening 75
Motherwort 54, 68, 128, 189, 190, 191, 288, 290, xxii
mucous 162
Mudras 267, 274, 275, 279, xxiv
Mullein 141, 192, 193, 194, 195, 197, 202, xxii
muscles 133, 185, 190, 255, 259, 261, 262, 263, 290

N

nausea 95, 132, 149, 185, 266, 279
Nettle 18, 54, 118, 128, 136, 196, 197, 198, 199, 205, 206, 213, 236, 242, xxii
neurotransmitters 254, 260
Nick Urata 39
NIMA 45, xx

O

oils 1, 59, 82, 115, 122, 123, 124, 131, 165, 192, 202, 203, 217, 234, 237, 240, 248, 267, 278, 281, 283, 285, 287, 292, 294, 295, 303, 328, 329, 330
Osha 114, 122, 200, 201, 202, 203, 226, 275, 276, 280, 288, xxiii
oxygen 73, 111, 245, 260, 261, 277, 346

P

pain 18, 29, 59, 137, 143, 149, 152, 162, 163, 164, 177, 190, 193, 197, 198, 199, 206, 253, 259, 262, 285, 286, 329, 362
Peace 11, 14, 17, 18, 21, 22, 29, 30, 47, 147, 209, 370, 371, 373, xvii, xx
Pineal Gland 224, 234, 277
Plantain 18, 101, 164, 197, 204, 205, 206, 207, xxiii
poison 52, 63, 122, 198, 205, 206, 237, 269, 300, 360
Pollinators 49, 53, 54, 60, 66, 87, 117, 126, 172, 207, 214, 217, xvi, xx
Potassium 93, 94, 95, 107, 142, 151, 155, 160, 162, 167, 173, 176, 180, 189, 196, 209, 216, 228, 238, 241, 260, 262, 263
Prayer 14, 27, 28, 29
Prebiotics 263
pregnancy safety iii, 287

Prepping 343, xxv
Probiotics 98, 160, 253, 254, 263, 264, 265
purifying 174, 201, 202, 238, 270, 332, 345
Purslane 68, 83, 207, 208, 209, 210, 211, 251, 252, 253, 304, xxiii

Q

Quercetin 155, 167, 173, 177, 189, 196, 216, 228, 238, 241, 265, 266, 267, 280

R

Rainbow 99, 136, ix, xi, xii, xxi, xxiv, xxv
rashes 136, 142, 156, 197, 242
raw food 19, 37, 62, 89, 255, 268, 269, xxiv
recipes 1, 3, 37, 58, 101, 103, 104, 105, 119, 136, 140, 154, 182, 185, 186, 189, 194, 199, 207, 225, 226, 256, 271, 281, 283, 318, 320, 322, 323, 327, 330, 331, 333
Red Clover 54, 127, 212, 213, 214, xxiii
retreats 37, 268
roots 74, 75, 96, 110, 123, 138, 143, 144, 149, 160, 161, 165, 167, 168, 169, 171, 176, 200, 202, 210, 226, 228, 242, 340
Rowan 69, 70, 71, 134, 287 (in utero), x, xx, xxi, xxiv, xxv

S

sachets 126, 143, 239
salt 181, 183, 195, 205, 235, 323, 327, 335, 345
salve 59, 156, 163, 164, 165, 259, 287, 360
Saturn 9, 146, 156, 163, 177, 180, 193, 217, 242
seaweed 109, 181
sedative 146, 149, 185, 213, 229
Self-Care 245, 246
sexual energy 203, 229, 293
Shepherd's Purse 125, 216, 217, 288, xxiii
skin 16, 19, 94, 124, 136, 141, 143, 144, 152, 157, 160, 162, 163, 164, 167, 173, 175, 177, 186, 191, 193, 196, 197, 205, 206, 209, 213, 220, 224, 242, 251, 252, 254, 255, 256, 257, 262, 263, 283, 286, 290, 306, 340, 363
sleep 22, 59, 126, 132, 135, 185, 190, 193, 209, 210, 224, 229, 259, 260, 278, 289, 290, 291, 292, 293, 353, 363
smoking 147, 178, 192, 201, 259, 267, 275
sneezing 59
soil 30, 67, 265
Sourdough 97, 100, 101, 102, 103, 104, 105, 264, xxi
Spirit 20, 21, 22, 23, 26, 30, 34, 77, 78, 80, 114, 138, 147, 148, 153, 168, 174, 188, 193, 201, 202, 203, 209, 217, 225, 227, 230, 233, 234, 239, 243, 297, 333, 369, 370, 371, x, xx
sprains 142, 143, 163, 164

stamina 93, 168, 199, 202, 233, 294
stimulant 146, 160, 163, 167, 190, 197, 201, 238
stress 64, 190, 229, 236, 252, 254, 259, 262, 264, 265, 282, 291, 306, 367, 374
sugar 19, 50, 58, 59, 90, 93, 94, 95, 104, 131, 160, 173, 174, 177, 180, 209, 220, 226, 238, 259, 262, 263, 264, 271, 278, 282, 284, 292, 293, 320, 322, 323, 335, 336, 354, 367
Sun 8, 22, 25, 86, 114, 159, 160, 165, 166, 167, 168, 171, 174, 184, 188, 193, 198, 201, 204, 219, 220, 221, 224, 235, 241, 256, 261, 292, 297, 325, 326, 330, 332, 340, 355, 356, xxiv, xxv
Sunflower 54, 65, 92, 123, 124, 141, 219, 220, 221, 222, 251, 252, 253, 257, 261, 262, 263, 266, 285, xx, xxiii
Superfoods 20, 62, 65, 251, 293, 319

T

Tarot 47, xiv, xxxiv, xxxv
teas v, 42, 50, 68, 114, 124, 129, 132, 143, 144, 147, 148, 152, 155, 157, 158, 160, 161, 162, 163, 165, 166, 167, 168, 169, 172, 173, 174, 177, 178, 180, 185, 187, 188, 189, 190, 191, 192, 194, 197, 198, 199, 201, 202, 205, 213, 216, 217, 221, 224, 225, 226, 230, 238, 239, 240, 242, 243, 278, 287, 290, 291, 315, 319, 326, 328, 332, xii
teeth 143, 177, 255, 260, 268, 271
testosterone 136, 173, 229, 256, 268, 270, 292
tinctures 328
Todd Rundgren 39, xx
tonic 99, 134, 136, 152, 156, 163, 167, 177, 185, 188, 190, 193, 197, 205, 209, 229, 231, 238, 242, 243, 273, 277, 307
toothaches 152
trauma 164, 174, 186, 191, 206

U

ulcers 59, 143, 162, 163, 177, 180, 185, 205, 224, 238, 273

V

vegan iii, 64, 65, 94, 95, 182, 220, xx
vegan protein iii, 65, 94, 95, 127, 146
veins 126, 129, 136, 141, 162, 163, 167, 172, 184, 189, 192, 197, 204, 226, 239, 242
Venus 131, 142, 160, 174, 185, 191, 206, 213, 224, 230, 234, 239, 300
Violet 136, 211, 223, 224, 225, 226, 227, 255, 282, xxiii
viral 19, 47, 115, 128, 144, 158, 185, 188, 226, 256, 280, 281
virus 18, 144, 280, 353
Vitamin A 93, 155, 167, 180, 205, 209, 216, 223, 241, 251, 252, 266, 276
Vitamin B 160, 216, 219
Vitamin C 12, 94, 95, 132, 136, 142, 156, 167, 173, 176, 181, 184, 189, 209, 210, 212, 216, 223, 232, 237, 248, 249, 254, 255, 257, 261, 278, 294, 331
Vitamin CBD 258

Vitamin D 255, 256, 260, 292, 293, xvii
Vitamin E 94, 195, 209, 219, 220, 256, 257, 331
Vitamin K 151, 167, 216, 257, 258, 264
vitamins 58, 63, 64, 89, 90, 93, 94, 95, 134, 137, 151, 173, 196, 205, 212, 228, 248, 250, 252, 276, 280
Volume Four 4, 60
Volume One 3, 37, 69
Volume Three F, 4, 24, 26, 278, 332, 345, 346, viii
Volume Two 1, 2, 3, 37, 203

W

wands 178
water 28, 54, 60, 68, 73, 74, 75, 82, 84, 86, 88, 89, 91, 92, 93, 94, 96, 100, 101, 103, 104, 105, 107, 110, 111, 113, 115, 116, 119, 126, 132, 137, 138, 141, 143, 144, 147, 151, 153, 154, 157, 161, 163, 165, 166, 167, 168, 174, 175, 177, 178, 179, 180, 185, 186, 187, 188, 190, 195, 197, 205, 207, 209, 216, 217, 222, 223, 225, 226, 230, 235, 243, 252, 254, 255, 259, 263, 266, 273, 276, 278, 284, 286, 299, 300, 307, 309, 317, 319, 322, 323, 324, 325, 326, 327, 328, 330, 331, 332, 335, 336, 337, 338, 339, 341, 343, 345, 346, 359, xvii, xx, xxii
weeds i, 53, 68, 85, 87, 99, 109, 119, 121, 134, 181
Wild Asparagus 230, xxiii
Wild Blueberry 232, 233, 234, 235, 236, xxiii
Wish You Were Pink 40, xx
World Peace 29, 47
wounds 19, 59, 134, 143, 152, 156, 160, 162, 163, 164, 168, 173, 174, 177, 185, 197, 201, 205, 206, 216, 221, 239, 240, 242, 256, 344

Y

Yarrow 54, 123, 124, 182, 183, 237, 238, 239, 240, 272, 288, xxiii
Yeast iii, 4, 65, 103, 104, 105, 252, 253, 256, 257, 259, 266, 285
Yellow Dock 18, 133, 197, 213, 241, 242, 243, 261, xxiii, xxiv

Z

Zinc 4, 93, 94, 95, 107, 142, 160, 167, 180, 196, 219, 220, 228, 248, 249, 266, 267, 280, 294

ABOUT THE AUTHOR

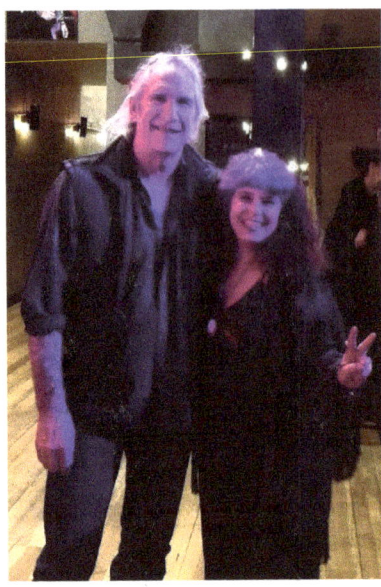

"A quiet secluded life in the country, with the possibility of being useful to people to whom it is easy to do good, and who are not accustomed to have it done to them; then work which one hopes may be of some use; then rest, nature, books, music, love for one's neighbor - such is my idea of Happiness."

~ Leo Tolstoy

Laura Lamun currently lives within the Big Trees of Tennessee, but will likely be on the move again soon. She is a Life-Lover, an Author, a Singer, a Tarot Therapist, an Earthologist, a Sound Healer and a Body Guide: an **Agent of Positive Change**. She is a Crusader for our Earth, tirelessly supporting GAIA and all the Gaian Kingdoms, Elements, Elementals and Beings. She is a Freedom of Information Warrior, seeking to help others open their minds and have access to many sources of Education. Her Mission is to spread Light, Love, Encouragement, and Knowledge.

She can be found playing music with her Beloved Dave Allen, playing with her Goldy kitty and puppy Ruby, staring off into space in her backyard talking to Spirits, laughing loudly while her purple hair blows in the wind, talking to the Plants and Trees, reading, doing yoga, chef-ing it up, playing with crystals, watching football, writing in notebooks, seeking deep companionship with Tarot cards, or sometimes just sitting still waiting for Butterflies to alight upon her. She lives a radically Blessed Life in our Wondrous Garden. Her deep Happiness is something she works at, and is grateful for, every day.

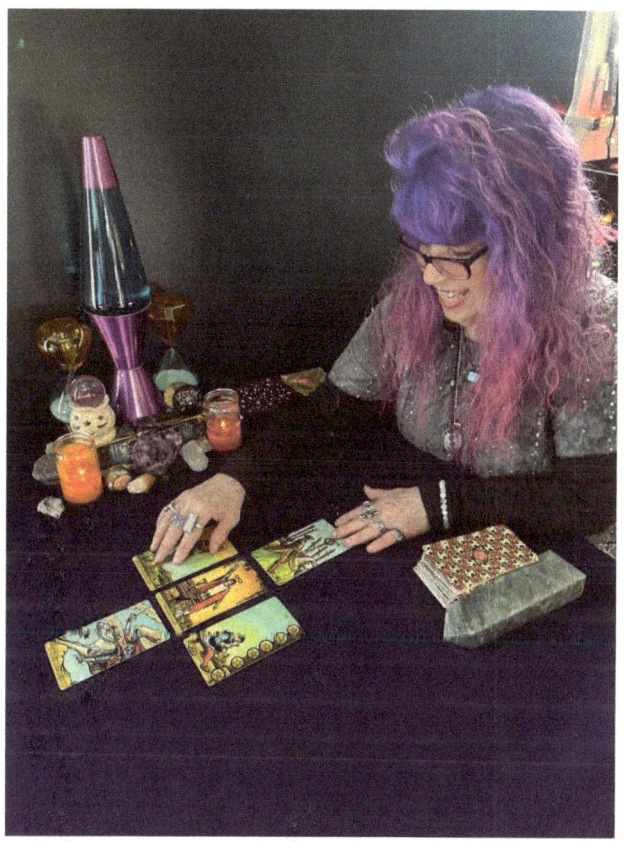

I'd LOVE to read Tarot for you!

Email me with requests, comments, desires or support at:

littlelauralamun@gmail.com

Look for *Volume Three*, and a great educational opportunity coming soon ~
The Garden of Earth School!

lauralamun.com

www.ingramcontent.com/pod-product-compliance
Lightning Source LLC
Chambersburg PA
CBHW062055290426
44110CB00022B/2602